TOWARDS SAFER CARDIAC SURGERY

TOWARDS SAFER CARDIAC SURGERY

EDITED BY

D. B. Longmore
Consultant Clinical Physiologist
The National Heart Hospital, London

Based upon the Proceedings of an International Symposium held at the University of York 8–10th April, 1980

MTP PRESS LIMITED · LANCASTER · ENGLAND
International Medical Publishers

Published by
MTP Press Limited
Falcon House
Lancaster, England

Softcover reprint of the hardcover 1st edition 1981

First published 1981

British Library Cataloguing in Publication Data

Towards safer cardiac surgery.
1. Heart – Surgery
I. Longmore, Donald
616'.412 RD598

ISBN-13: 978-94-009-8050-1 e-ISBN-13: 978-94-009-8048-8
DOI: 10.1007/978-94-009-8048-8

Typeset by Speedlith Photolitho Ltd., Manchester

Contents

List of Contributors ix

Introduction
D. B. Longmore 1

SECTION I ASPECTS OF CARDIAC SURGERY

1 Historical review and introduction
W. P. Cleland 7

2 Congenital heart disease
P. B. Deverall 13

3 Reviewing the pros and cons of myocardial preservation within cardiac surgery
H. J. Bretschneider, M. M. Gebhard and C. J. Preusse 21

4 Biological aspects of prosthetic materials
W. H. Wain 55

5 Clinical problems and aspirations of biological materials
D. N. Ross 65

6 Preoperative and postoperative echocardiographic assessment of left ventricular function
L. Cotter and D. G. Gibson 69

7 Changing aspects of surgical technique in coronary artery surgery
J. E. C. Wright 81

8 Re-emphasis of the importance of clinical observation
D. G. Julian 95

9 The importance and hazards of angiocardiography
J. B. Partridge 99

10 The mechanisms and hazards of echocardiography
P. N. T. Wells 109

11 The importance of echocardiography in preoperative diagnosis
L. Cotter and D. G. Gibson 139

12 The perioperative value of nuclear magnetic resonance
P. Mansfield 153

13 Computed tomography of the heart
J. J. K. Best 167

14 Nuclear imaging techniques in cardiology and cardiac surgery.
Part 1 Static imaging and myocardial blood flow
D. S. Dymond 179

15 Nuclear imaging techniques in cardiology and cardiac surgery.
Part 2 Dynamic imaging
D. S. Dymond 223

SECTION II ASPECTS OF CARDIOPULMONARY BYPASS AND ANAESTHESIA

16 Historical review and introduction
D. G. Melrose 259

17 Anaesthesia for coronary artery surgery
D. W. Bethune, J. M. Collis, I. Hardy and R. D. Latimer 267

18 Hyperthermic circulatory arrest in infants and children
G. Jackson Rees 281

19 Cerebral perfusion during cardiac surgery using cardiac bypass
J. C. Simpson 287

20 Towards safer cardiopulmonary bypass
Ch. R. H. Wildevuur 293

21 Haematological effects of cardiotomy suction
G. Wright 313

22 Gaseous microemboli during open heart surgery
D. T. Pearson, R. F. Carter, M. B. Hammo and P. S. Waterhouse 325

23 The value of prostacyclins in cardiopulmonary bypass
D. B. Longmore 355

24 Features of cardiac myocytes in culture: characterization of the failing cell
Jocelyn W. Dow and Elaine J. Walker 379

25 Factors influencing the origin and cycling of hydrogen ions in cardiac surgery
Jocelyn W. Dow, N. G. L. Harding, G. N. C. Kenny, M. A. Turner and P. G. Wallace 391

26 Which priming fluids?
M. A. Tobias and J. M. Fryer 401

27 Can cardiopulmonary bypass be a safe procedure?
D. R. Wheeldon 427

28 Toxins in open heart surgery
D. B. Longmore and Merilyn Smith 447

29 Long term extracorporeal membrane oxygenation (ECMO)
R. Wyatt 475

30 Why pulsatile flow during cardiopulmonary bypass?
K. M. Taylor 483

SECTION III ASPECTS OF POSTOPERATIVE CARE (I)

31 Introduction: emphasis of clinical assessment
D. J. Wheatley 503

32 Is inotropic stimulation outdated?
P. A. Poole-Wilson 513

33 Which electrolytes matter?
Eunice Lockey 531

34 Some applications of computers in postoperative care
S. Rao and D. B. Longmore 535

35 Is red cell potassium a prognostic indicator?
R. Wyatt 547

36 Nursing management
Joan E. Blundell 549

37 Nutritional care in cardiac surgery
R. K. Walesby 553

SECTION IV ASPECTS OF POSTOPERATIVE CARE (II)

38 Control of blood loss
H. Bentall 569

39 The horizontal dimension.
A patient from the intensive therapy unit 571

40 Pulmonary problems after cardiopulmonary bypass
J. W. W. Gothard 575

41 The aetiology, pathogenesis and prevention of prosthetic valve endocarditis
R. Freeman 583

42 Prevention and treatment of renal failure
F. D. Thompson 601

SECTION V THE BRAIN

43 Psychometric testing in the evaluation of the postoperative cardiac patient
D. W. Bethune 613

44 Brain damage following open heart surgery
G. Rodewald, P. Götze, J. Guntau, R. Janzen, H.-J. Krebber and H. Pokar 619

45 THE SIR THOMAS HOLMES SELLORS LECTURE
Preservation of the myocardium: some biological considerations
Winifred G. Nayler 627

Comment on Professor Nayler's lecture
H. J. Bretschneider, M. M. Gebhard and C. J. Preusse 648

Reply to Professor Bretschneider
Winifred G. Nayler 651

Conclusions
M. P. Holden 653

Index 661

List of Contributors

H. H. BENTALL
Royal Postgraduate Medical School
Hammersmith Hospital
London W12 0HS, UK

J. J. K. BEST
Department of Medical Radiology
University of Edinburgh
The Royal Infirmary
Edinburgh EH3 9YW, UK

D. W. BETHUNE
Thoracic Surgical Unit
Papworth Hospital
Papworth Everard
Cambridge CB3 8RE, UK

J. E. BLUNDELL
Recovery Ward
National Heart Hospital
London W1M 8BA, UK

H. J. BRETSCHNEIDER
Institute of Physiology 1
University of Goettingen
D-3400 Goettingen
Federal Republic of Germany

R. F. CARTER
Department of Cardiothoracic Anaesthesia
Regional Cardiothoracic Centre
Freeman Hospital
Newcastle upon Tyne NE7 7DN, UK

W. P. CLELAND
Department of Surgery
Cardiothoracic Institute
2 Beaumont Street
London W1N 2DX, UK

J. COLLIS
Thoracic Surgical Unit
Papworth Hospital
Papworth Everard
Cambridge CB3 8RE, UK

L. COTTER
Cardiac Department
Brompton Hospital
London SW3 6HP, UK

P. D. DEVERALL
Department of Cardiac Surgery
Guy's Hospital
London SE1 9RT, UK

J. W. DOW
Department of Biochemistry and Medical Cardiology
University of Glasgow
Glasgow G12 8QQ, UK

D. S. DYMOND
Department of Medicine
Mount Sinai Medical Center
Milwaukee
Wisconsin 53201, USA

R. FREEMAN
Department of Microbiology
Freeman Hospital
Newcastle upon Tyne NE7 7DN, UK

J. M. FRYER
Department of Anaesthesia
Wythenshawe Hospital
Manchester M23 9LT, UK

M. M. GEBHARD
Institute of Physiology 1
University of Goettingen
D-3400 Goettingen
Federal Republic of Germany

D. GIBSON
Cardiac Department
Brompton Hospital
London SW3 6HP, UK

J. W. W. GOTHARD
Anaesthetic Department
Brompton Hospital
London SW3 6HP, UK

P. GÖTZE
Department of Psychiatry
University of Hamburg
Hamburg
Federal Republic of Germany

M. B. HAMMO
Department of Cardiothoracic Anaesthesia
Regional Cardiothoracic Centre
Freeman Hospital
Newcastle upon Tyne NE7 7DN, UK

N. G. L. HARDING
Department of Pathological Biochemistry
University of Glasgow
Glasgow G4 0SF, UK

I. HARDY
Thoracic Surgical Unit
Papworth Hospital
Papworth Everard
Cambridge CB3 8RE, UK

M. P. HOLDEN
Regional Cardiothoracic Centre
Freeman Hospital
Newcastle upon Tyne NE7 7DN, UK

R. JANZEN
Department of Neurology
University of Hamburg
Hamburg
Federal Republic of Germany

D. G. JULIAN
Department of Cardiology
Freeman Hospital
Newcastle upon Tyne NE7 7DN, UK

G. N. C. KENNY
Department of Anaesthesia
University of Glasgow
Glasgow G12 8QQ, UK

H. -J. KREBBER
Department of Cardiovascular Surgery
University of Hamburg
Hamburg
Federal Republic of Germany

R. D. LATIMER
Thoracic Surgical Unit
Papworth Hospital
Papworth Everard
Cambridge CB3 8RE, UK

E. LOCKEY
Department of Chemical Pathology
Barnet General Hospital
Barnet, Herts. EN5 3BG, UK

D. B. LONGMORE
Department of Clinical Physiology
National Heart Hospital
London W1M 8BA, UK

P. MANSFIELD
Department of Physics
University of Nottingham
Nottingham NG7 2RD, UK

D. G. MELROSE
Department of Surgery
Royal Postgraduate Medical School
Hammersmith Hospital
London W12 0HS, UK

W. G. NAYLER
Department of Medicine
University of Melbourne
Austin Hospital
Melbourne
Victoria 3084, Australia

J. B. PARTRIDGE
Department of Radiology
Killingbeck Hospital
Leeds LS14 6UQ, UK

D. T. PEARSON
Department of Cardiothoracic Anaesthesia
Regional Cardiothoracic Centre
Freeman Hospital
Newcastle upon Tyne NE7 7DN, UK

H. POKAR
Department of Cardiovascular Surgery
University of Hamburg
Hamburg
Federal Republic of Germany

P. A. POOLE-WILSON
Cardiothoracic Institute
2 Beaumont Street
London W1N 2DX, UK

C. J. PREUSSE
Institute of Physiology 1
University of Goettingen
D-3400 Goettingen
Federal Republic of Germany

LIST OF CONTRIBUTORS

S. RAO
Department of Clinical Physiology
National Heart Hospital
London W1M 8BA, UK

D. JACKSON REES
Liverpool Paediatric Cardiological Unit
Royal Liverpool Children's Hospital
Liverpool L7 7DG, UK

G. RODEWALD
Cardiovascular Surgery
University of Hamburg
Hamburg
Federal Republic of Germany

D. ROSS
25 Upper Wimpole Street
London W1M 7TA, UK

J. C. SIMPSON
Anaesthesia Department
National Heart Hospital
London W1M 8BA, UK

M. SMITH
Department of Clinical Physiology
National Heart Hospital
London W1M 8BA, UK

K. M. TAYLOR
University Department of Cardiac Surgery
Royal Infirmary
Glasgow G4 0SF, UK

F. D. THOMPSON
St Peter's Group of Hospitals
Institute of Urology
Shaftsbury Hospital
London WC2, UK

M. A. TOBIAS
Department of Anaesthesia
Wythenshawe Hospital
Manchester M23 9LT, UK

M. A. TURNER
Cardiothoracic Unit
Western Infirmary
Glasgow G4 4NT, UK

W. H. WAIN
Homograft Department
National Heart Hospital
London W1M 8BA, UK

R. K. WALESBY
Cardiothoracic Unit
Hospital for Sick Children
Great Ormond Street
London WC1N 3JH, UK

E. J. WALKER
Cardiothoracic Unit
Hospital for Sick Children
Great Ormond Street
London WC1N 3JH, UK

P. G. WALLACE
Department of Anaesthesia
Western Infirmary
Glasgow G11 6NT, UK

P. S. WATERHOUSE
Department of Cardiothoracic Anaesthesia
Regional Cardiothoracic Centre
Freeman Hospital
Newcastle upon Tyne NE7 7DN, UK

P. N. T. WELLS
Department of Medical Physics
Bristol General Hospital
Bristol BS1 6SY, UK

D. J. WHEATLEY
Department of Cardiac Surgery
Royal Infirmary
Glasgow G4 0SF, UK

D. R. WHEELDON
Surgical Unit
Papworth Hospital
Papworth Everard
Cambridge CB3 8RE, UK

Ch. R. H. WILDEVUUR
Department of Experimental Surgery
University Hospital
9700 RB Groningen, The Netherlands

G. WRIGHT
W. E. Dunn Unit of Cardiology
University of Keele
Keele, Staffs. ST5 5BG, UK

J. E. C. WRIGHT
Department of Surgery
London Chest Hospital
London E2 9JX, UK

R. WYATT
Anaesthetic Department
The Groby Road Hospital
Leicester LE3 9QE, UK

Introduction

D. B. LONGMORE

The concept of the meeting on which this book is based is unique. There has never before been a multi-disciplinary meeting based entirely on the concept of making a major branch of surgery safer. Hopefully, this meeting will be archetypal and will set a precedent for similar attempts in other disciplines as well as future efforts to make cardiac surgery safer. Cardiac surgery is still a rapidly growing discipline even after a quarter of a century of experience. Like any new area of science, or medicine, initially there is an exponential growth of work, publications, meetings, options of available equipment and all the ancillary and peripheral disciplines associated with it. The ideas of the handful of original surgical pioneers, some of whom have contributed to this book, formed the basis of a still rapidly growing young branch of surgery with a whole new medical discipline of total extracorporeal circulation involving biochemical and haemodynamic control of a patient.

Unlike any other branch of surgery, progress is now completely dependent on large numbers of associated staff – the pump technician, the anaesthetist, the sister in charge of intensive care, the nurse at the bedside, the radiologist, the physiologist, the surgical assistant, the bioengineer, the cardiac diagnostician and many others. All these people make such a large contribution to the management of the patient that it is impossible to pinpoint which parts of the preoperative, operative and postoperative procedure contribute most importantly to the outcome – hopefully a patient with more than just a palliative operation but a person who can look forward to a normal life span with a high quality of life.

Cardiac surgeons were quick to recognise that surgical results can be adversely influenced by factors beyond the control of the medical and other staff. The equipment and the very plastics which are used in the extra corporeal apparatus may severely impair the prognosis of our patients. We are fortunate that the majority of equipment manufacturers are ethical and strive to produce safe and reliable apparatus to use directly on the patient and to monitor his progress. The pioneer cardiac surgeons had to develop new surgical techniques but in addition they had to produce new engineering designs for bypass equipment and to learn the new established techniques of post-operative management. Naturally at that stage surgeons were pleased if a proportion of their patients could be fought through the postoperative stage and discharged home fit.

Those of us who have been involved since the beginning of cardiac surgery and those who take the trouble to look at films which were made over 20 years ago showing cardiac surgical technique notice how little of what we do as routine today has changed in principle. PVC apparatus, the bubble oxygenator and silicone antifoam are still commonplace. The most common techniques enabling the chambers of the heart to be opened are only different in detail from those originally used. A modest degree of hypothermia is often still used, as are cold solutions to still the heart and to modify the myocardial cellular metabolism.

After the initial phase of surgery with the horrendous mortality rate there have been few fundamental, conceptual changes. There have been variations of the basic apparatus, which for a period became extremely complex. Many of the electronic autoregulators of bypass and the cumbersome screen roller and disc oxygenators have been discarded in favour of the well founded simpler earlier techniques. There have, however, been many refinements of technique with gradual increments of knowledge with a consequential improvement in surgical results. Death was replaced by severe multi-organ damage as the common postoperative complication. Cerebral devastation was a frequent occurrence in the early sixties, often associated with renal failure. Moderate cerebral impairment was, for a time, almost routine. Gradually the results have improved, so that now the mortality rates compare very favourably with routine, simple general surgical operations. The post-operative morbidity is remarkably low. Even operations involving the implantation of large prosthetic implants are not commonly infected. Failure to return to work and some degree of cerebral dysfunction remains as the most common complication. The frequency with which cerebral damage is diagnosed depends on the care when monitoring the patient's post-operative course. There are still sporadic outbreaks in most cardiac surgical units of serious cerebral and multi-organ complications. These intermittent problems usually disappear as soon as they are investigated, suggesting that attention to the adherence to accepted safety standards is all that is required.

The view could have been taken by the International Group of Cardiac Surgeons that the procedure had reached a plateau of safety from which there could always be an irreducible minimum of lethal and debilitating complications due to unavoidable accidents. Cardiac surgeons could have been forgiven for taking this view, especially when it is remembered that the most commonly performed operations in cardiac surgery are for a lethal disease, occlusive coronary vascular disease. The mortality rate for coronary vein grafting in the best units is comparable with the accepted mortality rate for appendicectomy. Happily, this has not been the view adopted by cardiologists, cardiac surgeons and others involved in the discipline. Cardiac surgeons still strive to make their procedures safer. There are as many different approaches to safety in cardiac surgery as there are cardiac surgical units. All depend on the intellectual honesty of the surgeon in overall charge of the patient, who has to recognise and admit the role of the procedure in the genesis of the postoperative illness of the patient. The surgeon starts with the basic premise that there is a great potential for iatrogenic disease in the whole open heart procedure, for example a patient who has an open mitral valvotomy is always more ill postoperatively than the patient who has a closed operation. Cardiac surgery undoubtedly presents the biggest single safety problem there has yet been in medicine. In addition to all the usual hazards of major surgery, powerful pre-operative medical therapy can cause fundamental electrolyte disturbances. Complex anaesthesia, sometimes massive blood transfusion and psychological stress are all added to the complications of extra-corporeal circulation. This is compounded by the multidisciplinary involvement which can lead to communication difficulties between the staff who have different backgrounds.

Cardiac surgery now attempts to cope with the problems of occlusive vascular disease. Thus it now potentially encompasses over half of all disease. It is the one branch of surgery which will continue to expand rapidly. In other forms of surgically treatable disease such as trauma or carcinoma, most patients receive surgical care. Only a few percent of patients with occlusive vascular disease are presently operated on. There are historical reasons for this treatment gap – insufficient open heart units and inadequate diagnostic procedures. Lack of understanding of the potential of bypass operations and the sometimes poor results all contribute. Non-invasive techniques for the early detection of heart disease are currently not widely available or adequate. If these were to become so it would be possible to monitor preventive measures to find which of these techniques are really beneficial, apply them with the aid of public education programmes and thus reduce the incidence of occlusive disease and the need for surgical treatment. Such a goal is not within sight. Even when the natural history of occlusive disease is known and when prevention is effective there will still be a time lag of a generation during which the existing diseased population will need treatment.

There are special groups of 'super-specialists' in cardiac surgery who concentrate on different aspects of the subject. The surgical group which specializes in correcting transposition of the great vessels will have little knowledge of the problems faced by the coronary vein grafting groups. For these reasons and because of the individuality of surgeons, throughout this book it may appear that there are differing views of how the discipline might be made even safer. The surgeon who is interested in the safety of a particular type of valve used by him may give the impression that he is concerned only about complications arising from prosthetic or homograft valves whilst another who is involved with coagulation studies will give the impression that he feels that the introduction of platelet stabilizing agents, such as prostacyclin, may be the only approach to revolutionize the safety aspects of open heart surgery. Of course, such views are much too simplistic. The success of the procedure depends on meticulous attention to detail of all aspects of the techniques involved and the overall safety of the patient depends as much on care as on the introduction of new technology. No excuse is made for the many different approaches to the problem of safety within the following chapters, nor has any attempt been made to rank the hazards to patients in order of potential severity of incidence.

Any person who undergoes cardiac surgery for virtually symptomless occlusion of one of his coronary arteries in order to possibly extend his useful life span, cannot entertain an operation which may render him unable to hold down his job or to live in normal harmony with his family and friends. Even the most rare and unlikely complication of cardiac surgery is, at the moment, occasionally capable of such a devastating consequence to an individual patient.

The contributions to this book have been chosen from the wide range of disciplines associated with cardiac surgery on the heart; including nurses, a patient, biochemists, perfusionists, computer scientists, intensivists and many others. They represent a proportion of those people striving to make cardiac surgery even safer than herniorrhaphy or appendicectomy. The feeling of urgency amongst cardiac surgeons and their colleagues about the subject of safety was so great that many other willing contributors who could have taken part in a larger meeting on this subject had to be left out of the programme. It became clear from the enthusiasm of those present that the meeting could have been many times longer and more comprehensive than it was. This book will doubtless be the first in a series on this vital topic.

Acknowledgements

I express the views of the authors in thanking the staff of Travenol for giving the organizing committee a free hand and generous help in setting up the meeting. Virtually all the chapters were received on time. This unprecedented effort must be indicative of the importance attached to the subject by the contributors.

There have been many books of varying value produced from the proceedings of symposia. The Editor and Publishers have produced previous books on cardiac surgery in which the contributors have concentrated on the teaching aspects of their subjects rather than the more usual surgical format usually designed to demonstrate the excellent results of the surgeon's favourite procedure. On this occasion the contributors have made even greater efforts to impart useful knowledge about safety and to set aside any opportunities of championing their favourite subject. Once more I thank them all for making such a great effort to help me to disseminate their unique knowledge.

SECTION I
Aspects of Cardiac Surgery

1
Historical review and introduction

W. P. CLELAND

In 1953, Melrose, Bentall and I, together with a group of keen technicians and devoted nurses, carried out our first operations using cardiopulmonary bypass. The initial procedures, which would now be described as supportive bypass, enabled us to carry out closed heart procedures (such as aortic valvotomy) on very sick patients with success.

Initial attempts to proceed to total cardiopulmonary bypass and open heart surgery failed, for reasons which today would appear to you to be quite obvious. It took us nearly 4 years of research and experimentation, and several trips to Rochester and Minneapolis, before we were able to perform successfully total cardiopulmonary bypass, initially only on right-sided congenital lesions.

In the decade 1958–67 following these beginnings no fewer than 1200 open heart operations were carried out at Hammersmith Hospital, and since then approximately 4000 further open heart procedures must have been performed.

It is now my wish to discuss some of the factors which have led to a vast increase in scope for open heart surgery and a steady improvement in results. These we can consider under four main headings: viz. physiological, anatomical, mechanical, and surgical.

PHYSIOLOGICAL

At the outset it looked as though the surgeon's ideals of a dry and motionless operating field and the absence of a time limit could be met with potassium citrate arrest. Time was limited, however, to about 30 min and this technique was used by us without troubles for the first 50–60 cases. Reports of myocardial damage from the potassium came from across the Atlantic, and we were obliged to abandon this favourable technique even though we had no positive evidence of damage in our own patients.

We then passed through a period of operating with the beating heart and trying out other means of myocardial handling, from simple aortic cross-clamping with or without hypothermia either general or local, and varying patterns of coronary perfusion and elective ventricular fibrillation.

In our hands, continuous coronary perfusion with DeBakey cannulae and with moderate hypothermia seemed to be the safest and best method of preserving the myocardium and giving the surgeon conditions suitable for operating, though it still had certain disadvantages – the coronary lines got in the way or they leaked – occasionally subendocardial ischaemia occurred for no obvious reason – and very occasionally there was trauma to the coronary vessels themselves.

We now reach the present era of cardioplegia with cold solutions of carefully selected agents all designed to maintain the myocardium in prime condition – the wheel has gone full circle – or nearly so.

The operating conditions are superb, and better than any achieved by the earlier procedures, but there still must be a time limit though this clearly varies from operation to operation.

Whilst on the topic of myocardial preservation one must mention the importance of having the left ventricle at complete rest and incapable of doing any work by LV venting, which also eliminates any possible risk of overdistension when the aortic clamp is removed.

I think the next most important step was the control of fluid and blood balances – a matter which became of greater importance as more and more haemodilution was employed. Initially we relied very much on central venous pressure as a guide for the final fluid balance coming off bypass, and a later check was carried out by whole-body weighing. The latter proved very cumbersome and unreliable and was soon abandoned as a means of control. Gradually we relied more and more on a carefully calculated fluid balance account and haematocrit estimations at repeated intervals.

This is perhaps a suitable moment to mention the tremendous advantages in having biochemical apparatus available on a moment-to-moment basis, both in the theatre and in the intensive care unit. The perfection of the acid–base and blood gas laboratories, and the Na and K analyser, have been of inestimable value to the surgical team. Gone are the days when we had a special team of runners carrying blood samples to the laboratories, which always seemed to be so far away.

ANATOMICAL

I would like now to turn to anatomical factors which have helped towards safer surgery. First, heart block comes to mind. This was a very real hazard in the early series of ventricular septal defects and tetralogy operations, and its production was bad news for the patient. Very few of those with persistent heart block survived for long, and in those with temporary block it often recurred.

Electrical methods for mapping the course of the bundle were not particularly helpful and had other logistic drawbacks, but the anatomists soon told us with some conviction the whereabouts of the bundle in the more usual varieties of congenital disease with which we were dealing. With this knowledge the surgeon was able to place sutures in tissue remote from the bundle and its branches and the bogey of heart block virtually disappeared. At the present time I imagine that heart block after closure of ventricular septal defect or Fallot repair is almost unknown – at least I hope so.

Another cause of embarrassment to the surgeon, and morbidity to the patient, was the discovery of unexpected abnormalities during surgery; particularly at a time when one was ill-prepared to deal with, say, an abnormal valve or a large patent ductus. The development of radiological anatomy during the past two decades has ensured that the majority of patients now come to the operating theatre with a complete and correct diagnosis, and no longer is the surgeon faced with an unexpected finding.

To illustrate these points I wish to refer you to a report we published in 1968[1] of experiences in the past 10 years at the Hammersmith Hospital. The following figures all refer to ventricular septal defects of which we had then operated on 227 patients with an 11% early mortality (Table 1). You will notice that many of the deaths occurred in complicated situations, the true nature of which was often not obvious when the operation was started. This would certainly never be the case today. Table 2 shows that we were still plagued by anatomical problems right through the decade, but that our handling of these and of the pulmonary hypertensive group steadily improved.

Table 3 analyses the various types of anatomical problems encountered in a group of 175 patients and how these complicating factors affected mortality.

Table 4 shows the early mortality from whatever cause, to underline that heart block and pulmonary hypertension were important factors, and finally, Table 5 the late follow-up shows that three out of five patients surviving the operation with heart block had subsequently died, and probably the remaining two succumbed later.

Table 1 Congenital ventricular septal defect (VSD)

Category	*No. of cases*	*No. of operative deaths*
Uncomplicated VSD	139*	3 (2%)
Complicated VSD		
Severe pulmonary vascular disease	31	10 (32%)
VSD with aortic regurgitation or sinus of valsalva fistula	30	7 (23%)
VSD with mitral valve disease	6	2
VSD with tricuspid regurgitation	2	1
Incomplete common ventricle, multiple defects, coronary artery anomaly or corrected transposition	19	3
TOTAL	227	26 (11%)

* Aged 2–56; male:female = 1.4:1

Table 2 Mortality in operations for ventricular septal defect (1958–66)

	Uncomplicated		*Physiological complications (pulmonary vascular disease)*		*Anatomical complications*	
Year	*Number*	*Mortality*	*Number*	*Mortality*	*Number*	*Mortality*
1958	16	0	7	4	3	1
1959	18	2	1	0	10	3
1960	27	0	4	2	3	0
1961	19	1	4	2	1	0
1962	17	0	2	1	4	0
1963	15	0	2	0	6	1
1964	11	0	2	0	5	3
1965	8	0	1	0	11	4
1966	8	0	8	1	14	1
	139	3	31	10	57	13

Table 3 Complicated ventricular septal defects (175 patients)

Aortic incompetence	11	(1 died)
Multiple defects	6	(2 died)
PDA	7	(1 died)
Absent pulmonary valves	3	
LV–RA shunt (Gerbode)		
Corrected transposition	2	(1 died)
Secundum ASD	3	
Mitral stenosis	3	
Common ventricle	5	(2 died)

RESPIRATORY

Finally I would like to mention the very important improvements in the handling of the lungs before, during, and after cardiac surgery.

An assessment of pulmonary vascular disease by haemodynamic and histological means has led to better selection of patients for surgery and a reduction in mortality and morbidity.

Better protection for the lungs during bypass – with the avoidance of either increased flow or pressure in the pulmonary circuit from whatever cause, be it back pressure from left-sided failure or overperfusion – has led to a happy decrease in the pump lung syndrome.

But perhaps the most important breakthrough came from the anaesthetists who accepted and eventually mastered the problems associated with artificial ventilation. Pulmonary complications were an important cause of

Table 4 Early deaths (175 patients)

Severe PHT (pulmonary hypertension)	4
Severe PHT + duct	1
Severe PHT + multiple defects	1
Heart block	2
After second operation	3
Anomalous coronaries	1
Aortic incompetence	1
Respiratory accidents	2
TOTAL	15

Table 5 Late follow-up (160 patients)

Permanent heart block (5)	died	3
	alive	2
Unrelated death (after anaesthetic)		1
Persistent shunt		17
Residual aortic incompetence		10
Alive and well		127
TOTAL		160

mortality in patients operated on in the 1950s and 1960s – usually recorded as 'respiratory failure'. Tracheostomy was frequently employed and even done prophylactically. But the problems were many – infection, mechanical breakdown, imperfect physiological control, and sheer ignorance – all contributed to many anxious moments on the part of the medical and nursing staff and often to mortality or morbidity for the patient. Of course the need for artificial ventilation has receded dramatically as a result of better perfusion, better surgery, and better knowledge; but when required today, it is carried out efficiently and effectively and with none of the terrors that it used to engender in the minds of the nursing and medical staff in those early days.

Finally, I think it is a good exercise to look into the future and try and define those areas most likely to make cardiac surgery safer and more reliable. I cannot see great advances being made in surgical techniques or instrumentation, but I believe that comprehensive data analysis of computerized material should help to pinpoint those areas which are weak or wanting. I would refer you to the recent Presidential address of Professor John Kirklin[2] to the American Association for Thoracic Surgery, and the 1980 Hammersmith Surgical Lecture delivered by D'Arcy Sutherland[3] both of which show how data analysis and the determination of incremental risk factors can determine better results.

References

1. Cleland, W. P., Goodwin, J. F., Bentall, H. H., Oakley, C. M., Melrose, D. G. and Hollman, A. (1978). A decade of open heart surgery. *Lancet*, **1**, 191
2. Kirklin, J. F. (1979). A letter to Helen. *J. Thorac. Cardiovasc. Surg.*, **78**, 643
3. Sutherland, H. D. (1980). The changing pattern of cardiac surgery in a closed community. 1980 Hammersmith Hospital Surgical Lecture. (To be published)

2
Congenital heart disease

P. B. DEVERALL

A safe operation is defined as a predictable procedure which can be performed with minimal risk at an optimal time in the natural history of the particular disease, and which gives optimal long-term benefit to the patient.

Predictability implies precise preoperative knowledge of the morphological and haemodynamic characteristics of the patient, and precise control of all the events occurring in the operative and perioperative period. The validity of the judgments exercised at these stages in the treatment programme can only be assessed by observing and analysing the subsequent long-term course of the patient.

The events occurring at the time of operation are *the* major determinants of mortality and early and late morbidity, but the events have also to be placed in the context of the natural history of the specific disease. Since the individual variations within a specific diagnostic entity are legion, it is obvious that in analysing any course of action all such variables have to be included.

The major determinants of a safe operation are listed below:

(1) disease and its assessment;
(2) age/size of patient;
(3) operative procedure;
(4) postoperative care;
(5) adaptation to survival;
(6) data analysis.

These factors will now be examined in more detail.

DISEASE AND ITS ASSESSMENT

The following factors are important in the assessment of disease:

(1) morphological and haemodynamic assessment;

(2) relationship between (1) and predictability of operation;
(3) relationship between (1) and (2) and subsequent result.

It is axiomatic with congenital heart disease that a complete morphological and haemodynamic evaluation precedes operation. Although non-invasive techniques facilitate analysis and will probably assume even greater importance, cardiac catheterization and selective angiocardiography remain the cornerstones of assessment. Recent advances in quality control, and the use of a range of projections, permit acquisition of detailed information regarding intracardiac and vascular morphology. Safer, more precise and expeditious intracardiac surgery directly correlates with this information.

It is generally accepted today that the problem of pulmonary vascular disease is mainly a problem of early infancy, in the sense that this is the period when the events causing vascular damage begin to be operative but are reversible. The onus is, therefore, the early recognition of the 'at-risk' group of patients and their treatment.

Table 1 illustrates the clinical conditions of tetralogy of Fallot and transposition of the great arteries, the spectrum of intracardiac structures and function, whose assessment is critically relevant to the choice, timing, and technique of operative intervention.

In the case of tetralogy of Fallot, the preoperative analysis documents the presence and size of the cardiac chambers, the morphology of the cardiac septa and atrioventricular valves, the ventriculo-arterial connections, the morphology of right ventricular to pulmonary arterial connection and the morphology of the major vessels and pulmonary blood supply. Anomalies such as a second ventricular septal defect, atrioventricular canal deformities, anomalous accessory tricuspid valve tissue, anomalous coronary artery distribution, patent ductus arteriosus or peripheral pulmonary arterial stenoses are all rare with tetralogy, but their presence can significantly influence the conduct and result of operative intervention. Each and all of

Table 1 Tetralogy of Fallot

Determinants of predictability
1 Ventricular septal morphology
2 Atrioventricular valve anomalies
3 Outflow 'tract' morphology
4 Relation between (3) and, e.g., transannular patching
5 Coronary arterial anomalies
6 Atrial septal patency
7 Aortopulmonary collaterals
8 Changes secondary to previous operations

Major questions
1 One- or two-stage repair?
2 If initial shunt – which?
3 Transannular patch or not?
4 Is a 'Pulmonary' valve mechanism required?

these anomalies should be recognized and considered at the preoperative decision-making time.

Although primary total correction of tetralogy in infants is successfully accomplished by some groups, this is not true in general, and the alternative course of two-stage treatment remains a valid alternative. There are some data to suggest that the need for transannular patch enlargement of the right ventricular outflow tract is an incremental risk factor in children in the first 2 years of life. It is probably possible to predict the need for such patching on the basis of angiocardiographic measurements of the structures of the outflow tract, and thus these measurements may assume major importance in developing 'safer treatment'. Major questions regarding tetralogy remain, and are tabulated in the second half of Table 1. Scrupulous follow-up of survivors and careful analysis of recorded data will, in time, answer these questions.

Transposition of the great arteries, whether simple or complex, represents a major continuing challenge. Although balloon atrial septostomy and atrial redirection of venous inflow operations have revolutionized life prospects for many patients, many problems of management and questions of the validity of policies of treatment at present in use, remain (Table 2). The widespread application of the Mustard technique of redirection of venous inflow, and the generally good early results in patients with transposition and intact ventricular septum, was one of the surgical landmarks of the late 1960s and 1970s. Yet now this operation has virtually been abandoned in favour of the Senning technique. There are, as yet, only few data to show that the latter procedure, though theoretically more attractive, is truly a safer operation, as defined at the head of this chapter.

Apart from arrhythmias, baffle complications and adaptations to growth in the reconstructed atria, both operations leave the geometrically and morphologically unsuitable right ventricle and tricuspid atrioventricular valve

Table 2 Transposition of the great arteries

Determinants of predictability
1 Ventricular function
2 Ventricular septal morphology
3 Left ventricular mass
4 Left ventricular outflow morphology
5 Pulmonary arterial connections and distribution
6 Coronary arterial anatomy
7 Pulmonary vascular resistance

Major questions
1 Simple or complex?
2 Venous redirection – Mustard or Senning?
3 Banding or complete repair in TGA/VSD?
4 Indications for arterial switch
5 How to manage TGA/LVOTO ± VSD
6 Late results

supporting the systemic circulation. Redirection of intracardiac flow at ventricular level, coupled with insertion of an external conduit to establish right ventricle to pulmonary artery continuity, has limited application to some complex transposition patients. Results of this approach in young children have remained unpredictable, and even in older patients (5 years or more) – although the operative risk is less – long-term problems related to the external conduit remain.

Arterial switching is an attractive alternative concept but, as yet, there are many unpredictable facets in this approach. The optimal reported results are in children with intact ventricular septum, but in whom left ventricular mass and function are adequate to support acutely the systemic circulation after operation. Banding of the pulmonary artery as a preliminary preparatory procedure has been advocated. A true ethical dilemma exists in this group of infants with transposition and intact ventricular septum, in whom a tried and tested and simpler technical alternative exists. The answers in this group of patients are not yet available.

Transposition with large ventricular septal defect is a complex problem. Although improved results from defect repair, coupled with atrial redirection of venous inflow, have been reported recently, the outcome of operation remains unpredictable. There is no doubt that improved understanding of the morphology of the septal defects has been a factor in the improved results, and further illustrates the principles outlined in Tables 1, 2 and 3. It is notable that the least satisfactory results of the arterial switch operation have been obtained in those sick infants in whom the risk of the more classical approach is also high. Early-onset pulmonary vascular disease may be a contributory factor in this equation.

These two conditions exemplify the complex interrelationship which exists between morphology, haemodynamics, clinical progress, and the choice, technique, complexity and results of operative intervention. Safer cardiac surgery follows improved comprehension of these relationships.

AGE/SIZE

Is the age and/or size of the patient an independent incremental risk factor?

There is no doubt that the highest risk of operation remains in the infant group. However, this is a highly selected group, presenting for treatment in infancy because of major morphological and haemodynamic disturbance.

Technical demands of treatment are great in small subjects, and the margin for error in management is minimal. Existing mechanical equipment, e.g., ventilators and heart–lung machines, are sophisticated but functioning at the limit of accuracy. Haematological and rheological balance is more difficult to achieve. There is at least some evidence that the newborn behaves in subtly different biological ways.

However, good results of major operations are achieved, even in the smallest infants, e.g., with intracardiac total anomalous pulmonary venous connection. It may be that this is because operation can achieve an immediate and dramatic improvement in haemodynamics. Less good results, in general, correlate with less dramatic haemodynamic change.

It is thus very difficult to know whether age/size is a true independent risk factor, but recent attempts to analyse this do favour a positive correlation between age/size and risk.

OPERATIVE INTERVENTION

Table 3 tabulates some of the important aspects of the operative intervention. Assuming accurate preoperative assessment and adequate postoperative care, it is the events at the time of operation which are *the* principal determinants of mortality and morbidity.

These events divide themselves into details of the technique of the intracardiac manipulation and details of the general supportive anaesthetic, metabolic, and extracorporeal perfusion systems. The two sets of details are interrelated. Protection of the myocardium is of major importance and an enormous advance has been the development of techniques of protection which simultaneously provide the surgeon with the ideal working conditions of a still, relaxed, bloodless, operative field. These conditions, plus detailed knowledge of normal and abnormal cardiac morphology and technical expertise, each contribute to predictable, expeditious safe surgery. It is not coincidental that complications, e.g. bleeding and arrhythmias, have become less common in recent years and that, in general, postoperative recovery has been smoother.

Cardiac output after operation has been shown to be closely correlated with mortality and morbidity – without doubt myocardial protections and the completeness of haemodynamic repair are the main determinants of this.

Table 3 Operative procedure

1	Planned controlled event
2	Technical expertise
3	Anatomical and physiological awareness, e.g. conduction tissue
4	Organ protection
5	Interrelation between operative events and postoperative complications

Table 4 Incremental risk factors of operation

1	Age/size
2	Preoperative condition/diagnosis
3	Perfusion system
	i ? membrane
	ii ? pulsatile flow
4	Myocardial protection
5	Residual haemodynamic abnormality
6	Cardiac rhythm

Quality and design of the components of the extracorporeal perfusion gas-exchange systems has improved gradually over the years. Theoretically, membrane systems are preferable to those incorporating a direct blood–gas interface, but there are no data clearly demonstrating an advantage to the membrane system in routine clinical practice and excluding the problem of prolonged perfusion. However rarely major postoperative lung dysfunction now occurs, it still does happen and, in the absence of causes such as residual intracardiac shunting or pulmonary venous hypertension, complex changes at capillary level within the lungs are probably occurring and may relate to damage to, or change in, blood components exposed to the direct blood–gas interface in the extracorporeal circulation. Membrane systems may well still prove to be safer.

Much interest in pulsatile perfusion exists. There appear to be data showing more normal tissue function if pulsatile flow is generated during the perfusion period. There are difficulties in transmitting extracorporeally generated pulsatility into the circulation of small individuals when small restrictive cannulae are used, and it is not immediately apparent what the ideal type of pulsatile system may be; this area is, however, likely to develop rapidly in the coming years.

POSTOPERATIVE CARE

Programmes of postoperative care may differ in detail, but are all based on continuous nursing and medical attention with monitoring of the various subsystems. The degree to which subsystem analysis can be quantitated varies, and the majority of groups still rely heavily on limited monitored data and regular clinical evaluation. The most sophisticated levels of monitoring with a degree of automated patient care and regular assessment of cardiac output are not generally applicable, but the lessons which can be learned from such experience can be applied.

Table 5 examines aspects of postoperative care and illustrates the way in which one, i.e. the circulatory subsystem, can be manipulated. Judgment in the postoperative situation remains a complex intellectual process based on available data, analysis of those data, experience, knowledge of the therapies available, and ability to relate decision-making to sometimes rapidly changing events.

A major and continuing problem is the elimination of error in postoperative management. It should be possible to minimize technical error and to devise safeguards against acting on erroneous data, but human frailty and variability remain a major problem. There is no disputing that different individuals have varying degrees of sensitivity to the often subtle clinical change in a patient's condition. Teaching reduces this variability and monitoring, and maybe a degree of automated care may reduce it further. Safer cardiac surgery, however, will occur generally by attention to methods which maximally utilize available high-level skills. There are major implications in recognizing this and these implications, e.g. reward for nursing skill has to be faced.

Table 5 Aspects of postoperative care

1 Elimination of variables:
  human
  technical
  input data analysis
2 Is (1) an indication for automated patient care?
3 Subsystem function
4 Analysis and treatment of subsystems
5 Data analysis

Subsystem function: How can we improve subsystem control? (circulatory subsystem)
1 Rhythm
2 Cardiac output
3 Contractility
4 Preload/afterload
5 Substrate utilization – metabolic control
6 Recognition of haemodynamics
7 Interrelation between pulmonary subsystem control and circulatory subsystem

INVASIVE TECHNIQUES IN POSTOPERATIVE ANALYSIS AND CARE

It is within the experience of all groups that valuable information is often obtained by invasive techniques. Intracardiac pressure monitoring, e.g., left atrial or right ventricular lines, atrial and/or ventricular pacemaker leads for pacing or electrography, or repeat cardiac catheterization as a means of analysing a difficult postoperative clinical situation, all may contribute in a major manner. Equally, all invasive techniques carry a risk and it is mandatory that the relative advantages and disadvantages of techniques be continually analysed.

Manipulation of a subsystem may involve giving potentially dangerous drugs. The theoretical advantage of substrate utilization may cause the administration of expensive regimes which are, in fact, of no value. As with invasive analysis, continual informed critical review of management programmes is likely to lead to safer, and often simpler, care.

ADAPTATION TO SURVIVAL AND DATA ANALYSIS

Detailed follow-up studies of survivors of surgically treated patients with congenital heart disease can alone evaluate the true results of that surgery and in turn influence the future evolution of treatment. Table 6 tabulates some of the facets of the adaptation to survival and the need to record, analyse, and report that experience.

Progression or resolution of pulmonary vascular disease has been analysed in patients undergoing repair of isolated ventricular septal defect in childhood, and the results have been a major influence in focusing attention, with

Table 6 Aspects of adaptation to survival imponderables

(a) Persisting haemodynamic abnormality, e.g. pulmonary regurgitation
(b) Late sequelae of morphological and/or haemodynamic abnormality, e.g. ventricular enlargement
(c) Rhythm
(d) Durability of 'materials'
(e) Adaptation to growth
(f) Pulmonary vascular disease

Data analysis
(a) Recording
(b) Analysing
(c) Sharing
(d) Problem of 'bad news'
(e) Prospective and/or retrospective studies
(f) Literature search
(g) Conclusions form data analysis and applicability

this disease, on the period of infancy. The recognition of the late incidence of complete heart block in tetralogy patients with electrocardiographic evidence of right bundle branch block and left hemiblock, and the correlation of this with even brief periods of complete heart block at the time of operation, has changed the management of at-risk patients. Late analysis of external conduit function is continuing to cause modifications of conduit design and techniques of insertion.

These are three examples ranging through haemodynamics, cardiac rhythm, and durability of materials, where safer cardiac surgery is evolving as a result of data analysis.

CONCLUSION

Safer cardiac surgery with congenital heart disease will result from meticulous attention to detail at all stages in management. This chapter has sought, in general terms, to identify some of the determinants which do and will influence this management.

3
Reviewing the pros and cons of myocardial preservation within cardiac surgery

H. J. BRETSCHNEIDER, M. M. GEBHARD AND C. J. PREUSSE

INTRODUCTION

Myocardial protection within cardiac surgery, in our definition, means the prolongation of the tolerance time of the whole heart to a total ischaemia. An aerobic continuous perfusion of the arrested heart using blood, haemoglobin solutions or even other oxygen-rich cardioplegic agents do not come within the terms of this definition. Nor does an intermittent coronary perfusion of the fibrillating heart where only the creatine phosphate content of the myocardium decreases slightly during the ischaemic interval, returning to normal values during the following perfusion period – the ATP content, however, remaining unchanged.

Myocardial protection, as defined here, has to be divided into the following phases:

(1) A preoperative basic medication or discontinuance of medication before the surgical intervention (e.g. β-blocking agents, nitrites, digitalis glycosides).

(2) The anaesthesia and, perhaps, a more specific premedication (e.g. neurolept analgesia and, additionally, calcium antagonists).

(3) The introduction and maintenance of a special cardioplegia as well as of a certain myocardial temperature (which may vary widely in the different areas of the heart). This phase we define as 'myocardial protection in the strict sense'.

(4) The extracorporeal circulation (ECC) before, during, and after the cardioplegia with the parameters flow-rate, perfusion pressure, temperature, degree of haemodilution, osmolality, pH, electrolytes, substrates, hormones, and drugs.

(5) The re-animation and recovery of the heart following the restoration of the coronary circulation, with the aid of ECC and, if necessary, of more distinctive measurements such as the employment of a special reperfusion solution.

(6) The postoperative recovery period of the patient in the intensive care unit with eventual support by pharmacological relief of the heart (e.g. sodium nitroprusside) or the use of a mechanical assistance.

The measures during these six phases only partially act in the sense of an 'obvious supplementation and additivity'; they often are intercorrelated in a rather complex way and therefore are to be considered as non-additive. The effectiveness of myocardial protection in the more general sense depends on the careful coordination of all measures, after extensive experimental proof of their mutual compatibility. Before a more detailed discussion, however, it must be pointed out that omissions during the first four phases, especially during the phase of proper myocardial protection, can seldom be made good even using intensive procedures during the post-ischaemic reperfusion period.

PRINCIPAL ASPECTS

The main problem in the study of living organisms is the mutual connection between functional ability, metabolic activity, and structure. For methodological reasons, we can only try *a posteriori* to reconstruct the physiological, biochemical, and morphological aspects as a whole.

The death of a cell or organism can be initiated by the destruction of substructures, by disturbance of metabolic functions, or even by overloading or unloading of certain functional activities. It is not possible to give one overall abstract and methodological summary, which satisfactorily considers all the changes in function, metabolism and structure. The most comprehensive and reliable one is given by the 'energy' approach, if one keeps in mind the fact that primary structural damage or primary metabolic toxins can lead to a disturbance of the cellular energy status and, consequently, can adversely effect the energy balance and cause an increasing energy deficit.

The following scheme of the energy approach to ischaemic anaerobiosis of the heart in detail covers five points:

(a) The determinants of the energy demand of the working heart.

(b) The function- and structure-related parts of the resting energy demand of the heart, and divergences between aerobic and anaerobic conditions.

(c) The energy production during anaerobiosis, glycogen reserves and glycolytic energy, given from glycogen and glucose, respectively.

(d) The high energy phosphates as 'energy reserves'; possibilities of optimizing the pre-ischaemic initial content of creatine phosphate (CP) and ATP; formal analysis of the anaerobic energy turnover.

(e) Differentiation between ischaemic anaerobiosis and anaerobic perfusion.

These factors will now be considered in more detail.

(a) Of the attempts to quantify the haemodynamic determinants of the energy demand of the working heart the most exact and generally valid one seems to be the equation first formulated in 1971[2,3]. As can be seen from Table 1, the total energy demand is additively composed of five terms:

- E_0 means the aerobic energy demand of the resting heart at normothermia, which is about 0.8 ml $O_2 \times$ 100 g ww per min;
- E_1 gives the frequency-dependent energy demand of the electrophysiological events within myocardial plasmalemma;
- E_2 gives the energy demand of the tension maintenance during the ejection phase, where an increasing pressure and a simultaneously decreasing ventricle volume result in a nearly constant fibre tension;
- E_3 gives the energy demand of the tension development during the isovolumetric contraction phase;
- E_4 gives the energy demand of the relaxation phase and is suggested to be equivalent to the calcium reabsorption work of the sarcoplasmic reticulum.

The derivation of these components would require a separate paper. Here only two are emphasized: (1) E_2 and E_3 are calculated according to the hypothesis that the elementary mechanical interactions of a myosin head with an actin filament must be described as force impact '$K \,.\, dt$' instead of work '$K \,.\, ds$'; (2) from E_2 and E_3 valid parameters can be derived by which the efficiency of pumping of the heart can be quantified and the principles of economy of the pumping performance can be deduced. The decisive determinants of a high energetic efficiency of the pumping of the heart are a high stroke volume and an optimal (not maximal) value of the quotient $dp/dt_{max}/P_{syst}$ (10–15 in the dog heart and 8–12 in the adult human heart). Therefore all principal energy effects of pharmacological or even mechanical relief of the heart can be deduced, provided that there is a sufficient coronary blood supply.

Table 1

$$E = E_0 + E_1 + E_2 + E_3 + E_4$$

$E_0 = k_0$	$k_0 = 8.0.10^{-1}$
$E_1 = t_{syst} \,.\, \mathrm{HR} \,.\, k_1$	$k_1 = 3.0.10^{-2}$
$E_2 = P_{syst} \,.\, (\mathrm{ESV}/100\,\mathrm{g})^{1/2} \,.\, \mathrm{sep} \,.\, \mathrm{HR} \,.\, k_2$	$k_2 = 2.0.10^{-4}$
$E_3 = dP/dt_{max} \,.\, \mathrm{HR} \,.\, k_3$	$k_3 = 1.2.10^{-5}$
$E_4 = d^2P/dt_{max} \,.\, \mathrm{HR} \,.\, k_4$	$k_4 = 1.0.10^{-8}$

E = total energy demand of the left ventricle (ml O_2/min.100 g)
E_0 = basal energy demand of the artificially arrested heart in normothermia
E_1 = energy demand of electrophysiologic processes
E_2 = energy demand of maintenance of tension during systolic ejection period
E_3 = energy demand of tension development during isovolumetric contraction
E_4 = energy demand of inactivation of the contractile system

(b) The aerobic energy demand of the resting heart, previously called E_0, has up to now been considered to be a constant, only temperature-dependent value. Figure 1 shows the aerobic energy requirement of the arrested heart between 35 °C and 5 °C according to Bonhoeffer[4], based on work done in 1967 by our team at the Department of Experimental Surgery in Cologne. The aerobic coronary perfusion was carried out with the sodium-poor, calcium-free, procaine-containing cardioplegic solution being introduced at that time[5]. Under these conditions, the O_2 consumption at normothermia is only 0.8 ml/min × 100 g, that is about one-tenth of that required by a heart working at basic turnover conditions of the whole organism. Although the analyses were done during perfect steady-state conditions, newer experiences call for a more differentiated view in several respects:

(1) The aerobic resting O_2 consumption can vary widely, dependent on the 'pre-ischaemic stress of the heart', substrate and hormone availability, and the electrolyte composition of the cardioplegic solution used. The variation in absolute values, nevertheless, is low compared with the range of energy turnover of the working heart; an example is taken from a paper of Isselhard[6,7] (Figure 2).

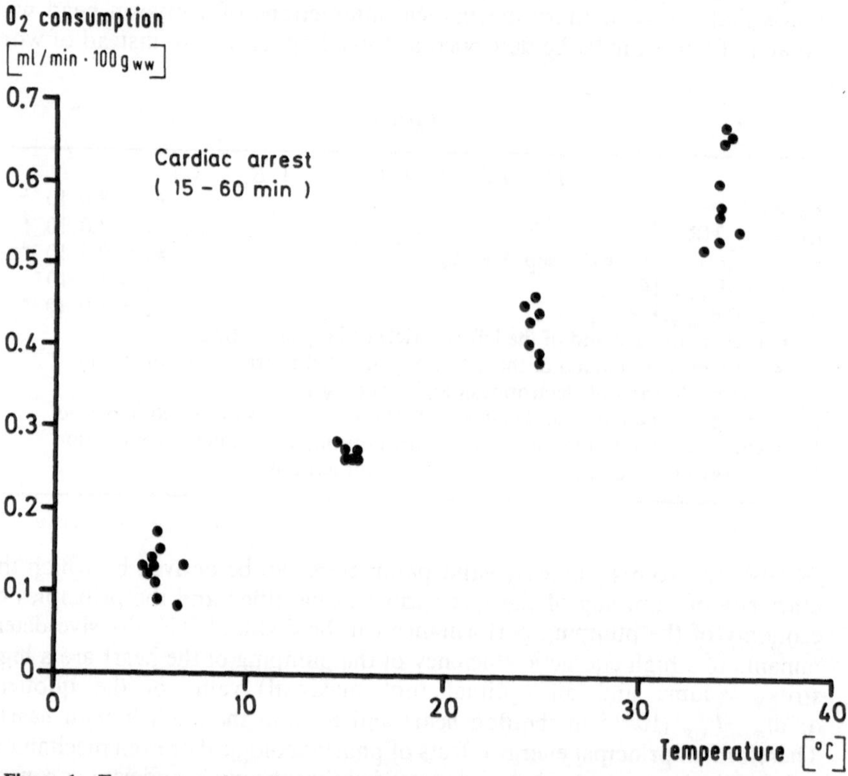

Figure 1 Temperature-dependence of myocardial O_2 consumption within the first hour of cardioplegic arrest

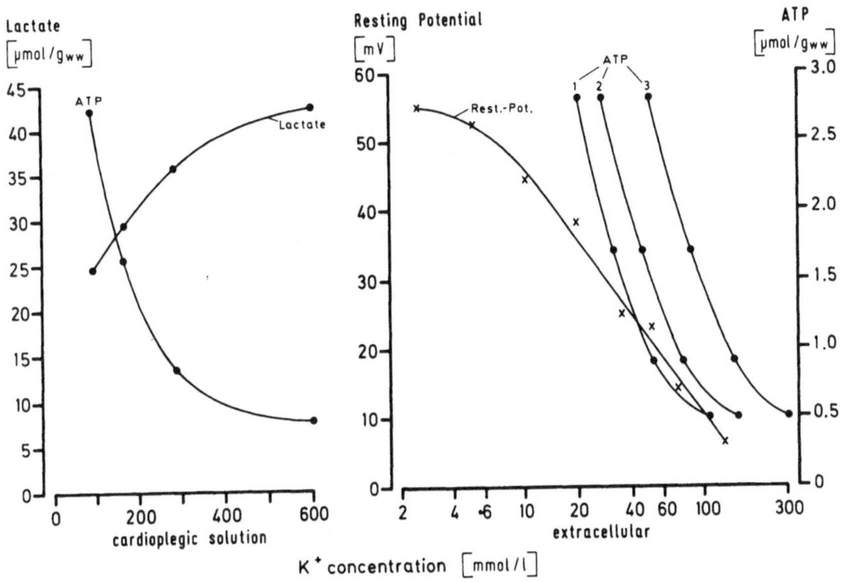

Figure 2 Lactate (left ordinate) and ATP concentration (right ordinate) and resting potential (median ordinate) in dependence of different K^+ concentrations of the cardioplegic solution. Lactate and ATP were analysed in the myocardium of guinea pig hearts after ischaemia (15 min) at 37 °C, while the resting potential was determined at the atrium of cat heart. The ATP curves 1, 2, 3 were calculated from the left ATP curve by varying the fraction of the intravascular capillary volume of the total extracellular space

(2) For a better elucidation of the range of resting O_2 consumption at least four energy-demanding compartments of heart muscle cell must be mentioned: the plasmalemma, the contractile system, the mitochondria, and the sarcoplasmic reticulum.

(3) The aerobic resting energy turnover may not be equated with the structure maintaining energy demand. The latter is to be defined as: 'the minimal resting energy turnover, at which – depending on temperature – all structures can be just kept intact'.

(4) The anaerobic (resting) energy turnover of the heart may vary within wide margins, depending on anamnesis; drugs, substrate- and hormone-supply; as well as on the composition of the cardioplegic solution. Exceptionally, the anaerobic resting energy turnover can be higher than the resting energy turnover during the preceding aerobiosis. Moreover, after an initial phase which may correspond to the phase of creatine phosphate breakdown, in any case the anaerobic energy supply is too low to cover the energy requirement of structure maintenance, as can be seen from the more or less protractedly increasing structure destruction, as well as from the decrease of the energy potential (high energy phosphate, electrolyte gradients) during any myocardial ischaemic anaerobiosis. Figure 3 is a first attempt to graphically describe these connections for a positive 'anamnesis'.

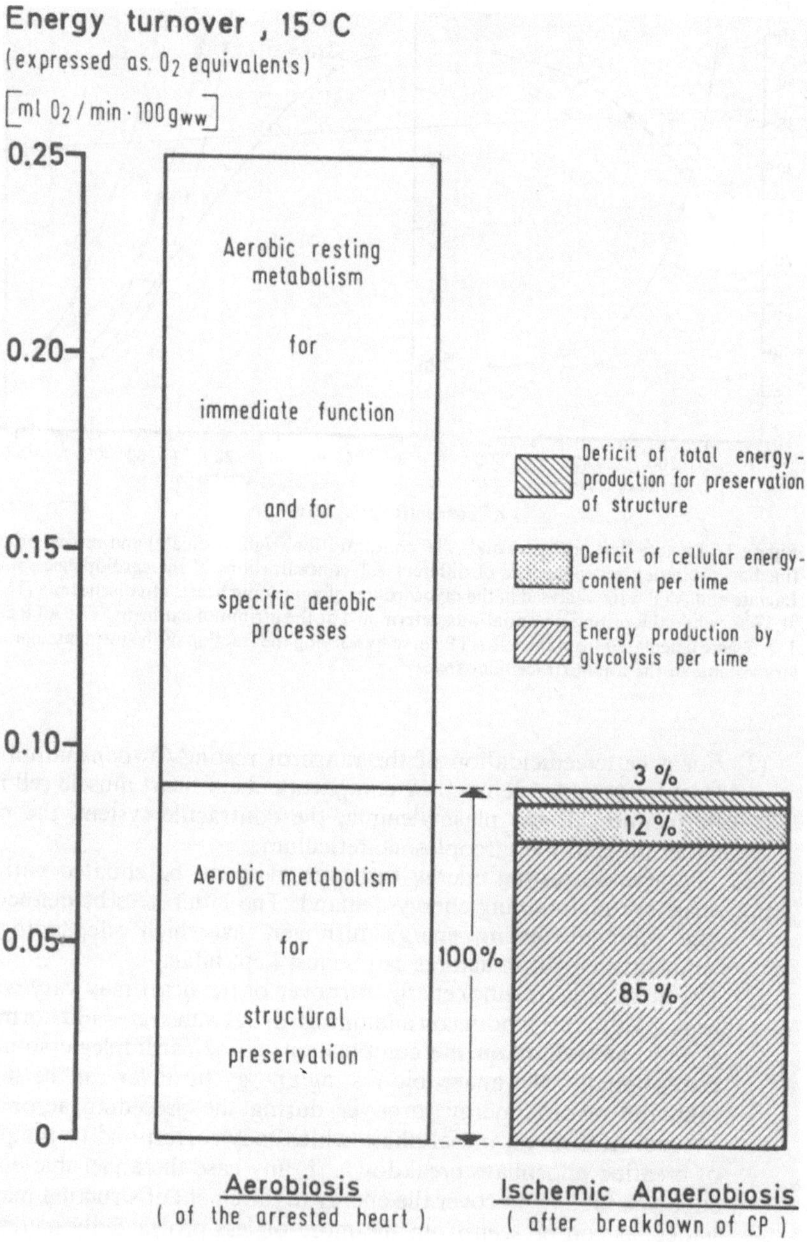

Figure 3 Schematic representation of the components of the myocardial energy turnover of the cardioplegically arrested heart during aerobiosis and anaerobiosis

(c) The energy supply of the heart during ischaemic anaerobiosis comes almost completely from myocardial glycolysis (Table 2). The ATP gain is higher from glycogen than from glucose, and amounts to 1.5 and 1.0 moles per mole lactate respectively. Therefore, and because of a possible retardation of acidification, it seems more favourable to increase the myocardial glycogen reserves pre-ischaemically than to give glucose just before, or even during ischaemia.

The limitation of glycolytic energy gain from glycogen and/or glucose in the myocardium in general is not due to deficiency of substrates, but is based on self-inhibition of the glycolysis by the inevitably increasing acidification. There are two ways to delay the glycolysis-induced intracellular acidosis:

(1) A washout of the protons by intermittent or continuous coronary perfusion[8]; in this case, however, from a rational point of view one would perfuse aerobically.
(2) An additional buffering of the myocardial extracellular space (Table 3).

The efficiency of the latter principle depends on the following points:

(i) good compatibility and solubility of the buffer substance even in higher concentrations;
(ii) appropriate pH value of the buffer substance compared to the normal, as well as to the critical, cellular pH of the myocardium;
(iii) optimal 'dilation' of the extracellular space and homogeneous equilibration, also of the interstice, with the buffer solution;
(iv) high permeability of the myocardial cell membrane to H^+ as well as lactate ions[9];
(v) an osmotic margin within the cardioplegic solution as high as possible without becoming hyperosmotic.

The latter can only be reached by combining the buffer concept with the principle of a cardioplegia by a low-sodium and calcium-free solution. The conditions 'appropriate pK value' as well as 'high water solubility', 'compatibility', and, last but not least, a tolerable price seem only to be fulfilled

Table 2 Postulates for optimizing myocardial protection

Aspects of energetics

4. The decisive energetic principles for a prolongation of ischaemia tolerance of the heart are:
   (a) minimization of the anaerobic *energy requirement* (contractile system, plasma membrane, sarcoplasmic reticulum, mitochondria)
   (b) maximization of anaerobic *energy reserves* (ATP, CP, glycogen)
   (c) optimalization of anaerobic *energy turnover* (quotient of Δ ATP/Δ time, quotient of Δ lactate/Δ time)
   (d) optimalization of the effectiveness of the anaerobic *energy production* (ATP regeneration, quotient of Δ lactate/$\Delta \sim P$)

Table 3 Postulates for optimizing myocardial protection

Aspects of metabolism

1. Maximal reserves of CP and ATP most certainly are obtained by lowering the energy requirement and slowing down the energy turnover by an extensive inactivation of the heart *before* anaerobiosis

2. An optimalization and a prolongation of the anaerobic energy production in the heart is reached by retardation of the autoinhibition of glycolysis by the lactate acidosis. This, principally, becomes possible by an intermittent or continuous coronary perfusion or by raising the extracellular buffer capacity of the heart

by histidine/histidine-HCl[10,11] (Table 4). This buffer system also has the virtue that its p*K* value, with decrease of temperature, increases parallel to the neutral point of water (Figure 4). It can be expected that the addition of a buffer substance of a slightly higher p*K* value – the p*K* of histidine is 6.1 at 25°C – would improve the whole-buffer effectiveness even further.

(d) The energy reserves in the high-energy phosphate content are not to be seen as substrates of the energy protection supply in a strict sense. Nevertheless, they contribute to the energy supply of the cell although with a decimation of the cellular energy charge. Their contribution is higher if the pre-ischaemic starting values are high.

The pre-ischaemic creatine phosphate content is very closely allied to the degree of inactivation and relaxation of the contractile system. Hence a complete relaxation of the myocardium does not only promote a low resting energy turnover but also promotes a high starting creatine phosphate reserve[12].

The pre-ischaemic ATP content seems to be determined by more complex regularities. Under optimal cardioplegic conditions in the dog myocardium we reached values up to 7 μmol/g ww with a total adenine nucleotide content of nearly 9 μmol/g ww. Lower values may result from a non-optimal premedication and anaesthesia, as well as from a disadvantageous membrane effect of the cardioplegic agent. To date, there are no practical methods to increase the myocardial ATP content beyond the mentioned limit of 7 μmol/g ww.

Table 4 Postulates for optimizing myocardial protection

Aspects of metabolism

1. Up to now from all tested buffer substances only histidine/histidine-HCl showed, at the required concentrations no toxicity, sufficient solubility, and good usefulness. At histidine concentrations between 150 and 200 mmol/l the buffer capacity of the myocardium is doubled within the critical pH range

2. The maximally obtainable concentration of lactate in the anaerobic myocardium is raised up to 60 μmol/g ww using this buffer, i.e. it is doubled in comparison with usual values

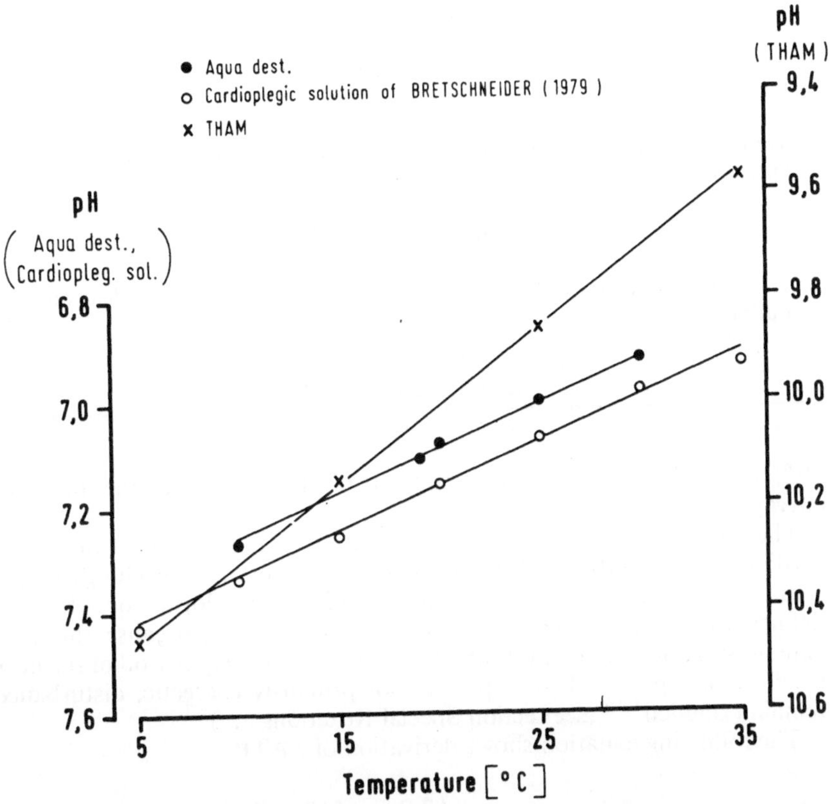

Figure 4 Shifting of pH values of water, histidine-buffered cardioplegic solution, and THAM in dependence of temperature

The sum of the energy equivalents per unit of time, coming from the decrease of the high-energy phosphate and the production of lactate, yields the 'anaerobic whole-energy turnover'.

$$\dot{E}_{\text{anaerobic}} = \frac{\Delta \sim p}{\Delta t} + 1.5 \times \frac{\Delta \text{lactate}}{\Delta t}$$

The ratio 'anaerobic glycolytical energy gain' (from glycogen): 'anaerobic whole-energy turnover' we define as 'efficiency of the anaerobic energy production' (see also Table 5).

$$\eta = \frac{1.5 \times \Delta\, \text{lactate}}{\Delta \sim p + 1.5 \times \Delta\, \text{lactate}}$$

An effective buffering of the myocardial extracellular space, together with an appropriate electrolyte composition of the extracellular space, increase the effectiveness of the anaerobic energy supply from 70 %[8] up to 85 %[9]; that means, the uncovered part of the energy demand, which becomes apparent in proportion to the increasing energy deficit, can be reduced from about

Table 5 Energetic determinants of ischaemia tolerance of the heart

1. *The energy pool* available during ischaemia (high-energy phosphates, substrates for glycolysis)

2. *The energy demand* during ischaemia (assumed to be identical with the ischaemic energy turnover):

$$\dot{E} = \frac{\Delta \sim P}{\Delta t} + \frac{\Delta \text{ lactate} \times 1.5}{\Delta t}$$

3. *The energy production* by anaerobic glycolysis, related to the energy demand during ischaemia:

$$\eta = \frac{\Delta \text{ lactate} \times 1.5}{\Delta \sim P + \Delta \text{ lactate} \times 1.5}$$

30% to nearly 15% by an optimization of effectiveness of the anaerobic energy gain.

The tolerance time to a certain ischaemic stress (temperature, anamnesis, cardioplegic method) is best characterized by the time until reaching a certain critical ATP content; as 'ATP-time' (*t*-ATP) in the dog myocardium we defined this as the time until reaching 4 μmol/g ww, because this ATP content still allows a tolerable and reproducible recovery period of the heart of 20–30 min provided that specific, not primarily energetic, disturbances remain excluded[5,13] (see section Special Reactions . . .).

The following equation shows derivation of *t*-ATP:

$$t\text{-ATP} = \frac{[\text{ATP}_\text{I}] - [\text{ATP}_\text{cr}]}{\Delta[\text{ATP}]/\Delta t}$$

where ATP is the pre-ischaemic initial ATP content; ATP_cr the critical ATP content as defined above; and $\Delta\text{ATP}/\Delta t$ the mean decrease velocity of ATP. Using the previously introduced terms '$\dot{E}_\text{anaerobic}$' and $\eta_\text{anaerobic}$', $\Delta\text{ATP}/\Delta t$ can also be expressed as '$\dot{E}$'. $(1 - \eta)$; therefore:

$$t\text{-ATP} = \frac{[\text{ATP}_\text{I}] - [\text{ATP}_\text{cr}]}{\dot{E}.(1 - \eta)}$$

According to this idea the ischaemic tolerance time is larger if the anaerobic energy turnover is smaller and the efficiency of the glycolytical energy gain is higher. An optimum of *t*-ATP is reached at a minimum of denominator product, not, however, at an 'absolute minimum of "$\dot{E}$"' or at an 'absolute maximum of "η"'.

(e) Concluding the energy aspects, some fundamental differences of the ischaemic compared to the anoxic, non-ischaemic anaerobiosis should be noted, because a lot of experiments on myocardial protection are done in the small-animal heart model using anaerobic perfusion techniques. Besides the considerable species differences, three other decisive differences must be emphasized:

(1) The washout of glycolytically produced lactate and thereby a relative constancy of the intracellular pH.
(2) The maintenance of the extracellular electrolyte, as well as H^+, concentration.
(3) The permanent supply of small but non-negligible amounts of oxygen; at a minimal arterial PO_2 of about 6–10 mmHg, and a flow rate of 4 ml/min × g at normothermia continuously 0.08–0.12 ml O_2/min × 100 g are available to a small animal heart.

Taking into account the usually higher flow rates as well as a possible additional O_2 diffusion into the perfusate during passage through the thin tubing of the perfusion system, then the arterial oxygen supply during the presumed anaerobiosis reaches 15–20% of the anaerobic energy demand. From these considerations the isolated perfused small animal heart is well appropriate for screening tests, but not for reliable quantifications of ischaemia or even anoxia tolerance of the myocardium.

Special reactions of endogenous H^+, Ca^{2+}, tissue hormones, substrates of lipid metabolism as well as osmolality variation on energy turnover of ischaemic anaerobiosis

As discussed in the previous section under the key-word 'energy aspect' one cannot suppose that the ratio of energy demand to energy supply remains unchanged through all the phases of ischaemic anaerobiosis. An imbalance during the first phase of ischaemia, the creatine phosphate decay ('CP phase'), can be improved, in the sense of a better coverage of the energy demand, in that further energy-requiring processes become suppressed. This seems to occur relatively often at the beginning of the second phase of ischaemia, the slow ATP decay ('ATP phase'). However, the imbalance also can become progressively worse in that the efficiency of glycolysis decreases with increasing intracellular acidification.

Both changes could also be considered systematically under the energy aspect. A new aspect, however, is introduced when at a certain critical degree of intracellular acidification compartment barriers break up or disintegrate entirely and thereby cause an 'avalanche-like' excitement of energy requirement or another destructive 'vicious circle'. By way of example, catecholamines and secondarily, or even primarily, Ca^{2+} could be released from intramyocardial stores. This hypothesis is supported by the protective effect of a premedication with β-blocking as well as Ca^{2+}-antagonistic drugs[14,15]. Moreover, it could be an explanation for the protective effect of potent extracellular buffering. The hypothesis is also compatible with the experience that the margin of normothermic ischaemia tolerance by pretreatment with β-blockers or Ca^{2+} anatagonists, in the ischaemic arrest as well as in insufficient myocardial protection, only amounts to a few minutes. In combination with our new cardioplegic method, however, it reaches 30 min; in both cases the additional protective effect can be estimated to be about 20%. A combination of β-blocking and Ca^{2+} antagonistic pretreatment hitherto has not been tested, and for clinical use is highly problematic.

The analysis of the products of lipid metabolism, which appear with increasing ischaemic stress, is not yet fully understood. It cannot be excluded that detergents – like metabolites, e.g. lysolecithins – could accelerate the above-mentioned avalanche processes by membrane disaggregation and may be formed parallel with the progression of energy deficiency and acidification, or may be partially independent of it. Convincing experimental indications for a therapeutically useful interference in the ischaemic lipid metabolism – in the sense of further enhancement of ischaemic tolerance of the heart – show that all previously discussed determinants of the ischaemia tolerance have been optimized and standardized. The lipid metabolism probably cannot be influenced decisively by the electrolyte composition of the cardioplegic solution itself; practicable possibilities of influencing the lipid metabolism are more likely to be found in the pre-ischaemic modification of myocardial metabolism.

The optimal osmolality of the cardioprotective solution has to be seen in connection with the normal intracellular osmolality and its change during an ischaemic stress. If the heart–lung machine is filled normotonically, oxygen supply is sufficient and higher doses of osmotically active diuretics and other hypertonic infusions are avoided before cardioplegia; in general one may suppose a physiological intracellular osmolality in the myocardium. In this case normotonicity, about 290 mosmol/l, of the cardioplegic solution gives the best results. Deviations up to $\pm 5\%$ are of no clear effect, a significant hypotonicity as well as a strong hypertonicity, however, act negatively: Hypotonicity of the protective solution causes cell edema and thereby: (1) an initial swelling of subcellular as well as cellular parts, the membranes of which otherwise become stressed by ischaemia-caused increasing osmotic gradients; and (2) a reduction of the available extracellular buffer space. A higher hypertonicity of the cardioplegic agent initially counteracts the ensuing swelling of cellular structures, but thereby reduces the intracellular and cellular exchange surfaces. A diminution of the available buffer space, however (as well as an impairment of permeation conditions within and outside the cell), obligatorily decreases the effectiveness of an extracellular buffer.

In principle the cellular and subcellular swellings that occur during severe ischaemic stress do not result from an inappropriate osmolality of the cardioplegic solution, but indicate osmotic gradients no longer being compensated. The ischaemic anaerobiosis unavoidably leads to an increased intracellular accumulation of low molecular substances. Their osmotic effect causes destruction in the long run which can only be reduced in two ways (without the disadvantages of an initial shrinking) (1) by good conditions of permeability that will not influence the numerical increase of osmoles per unit of time, but will delay the development of gradients; (2) by numerical decrease of the produced osmoles per unit of time, that means, decreasing the glycolytic turnover. The last aspect offers an additional argument not to consider the expression '$\dot{E} \,.\, (1 - \eta)$' discussed in the previous section as requiring a maximal η and thus a maximal glycolytic turnover. A smaller glycolytic intensity formally leads to lower but more advantageous values of $\dot{E}$;

probably it will reduce the osmotic gradients, too, and will delay the development of the acidosis in any case. At a critical point both processes may additionally inaugurate, as mentioned above, deleterious procedures, e.g. release of catecholamines and Ca^{2+}.

Effects of temperature on methods of myocardial protection

It is generally accepted that a drop in temperature will reduce the aerobic and anaerobic metabolic intensity and thereby lead to a prolongation of the myocardial ischaemia tolerance. To date a coefficient of change in temperature for 10°C–Q_{10} value – of about 2 had been observed; lowering the temperature by 30°C you may calculate a factor $2^3 = 8$. The absolute value for the prolongation of the tolerable myocardial ischaemic time obviously depends on the magnitude of the normothermic basic turnover. It may be much smaller in the case of a thyrotoxicosis than in a hypothyreosis.

Our more recent results demonstrate that the conceptions about the temperature-range between 35°C and 5°C must be extended and partly corrected. The most surprising fact is that the critical extracellular pH value – most probably the critical intracellular pH as well – is independent of temperature. In our cardioplegic method the critical extracellular pH value is about 6.0 over the temperature range of interest; consequently the critical extracellular pH value is not involved in the shifting of the neutral point at a decreasing temperature (see Figure 4), but the critical, absolute H^+ concentration remains constant. With decreasing temperature supplementary 'buffer reserves' will be made intracellularly and extracellularly accessible, and which will make possible much higher total lactate concentration until reaching the critical pH value, unless the extracellular pH value is systematically adjusted to the temperature. Moreover with a drop in temperature the metabolic activities decrease much more (according to the higher temperature coefficient) – especially the glycolytic turnover – than the pure physical processes of permeation and diffusion, even taking into account a 'loss of fluidity' of the membranes with decreasing temperature. The organ-protective effects of a drop in temperature may be differentiated as follows:

(1) Reduction of the energy demand, of the glycolytic intensity and of the production of protons.
(2) Provision of a supplementary 'buffer reserve' by shifting the neutral point of water and the p*K* values of buffers to the alkaline side at a nearly constant critical pH value.
(3) Improvement of the ratio of permeability to substrate accumulation because of the greater temperature-dependency of biochemical processes compared to pure physical processes.

Therefore it is reasonable that the protective effect of a drop in temperature cannot be calculated from the temperature-dependency of various individual 'limiting processes'. Certain ion combinations may act in a relatively advantageous manner in hypothermia while they act contrarily in normothermia.

The opposite is true for pure ischaemic cardiac arrest, because the cold-induced depolarization of the sarcolemma is followed by an increase of the tonus and also of the energy demand if there is a normal extracellular ionic composition. Therefore the temperature coefficient between 35 °C and 5 °C (Q_{30} value) is relatively small in the case of pure ischaemic arrest: it is about 8 for the canine heart during neurolept analgesia. Using our buffered cardioplegic solution we reached Q_{30} values of about 13. This gain will become particularly evident at lower temperatures, which has some advantage for organ preservation.

The regularities described are not restricted to the myocardium, they must be valid for all organs with high metabolic activity. First experimental investigations for kidney preservation in our institute have shown that the fundamental considerations described are completely transferable to the kidney, although no creatine phosphate, and only a low mean ATP content, are present; the kidney has other functions and is structured very heterogeneously.

METHODICAL REALIZATION OF THE ENERGETIC AND SPECIAL ASPECTS FOR PROLONGATION OF ISCHAEMIA TOLERANCE OF THE HEART

Setting aside the cardiac mechanical performance brings the highest absolute reduction of myocardial energy requirement. Thus often the terms 'cardioplegia' and 'myocardial protection' are employed as synonyms. From the modern view 'myocardial protection' is the superordinate category and 'cardioplegia', the artificial cardiac arrest, is one method of ameliorating myocardial protection. A fully reversible and immediately effective cardioplegia can be reached in different ways. The mostly relevant ones are (see also Table 6):

(a) Depolarization by increase of extracellular K^+ concentration.
(b) Electromechanical uncoupling by reversible extracellular Ca^{2+}-withdrawal.
(c) Suspension of electrical activity by drastic reduction of extracellular Na^+ concentration.
(d) Suppression of excitability by inactivation of the fast Na^+ canal and general 'membrane stabilization' by extracellular local anaesthetic agents, respectively.
(e) Membrane stabilization and suppression of excitability by high extracellular Mg^{2+} concentrations.
(f) Reduction of excitability by deep local hypothermia.
(g) Depletion of creatine phosphate reserves by disconnection of coronary circulation (ischaemic cardiac arrest).

Apart from ischaemic cardiac arrest, which is not suitable for a myocardium protection, and from acetylcholine arrest[17], which does not relieve excitability of the unspecific myocardium, the above-mentioned methods can be com-

Table 6 Methods of artificial cardiac arrest

1. Complete ischaemia of the heart at body temperature
2. Deep hypothermia of the heart by either topical or systemic cooling
3. Depolarization of the myocardium by high extracellular potassium concentrations
4. Suspension of the electrophysiological processes by low extracellular sodium concentrations
5. Electromechanical uncoupling by removal of the extracellular calcium
6. Suspension of the electromechanical activity by high extracellular magnesium concentrations
7. Pharmacological suppression of the electrophysiological processes, especially by anti-arrhythmic drugs
8. Suppression of the pacemaker automaticity by acetylcholine or corresponding agents, or by topical cooling
9. Electrically induced depolarization
10. Combinations, especially of methods, 2, 4, 5, 6, and 7

bined in manifold ways. By a well-considered combination unsuitable influences of the extracellular ion concentrations required for the cardiac arrest, on plasmalemma and metabolism of myocardial cells, can be avoided; also the interval between introduction of cardioplegic solution and incidence of cardiac arrest thereby can be varied. In nearly all presently applied cardioplegic methods the additional protection effect of hypothermia is used and the myocardium is at least initially cooled down to 10–20 °C by introducing cooled cardioplegic solution.

The first method of cardiac arrest by potassium citrate introduced by Melrose in 1955 was an original combination of potassium and calcium-withdrawal arrest[18]. The method showed the disadvantage that the calcium withdrawal was too late and too incompletely reversible; his principles, however, are useful to this day, as can be seen in the combination of potassium arrest and calcium antagonistic pretreatment. Even the concept we introduced in 1964[5], which combines the extracellular calcium withdrawal and sodium reduction, was decisively stimulated by the method of Melrose. The additional employment of procaine, which we used at that time, brings the following advantages:

(a) A prolongation of ischaemia tolerance of about 25 %.
(b) An immediately resulting maximal coronary dilation.
(c) Fast incidence of cardioplegia.
(d) Anti-oedema effect in protracted cardioplegic perfusion.

Against this, current knowledge indicates several disadvantages of procaine in cardioplegia which must be mentioned:

(a) Procaine hinders the permeation of H^+ and lactate ions into the extracellular space and thereby reduces its potential buffer effectiveness decisively[10].

(b) In longer or continually repeated perfusions procaine in concentrations of about 0.1 % and higher may act toxically on the cells of the excitation conduction system, which becomes manifested by post-ischaemic arrhythmias.

(c) Procaine accelerates the rate of cardiac arrest considerably. The achievement of equilibrium via the last pre-ischaemic contractions is thereby eliminated, which is of special importance in hypertrophic or coronary stenotic inhomogeneous perfused hearts, and increases the risk of insufficiently protected myocardium areas.

It would lead too far afield to discuss the pros and cons of all possible, or even only of all presently employed, combinations of cardioplegic methods; five clinically used and often discussed methods will be compared in the next section of this paper, 'Experimental Results'. Two general important practical points, however, can be summarized:

(i) One must not examine a cardioplegic agent or a cardioprotective solution in isolation, but must consider in every case the whole cardioplegia and protection procedure (including temperature, perfusion pressure, perfusion rate and application time).

(ii) A cardioplegic and myocardium-protective solution cannot be optimized by a summation of the special virtues of its diverse components. The interactions between the various effects are generally not simply additive, and in many cases cannot be quantitatively explained by the ion theory of excitation; all the more since, for example, actions of drugs or temperature may be superimposed.

On the first point, cardioplegic agent and application made, some comments seem to be indicated, because of several general misunderstandings:

(i) A sodium-poor, calcium-free solution has to be applied cold; with warm application a calcium paradox may be evoked whereas at 15 °C a 120 min continuous perfusion is without risk (Figures 5 and 6)[19].

(ii) Equilibration of the interstitial space requires much more time than wash out of the coronary system; according to our experimental results at 10°C in normal coronary system at least 7–10 min are needed. A single or even repeated injection of 200 ml of a cardioplegic agent is insufficient to achieve a new steady state of extracellular electrolyte concentrations. Moreover, according to calorimetric calculations, 200 ml of an 0°C solution reduces the temperature of a 400 g heart by 10 °C, that is from normothermia to 25 °C, at most.

A further argument, closely connected with those mentioned above, is that the relatively high energy demand of the beating heart graduates into resting energy demand; during this transition period energy reserves in ATP and CP, especially, accumulate, provided that aerobiosis is covered. This, in detail, is shown in Figure 7. Here the course of equilibration during perfusion with our solution at 200–250 ml/min × 100 g ww is demonstrated by means of the parameters perfusion pressure, myocardial temperature, CO_2 and O_2 partial pressure, and O_2 consumption of the heart. It becomes evident that a cardioplegic perfusion time, shorter than 7–10 min, would be equiva-

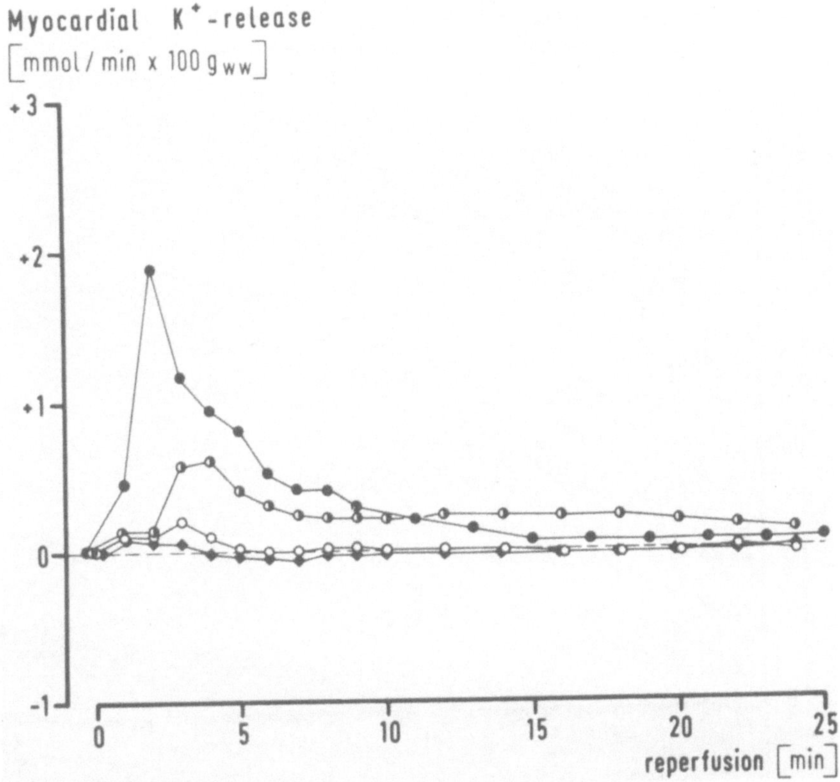

Figure 5 K^+-release of the empty-beating dog heart during Tyrode-solution reperfusion at 35 °C after continuous long-time application of the Ca^{2+}-free cardioplegic solution (Bretschneider, 1979):

●——● Cardioplegic perfusion: 60 min at 35 °C
◐——◐ Cardioplegic perfusion: 30 min at 35 °C
○——○ Cardioplegic perfusion: 30 min at 25 °C
◆——◆ Cardioplegic perfusion: 60 min at 25 °C

lent to an energy waste. At the beginning of the 10 min cardioplegic perfusion the perfusion pressure is between 80 and 70 mmHg, after 2 min about 60 mmHg, and at the end of the perfusion it is about 40 mmHg; the coronary flow is held nearly constant and is adjusted – after estimation of the heart weight – to 200–250 ml/min and 100 g. Probably the diminution of the coronary resistance to nearly half of the initial value – in spite of the increased viscosity of the cardioplegic solution as a function of the decreasing temperature – depends predominantly on an increasing myocardial relaxation as a result of the proceeding reduction of the 'myocardial component of the coronary resistance'. The oxygen supply–at least 200 ml/min and 100 g × 0.5 vol. % = 1.0 ml O_2/min and 100 g, maximally 250 ml/min and 100 g × 0.6 vol. % = 1.5 ml O_2/min/100 g– is sufficient to cover the oxygen demand after the first minute of perfusion, although the solution is not equilibrated with pure

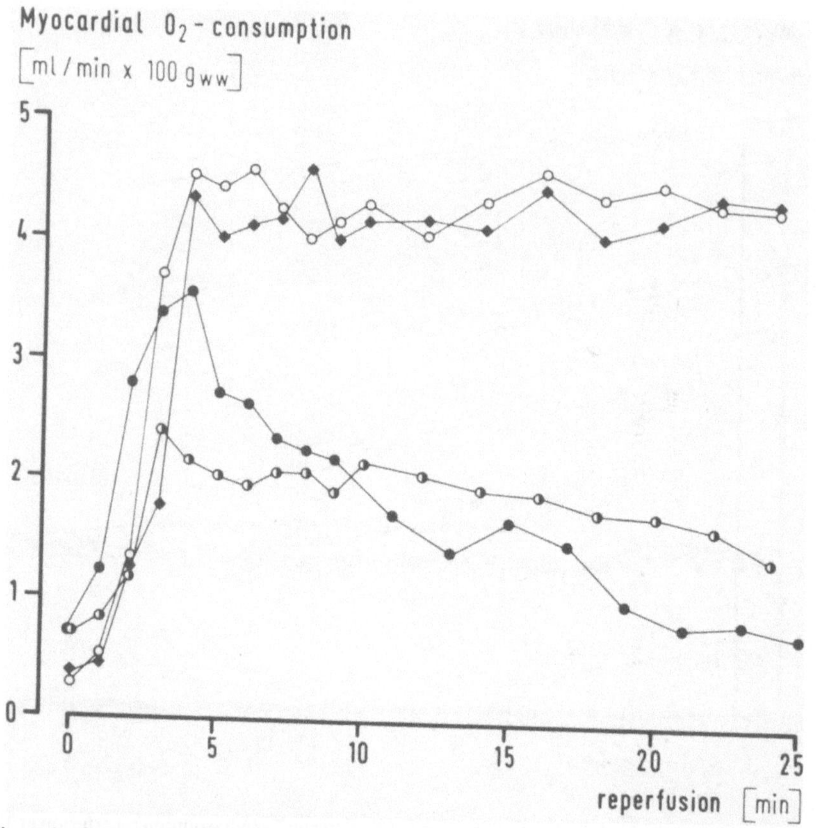

Figure 6 O_2-consumption of the empty-beating dog heart during Tyrode-solution reperfusion at 35 °C after continuous long-time application of the Ca^{2+}-free cardioplegic solution (Bretschneider, 1979):

●——● Cardioplegic perfusion: 60 min at 35 °C
◐——◐ Cardioplegic perfusion: 30 min at 35 °C
○——○ Cardioplegic perfusion: 30 min at 25 °C
◆——◆ Cardioplegic perfusion: 60 min at 25 °C

oxygen. This can be achieved by: (a) the low viscosity of the solution and the high flow rate; (b) the rapid cooling of the myocardium with the 8–10 °C cold solution in combination with the high flow rate; (c) the electrical and mechanical inactivation of the heart within the first minute after perfusion onset.

EXPERIMENTAL RESULTS (CANINE HEART) OF SIX DIFFERENT METHODS OF MYOCARDIAL PROTECTION

Table 7 represents the most important data concerning the composition of four cardioplegic solutions being currently employed in clinical practice. The 'Kirklin solution' is exemplary for a pure potassium-induced cardiac

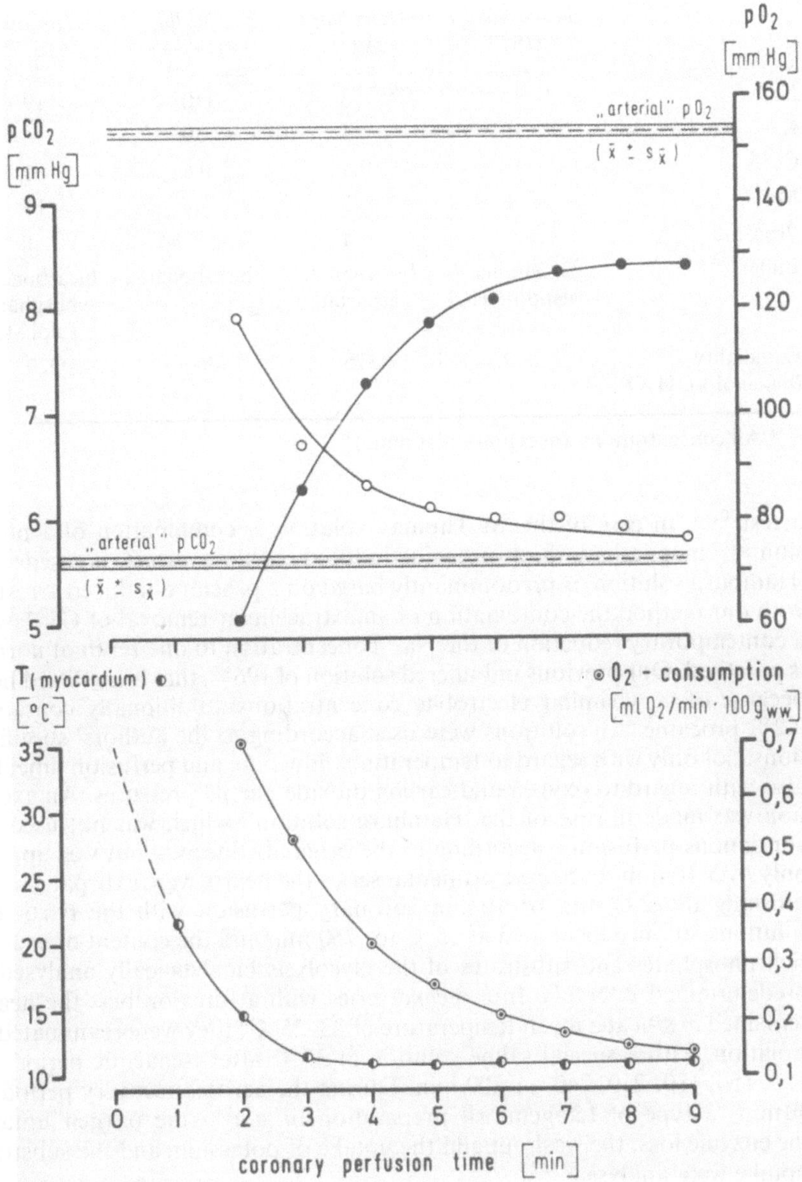

Figure 7 Myocardial equilibration with regard to coronary perfusion pressure, temperature, PO_2, PCO_2 and O_2 consumption ($\dot{V}_{O_2}$) during coronary perfusion with the histidine buffered cardioplegic solution

Table 7 Cations* and buffer substances at various cardioplegic solutions

	Bretschneider (1979)	*Cardiac Surg.* (*Hamburg*) (1975)	*Kirklin* (1977)	*St Thomas' Hospital* (1977)
Na^+	15	50	110	119
K^+	10	5	30	16
Ca^{2+}	–	0.5	0.5	1
Mg^{2+}	8	2	–	16
Procaine	–	4	–	1
Buffer	histidine, histidine-HCl	bicarbonate, aspartate	bicarbonate	bicarbonate, phosphate, sulphate
Osmolality (mosmol/kg H_2O)	300	375	360	320

* All concentrations are expressed as mmol/l.

arrest[20,21], in case of the 'St Thomas' solution' a combination of a potassium[22], magnesium, and procaine-induced cardiac arrest is used; the 'Hamburg solution' is predominantly based on a procaine-induced arrest[23]; with our method the combination of an extracellular removal of Ca^{2+} with a contemporary reduction of the Na^+ concentration to one-tenth of normal is practised. Our previous unbuffered solution of 1964[5], that is not listed here, because of very similar electrolyte concentrations, additionally contained 0.2% procaine. All solutions were used according to the authors' specifications, not only with regard to temperature, flow rate, and perfusion time, but also with regard to oxygen and carbon dioxide partial pressures. An exception was made in case of the 'Hamburg solution', which was not used for continuous perfusion – according to the original concept – but was applied only over 10 min. In *one* experimental series the hearts were extirpated after finishing the 2–3 min or 10 min coronary perfusion with the particular solutions, at once incubated at 15 °C for 750 min and the content of energy-rich phosphates and substrates of the glycolysis biochemically analysed at predetermined intervals. In a *second* series with a function bias the hearts remained *in situ* at a mean temperature of 23–25 °C; they were reanimated in isolation, with a special saline solution at 35 °C after ischaemic periods of 120, 150, 180, 210, 240, or 300 min. During the aerobic recovery period of 30 min – a type of Langendorff preparation *in situ*[24] – the oxygen uptake, the enzyme loss, the washout and the uptake of potassium and the substrate uptake were analysed[21,25].

The results of the first series are summarized in Figures 8–10. Figure 8 represents comparative biochemical results of the St. Thomas' method and the Kirklin method. The time intervals until reaching the 'critical' ATP value of 4 μmol/g ww are nearly equal, although the CP breakdown is distinctly faster in case of the Kirklin method. This result is of principal importance:

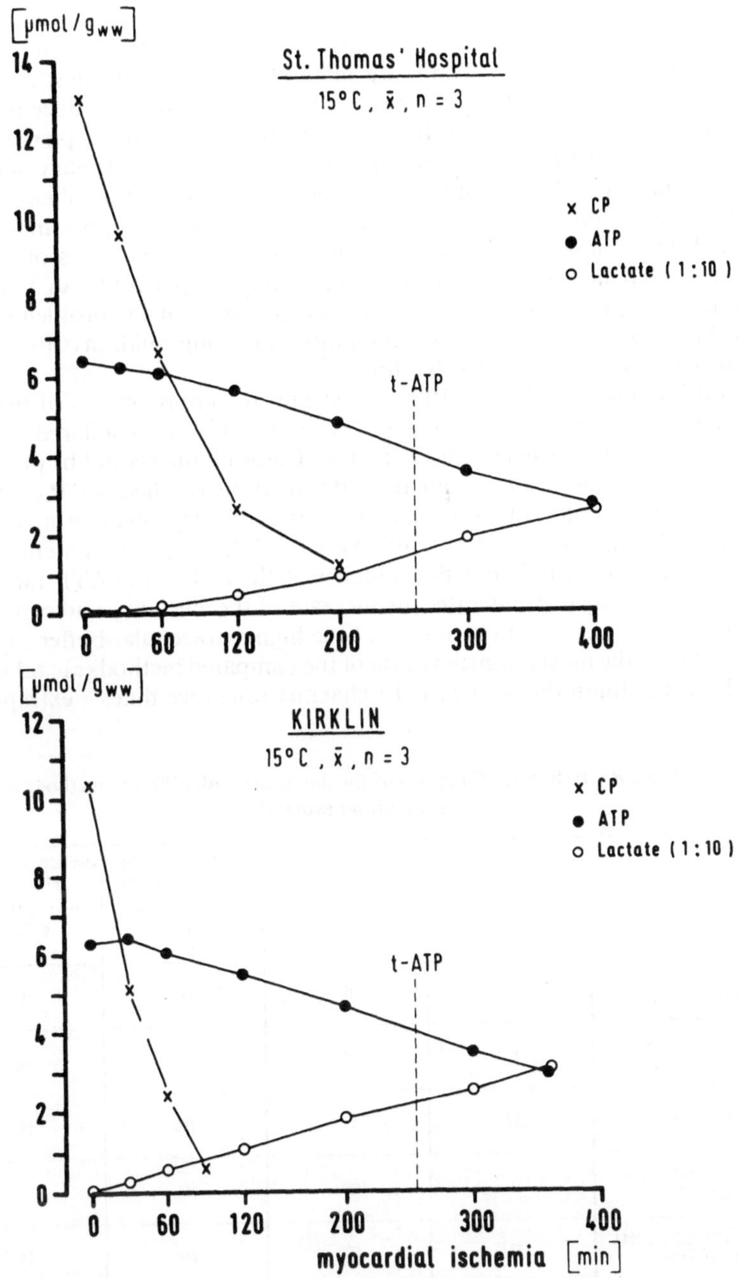

Figure 8 Biochemical analyses(mean) (CP ×, ATP ●, lactate ○) during myocardial ischaemia at an incubation temprature of 15 °C. The hearts were arrested with the cardioplegic solution of St Thomas's Hospital (n = 3) and of Kirklin (n = 3)

the velocities of CP breakdown and ATP breakdown can be influenced in a large range independent from one another.

In Figure 9 the myocardial ischaemia tolerance at 15 °C after myocardial protection with the 'Hamburg solution' is compared with pure myocardial ischaemia. Although the 'Hamburg method' shows the shortest ATP time of the recent methods, the prolongation of the ischaemia tolerance time to a factor of 3 is very impressive. In this connection it must be emphasized that the 'Hamburg method' was developed for a continuous coronary perfusion and for this it is also very suitable, because of its composition of electrolytes and its normal oncotic pressure. On the occasion of the symposium on Myocardial Protection in Cologne we pointed out the consequences of the high viscosity that may occur in hearts with extreme hypertrophy or with very inhomogeneous coronary circulation, and pointed out the problems of the sensibility to procaine in the case of infants and young children (substantially smaller radius of the myocardial fibre)[26].

In this connection Figure 10 demonstrates the improvement of the myocardial protection that was reached with the histidine-buffered solution compared to our former method of 1964. The ATP time could be prolonged to more than a factor of 2, while the CP time (time reaching a CP content of 3 μmol/g ww) could only be extended by 50 %. The glycolytic turnover – the quotient Δlactate/Δt – does not differ very much from the other methods, but the lactate content is 2 to 3 times higher at the end of the ATP time. This finding obviously demonstrates the increase of the efficiency and capacity of the glycolytic energy gain by means of the high extracellular buffer capacity.

In Table 8 the most important data of the compared methods are tabulated. In the last column the myocardial ischaemia tolerance times – extrapolated

Table 8 Ischaemia tolerance of the dog heart with different methods of myocardial protection

Myocardial Protection	Lactate Content at "t - ATP" (4 μmol ATP/g ww) at 15 °C [μmol/g ww]	"Survival Time" "t - CP" (3 μmol CP/g ww) at 15 °C [min]	Exper. Usable Time of Ischemia: "t - ATP" (4 μmol ATP/g ww) at 15 °C [min]	Clinically Usable Time of Ischemia (≈ 5 μmol ATP/g ww) at 30 °C [min]
Ischemic cardiac arrest	17	10	60	12
Cardiac surgery Hamburg, 1975	14	80	200	40
KIRKLIN, 1977	22	55	260	50
St. Thomas' Hospital London, 1977	16	120	280	55
BRETSCHNEIDER, 1964 with procaine	17	120	280	55
BRETSCHNEIDER, 1979 propranolol-pretreatment	48	180	600	120

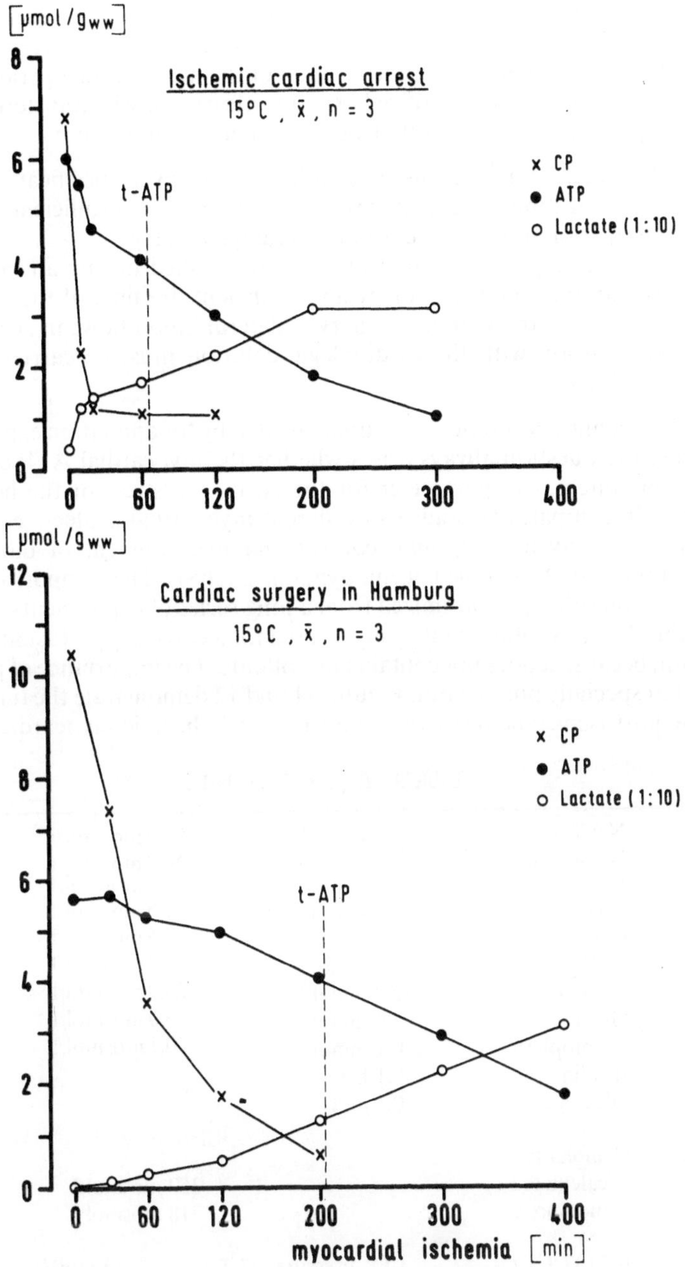

Figure 9 Biochemical analyses (mean) (CP ×, ATP ●, lactate ○) during myocardial ischaemia at an incubation temperature of 15 °C. The hearts were arrested without any protection ('ischaemic cardiac arrest') ($n = 3$) and with the 'Hamburg cardioplegic method' ($n = 3$)

to 30°C and an ATP content of 5 μmol/g ww – for the different cardioplegic methods are listed. These tolerance times can also be considered as the clinically useful times where the recovery time of more than 20 min is not necessary. These data contain a certain safety factor which is very advisable in view of the unpredictable precondition of the hearts to be operated upon. The data of our well-standardized experiments can only be transferred to the clinical practice under the following fundamental conditions:

(1) The method must be used according to the given specifications.
(2) Even an inhomogeneous myocardium with an insufficient coronary circulation must be equilibrated homogeneously.
(3) The cardioplegic solution may not be washed out by an incomplete isolation of the heart, or by an insufficient draining of the ventricles, or by an extreme non-coronary collateral blood flow; in such cases a reperfusion with the cardioplegic colution must be carried out immediately.

The 'biochemical test series' was supplemented by 're-animation experiments' because the question always arises whether the myocardial ATP content is a reliable integrative parameter for the ischaemic stress of the heart – especially in comparative studies of different myocardial protective methods. Priority was given to optimal control and measurement of biochemical data at the cost of a detailed haemodynamic analysis. The composition of the 'reperfusion solution', optimized from a long series of experiments, is shown in Table 9[27]; this solution may only be used for a coronary perfusion of about 30 min, because it does not contain any colloids. The importance of glucagon may be especially pointed out. Figures 11 and 12 demonstrate the time course of the post-ischaemic heart rate and the post-ischaemic myocardial oxygen

Table 9 Reperfusion solution

NaCl	146.0 mmol/l	292.0 mosmol/l
Na lactate	5.0 mmol/l	10.0 mosmol/l
KCl	4.0 mmol/l	8.0 mosmol/l
$MgCl_2$	0.5 mmol/l	1.5 mosmol/l
$CaCl_2$	2.5 mmol/l	7.5 mosmol/l
NaH_2PO_4	0.5 mmol/l	1.5 mosmol/l
$NaHCO_3$	12.0 mmol/l	24.0 mosmol/l
Glucose	5.0 mmol/l	5.0 mosmol/l
Tryptophan	0.1 mmol/l	0.1 mosmol/l
Insulin	0.1 E/l	
Glucagon	0.1 μg/l	
Osmolality		
calculated		350 mosmol/l
measured		318 mosmol/l
pH (37°C) 7.4	CO_2 pressure (37°C)	15 mmHg
O_2 content 1.7–1.9 vol. %	O_2 pressure (37°C)	540–600 mmHg

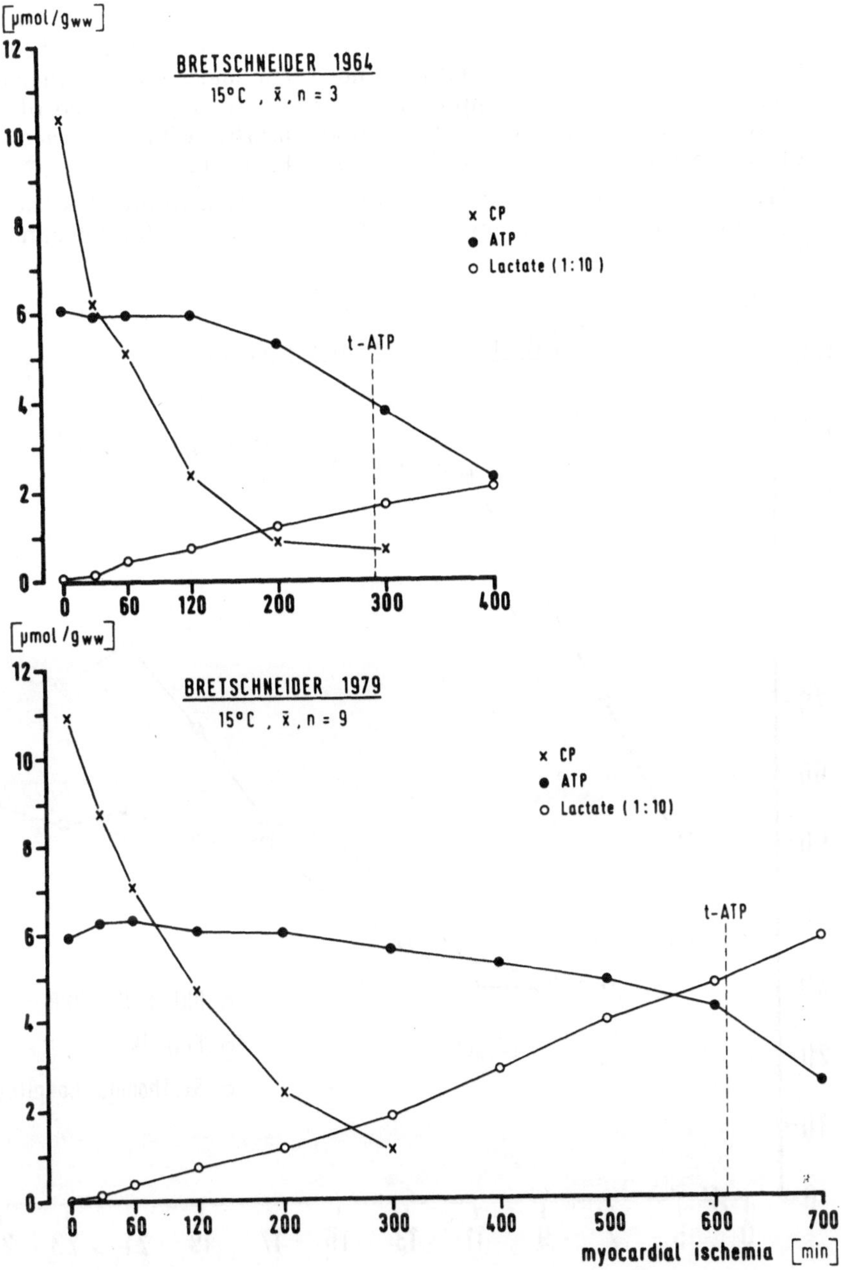

Figure 10 Biochemical analyses (mean) (CP ×, ATP ●, lactate ○) during myocardial ischaemia at an incubation temperature of 15 °C. The hearts were arrested with the unbuffered, procaine-containing cardioplegic solution of Bretschneider (1964) ($n = 9$)

uptake at 35 °C. At the end of the reperfusion period of 30 min the myocardial contents of CP, ATP, and lactate were determined. The post-ischaemic ATP contents (Figure 13) were in very good relation to those ATP values, being extrapolated from the biochemical test series; this may result from the fact that a *de-novo* synthesis of ATP does not occur under our experimental conditions. Since the total impression of the recovery period and of the ability for recovery does correlate – almost linearly – with the decreasing ATP content, the following assertions seem to be justified:

(1) The ATP content is a very good indicator for myocardial ischaemic stress and the ability for myocardial recovery, even for comparative

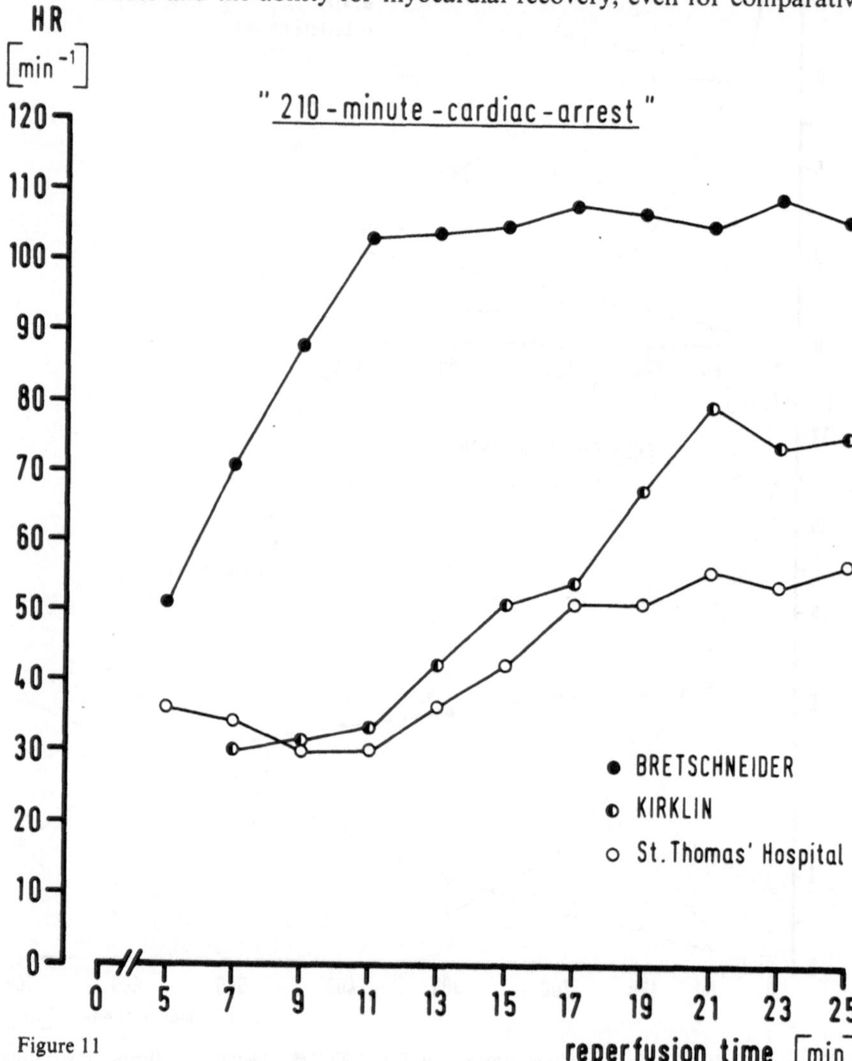

Figure 11

Figures 11 and 12 Post-ischaemic heart rates and O_2 consumptions (mean) at 35 °C after 210 min of cardiac arrest induced by different cardioplegic solutions experiments with very different methods of myocardial protection – an exception must be made, of course, in the case of a specific myocardial poisoning.

(2) The 'initial or functional recovery period' of the heart is almost linearly extended between an ATP content of 6.0 and 4.5 μmol/g ww; at an ATP content of 4 μmol/g ww it lasts about 30 min (Figure 14).

(3) The 'complete or energetic–metabolic recovery period' may only correspond to the initial recovery demand at an ATP content of more than 5.5 μmol/g ww, because the *de-novo* synthesis of a distinctly

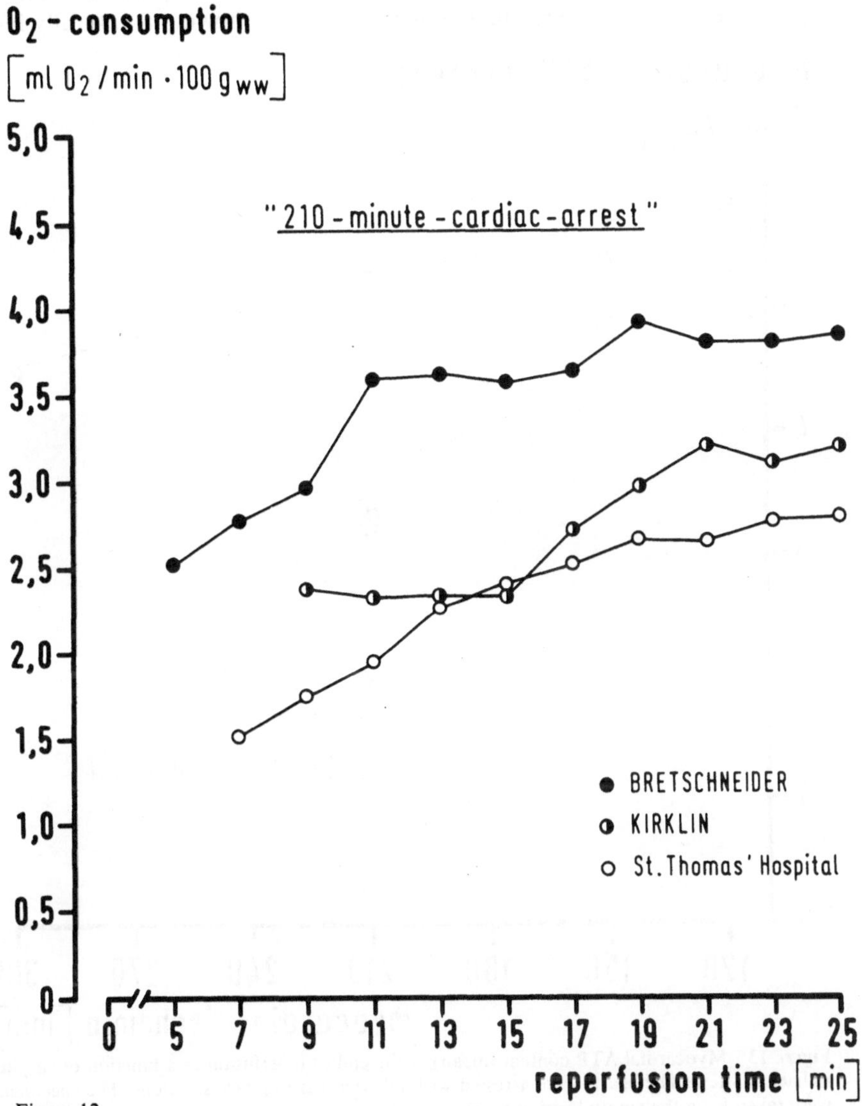

Figure 12

reduced ATP content requires much more time, in certain cases several days (Figure 14)[28-30].

(4) A distinctive functional analysis can reveal certain strong or weak points of different cardioplegic methods with regard to the myocardial conduction system and the myocardial contractile system; therefore it is necessary for comparison purposes to avoid the preferred technique of an electrical pacemaker. Our experiences until now suggest that the St. Thomas' solution protects the myocardial contractile system particularly well, while the Kirklin solution does the same for the myocardial conduction system. Perhaps one may assume that the tissue of the myocardial conduction system, showing a naturally high

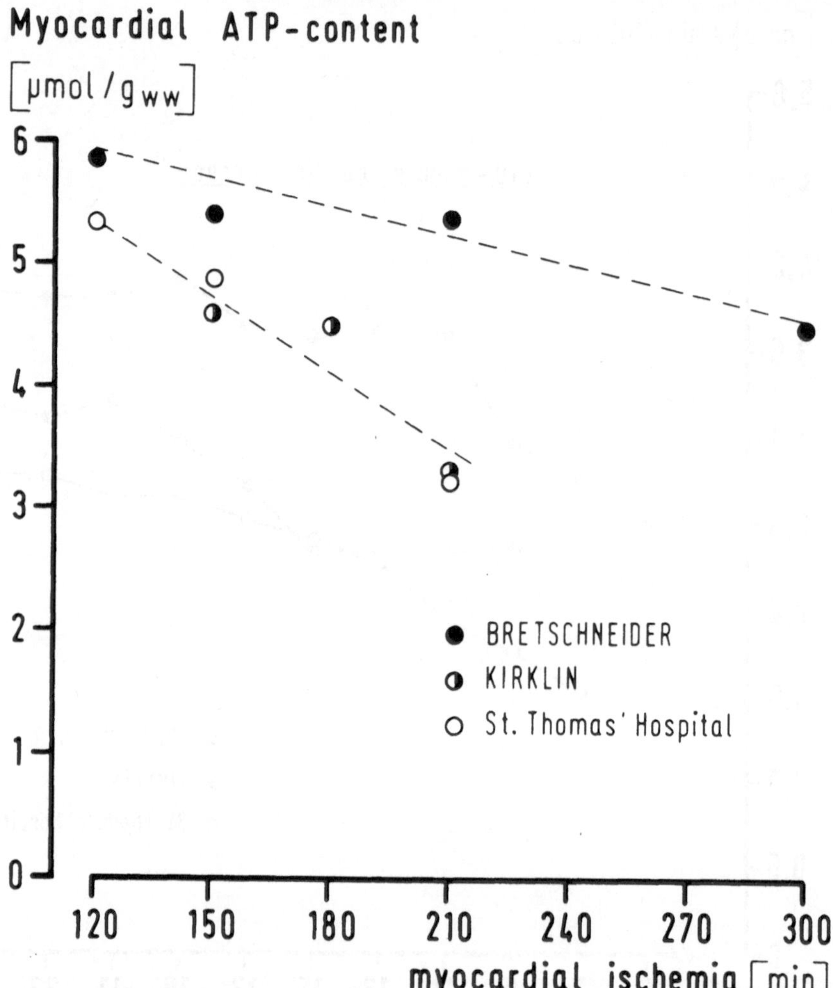

Figure 13 Myocardial ATP content (mean) at the end of reperfusion as a function of varying ischaemic stress. The hearts were arrested with different cardioplegic solutions. The specimens were taken from the empty-beating hearts at 35°C

glycolytical capacity, will not be sufficiently protected by methods with distinctly reduced glycolytic turnover (see Table 8, column 1).

DISADVANTAGES OF MYOCARDIAL PROTECTION

In our opinion there are no longer decisive disadvantages of myocardial protection. Nevertheless, the following risks are not unimportant:

(1) A slight overdilatation of the very flaccid myocardium, which leads to the necessity of a sufficient ventricular drainage.

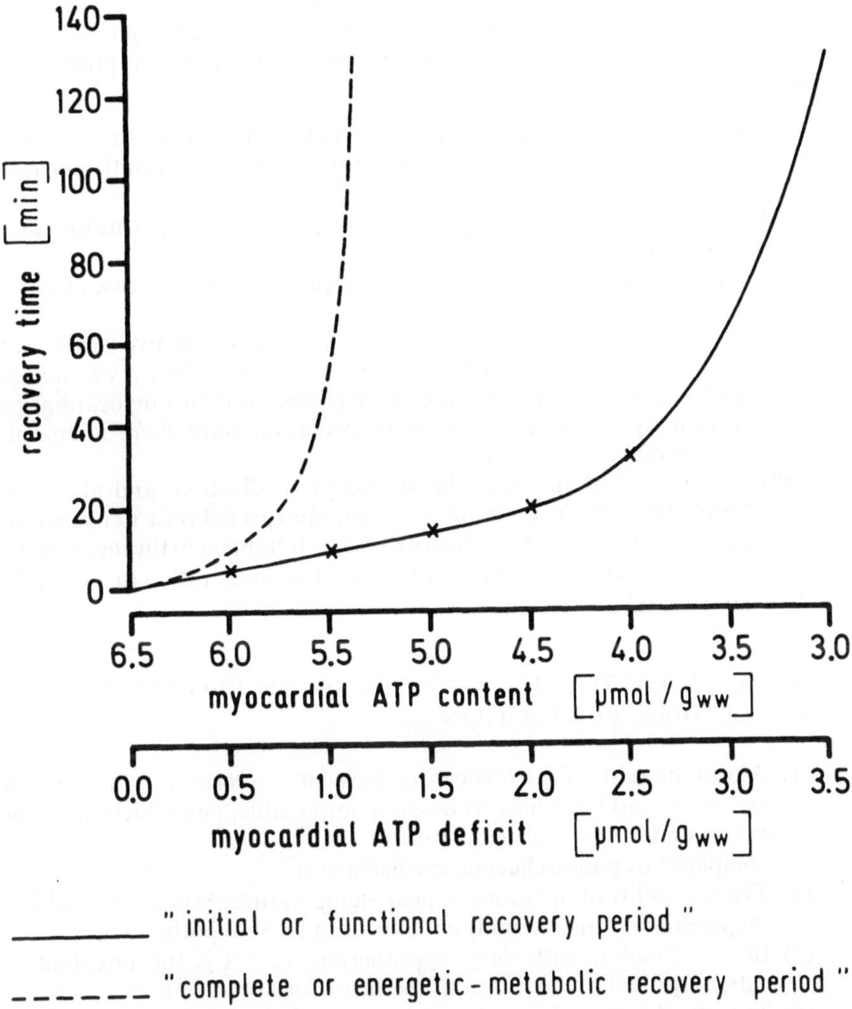

Figure 14 Schematic representation of the required time for the 'initial or functional recovery period' and the 'complete or energetic–metabolic recovery' after cardiac arrest as a function of the amount of the ATP deficit after complete myocardial ischaemia

(2) A delay in the intra-operative function control, e.g. of special parts of the conduction system.
(3) To some extent an uncertainty of the still available ischaemic tolerance of the heart, if there are indications for the washout of the protective solution.

The first two disadvantages mentioned above must be accepted for every good cardioplegia. The third disadvantage does not exist in case of the 'Hamburg method', because of the continous perfusion. But it may be possible to develop methods for intra-operative control of the 'ischaemic stress' or of the 'reserve of the possible ischaemic tolerance', for example with micro-pH electrodes or with similar physical measurements.

Disadvantages can be seen in the following points, although these disadvantages are more factors requiring a reorientation in current practice than they are real problems:

(4) The inevitable readjustment to a different flaccid consistency of the organ and, eventually, to another chronological order of the operating steps.
(5) The 'time loss' for the first cardioplegic coronary perfusion via the aortic root.
(6) The need for a reperfusion with cardioplegic solution in case of a major non-coronary collateral flow.
(7) The 'three-steps procedure' in the case of distinctive aortic valve insufficiency: (i) incomplete cardiac arrest by perfusion via the aorta and external cooling; (ii) coronary canulation; (iii) myocardial protection by cardioplegic coronary perfusion until there is complete myocardial equilibration.
(8) Adjustment of the anaesthesia and premedication, and also of the termination of the anaesthesia (to an unexpected post-ischaemic output capacity of the heart) and of the after-treatment in the intensive-care unit (electrolyte-substitution), taking into consideration the methods of myocardial protection.

SUMMARY OF THE ADVANTAGES OF AN EFFECTIVE MYOCARDIAL PROTECTION

(1) A prolongation of the myocardial ischaemia tolerance, which 20 years ago we would have held to be quite impossible, and which in the dog heart, under identical temperature conditions, reaches a factor of 10 compared to pure ischaemic cardiac arrest.
(2) The possibility of operating at heart-temperatures between 15 and 25 °C (depending on the method) without deep local hypothermia.
(3) In combination with deep hypothermia (2–5 °C), the possibility of extracorporeal preservation of the heart for about 20 h.
(4) The avoidance of haemolysis, which in the case of a continuous or intermittent blood perfusion of the heart is caused by the coronary sucker.

(5) A sparing of the coronary orifices because of the possible renunciation of coronary canules under most circumstances.
(6) The improvement of the general operating condition on the flaccid, bloodless hearts, among other things also an enlarging of the ventricular volume of the infant heart by relaxation.
(7) The possibility of microsurgical interventions with the aid of optical devices (e.g. in coronary heart surgery).
(8) A better training of young surgeons without time stress. The lengthening of the available time makes it possible to perform a better survey of any complicating circumstance, especially with complex congenital organic heart defects.
(9) A short myocardial recovery time because of the nearly homogeneous protection of the total myocardium and the relatively high energy and ATP reserves at the end of the ischaemia.
(10) In many cases a decrease of the total bypass time, and thereby a decrease of the ECC trauma because of the short post-ischaemic myocardial recovery time.
(11) A decrease of the postoperative complications, and of the indications for a postoperative assisted circulation.
(12) A decrease of the postoperative stay in the intensive care unit, and thereby a considerable saving in finance, personnel and bed-space.

Acknowledgments

The authors would like to thank Mrs R. Hähn, Mrs I. Hagemann, Mrs I. Markmann, Mrs E. Neumeyer, Mrs M. Rubbert, Mrs G. Sander and Mrs H. Schuchardt for their technical assistance during the experiments, and for the preparation of the figures.

This work was supported by the Deutsche Forschungsgemeinschaft, SFB 89–Cardiology, Goettingen.

References

1. Folette, D., Fey, K., Livesay, J., Maloney, J. V. and Buckberg, G. D. (1977). Studies on myocardial reperfusion injury. I. Favorable modification by adjusting reperfusate pH. *Surgery*, **82**, 149
2. Bretschneider, H. J. (1971). Die hämodynamischen Determinanten des myokardialen Sauerstoffverbrauchs. *Drug Res.*, **21**, 1515
3. Baller, D., Bretschneider, H. J. and Hellige, G. (1979). Validity of myocardial oxygen consumption parameters. *Clin. Cardiol.*, **2**, 317
4. Bonhoeffer, K. (1967). *Der Sauerstoffverbrauch des normo- und hypothermen Hundeherzens vor und während verschiedener Formen des induzierten Herzstillstandes.* (Basel–New York: Karger; Bibl. Cardiol. Fasc. 18)
5. Bretschneider, H. J. (1964). Ueberlebenszeit und Wiederbelebungszeit eines Herzens bei Normo- und Hypothermie. *Verh. Dtsch. Ges. Krieslaufforsch.*, **30**, 11
6. Isselhard, W. (1964). 'Vergleich des Herzstoffwechsels bei verschiedenen Methoden des Künstlichen Herzstillstandes und bei anschliess ender Reperfusion'. Habilitationsschrift
7. Isselhard, W., Merguet, H. and Aengenvoort, J. (1965). Vergleich des Herzstoffwechsels bei verschiedenen Methoden des künstlichen Herzstillstandes. *Pflügers Arch.*, **286**, 336

8. Kübler, W. (1969). *Tierexperimentelle Untersuchungen zum Myokardstoffwechsel im Angina-pectoris-Anfall und beim Herzinfarkt.* (Basel–New York: Karger; Bibl. Cardiol. Fasc. 22)
9. Preusse, C. J., Bretschneider, H. J., Kahles, H., Nordbeck, H. and Spieckermann, P. G. (1976). Use of myocardial extracellular space for prolongation of ischemic tolerance of the heart by variation of myocardial permeability and extracellular buffer capacity. *Pflügers Arch.*, **365**, R3
10. Bretschneider, H. J., Gebhard, M. M. and Preusse, C. J. (1980). Optimization of myocardial protection. In Heiss, H. W. (ed.) *Advances in Clinical Cardiology*, Vol. I. pp. 581–91 (New York: G. Witzstrock Publishing House Inc.)
11. Bretschneider, H. J., Preusse, C. J., Kahles, H., Nordbeck, H. and Spieckermann, P. G. (1975). Further improvement in artificial cardiac arrest with subsequent anaerobiosis by combination of various parameters. *Pflügers Arch.*, **359**, R13
12. Kübler, W. (1967). Nutzbare Ischämiedauer des Herzens in Abhängigkeit von der energetischen Ausgangslage des Myokards, der Kardioplegieform und der Temperatur. *Langenbecks Arch. Chirur.*, **319**, 648
13. Bretschneider, H. J., Hübner, G., Knoll, D., Lohr, B., Nordbeck, H. and Spieckermann, P. G. (1975). Myocardial resistance and tolerance to ischemia: physiological and biochemical basis. *J. Cardiovasc. Surg.*, **16**, 241
14. Nayler, W. G., Fassold, E. and Yepez, C. E. (1978). Pharmacological protection of mitochondrial function in hypoxic heart muscle: effect of verapamil, propranolol, and methylprednisolone. *Cardiovasc. Res.*, **12**, 152
15. Nayler, W. G., Yepez, C. E. and Fassold, E. (1978). Experimental studies on the effect of beta-adrenoceptor antagonists on hypoxic heart muscle. In Mäurer, W., Schömig, A., Dietz, R. and Lichtlen, P. R. (Eds.). *Beta-Blockade* 1977 pp. 32–49. (Stuttgart: Georg-Thieme Verlag)
16. Spieckermann, P. G. (1973). Ueberlebens- und Wiederbelebungszeit des Herzens. In Frey, R., Kern, F. and Mayhofer, O. (Eds.). *Anaesthesiologie und Wiederbelebung*, Bd. 66. (Berlin–Heidelberg–New York: Springer Verlag)
17. Lam, C. R., Gahagan, R. and Lepore, A. (1955). Induced cardiac arrest for intracardial surgical procedures. *J. Thorac. Surg.*, **30**, 620
18. Melrose, D. G., Dreyer, B., Bentell, H. H. and Baker, J. B. (1955). Elective cardiac arrest: preliminary communication. *Lancet*, **2**, 21
19. Gebhard, M. M., Bretschneider, H. J., Mezger, V. A., Preusse, C. J. and Spieckermann, P. G. (1980). Principles to avoid the Ca^{++}-paradox in myocardial protection. *Myocardial Protection for Cardiovascular Surgery.* International Symposium, Köln, 2–4 October 1979. (München: Pharmazeutische Verlagsgesellschaft)
20. Kirklin, J. W., Conti, V. R. anf Blackstone, E. H. (1979). Prevention of myocardial damage during cardiac operations. *N. Engl. J. Med.*, **301**, 135
21. Preusse, C. J., Gebhard, M. M. and Bretschneider, H. J. (1980). Comparison of cardioplegic methods of Kirklin, Bretschneider and St Thomas' Hospital by means of biochemical and functional analyses during the postischemic aerobic recovery period. *Myocardial Protection for Cardiovascular Surgery.* International Symposium, Köln, 2–4 October 1979. (München: Pharmazeutische Verlagsgessellschaft)
22. Jynge, P., Hearse, D. J. and Braimbridge, M. V. (1977). Myocardial protection during ischemic cardiac arrest: a possible hazard with calcium-free infusates. *J. Thorac. Cardiovasc. Surg.*, **73**, 848
23. Beleese, N., Döring, V., Kalmar, P., Pokar, H., Polonius, M. J., Steiner, D. and Rodewald, G. (1978). Intraoperative myocardial protection by cardioplegia in hypothermia. *J. Thorac. Cardiovasc. Surg.*, **75**, 405

24. Langendorff, O. (1895). Untersuchungen am überlebenden Säugetierherzen. *Pflügers Arch. Physiol.*, **61,** 291
25. Preusse, C. J., Gebhard, M. M. and Bretschneider, H. J. (1979). Recovery of myocardial metabolism after a 210-minute-cardiac-arrest induced by Bretschneider cardioplegia. *J. Mol. Cell. Cardiol.*, **11,** Suppl. 2, 46
26. Bretschneider, H. J., Gebhard, M. M. and Preusse, C. J. (1980). Amelioration of myocardial protection by improvement of capacity and effectiveness of anaerobic glycolysis. *Myocardial Protection for Cardiovascular Surgery.* International Symposium, Köln, 2–4 October 1979. (München: Pharmazeutische Verlagsgesellschaft)
27. Preusse, C. J., Gebhard, M. M. and Bretschneider, H. J. (1979). Die Zusammensetzung des extrakorporalen Füllvolumens vom Aspekt der Wiederbelebung des Herzens nach künstlichem Herzstillstand mit Anaerobiose. *Z. Kardiol.*, **68,** 268
28. Isselhard, W., Mäurer, W., Stremmel, E., Krebs, J., Schmitz, H., Neuhof, H. and Esser, A. (1970). Stoffwechsel des Kaninchenherzens in situ während Asphyxie und in der postasphyktischen Erholung. *Pflügers Arch.*, **316**, 164
29. Zimmer, H.-G. and Gerlach, E. (1978). Stimulation of myocardial adenine nucleotide biosynthesis by pentoses and pentitols. *Pflügers Arch.*, **376,** 223
30. Zimmer, H.-G., Trendelenburg, C., Kammermeier, H. and Gerlach, E. (1973). De novo synthesis of myocardial adenine nucleotides in the rat. *Circ. Res.*, **32,** 635

4
Biological aspects of prosthetic materials

W. H. WAIN

This is an account of biological materials used as prostheses or replacements in cardiac surgery. They can be used for valve replacements[1], septal defect patches[2], intracardiac baffles[3], extracardiac conduits[4], coronary artery by-pass grafts[5], and small gussets and patches (Figure 1). Some of the biological materials used in this way have special properties and problems, whereas many of the properties and problems are common to all biological materials used for cardiac surgery. In general this account will describe the properties and problems of biological valve replacements, with occasional references to other materials and procedures where relevant (Figure 2: Table 1).

In fact, there are four major problems associated with all biological materials used in cardiac surgery. These may be listed as: (1) autolysis (and pre-surgical storage); (2) microbial contamination; (3) immunological rejection; and (4) long-term or more correctly, late-onset degeneration (Figure 3). In general, biological materials used in cardiac surgery are not associated with thromboembolic phenomena[6] although there is increasing concern about the necessity for anticoagulation with glutaraldehyde-treated porcine xenograft valves.

AUTOLYSIS

The potential for self-destruction or autolysis is initiated as the tissue dies, when the control of cellular metabolism fails and intracellular hydrolytic enzymes attack the structural components of the cell. This eventually destroys the integrity of the tissue, changing morphology and reducing strength. This morbid autolytic process can be slowed or stopped by a variety of preservation methods, some of which have been used by the food industry for thousands of years – that is, if simple procedures by nomadic cooks can be termed 'the food industry' without offending the high standards of today's gigantic food-processing companies.

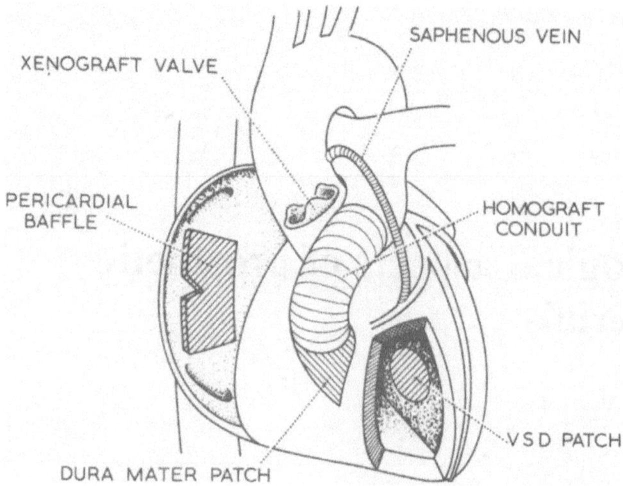

Figure 1 Diagram of some applications of biological tissues at different regions within and around the heart

The most effective method of stopping autolysis is to destroy all the proteins in the cell including the autolytic enzymes. Early man did this by heating or boiling, which is a rather drastic step for any tissue intended for subsequent cardiac surgery. A chemical alternative was introduced by the pathologists and histologists when they wished to examine the microscopic details of tissue. They introduced the technique of fixation, usually by formaldehyde[7], in order to arrest autolysis and to 'fix' the tissue in the state in which it was removed. Formaldehyde has been used to preserve biological tissues for cardiac surgery[8], but unfortunately it causes some shrinkage of

Table 1 The different biological tissues used for cardiac surgery in the last 20 years, indicating the source of the tissue as autograft, homograft, or xenograft

Biomaterial	*Autograft*	*Homograft or allograft*	*Heterograft or xenograft*
Aortic valve	—	×	×
Pulmonary valve	×	×	—
Mitral valve	—	×	—
Fascia lata	×	×	—
Dura mater	—	×	—
Pericardium	×	—	×
Saphenous vein	×	—	—
Umbilical vein	—	×	—
Carotid artery	—	—	×
Internal mammary artery	×	—	—

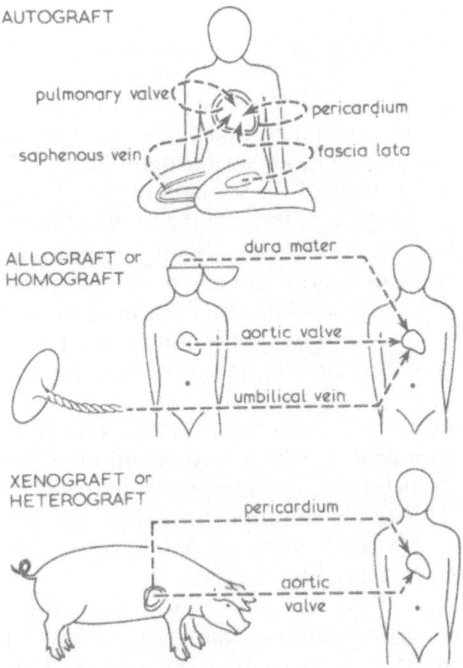

Figure 2 Diagram to illustrate the differences between autograft, homograft and xenograft tissues, with examples of each

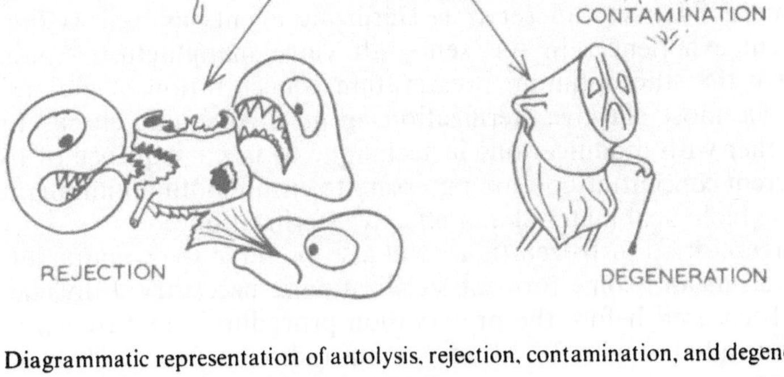

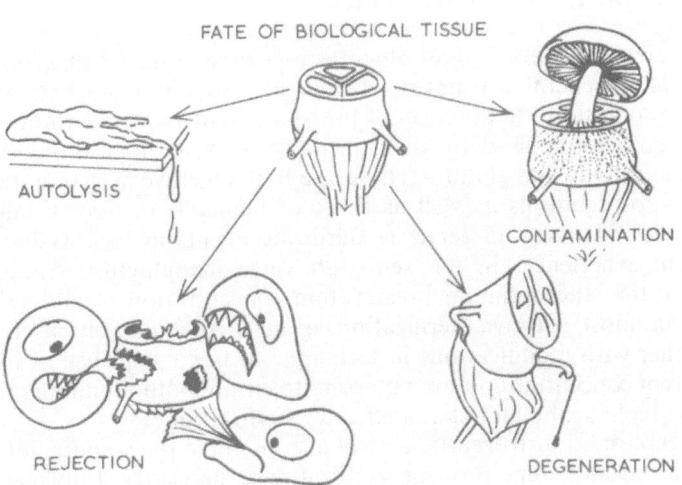

Figure 3 Diagrammatic representation of autolysis, rejection, contamination, and degeneration

the tissue and produces a less flexible, more brittle material than the original tissue. It has not been used as the principal preserving agent for biological valves since the 1960s. Glutaraldehyde is another histological fixative, used especially for preserving fine detail for electron microscopy[9]. It is also used as a tanning agent in the leather industry. In addition to arresting autolysis, glutaraldehyde produces a more flexible material than formaldehyde-treated tissue with better retention of the strength of the material. Other methods of preservation are more akin to those of the food industry. These include deep-freezing, to $-70\,^{\circ}C$[10] or $-196\,^{\circ}C$[11], with or without the cryopreservatives used for the storage of spermatozoa[12] or erythrocytes[13] and freeze-drying or lyophilization[14]. Glycerol has also been used for tissue preservation[15] in an analogous way to fruit-preservation in syrup. The glycerol is thought to replace the water within the cells and so prevent the autolytic enzymes from working.

Finally, the most extensive series of homograft valve replacements have been preserved by a process which retards autolysis, by suspension in tissue culture medium which is intended to permit tissue or organ maintenance at a low level[6,16]. This tissue culture maintenance at $4\,^{\circ}C$ reduces autolysis to an acceptable level without imposing the harsher restrictions of complete arrest of autolysis produced by chemical fixatives.

Those procedures which use autologous tissue from the patient, such as saphenous veins[5] or the internal mammary artery[17] for coronary artery bypass grafts, fascia lata for valve construction[18] or pulmonary valves switched into the aortic position[19], do not require any of these preservation methods, since the degree of autolysis during 60 min of surgery will be small when compared to the processing delay for animal tissue from slaughter-houses.

MICROBIAL CONTAMINATION

Apart from the group of autologous tissues mentioned at the end of the last section, in general, it is not practicable to obtain biological materials under sterile conditions. Some form of post-procurement sterilization is therefore necessary to cope with the inevitable microbiological contamination. Formaldehyde and glutaraldehyde are both effective at 'fixing' the proteins of micro-organisms as well as those of mammalian tissues, and so these chemical fixatives can serve as sterilizing agents as well as preservatives. Recent experiences in the xenograft valve manufacturing industry have shown that the optimum preservation concentration of glutaraldehyde is not the most effective sterilization agent[20]. Adequate checks for sterility, together with modifications in technique to use a sequence of fixatives, or different concentrations, are necessary to ensure both optimum preservation of the biological material and effective sterilization[21].

Freeze-dried or frozen tissue will also preserve the contaminating micro-organisms and some form of sterilization is necessary. Ethylene oxide gas has been used before the preservation procedure[14] and frozen valves have been irradiated with 2.2 Mrad gamma radiation from a ^{60}Co source[10], or with high energy electron beams[22]. The same problem of microbial preservation arises with thick-walled micro-organisms such as fungi in glycerol and with tissue culture maintenance. An adequate degree of antimicrobial treatment, as opposed to 'sterilization' can be achieved in both cases with complex mixtures of antibiotics and antifungal agents[23].

Micro-organisms which grow slowly, if at all, under test conditions for biological tissue, such as *Mycobacteria*[24], and unsuspected viruses, such as rabies virus reported in corneal grafts in 1979[25], still pose problems of microbial contamination. However, continued vigilance and different combinations of antimicrobial treatments have effectively reduced infection consequent upon biological material implantation essentially to a problem of theatre hygiene rather than product contamination, as with the autoclavable mechanical valve replacements and textile conduits.

IMMUNOLOGICAL REJECTION

Cardiac sites for the implantation of biological material seem to have a relatively privileged immunological status in that acute rejection of unmatched allograft valve replacements does not occur. This may also be partly due to the relatively low vascularity of the implanted valve, and to the fact that there are no specific revascularization procedures for the implanted tissue. It has been assumed that any nourishment and maintenance of the implanted tissues would come from the blood flowing through the implanted valve, rather than from specific implant revascularization. Obviously with the autologous tissues of fascia lata[18], saphenous vein[5] and pulmonary valve[19] there will be no possibilities for rejection. All the evidence to date suggests that allograft tissues can be implanted with similar acceptability to the host[6].

Xenograft tissue (animal to man) will invoke an immunological reaction unless the xenograft tissue is treated to reduce the antigenicity to an acceptable level.

Glutaraldehyde has this additional ability to reduce the antigenicity of xenograft tissue to a level at which such valves can be implanted into the heart without overt immunological reaction. In fact, studies with homogenates of valves have shown that the remaining low level of antigenicity after glutaraldehyde treatment can be reduced even further by subsequent treatment with formaldehyde[26]. This additional step obviously does not affect the acceptability of glutaraldehyde-treated valves in terms of acute immunological rejection phenomena. It may be, however, that subtle immunological reactions to antigenically weak allograft or treated xenograft valves may predispose the material to earlier, rather than later, late-onset problems of calcification and degeneration.

LATE-ONSET DEGENERATION

'It is a truth, universally acknowledged . . .'[27] that all biological valve replacements will eventually wear out. The question that remains is one of 'when?'

rather than 'whether?'. There are no obvious procedures to reduce, delay, or prevent late-onset degeneration or attenuation. It is the intention of all the methods of arresting autolysis, controlling contamination, and avoiding antigenic reactions to provide a biological material with a prolonged function as a cardiac prosthesis. This is a reasonable concept with the glutaraldehyde treatment since the tanning action to produce a stabilized material such as leather confers some functional stability on the leather when compared with rawhide. However, homograft valves do continue to function for over 10 years[6] (Figure 4), and such valves kept in the antibiotic solution at 4°C do not autolyse completely during 1 or 2 years' storage, although they are only stored clinically for up to 2 months[28].

Accelerated laboratory simulations can detect problems of wear due to mechanical or design defects and are very useful as an adjunct to preliminary animal experiments for the evaluation of new ideas. However, the intra-cardial milieu is a very demanding one, with high pressure variations, variable flows and repetitive flexing in the relatively hostile environment of blood. The effectiveness of the cumulative preservation and sterilization procedures in terms of affecting late-onset degeneration can only be assessed in terms of

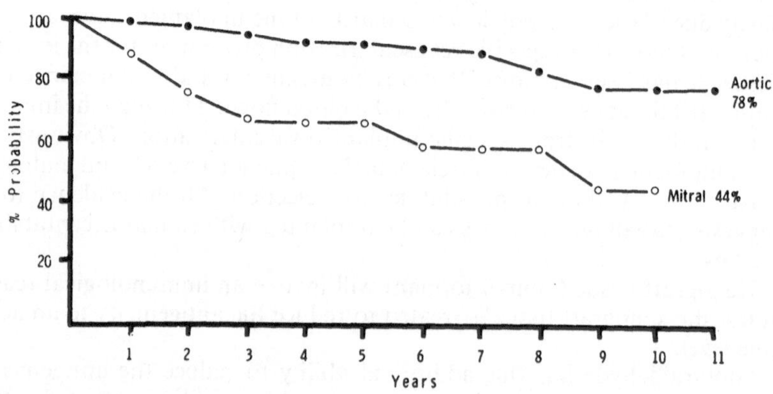

Figure 4 Probability of survival without complications of flash-frozen homograft valves used for isolated aortic or mitral valve replacement followed for 11 years

long-term function. A '10-year biological valve' may be regarded as a product with a satisfactory index of durability. However, durability is not the only criterion for satisfactory valve performance since over a 10-year period nearly 50% of patients with a 'totally durable' mechanical valve will have died or experienced one or more embolic episodes, some with major sequelae. On such a basis for comparison a 10-year biological valve with no history of emboli[6] can 'cock a snook' at any comments about durability (Figure 5).

However a 10-year valve is a bit like a man of 'three score years and ten'[29]. It is an average figure and it may be more accurate to talk of a '50% 10-year valve' when 50% of the original valves are still functioning after 10 years (Figure 6). Even then, the spread or scatter of valves about that 50% may show no valves after 12 years or 25% after 15 years.

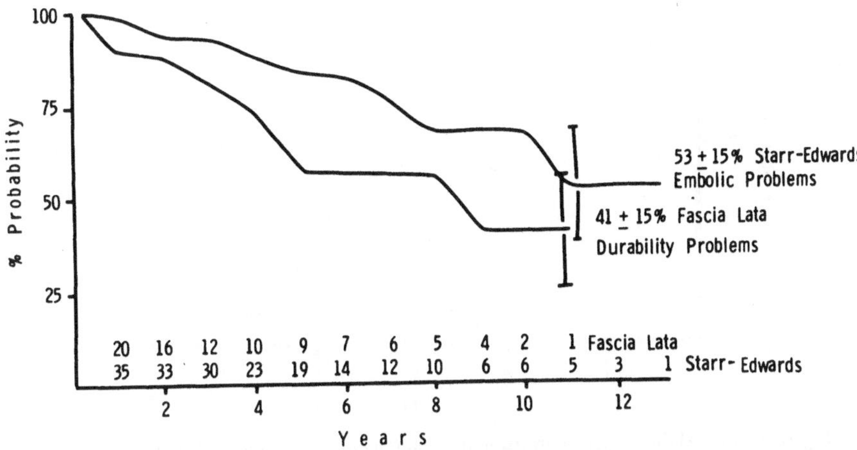

Figure 5 Probability of freedom from any complications for mitral valve replacements with Starr–Edwards caged ball prosthesis or frame-mounted fascia lata valve followed for 11 years

It is thus difficult to evaluate and express the effectiveness of different procedures to retard late-onset degeneration and attenuation. Adverse events in the first 5 years after implantation are more readily appreciated, and efforts can be reasonably made towards avoiding or preventing them.

Calcification within 5 years is a case in point[30], although the causes are still obscure and possibly of immunological origin. Another problem affecting long-term performance is the particular site within the heart. Identical valves implanted in the aortic and mitral regions of the same patient shows a marked difference in their long-term performance[31] regardless of the preservation and sterilization procedures (Figure 7).

Finally, at an anecdotal level, two patients seen in 1979 showed examples of the long-term functional durability of biological material. One man

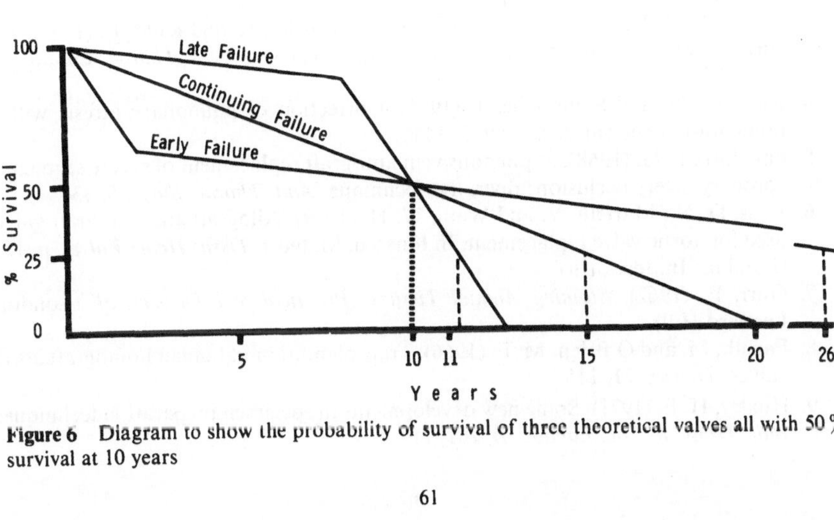

Figure 6 Diagram to show the probability of survival of three theoretical valves all with 50% survival at 10 years

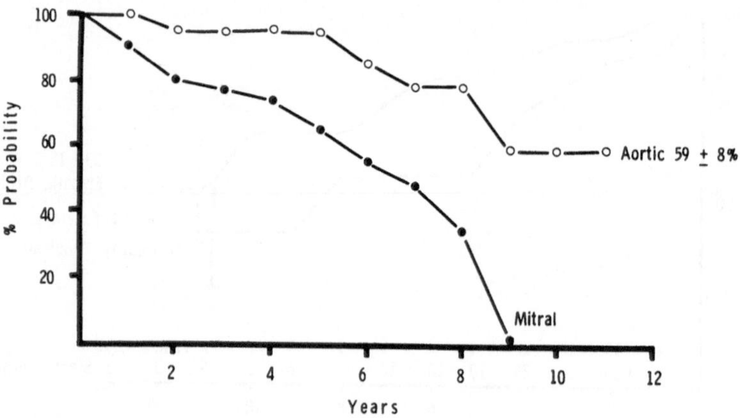

Figure 7 Probability of freedom from any complication for homograft valves used as double aortic and mitral valve replacement followed for 11 years

received his freeze-dried ethylene oxide sterilized aortic homograft valve in June 1965 and on 5 December 1979 was fit and well without any evidence of valve failure. The second man was not strictly a cardiac patient in the sense of the foregoing account. In 1955 he received a homograft aortic segment for relief of coarctation of the aorta. This homograft segment failed in 1979 and was replaced after 24 years. During this quarter century the patient had 'grown' from a boy of 8 years to a man of 32 years of age. Truly it is a question of 'when?' rather than 'whether?' for the eventual failure of biological materials used for cardiac surgery but 'when?' can and should take a long, long time.

References

1. Ross, D. N. (1962). Homograft replacement of the aortic valve. *Lancet*, **2,** 487
2. Ross, J. K. (1961). The fate of autogenous tissue grafts in the heart. *Ann. Rev. Coll. Surg.*, **29,** 275
3. Mustard, W. T., Keith, J. D., Trusler, G. A., Fowler, R. and Kidd, L. (1964). The surgical management of transposition of the great vessels. *J. Thorac. Cardiovasc. Surg.*, **48,** 953
4. Ross, D. N. and Somerville, J. (1966). Correction of pulmonary atresia with a homograft aortic valve. *Lancet*, **2,** 1446
5. Favoloro, R. G. (1968). Saphenous vein autograft replacement of severe segmental coronary artery occlusion: operative technique. *Ann. Thorac. Surg.*, **5,** 334
6. Ross, D. N., Martelli, V. and Wain, W. H. (1979). Allograft and autograft valves used for aortic valve replacement. In Ionescu, M. (ed.). *Tissue Heart Valves*, p. 127. (London: Butterworth)
7. Gurr, E. (1962). *Staining Animal Tissues: Practical and Theoretical*. (London: Leonard Hill)
8. Paneth, M. and O'Brien, M. F. (1966). Transplantation of human homograft aortic valves. *Thorax*, **21,** 115
9. Huxley, H. E. (1971). Some new developments in specimen preparation techniques. *Phil. Trans. R. Soc. London, B*, **261,** 119

10. Ingegneri, A., Wain, W. H., Martelli, V., Bodnar, E. and Ross, D. N. (1979). An 11 year assessment of 93 flash frozen homograft valves in the aortic position. *Thorac. Cardiovasc. Surg.*, **27,** 281
11. Parker, R., Nandakumaran, K., Al-Janabi, N. and Ross, D. N. (1977). Elasticity of frozen aortic valve homografts. *Cardiovasc. Res.*, **11,** 156
12. Polge, C., Smith, A. V. and Parkes, A. S. (1949). Revival of spermatozoa after vitrification and dehydration at low temperatures. *Nature* (*London*), **166,** 666
13. Solvitev, H. A. (1951). Recovery of human red blood cells after freezing. *Lancet*, **1,** 823
14. Longmore, D. B., Lockey, E., Ross, D. N. and Pickering, B, N. (1966). The preparation of aortic valve homografts. *Lancet*, **2,** 463
15. Pigossi, N. (1967). Implantacao de dura-mater homogena conservada em glycerina. *Revista do Hospital das Clinicas Faculdade de Medicina Universidade de São Paulo*, **22,** 204
16. Barratt-Boyes, B. G. (1979). Cardiothoracic surgery in the Antipodes. *J. Thorac. Cardiovasc. Surg.*, **78,** 804
17. Kolessov, V. I. (1967). Mammary artery–coronary artery anastomosis as a method of treatment for angina pectoris. *J. Thorac. Cardiovasc. Surg.*, **54,** 535
18. Senning, A. (1967). Fascia lata replacement of aortic valves. *J. Thorac. Cardiovasc. Surg.*, **54,** 465
19. Ross, D. N. (1967). Replacement of aortic and mitral valves with a pulmonary autograft. *Lancet*, **2,** 959
20. Tyras, D. H., Kaiser, G. C., Barner, H. B., Laskowski, L. F. and Marr, J. J. (1978). Atypical mycobacteria and the xenograft valve. *J. Thorac. Cardiovasc. Surg.*, **75,** 331
21. Koorajian, S., Frugard, G. and Stegwell, M. J. (1979). Sterilization of tissue valves. In Sebening, F., Klovekorn, W. P., Meisner, H. and Struck, E. (eds.). *Bioprosthetic Cardiac Valves*, p. 373. (Munich: Deutches Hertzzentrum Munchen)
22. Malm, J. R., Bowman, F. O. Jr., Harris, P. D. and Kovalik, A. T. W. (1967). An evaluation of aortic valve homografts sterilized by electron beam energy. *J. Thorac. Cardiovasc. Surg.*, **54,** 471
23. Wain, W. H. (1979). Antimicrobial treatment of allograft valves. In Longmore, D. B. (ed.). *Modern Cardiac Surgery*, p. 103. (Lancaster: MTP Press)
24. Anyanwu, C. H., Nassau, E. and Yacoub, M. (1976). Miliary tuberculosis following antibiotic sterilisation of heart valve allografts. *Thorax*, **32,** 740
25. Houff, S. A., Burton, R. C., Wilson, R. W., Henson, T. E., London, W. T., Baer, G. M., Anderson, L. J., Winkler, W. G., Madden, D. L. and Sever, J. L. (1979). Human to human transmission of rabies virus by corneal transplant. *N. Engl. J. Med.*, **300,** 603
26. Slanczka, D. J. and Bajpai, P. K. (1978). Immunogenicity of glutaraldehyde treated aortic and pericardial tissue. *Clin. Res.*, **26,** 1249
27. Austen, J. (1813). *Pride and Prejudice*, p. 1. (London: T. Egerton)
28. Bodnar, E., Wain, W. H., Martelli, V. and Ross, D. N. (1979). Long term performance of 580 homograft and autograft valves used for aortic valve replacement. *Thorac. Cardiovasc. Surg.*, **27,** 31
29. Psalm 90, verse 10.
30. Geha, A. S., Laks, H., Stansel, H. C., Cornhill, J. F., Kilman, J. W., Buckley, M. R. and Roberts, W. C. (1979). Late failure of porcine valve heterografts in children. *J. Thorac. Cardiovasc. Surg.*, **78,** 351
31. Ross, D. N., Shabbo, F. P. and Wain, W. H. (1979). Long term results of double valve replacement with aortic homografts. In Sebening, F., Klovekorn, W. P., Meisner, H. and Struck, E. (eds.). *Bioprosthetic Cardiac Valves*, p. 143. (Munich: Deutches Hertzzentrum Munchen)

5
Clinical problems and aspirations of biological materials

D. N. ROSS

The use of biological materials in cardiac surgery goes back many years and probably had its earliest application in replacing segments of aorta in the treatment of coarctation. For this surgery, and later for the replacement of the abdominal aorta, segments of homologous cadaver aorta were used. These were removed under sterile conditions shortly after death and preserved in balanced salt solution or buffered formalin. Although these segments invariably underwent calcification and atheromatous degeneration, many have performed well as blood conduits for 10–20 years.

In the intervening period a variety of biological tissues have been used and continue to be used, and probably the best-known example is in the use of freshly removed autologous vein grafts for bypassing the diseased coronary arteries. Here we are dealing with living bio-compatible tissues acting as simple conduits, and it is perhaps not surprising that their long-term results are impressively good.

In simple reparative surgery, like the closure of atrial septal defects and repair or enlargement of blood vessels and valve segments, living autologous pericardium removed at the time of surgery is an ideal biological membrane, combining a smooth endothelial surface with excellent stretch-and-recovery characteristics.

It is when we look for a source of readily available stored biological material collected from cadaver human or animal source that we come up against problems. These include sterilization, preservation, and storage difficulties and later the problem of degeneration – including wear and tear or calcification – and immunological rejection.

Curiously enough, however, woven Dacron tubes have proved the ideal conduit for replacement of the larger blood vessels, largely I believe due to their affinity for the ingrowth of autogenous tissue. In this way they represent a truc bioprosthesis. The plastic supplies only the background matrix or artificial collagen within which living tissue becomes enmeshed, and much of our present striving is towards such a happy 'coming together' of human and man-made fibres.

Turning to the heart-valve problem our difficulties are compounded by the unavoidable feature that the leaflets are stressed or flexed repeatedly at something like 50 million times a year. It seems doubtful whether the designers of Concorde were faced with stresses of this order of magnitude.

An obvious solution which has followed has been the move towards using the naturally occurring heart valves where the problem was solved many thousands of years ago. This was the basis of our initial approach in using a human aortic valve removed from a cadaver as a replacement for the aortic valve. The first of these operations was carried out in 1962 and the overall results have been rewarding.

These results are perhaps not too surprising, since both design and structure are perfect – having been conceived by a Master designer. Additional benefits derive from the fact that these natural valves are not traumatic or blood-destructive, and that they incorporate a unique central flow design. As with the normal valve there is no risk of embolism and this has been confirmed in over 1500 cases.

The main problem with these cadaveric homografts, as far as can be ascertained, lies in the fact that they are non-viable and therefore lack that unique quality of living tissue that is the ability to replace and maintain its structure from its living cellular components. In other words they are subject to the ordinary processes of wear and tear common to all inanimate structures. The problem can be summed up as lack of durability.

One answer is to borrow an identical living valve from the patient himself and transplant this within the aortic orifice. This becomes possible since the pulmonary and aortic valves are structurally and functionally identical. This operation of transplantation of the living pulmonary valve has been carried out in 200 patients and there is no doubt that these valves continue to live and function in their new position without degenerative problems. The important features about this valve is that it is *living*, *autogenous* and of *perfect design*. The technique, however, has obvious limitations and can only be applied at one site.

Still using living autogenous tissue, our next move was to use fascia lata taken from the patient's thigh at the time of surgery and from this tissue a valve or valves were manufactured and attached to a rigid frame. The idea was to combine correct design with ready availability and living autogenous tissue. However, the results were not encouraging and one reason relates to less than perfect design characteristics.

Immediately we were up against problems relating to technical imperfections in our crude manufacturing techniques and the stresses involved in attaching a flexible living membrane to a rigid metal frame, so that the cusps tended to tear away.

However another unexpected feature was that the markedly enriched biological environment of being totally immersed in blood made this tissue grow and distort in its attempts to conform to its new stresses. An interesting side to this experience was the fact that three cusp valves inserted in the mitral area tried vainly to change from a tricuspid structure to the bicuspid mitral structure that had evolved over the preceding thousands of millions of years of evolution. Clearly nature was offering a helping hand with our design imperfections.

At that stage we realized that, given a choice between viability and perfect design characteristics, something had to be sacrificed; and rightly or wrongly we and others have sacrificed viability – for the present – in favour of better design and possibly improved durability.

The result has been to take a cue from the leather industry and apply the technique of tanning or cross-linking of the collagen in our biological tissue with glutaraldehyde, with a view to strengthening the structure to form a sort of supple leather. This is currently the most popular technique both for preserving animal (porcine) valves and for valves wholly man-made, e.g. pericardium.

Unfortunately distressing features like calcification and simple wear and tear have not been eliminated by the glutaraldehyde tanning method and it is difficult to see how we are to overcome this unless the viability and original structure of the collagen and elastin are preserved.

Apart from knowing more about the molecular structure of collagen we need to know about the obscure and complex chemistry of the calcification process in biological tissues. Unfortunately calcification seems to be an important final process of degeneration in all biological membranes, especially in children where the calcification process is active. Once calcification occurs in a valve, the resulting rigidity of the tissue accelerates the process of destruction.

Mechanical valves offer outstanding durability but they are of relatively crude design and lack safety, particularly from the point of view of emboli. One is faced with the paradox of having a safe biological valve lacking in durability and precisely the opposite features in their mechanical counterpart, i.e. durability with less safety. In other words the mechanical valve may have the potential to last 50 years but the patient will not be there to enjoy it. Also although durability is the boast of mechanical valves, not all their components last.

This compromise between durability and safety is the dilemma still facing each surgeon when he does a valve replacement. In fact there has been no fundamentally new or significant development in the valve replacement field since 1962 when mechanical and biological valves were first introduced.

Looking hopefully to the future I would say that immunology has been largely ignored in this whole field of cardiac valve replacement, and it seems to me that if we are to make further advances with biological tissue this aspect cannot be left out of our calculations.

Cornea is transplanted regularly and successfully and the avascular cornea like the avascular aortic valve cusp is only weakly antigenic. Nevertheless it has been repeatedly demonstrated, both experimentally and clinically, that there is a well-defined immune reaction in the cusps of transplanted valves at about 10 days and the severity of the rejection will depend on the degree of tissue incompatibility.

With this in mind I would like us to re-explore and re-examine the prospect of using fresh, living homologous cadaver valves or biological membranes like pericardium removed at death under sterile conditions and maintained in a viable state until used, just as with other forms of organ transplantation – for example, kidneys.

Combined with conventional but low-dose modern immunosuppression I would hope that these tissues populated with living cells would then survive, function and continue to service their collagen matrix as permanent valve replacements and biological membranes.

Certainly the valves in transplanted animal and human heart show no evidence of degeneration thus far, and if I am correct in thinking that viability is of paramount importance then a study of the use of immunosuppressed living membranes as cardiac valve substitutes seems to be our next obvious step towards a safe long-term cardiac valve replacement.

6
Preoperative and postoperative echocardiographic assessment of left ventricular function

L. COTTER AND D. GIBSON

The performance of the left ventricle in patients with heart disease is complex and cannot be easily expressed or uniquely quantified by any single number. Instead, we would suggest that in clinical practice, left ventricular function may result from a number of independent disturbances. These may occur singly or in combination and may differ in their relative contribution from patient to patient[1]. Echocardiography has proved particularly suitable for undertaking this type of analysis of left ventricular function, and indeed for some of them it appears the investigation of choice.

Among the abnormalities which can be determined are:

(1) Changes in cavity size and architecture.
(2) Changes in velocity of wall movement.
(3) Changes in coordination of contraction and relaxion.
(4) Changes in filling and diastolic function.

LEFT VENTRICULAR CAVITY SIZE AND ARCHITECTURE

Enlargement of the ventricular cavity is a common manifestation of left ventricular disease and it can be well demonstrated by cross-sectional echocardiography. This method also allows cavity shape to be assessed so that left ventricular aneurysms and the abnormal cavity configuration of congestive and hypertrophic cardiomyopathies can be detected (Figure 1). Accurate measurements of the cavity dimension are less satisfactory using this method due to rather poor ability to visualize endocardium in stop frames and for this purpose the M-mode echocardiogram is more useful[2]. The repetion rate of the M-mode echocardiogram is 1000/s compared with 50/s for the cross-sectional echocardiogram and its resolution in depth is 1 mm. This allows the left septal and free wall endocardial surfaces to be

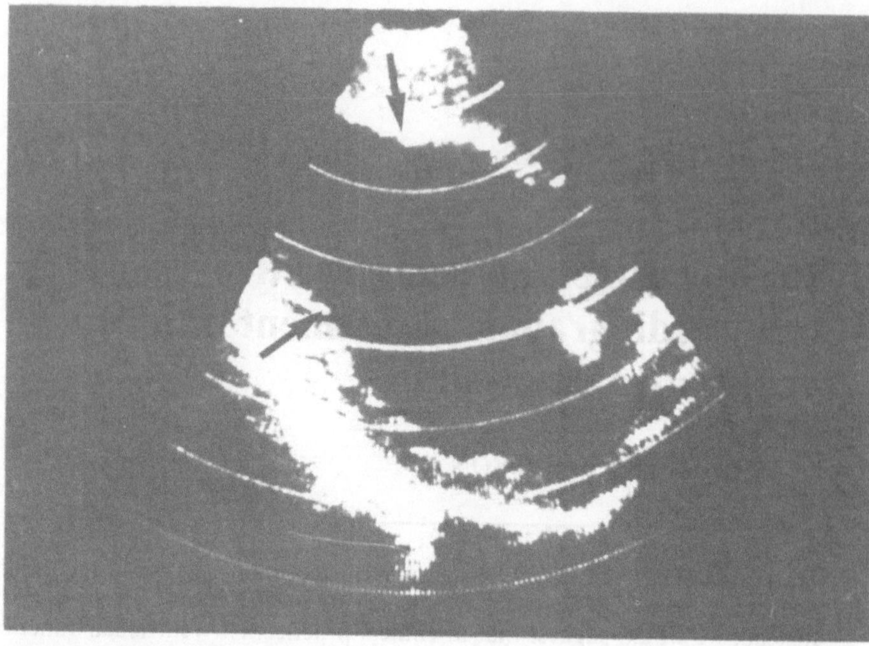

Figure 1 Cross sectional echocardiogram of patient with ischaemic heart disease showing a clear line of demarcation (arrowed) between a dilated ventricle and an apical aneurysm (scale marks are 2 cm apart).'(Courtesy of the Editor of the *British Heart Journal*)

determined with precision unrivalled by other techniques, including angiography, and facilitates the unambiguous measurement of the transverse dimension of the ventricle (Figure 2), even at times of rapid wall movement.

Attempts have been made to estimate left ventricular volumes from measurements of the short axis and a number of regression equations used. All such calculations require assumptions to be made about the shape of the normal left ventricle and uniformity of contraction about the whole perimeter of the ventricle during the cardiac cycle.[3] These assumptions have limitations even when applied to the normal ventricle and may be seriously misleading with the abnormal. In addition they are particularly sensitive to small errors in the measurement of dimension since values must be cubed at some stage during the calculations. It seems reasonable therefore, to avoid all these volume calculations along with derived quantities such as ejection fraction and stroke volume, and to speak only in terms of the dimension which has actually been measured.

The degree of short axis dimension change can be measured directly and is expressed as the shortening fraction, defined as:

$$\frac{(Dd - Ds)}{Dd}$$

where Dd is end diastolic dimension and Ds is end systolic dimension. The shortening fraction so derived correlates well with measurements of ejection fraction provided that contraction is coordinate[4]. However, it is based on measurements made on only two occasions within the cardiac cycle, at end-diastole and end-systole, and gives no information about wall motion between.

LEFT VENTRICULAR WALL MOVEMENT

Since the position of the left side of the septum and the posterior wall endocardium can be defined 1000 times per second using standard equipment it should be possible to measure the alteration in minor axis continuously along with its rate of change of dimension. When echocardiograms of sufficient quality are available, this can be achieved using a simple digitizing technique to extend the information obtainable[5]. The echocardiogram is placed on a digitizing table and a cursor is run manually over the traces representing echoes from the left side of the septum and the endocardium of the posterior wall. Subtraction of coordinates corresponding to these two lines yields a continuous trace of left ventricular dimension which can be differentiated to give its rate of change (Figure 3). The latter can be divided

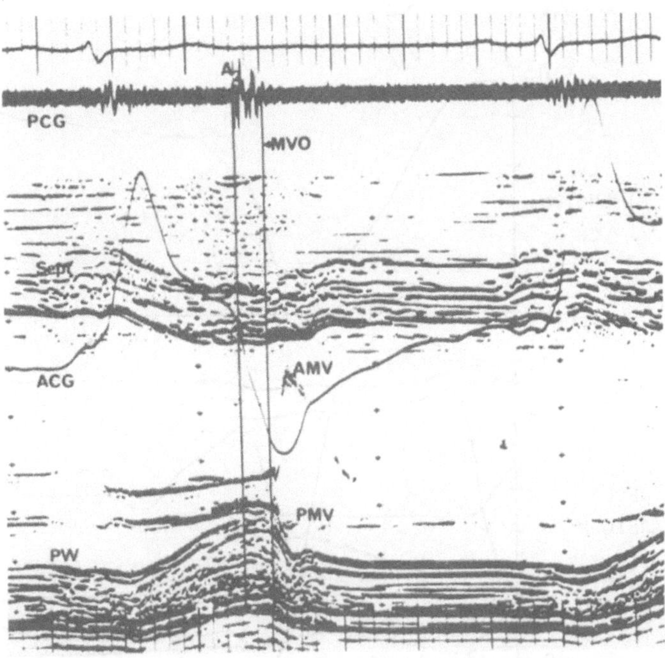

Figure 2 M-mode echocardiogram of left ventricular cavity of normal subject with simultaneous apex and phonocardiograms. (PCG = phonocardiogram, ACG = apex cardiogram, Sept = septum, PW = posterior wall, AMV = anterior mitral valve leaflet, PMV = posterior mitral valve leaflet, A2 = aortic component of second sound, MVO = mitral valve opening). (Courtesy of the Editor of the *British Heart Journal*)

by the simultaneous end-diastolic dimension to derive a normalized rate of dimension shortening during systole, sometimes spoken of as the 'velocity of circumferential fibre shortening' or VCF. The peak VCF obtained in this fashion can be shown to correlate closely with the peak rate of rise of the left ventricular pressure (peak d*P*/d*t*) for the same beat, if contraction is co-ordinate and there is no mitral regurgitation[6].

When left ventricular pressure is measured simultaneously with an echocardiogram showing transverse dimension and wall thickness, all the information required to estimate circumferential wall stress is available. This may be plotted during systole or diastole or left ventricular power may be derived as the product of wall stress and shortening rate[6].

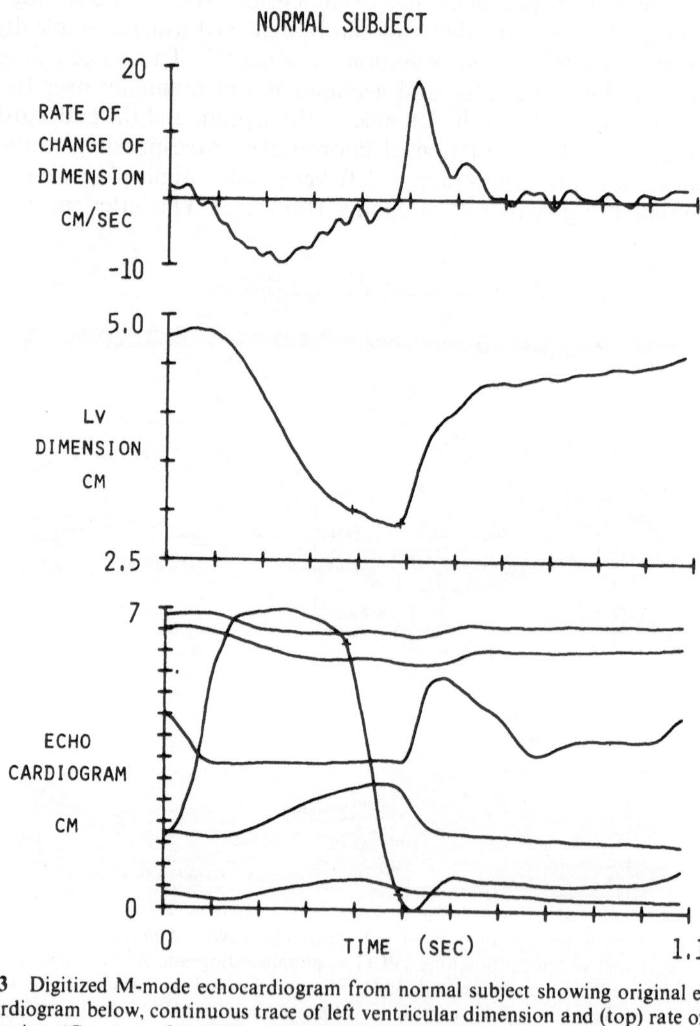

Figure 3 Digitized M-mode echocardiogram from normal subject showing original echo and apex cardiogram below, continuous trace of left ventricular dimension and (top) rate of change of dimension. (Courtesy of the Editor of the *British Heart Journal*)

COORDINATION OF LEFT VENTRICULAR CONTRACTION

Simultaneous measurement of the left ventricular pressure with echocardiographic measurement may also give information about the coordination of contraction. Synchronous contraction and relaxion of the ventricle imply a normal relationship between the pressure changes reflecting overall left ventricular function, and the echocardiographic dimension reflecting local function. This relationship between the pressure trace and dimension can be displayed as a pressure–dimension loop (Figure 4). The normal pressure–dimension loop is approximately rectangular with little change in the upstroke and downstroke – the limbs representing isovolumic contraction and

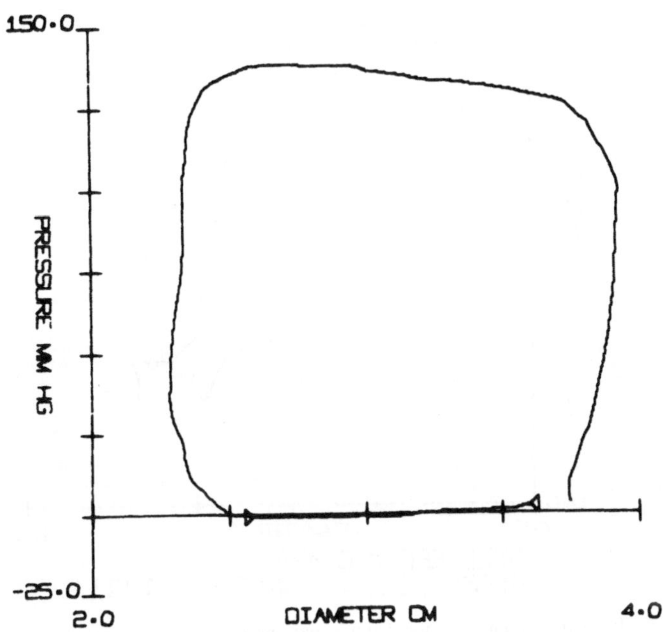

Figure 4 Normal left ventricular pressure-dimension loop showing near-rectangular configuration with little change in dimension during periods of isovolumic contraction (upstroke) and isovolumic relaxation (downstroke). Cycle efficiency is 85 %. (Courtesy of the Editor of the *British Heart Journal*)

isovolumic relaxation. The external work performed by that part of the myocardium on the circulation is shown graphically as the area within the loop. The maximum amount of work possible by the myocardium working over the observed pressure and dimension range is the product of the two, represented graphically as the rectangle which just contains the loop. Thus the efficiency of energy transfer from myocardium to the circulation is given by the ratio of the area within the loop to that of the rectangle, and in this way normal left ventricular function can be shown to be 75–90 % efficient.

By contrast, in Figure 5, is shown the pressure–dimension loop from a patient with coronary artery disease. It will be seen that abnormal dimension changes have occurred during isovolumic contraction and relaxion causing efficiency to drop below 50 %. This has proved to be the main cause of reduced cycle efficiency in left ventricular disease. It is thus convenient that the upstroke and downstroke of the left ventricular pressure trace is virtually synchronous with the upstroke and downstroke of the apex-cardiogram[7]. It is therefore possible to determine changes during the isovolumic periods non-invasively by substituting the apex-cardiogram for the left ventricular pressure[8]. Changes in dimension during the upstroke of the loop (the period

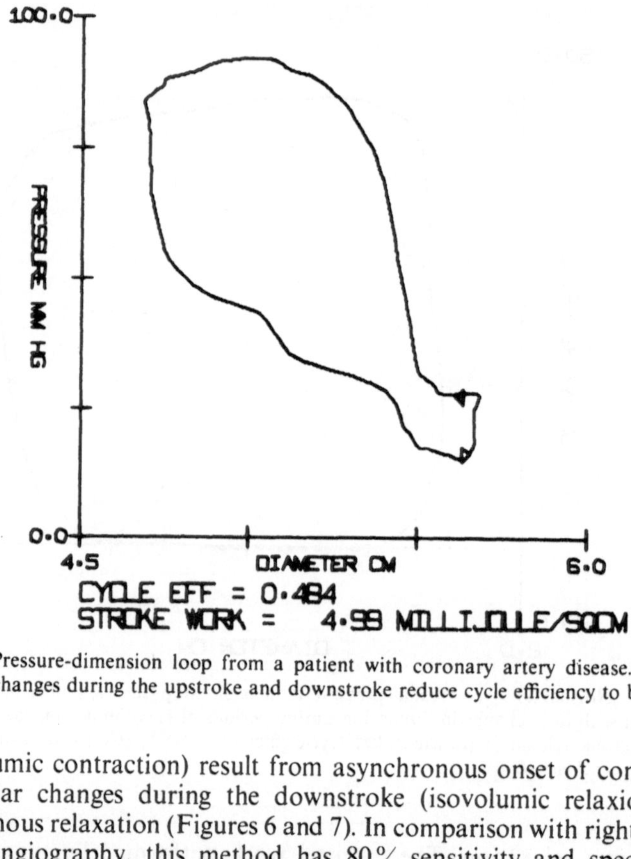

Figure 5 Pressure-dimension loop from a patient with coronary artery disease. Abnormal dimension changes during the upstroke and downstroke reduce cycle efficiency to below 50 %

of isovolumic contraction) result from asynchronous onset of contraction, and similar changes during the downstroke (isovolumic relaxion) from asynchronous relaxation (Figures 6 and 7). In comparison with right anterior oblique angiography, this method has 80 % sensitivity and specificity in detecting these abnormalities regardless of their position in the ventricle[9]. This sensitivity of M-mode echocardiography in detecting abnormalities outside the beam of ultrasound is not really surprising since isolated, localized wall movement during the isovolumic periods is not possible, any change in dimension in an ischaemic area must be accompanied by a similar net change in movement in the opposite direction elsewhere, since fluid is incompressible and both aortic and mitral valves are closed during these isovolumic periods. It is thus the latter, compensatory movement in otherwise normal regions that is detected by echocardiography. Such changes in the coordination of contraction and relaxation are common in all forms of heart disease including ischaemic heart disease, in which they may be reversed following coronary bypass grafting. They are also an almost invariable finding following cardio-pulmonary bypass even if less sensitive indicators show no signs of disturbance. All of 30 patients with aortic regurgitation studied following aortic valve replacement had such abnormalities[8]. They were maximal at 2–3 days, but still detectable after 10 days. These changes are not without clinical significance. In patients studied up to 8 years following aortic valve replacement for aortic regurgitation, post-operative symptoms were found to correlate well with isovolumic contraction abnormalities, poorly with cavity dimension and not at all with peak rates of systolic wall movement[10]. The cardiac effects of drugs such as propranolol are significantly influenced if asynergic contraction is present[11]. It may be that the choice of medical therapy should be influenced by their presence.

LEFT VENTRICULAR FILLING AND DIASTOLIC FUNCTION

It is axiomatic that it is as much a function of the left ventricle to fill as it is to empty, but nevertheless diastolic function has received much less attention than the systolic function of the ventricle. Diastolic abnormalities, however, can severely limit cardiac performance, particularly at high heart rates when the time available for filling is short. Echocardiography is an ideal tool for studying diastole and it is likely that more attention will be paid to this part of the cardiac cycle in the future.

The characteristic changes in the volume of the left ventricle were well described by Henderson and his colleagues[12], as comprising an early diastolic period of rapid filling followed by a period of diastasis or reduced inflow. This pattern in normals is reflected in the rates of change of dimension measured echocardiographically[13], and both are disturbed in mitral valve disease. In pure mitral stenosis the peak rate of increase in left ventricular dimension is reduced and there is no early period of rapid increase in dimension, the low rate of dimension increase continuing throughout diastole. In contrast, in pure mitral regurgitation the peak rate of increase of dimension is greater than normal. The left ventricular filling pattern of patients with prosthetic mitral valves is similar to that of patients with mitral stenosis. Observations of these patterns of filling have been used to compare the performance of different prostheses and to identify prosthetic malfunction[14].

Left ventricular hypertrophy, due to HCM or secondary to other disorders, also results in abnormalities of diastolic function[15,16]. Peak rate of dimension increase may be reduced and the period of early diastolic dimension increase altered in a similar way to patients with mitral stenosis. The abnormal diastolic properties of such ventricles are further indicated by prolongation of isovolumic realxation and delay in mitral valve opening with respect to the timing of minimum dimension. The latter appears to be evi-

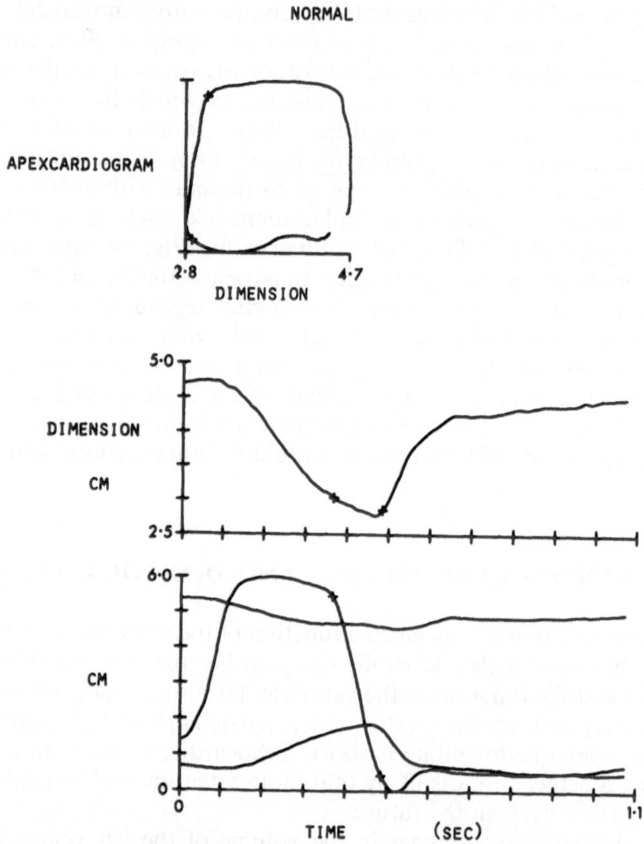

Figure 6 Normal apex cardiogram-dimension relations with little change in dimension during upstroke and downstroke. (Courtesy of the Editor of the *British Heart Journal*)

dence of incoordinate rather than simply prolonged relaxation in these ventricles.

In ischaemic heart disease, when segmental abnormalities of contraction are present, disturbances of relaxation are also common[17]. As in left ventricular hypertrophy, outward wall movement may precede mitral valve opening and, therefore, the onset of filling, although isovolumic relaxation is not usually prolonged. This abnormality is closely correlated with incoordinate wall motion during isovolumic contraction, and so probably represents asynchronous termination of systole rather than a primary abnormality of relaxion as in left ventricular hypertrophy. Delayed mitral valve opening is associated with changes in cavity shape during isovolumic relaxation, and thus with distortion of the pressure–dimension and apex–dimension loops.

Using digitized echocardiograms of the ventricle, continuous values for cavity dimension and wall thickness throughout diastole can be generated. When these are combined with information from a simultaneous cavity pressure trace measured with a catheter tip micromanometer, values for mean circumferential wall stress can be calculated. The stress–strain relations of areas of myocardium can then be derived throughout diastole. However although such measurements are interesting and shed light on the great complexity of diastole, their significance to clinical situations has not been fully evaluated.

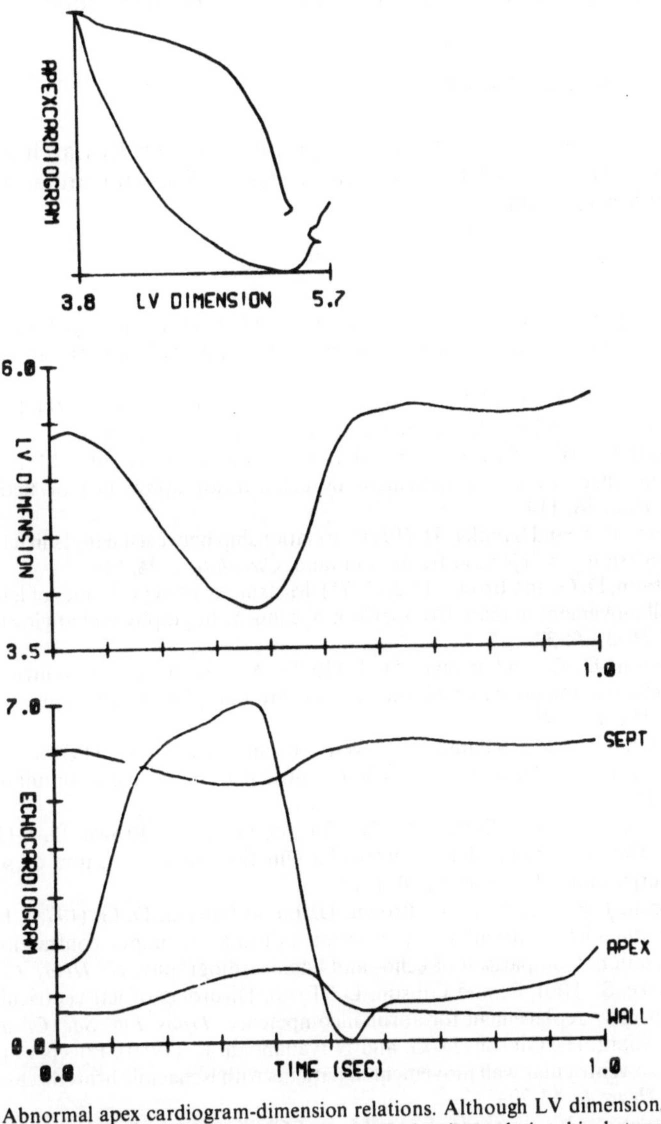

Figure 7 Abnormal apex cardiogram-dimension relations. Although LV dimension, extent of wall movement and apex cardiogram appear normal, the time relationship between them is disturbed. There are large dimension changes during the periods of isovolumic contraction and relaxation. (Courtesy of the Editor of the *British Heart Journal*)

CONCLUSIONS

Abnormalities of left ventricular function can be detected and quantified echocardiographically. The range of disorders which can be recognised is greatly extended by combining M-mode echocardiography with other measurements reflecting the function of the ventricle as a whole, particularly if digitizing techniques are used. For the assessment of some disturbances of left ventricular function such techniques may be the methods of choice.

ACKNOWLEDGEMENTS

This work has been supported by grants from the Research Fund of the National Heart and Chest Hospitals, and the Special Cardiac Fund of the Brompton Hospital.

References

1. Gibson, D. G. (1977). Clinical assessment of left ventricular function. In Hamer, J. (ed.) *Recent Advances in Cardiology*. Vol. 7, pp. 315–348. (London: Churchill-Livingston)
2. Fortuin, N. J., Hood, W. P., Sherman, M. E. and Craige, E. (1971). Determination of left ventricular volumes by ultrasound. *Circulation*, **44,** 575
3. Linhart, J. W., Mintz, G. S., Segal, B. L., Kawai, N. and Kotler, M. N. (1975). Left ventricular volume measurement by echocardiography: fact or fiction? *Am. J. Cardiol.*, **36,** 114
4. Lewis, R. P. and Sandler, H. (1971). Relationship between changes in left ventricular dimensions and ejection fraction in man. *Circulation*, **44,** 548
5. Gibson, D. G. and Brown, D. J. (1975). Measurement of peak rates of left ventricular wall movement in man. Comparison of echocardiography and angiocardiography. *Br. Heart J.*, **37,** 677
6. Gibson, D. G. and Brown, D. J. (1976). Assessment of left ventricular systolic function in man from simultaneous echocardiographic and pressure measurements. *Br. Heart J.*, **38,** 8
7. Manolas, J., Rutischauser, W., Wirz, P. and Arbenz, U. (1975). Time relation between apex cardiogram and left ventricular events using simultaneous high-fidelity tracings in man. *Br. Heart J.*, **37,** 1263
8. Venco, A., St John Sutton, M. G., Gibson, D. G. and Brown, D. J. (1976). Non-invasive assessment of left ventricular function after correction of severe aortic regurgitation. *Br. Heart J.*, **38,** 1324
9. Doran, J. H., Traill, T. A., Brown, D. J. and Gibson, D. G. (1978). Detection of abnormal left ventricular wall movement during isovolumic contraction and early relaxation. Comparison of echo- and angiocardiography. *Br. Heart J.*, **40,** 367
10. Clarke, S., Hall, R. and Gibson, D. (1978). Disorders of left ventricular function after valve replacement for aortic incompetence. *Trans. Eur. Soc. Cardiol.*, **1,** 8
11. von Bibra, H., Gibson, D. G. and Nityanandan, K. (1980). Effects of propranolol on left ventricular wall movement in patients with ischaemic heart disease (abstract). *Br. Heart J.*, **43,** 293
12. Henderson, Y., Scarbrough, M. M. and Chillingworth, F. P. (1906). The volume curve of the mammalian heart, and the significance of this curve in respect to the mechanics of the heart beat and the filling of the ventricles. *Am. J. Physiol.*, **16,** 325

13. Gibson, D. G. and Brown, D. (1973). Measurement of instantaneous left ventricular dimension and filling rate in man, using echocardiography. *Br. Heart J.*, **35,** 1141
14. St John Sutton, M. G., Traill, T. A., Ghafour, A. S., Brown, D. J. and Gibson, D. G. (1977). Echocardiographic assessment of left ventricular filling after mitral valve surgery. *Br. Heart J.*, **39,** 1283
15. Sanderson, J. E., Traill, T. A., St John Sutton, M. G., Brown D. J., Gibson, D. G. and Goodwin, J. F. (1978). Left ventricular filling and relaxation in hypertrophic cardiomyopathy. *Br. Heart J.*, **40,** 596
16. Gibson, D. G., Traill, T. A., Hall, R. J. C. and Brown, D. J. (1979). Echocardiographic features of secondary left ventricular hypertrophy. *Br. Heart J.*, **41,** 54
17. Upton, M. T. and Gibson, D. G. (1978). The study of left ventricular function from digitized echocardiograms. *Prog. Cardiovasc. Dis.*, **20,** 359

7
Changing aspects of surgical technique in coronary artery surgery

J. E. C. WRIGHT

The changing aspects of surgery for coronary artery disease will be a conventional presentation and will use the experience that we have at the London Chest Hospital to highlight some of the changes that we have noted and have participated in over the last 8 or 9 years. At the end I shall be giving some of my personal feelings on the safety aspects.

Table 1 shows the number of operations performed at the London Chest until December 1979. The overall mortality for elective vein graft procedures is 2.3 %. We have included all patients receiving vein grafts only, whether it be one, two, three, four or five grafts, and irrespective of the state of the left

Table 1 Coronary artery bypass graft surgery (London Chest Hospital 1971–1979)

	Number	*Hospital deaths*	%
Total CABG	1442	44	3.0
Isolated elective	1228	28	2.3
Other	214	16	7.5

ventricle. Of course, mortality rates can be broken up to show that for isolated vein grafts, single and double, the mortality is almost zero. The determinant of mortality in our experience is the state of the left ventricle, as one would expect. When operating on patients with an ejection fraction of around 15 or 20 %, not surprisingly the mortality increases to several per cent. I feel, when looking from one unit to another, the only sensible figure to look at is the one that has not been picked over too much, which is the overall mortality for coronary artery grafting.

Of course with associated procedures, which I shall delineate further on, it goes up to 7 %.

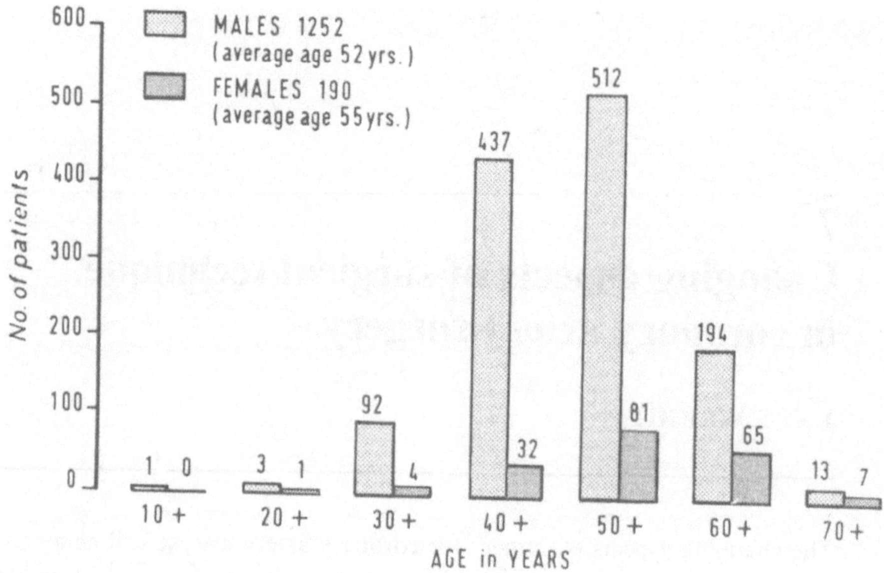

Figure 1

Figure 1 shows age and sex of patients. With increasing confidence we did feel that the upper age limit could be lifted above its initial 60–65, and nowadays even occasionally into the 70-plus. However, I am very loth to operate on patients over 70 for obvious reasons.

Figure 2 shows that the numbers of operations done per year, as in most units, has shown a dramatic increase. Starting with our early learning experience, in the first few years numbers rapidly escalated, apparently reaching a maximum in 1977. Since then, the numbers that we have been able to perform have been determined more by economic factors and financial restriction rather than the supply of patients. What I should really show, to go along with this data, is what has happened to the waiting list, which until a few years ago was in the region of a few weeks. A year ago the waiting was a year, and at present – April 1980 – our waiting list for a routine coronary graft is over 2 years. As the waiting list has gone up, clearly the morbidity on the waiting list has increased, and there is now about a 10 or 15 % annual myocardial infarction rate on the waiting list. In fact, the waiting list mortality exceeds the hospital mortality.

Immediately we get into logistic problems. I have in my hand the book, *Returns for UK Cardiac Surgery*. At the back of this book it shows that the mortality for coronary artery disease is lowest in the units that happen to do most operations, and that the mortality rates that are highest are – not unexpectedly – in those units that do very few. There are exceptions, but there is a good correlation running through that graph. Unfortunately, should any patient decide to patronize the hospital with the lowest operative mortality, he will also be patronizing the hospital with the highest waiting list,

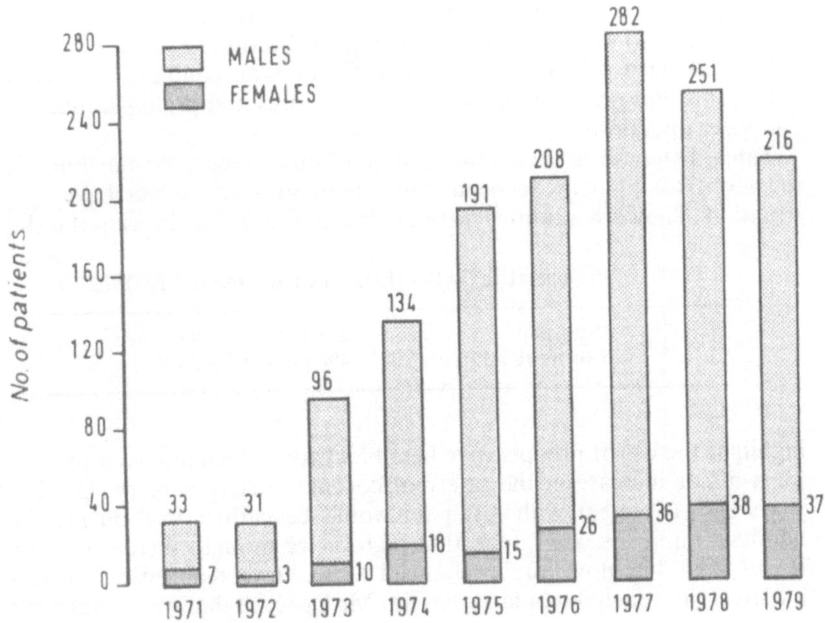

Figure 2

and the chances of dying on the waiting list are even higher. It is rather a difficult decision to make!

Table 2 shows associated procedures: 15% of all cases. The commonest associated procedure is the left ventricular aneurysm, which is hardly surprising when 34% of our patients had had previous myocardial infarcts.

Table 2 Other cardiac operations at time of CABG (London Chest Hospital 1971–1979)

Operation	*No.*
Left ventricular aneurysm	103
Aortic valve replacement	52
Mitral valve replacement	29
Mitral valve repair	28
Infarctectomy	11
Ruptured septum	6
Pacemaker	6
Aortic aneurysm	2
Atrial septal defect	1
Tricuspid valve replacement	1
Tricuspid valve repair	1
Total = 240 operations on 214 patients = 15%	

A word on the use of cardioplegia. I do not use cardioplegia for routine vein grafts but I do use it for all associated procedures. To my mind cardioplegia has been primarily responsible for making combined procedures – aneurysms and grafts, multiple valve procedures and grafts – a much easier and safer operation.

Table 3 shows the preoperative state of our patients. At our unit we use the term rest pain to delineate those patients who do not have a stable situation. They are admitted with angina at rest. I am showing the slide to

Table 3 Pre-operative CABG (London Chest Hospital 1971–1979)

'Rest pain'	251 patients	17%
1 or more infarcts	490 patients	34%

highlight the use of preoperative beta blockade, which has been responsible for a major increase in the safety of coronary artery surgery. Until a few years ago, a patient with rest pain would be catheterized on the day of admission and operated upon that night if we thought there was a critical lesion. This has now totally changed as we have realized that this is an incorrect approach. I would agree with Mr Deverall that we want the patient brought to theatre in a stable condition, and the use of preoperative beta blockade in unstable patients with rest pain has made a tremendous difference. I would now say almost categorically that there is no place for emergency coronary artery surgery except for following the occasional catheter room disaster, which is fortunately very rare.

Another aspect that has changed is that the number of vein grafts inserted into each patient has increased. Figure 3 shows that we soon realised in our early experience that some patients came back with angina. This was partly because we were not bypassing stenoses less than 60 or 70%. In other patients, restudy revealed that stenoses that were originally 40% were now 70%. Again, in early days we had no means of attacking a diffusely diseased artery. We were under-revascularizing. We soon learnt the lesson. By 1975, three or more grafts became the order of the day.

Having mentioned the diffusely diseased coronary artery, by 1973 and 1974 we felt that we could not ignore these arteries. We had to do something to them, so we developed the ability to perform endarterectomy, initially with rather reluctant cardiologist agreement. Following our initial experience, where we found that endarterectomy increased the mortality not at all, and with patency rates that were the same, we became very enthusiastic, and there was a great increase in the number of endarterectomies done. Around 30% of our patients required an endarterectomy (Figure 4).

Figure 5 shows the site of endarterectomy. As in most units, it is usually the right coronary, but we would attack any diffusely diseased artery irrespective of site, as it does not make any difference.

Figure 6 is included to show that not all endarterectomies are as successful as we might wish. Although the patency rate with endarterectomies is 90%, the same as for vein grafts, in about one-third of the endarterectomized

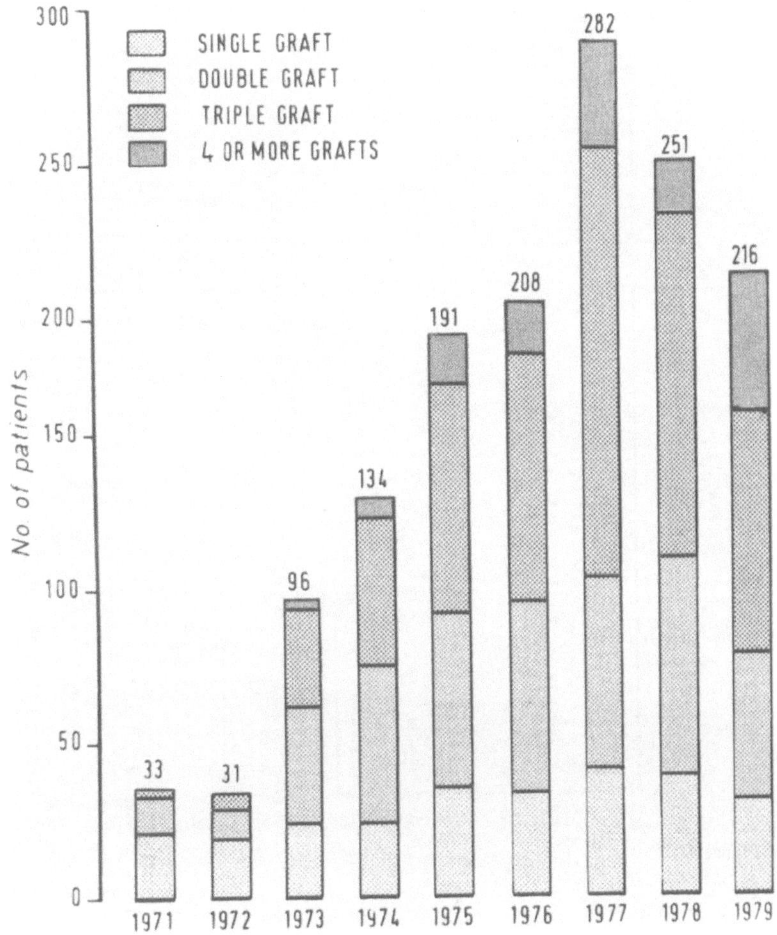

Figure 3

patients the run off is unsatisfactory. Figure 6 shows the vein graft running into a typical endarterectomized vessel, but the run off here has in fact closed.

So all patent grafts are not necessarily successful ones. Figure 7 is included to illustrate the problem. It shows a right coronary artery diffusely diseased at its bifurcation, effecting both the posterior descending, and further over, the left ventricular branch.

How should the problem be attacked? There are three methods. The bifurcation could be endarterectomized, and perhaps a few years ago I would have done that. But because of the poor run off that sometimes occurs, two single vein grafts may be put in; one into each branch. But of course currently in vogue is the use of the jump or snake graft which I shall now illustrate.

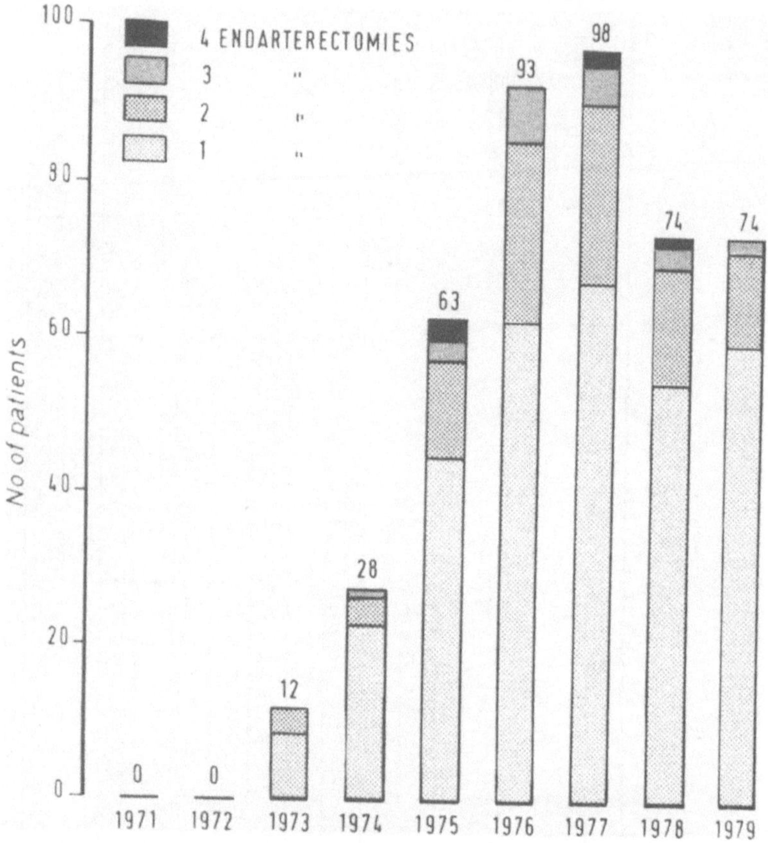

Figure 4

Figure 8 presents diagrammatically a right coronary diffusely diseased with significant stenosis by the marginal, and other plaque beyond the posterior descending. Two grafts can be put in, or the currently fashionable jump graft may be used where there is a side-to-side anastomosis followed by an end-to-side.

Figure 9 shows a procedure I am particularly fond of, which I use mostly in the diagonal LAD system. Early experience showed that the diagonal, being a small vessel and having a small run off, would only yield about a 50 % vein graft patency rate with single grafts. By using the jump graft, this can be increased, since the large flow going into the anterior descending will carry the small flow going down the diagonal. I am sure this is the operation of choice in this situation, with one reservation. Sometimes, to get a good lie with a jump, one is forced to put the LAD graft into a site which might not normally be desirable. Using a single graft, it could be inserted higher, where the artery is larger.

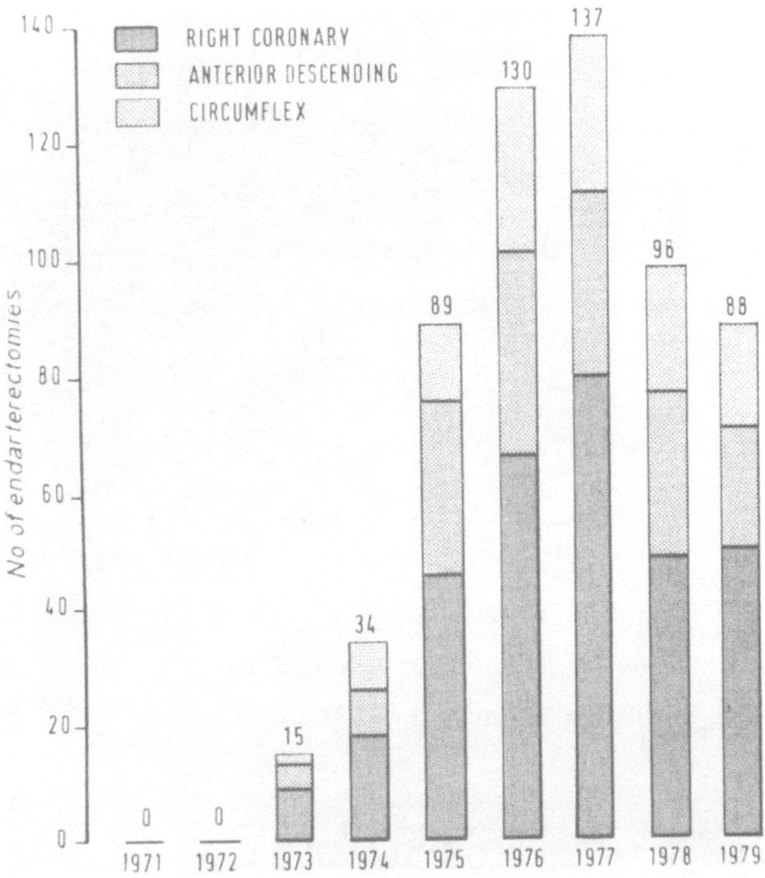

Figure 5

Figure 10 shows another variety of the jump, which might be called a snake, since it has a bent head. I have used it, but do not like it. To get a good lie onto the final artery, the graft can be bent round and brought in retrogradely. My experience with this is that it is something difficult to measure. There can be kinking on the apex, and what the effect of retrograde flow out of the graft is, I have no idea.

Figure 11 shows that jump grafts do work. It demonstrates a graft inserted into first the lateral circumflex and then into the posterior descending.

Figure 12 shows an example that I find even less attractive. This is the so-called transverse anastomosis with a diamond incision; a very small anastomosis that will, I am sure, cause trouble in the future. I have never used a transverse jump and do not like it.

The follow-up that is available can be looked at ˙n two ways. Table 4 shows the overall picture on our follow up: 82% asymptomatic. After all, most of our patients are operated on for pain at the present time.

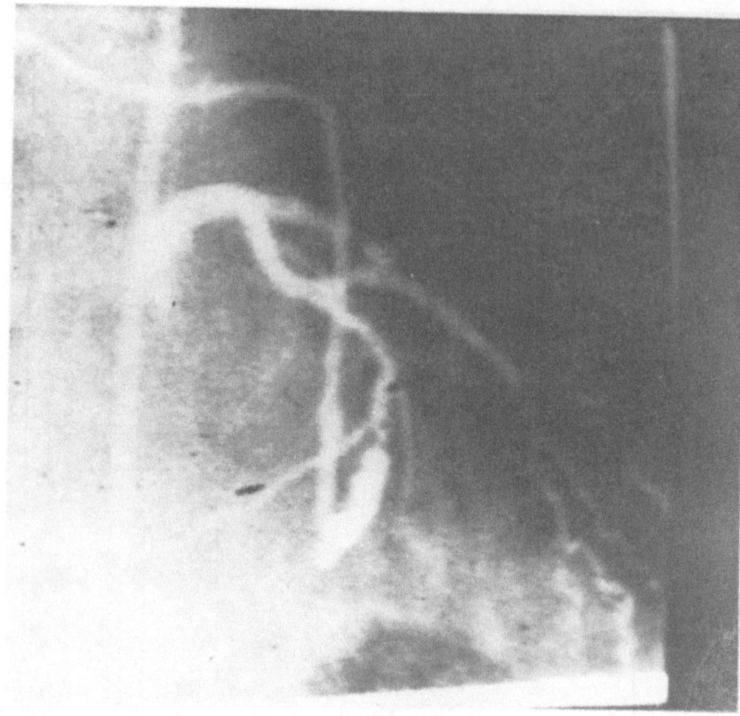

Figure 6

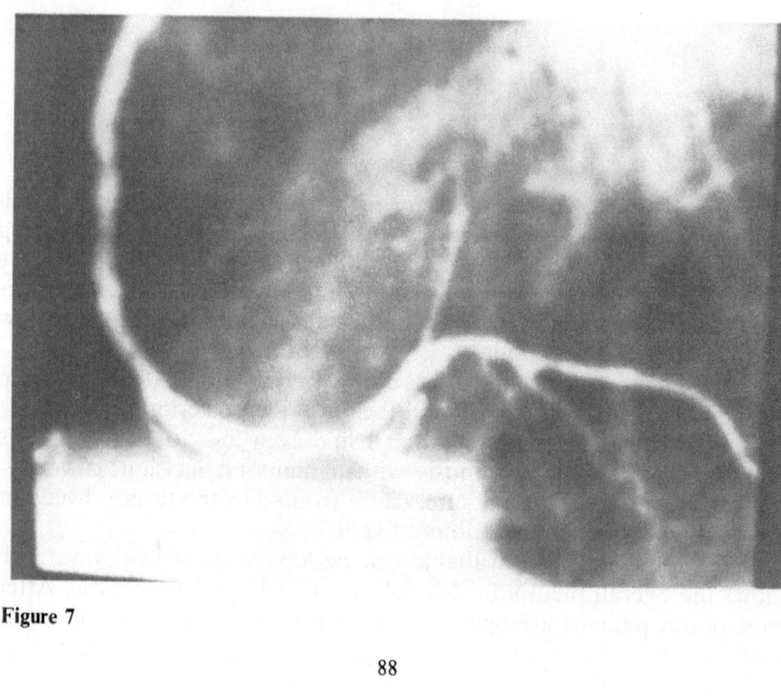

Figure 7

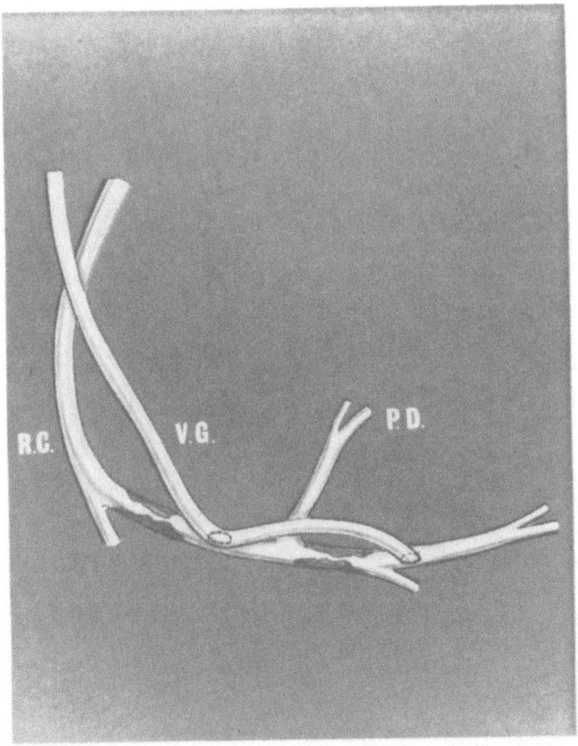

Figure 8

A better way of looking at it, as has already been pointed out, is to use a computer. Like most computers it is not fully up-to-date because it has not been programed up to date. The print out, on Figure 13, shows the percentage of patients asymptomatic each year following operation. At the end of the first year, 90% are asymptomatic. As the years go by, the percentage asymptomatic drops off, until at 5 years, the numbers are insignificant. The reason for this is twofold. In earlier days perhaps we were not doing an adequate number of grafts, and recurrent angina, which I shall not discuss, is now rearing its head.

Table 4 Postoperative follow-up (London Chest Hospital 1971–1979)

	(815 patients followed up for at least 1 year) *1 year–9 years*	
Asymptomatic	669 patients	82%
Improved	90 patients	11%
Same or worse	56 patients	7%
Total	815 patients	

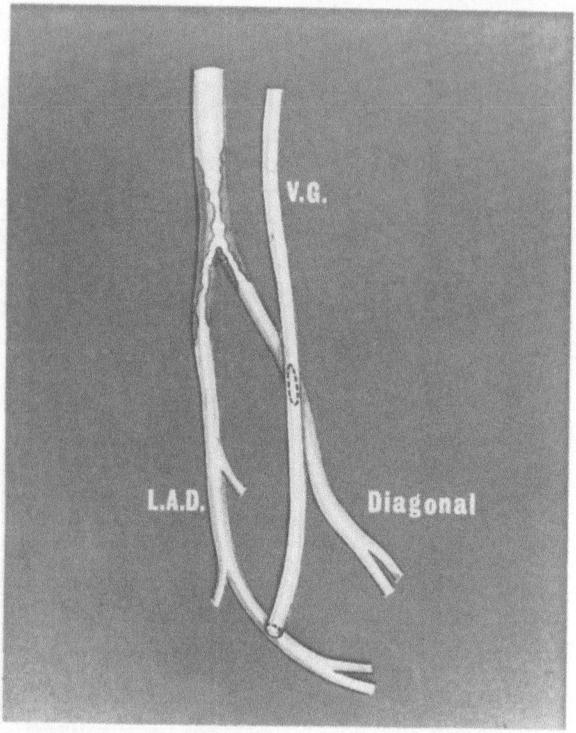

Figure 9

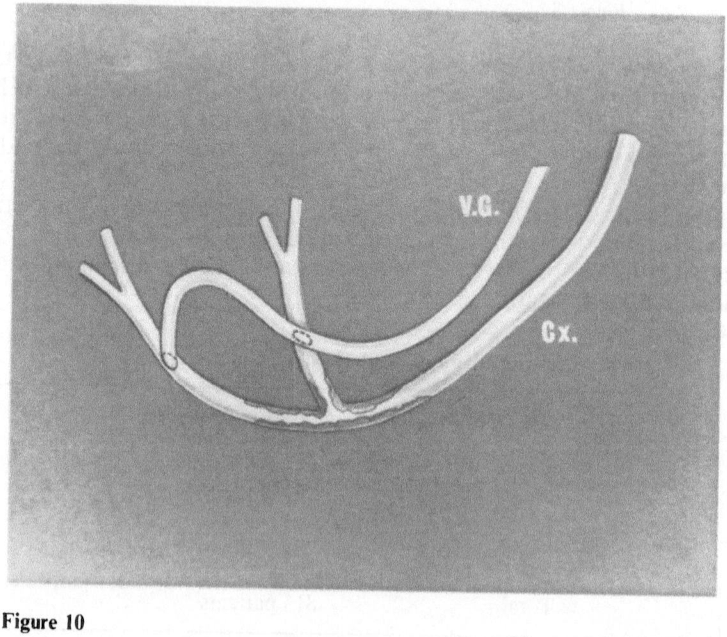

Figure 10

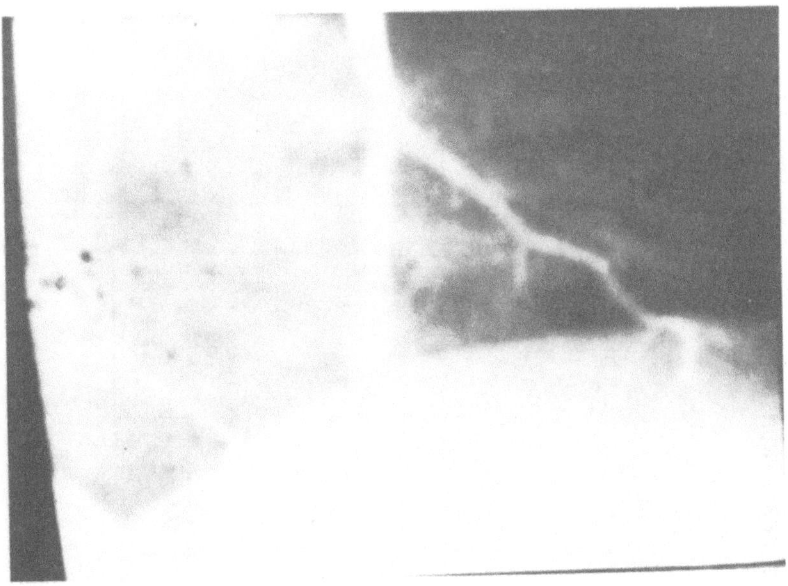

Figure 11

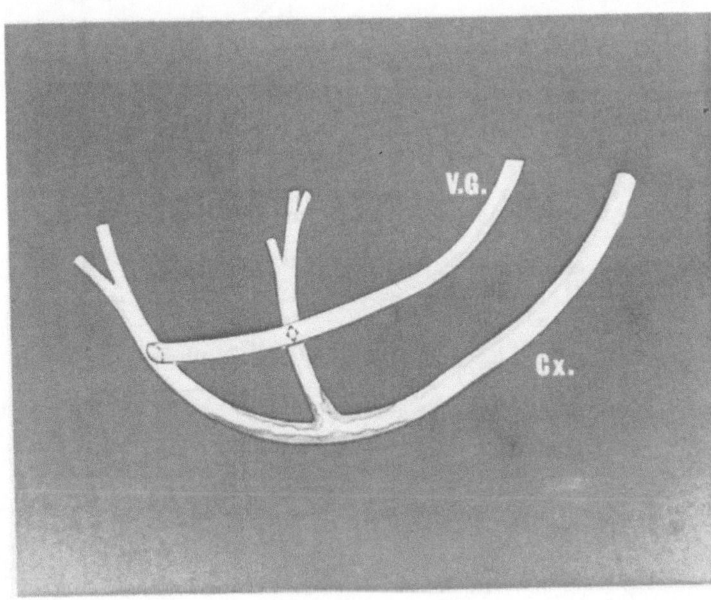

Figure 12

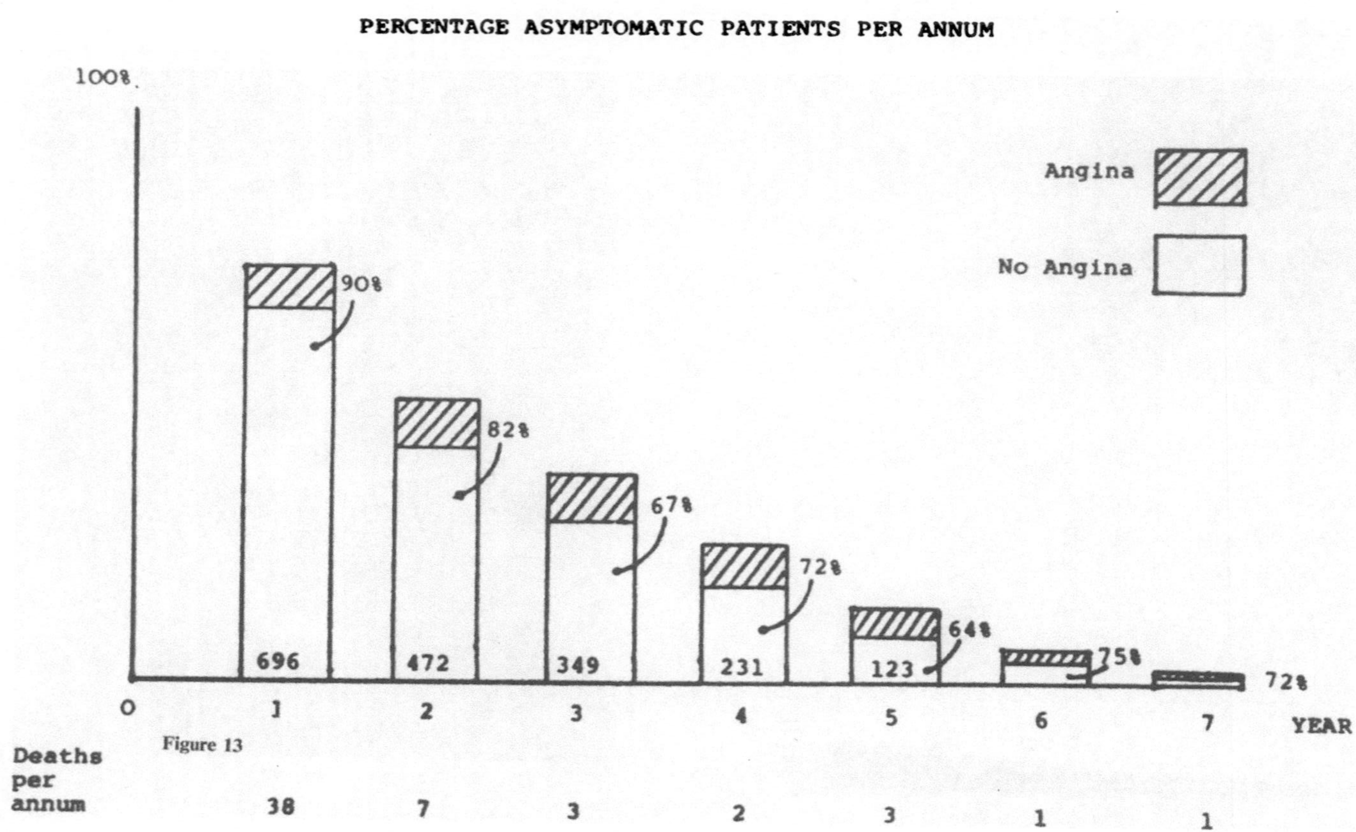
PERCENTAGE ASYMPTOMATIC PATIENTS PER ANNUM
100%
Angina
No Angina
90%
82%
67%
72%
64%
75%
72%
696
472
349
231
123
0
1
2
3
4
5
6
7
YEAR
Deaths per annum
38
7
3
2
3
1
1

Figure 13

ANNUAL RECURRENCE OF ANGINA IN ASYMPTOMATIC PATIENTS

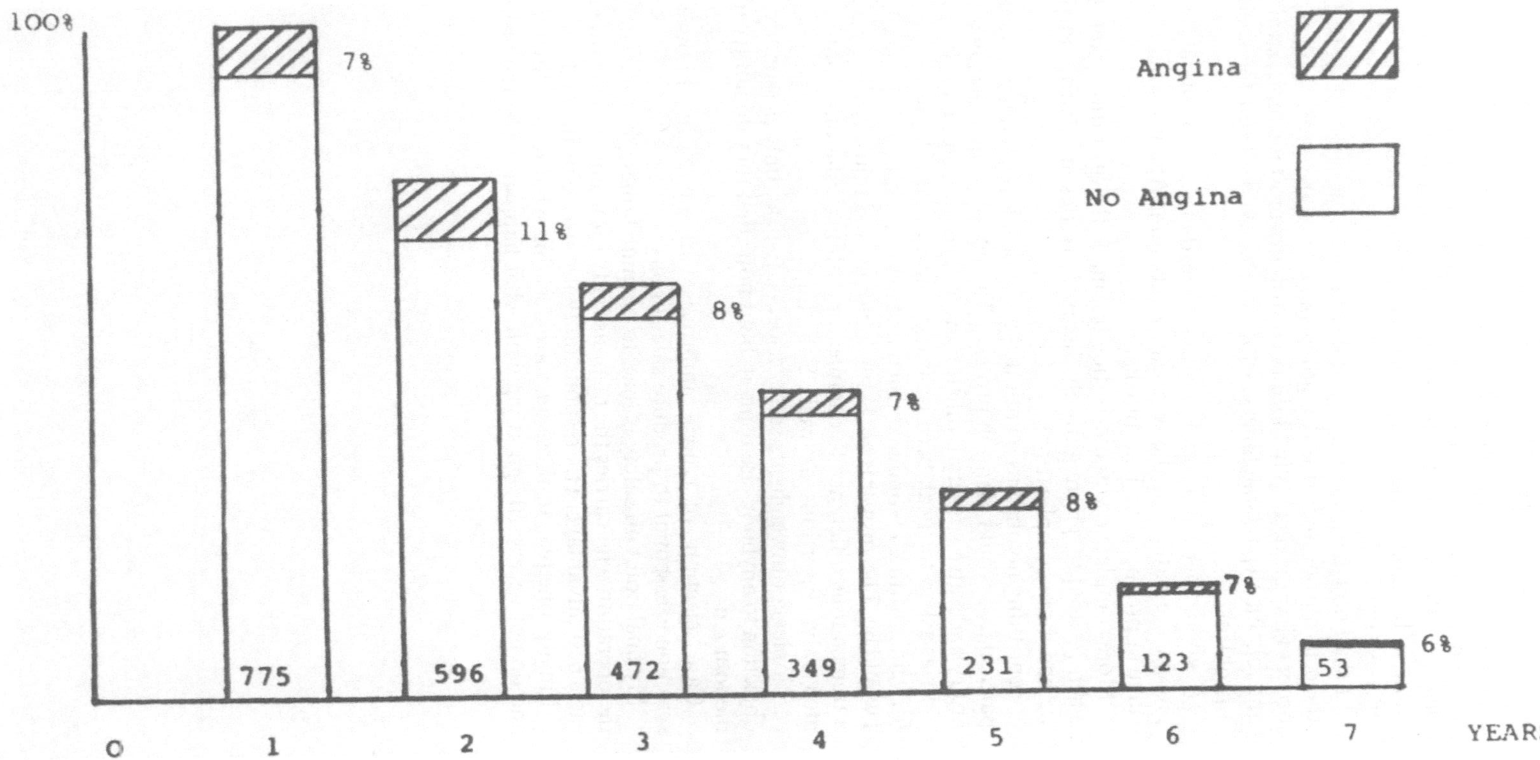

Figure 14 shows another way of looking at it. How many patients will develop recurrent angina if they are asymptomatic at the beginning of the year? As the years go by, about 7, 8 or 9% of patients who were asymptomatic will develop angina each year. The recurrent angina rate in our experience is about 7%.

I shall now pass a few anecdotal comments on safety aspects. I would put them in chronological order going back over the years, not necessarily in order of importance. What I think contributes most is simple, straightforward and reliable bypass machinery, which is now available off-the-shelf and is not a problem.

A good anaesthetic and a good anaesthetist is absolutely essential to present the patient in the way one wants him. Again I would mention the value of preoperative beta blockade.

More complete revascularization has made the operation safer. In the days when we used to ignore diffusely diseased arteries, it is hardly surprising that we had more complications.

Something no one has mentioned is the development of good materials. In particular, I would mention prolene. The use of prolene has made coronary artery and valve surgery a much more relaxed, easier and safer procedure.

I was asked to speak because it was known that I did not use cardioplegia for vein grafting. I wondered when first asked a year ago whether by this time I would be. The answer is no. I still do not use it. I think cardioplegia has made a tremendous difference to complex operations, long operations and associated valve insertions as well. For simple operations, the complexity of cardioplegia outweighs its safety aspects. I speak only personally. I have no objection to anybody else using it, but I hope that they do not try to convince me to use it.

Case selection, of course, improves with increasing knowledge. Case selection is essential to produce safe surgery.

My final point on safety is that, to be quite honest, it is the surgeon doing the operation who carries the responsibility for using all these other things to their best advantage. His responsibility it must be in the end.

Finally, one plea to those who are deciding what to use. Stick to the facts and do not necessarily go along with what happens to be the fashion.

8
Reappraisal of the value of clinical observation

D. G. JULIAN

It would now be true to say that in most good cardiothoracic centres the quality of anaesthesia, surgery and postoperative care is such that the chief determinant of successful surgery is the quality of clinical material presented to the surgeon. In this, the physician or cardiologist is the hero or the villain for it is he who is largely responsible for selecting the time during the natural course of the disease when the patient is considered for operation.

Many patients are sent to surgery too late in the natural history of their disease, whilst others are sent inappropriately or too early. The fact that prosthetic valves, whether biological or mechanical, are associated with serious complications and a limited lifespan means that to commit an asymptomatic individual with mitral or aortic regurgitation too early may be to impose totally unnecessary disability or death upon him. Likewise, the fact that a second coronary artery bypass graft operation is more difficult and less likely to be successful than the first, must be a factor in determining at what time the patient with little or no angina should be committed to surgery for the benefit of prognosis.

On the other hand, the very successes that have recently taken place in the medical management of angina pectoris and cardiac failure may mean that while the patient's symptoms are kept under control, his myocardium is being allowed to deteriorate beyond the point at which surgery is likely to help him.

It therefore behoves the physician to bear these factors in mind constantly in the several years in which it is often the case that he keeps the patient under review before surgery is contemplated. Whilst there is little doubt that both invasive and non-invasive techniques of investigation are obligatory in most cases prior to surgery, the expense and time they involve, as well as the discomfort which may be engendered, must make simple clinical observations, amongst which we must include radiology and electrocardiography, important. Indeed, it has always been the case that as investigatory techniques and surgery have advanced, they have led not to the abandonment of clinical observations but to their reappraisal. Thus, in the early days of cardiac surgery, the development of mitral valvotomy led to a rediscovery of the auscultatory features of mitral stenosis which had been previously largely ignored except in the French literature. When I was a student, we were taught nothing about the opening snap, even by a distinguished cardiologist. Now, even the most junior student is aware not only of its physiological significance but also of its implications with regard to surgery.

Over the succeeding years, many physical observations have been discovered or rediscovered in the light of new advances. The ability to close atrial septal defects led to an appreciation of the importance of the splitting of the second heart sound. Developments in angiography and echocardiography led to the finding that a mid-systolic click and late systolic murmur signified mitral valve prolapse, a condition which was not recognized until relatively recently. Not so long ago one would have thought that an atrial septal defect and mitral valve prolapse required invasive investigations for their diagnosis, but now the most junior registrar or resident can recognize them literally with his eyes shut.

Nowadays, clinical observation is of particular value in those situations in which surgery is indicated for prognostic as opposed to symptomatic reasons. Thus, timely intervention by surgery is important in aortic stenosis, in aortic regurgitation and in coronary artery disease in appropriate cases in the presence of few or even no symptoms. It is clearly undesirable to submit patients recurrently to cardiac catheterization to see whether the lesion has progressed to a point where surgery is indicated. While there is no question that when aortic valve disease gives rise to symptoms, surgery should be undertaken, the criteria for surgery in the asymptomatic are far from clear. However, the detection of a fourth heart sound in an aortic stenotic enables one to diagnose with some confidence that the gradient across the aortic valve is 75 mmHg or more and the end-diastolic pressure 20 mmHg or more, indications in themselves for surgery. The situation is less clear in aortic regurgitation but progression of the ECG and X-ray are certainly suggestive of impending deterioration. Perhaps the best index of deterioration at present is the demonstration of an increase in ejection fraction on exercise, as can be determined by echocardiography or nuclear imaging. It may well be that we will be able to find clinical correlates.

In the case of coronary artery bypass surgery, our search must be for techniques which may enable us to determine those whose bad prognosis can be improved by surgery. There is now no doubt of the relationship between left main disease or proximal triple vessel disease and a bad prognosis nor of its improvement by surgery. How can we identify such patients non-invasively? Undoubtedly, here, the value of the exercise test has been rediscovered. This applies not only to changes in the ST segment, but also to the work load that can be achieved and the haemodynamic response in terms of heart rate and blood pressure.

Another important facet of coronary disease which has been revealed by coronary arteriography is the existence of coronary arterial spasm. Clearly, it is undesirable for patients to be submitted to surgery who have coronary spasm as their major lesion rather than occlusive coronary atherosclerosis.

Most of these patients can be detected non-invasively by observation of the ECG during an episode, whether spontaneous or provoked by ergometrine.

Thus, over many years simple clinical investigations are seen to yield sufficient information to allow reliable conclusions and decisions to be made. They in no way diminish the importance of the more sophisticated techniques, but they allow them to be used more selectively and economically.

9
The importance and hazards of angiocardiography

J. PARTRIDGE

INTRODUCTION

An adequate delineation of the disordered anatomy is an essential preliminary to successful cardiac surgery. Sometimes the physical signs alone are adequate, as in an uncomplicated patent ductus arteriosus. Mostly, some form of imaging is required. The inherent simplicity and clarity of the basic radiographic image, which is no more than a shadow image cast in X-rays rather than light, has made angiocardiography the yardstick of anatomic demonstration against which newer methods of investigation are measured. Despite the notable advances in ultrasonics, nuclear medicine and CAT scanning, whose great value as an adjunct or preliminary to angiocardiography is not questioned, still very few surgical cases come to theatre without some invasive radiology.

THE IMPORTANCE OF ANGIOCARDIOGRAPHY

The importance of angiocardiography can be absolute; for example, coronary artery surgery cannot be performed without an angiogram, nor can correction of complex congenital heart disease. A look at some of the areas where non-invasive techniques are displacing the angiogram will be of greater interest.

Atrial septal defect

Many centres will repair a secundum atrial septal defect provided its presence is confirmed, its size estimated, and a primum defect excluded; all these questions can be answered by echocardiography. Some centres will also undertake the repair of a primum defect on clinical and echocardiographic evidence alone, whereas most would require an angiogram in order to accurately quantify 'mitral' regurgitation and exclude any ventricular septal defects. Thus the importance of the angiogram depends on local surgical attitudes.

Adult aortic valve disease

It is probably true that in selected cases aortic valve replacement can be carried out with acceptable mortality and morbidity without a cardiac catheterization or coronary angiography. The premise here is that echocardiographic evidence of satisfactory left ventricular function precludes significant coexistent coronary artery disease. This is probably so, but here again, surgical opinion will determine whether or not an angiogram is done, and the question the surgeon must ask is whether or not the *need* for valve replacement has been demonstrated.

Mitral valve surgery

Present interest in mitral valve repair rather than replacement enhances the need for close assessment of both the valve and its chordal attachments. Whilst there is no doubt that the echocardiogram provides accurate information, it and the left ventricular angiogram together yield a more accurate overall picture. Whether the echocardiogram alone will suffice is another instance where the attitude of the surgeon has much influence.

These examples show how surgical attitudes can influence the degree of investigation. It is therefore important for all concerned to appreciate the amount of information that can be obtained by angiography, particularly in view of improving standards of X-ray equipment, contrast media (see below) and radiographic techniques[1,2]. Space does not permit a comprehensive review, but a few salient topics are:

(a) The full delineation of coronary anatomy with selective injections even when there is abnormal coronary anatomy.
(b) A complete search for central pulmonary arteries in pulmonary artesia, including wedged pulmonary venography[3] (Figure 1).
(c) A complete delineation of pulmonary and coronary anatomy in tetralogy of Fallot (Figures 2 and 3).
(d) The ability to consistently sample pulmonary artery pressure in transposition of the great arteries and other complex disorders of chamber connection (Figure 4).
(e) The complete delineation of the various features of the spectrum of atrioventricular (canal) defects.

The completeness of this approach has not led to any significant increase in investigation time since modern catheter techniques allow a swifter procedure. For example, quite often a complete study can be performed from the transvenous route even when the pathology is left-sided (Figure 5).

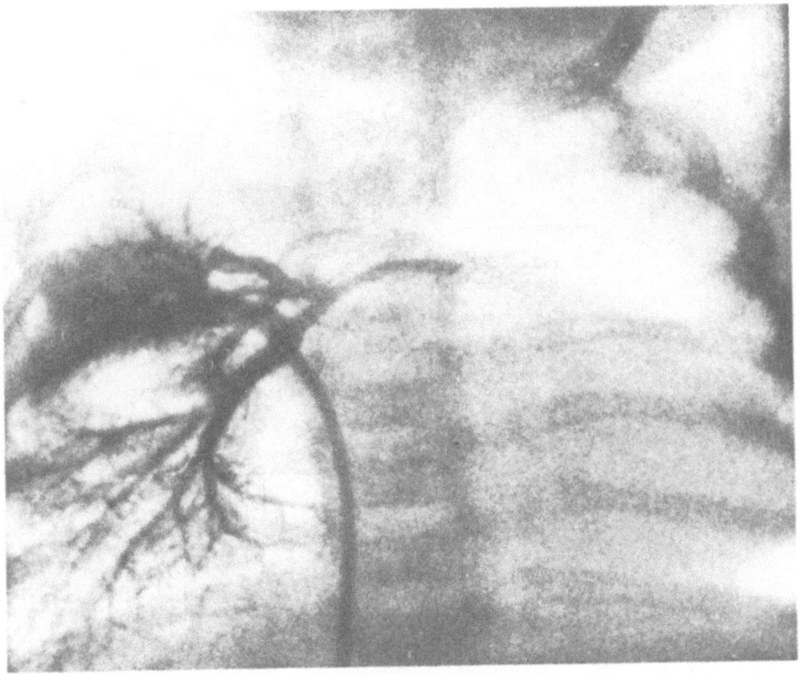

Figure 1 Demonstration of the central pulmonary arteries in pulmonary atresia by wedged pulmonary venography. The catheter is wedged in the right upper pulmonary vein and its tip is surrounded by capillary blush. All the vessels on this frame are true pulmonary arteries

THE HAZARDS

To all patients

In the case of a patient in good clinical condition, and with due regard to his comfort, it is a reasonable attitude to perform as much angiocardiography as is required to achieve a satisfactory demonstration of the pathology, within the limits of contrast dosage. In other words, the hazards of radiation exposure, arterial or venous catheterization, intracardiac catheter manipulation and of allergic reaction to the contrast medium, are small enough so as not to be a contraindication to the procedure. Clinical experience bears this out; for example, routine coronary arteriography now has a mortality of less than 0.3%. Improvements in techniques of catheter insertion, tubing material, and prophylactic heparinization have contributed to this satisfactory trend. Modern radiological equipment is constantly improving the quality and comfort of the procedures. The only factor of concern here is the escalating cost of these procedures, and we can all help alleviate this by encouraging the policy of maintaining units with a high turnover; this will also encourage higher standards of operator skill (Figure 6).

Routine contrast media, when used without incident, are usually considered to have been without long-term harmful effect. However, these media

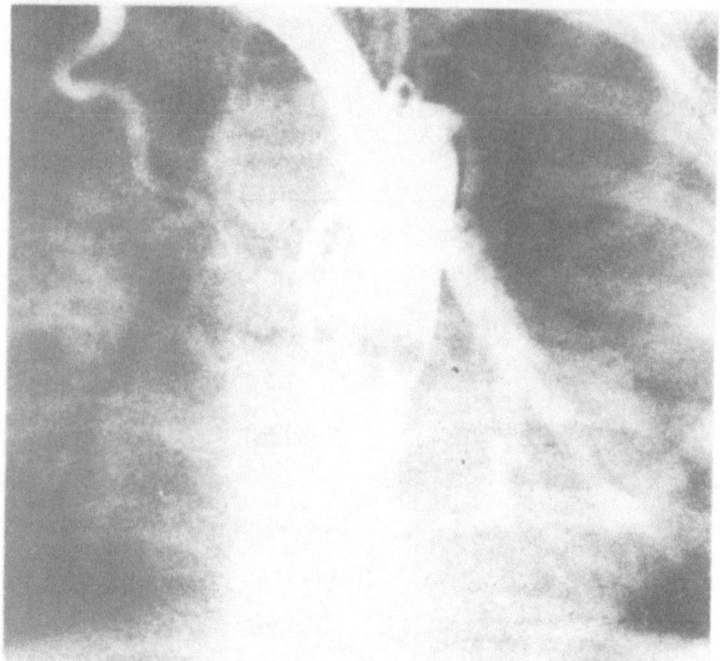

Figure 2 Aortogram using an inflated balloon catheter to optimize brachiocephalic filling. The stenosed left Blalock shunt and the left pulmonary artery were not adequately delineated by routine angiography

are ionic, hyperosmolar solutions which have some consistent effects on endothelial surfaces. There is considerable incidence of fresh thrombus forming *after* phlebography, 48 % in one series[4]; there is always evidence of disruption of the aortic endothelium after aortography[5], and functional disturbances of the blood–brain barrier can be demonstrated[6,7]. The significance of these universal effects is uncertain, but to both minimize them and to lessen general toxicity, non-ionic media of low osmolarity have recently been developed[8] (Figure 7).

The hazards to the patient in poor condition

A number of factors can terminate an investigation before full angiography has been achieved. The less toxic non-ionic media should help greatly in this respect.

Low-output and cyanotic conditions

In general, patients who are in poor condition but do not have any actual or incipient pulmonary oedema can be adequately studied. For example, coronary arteriography in low-output cardiogenic shock after myocardial infarction is a recognized procedure (Figure 8); most congenital severely-

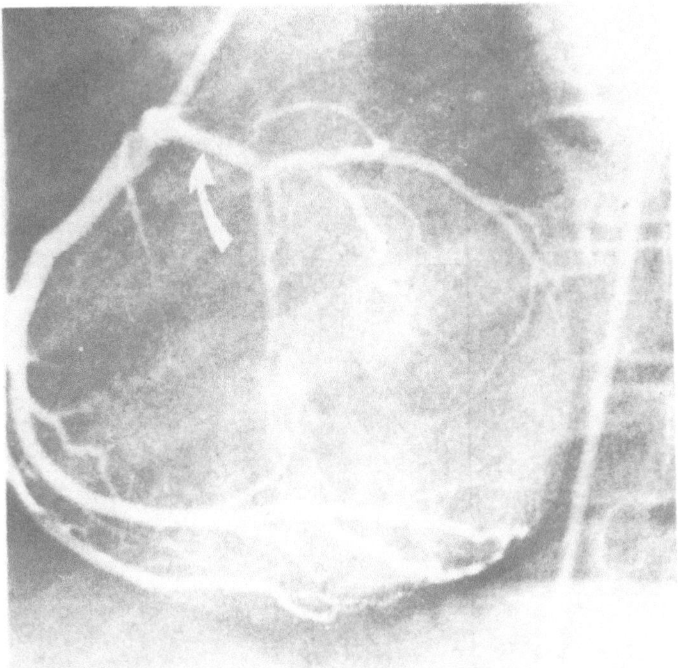

Figure 3 Coronary artery anomaly in tetralogy of Fallot. A selective right coronary injection in this 8-year-old child shows the left coronary artery (arrowed) arising from it and passing leftwards in front of the right ventricular infundibulum (left anterior oblique view)

cyanotic heart disease can be safely investigated; patients with dissecting aneurysm should tolerate two or three angiograms. One exception is the patient with obliterative pulmonary vascular disease in whom a fatal rise in pulmonary resistance may occur. This is another contrast-induced change that the non-ionic media should alleviate[9].

Conditions with actual or incipient pulmonary oedema
Patients who are severely dyspnoeic may not tolerate investigation in the supine position long enough for even one angiogram. In this group it is best to assume that only one injection of contrast will be tolerated, and to plan its site and timing carefully.

Incomplete examinations due to anatomy

Despite the sophistication of modern catheter techniques, some pathologies remain a problem. Aortic valve disease, and valve prostheses, can frustrate efforts to enter the left ventricle; reports of percutaneous angiography have appeared. Total anomalous pulmonary venous drainage can be difficult to demonstrate if a patent ductus 'steals' contrast from a pulmonary angiogram. In these cases, failure is no fault of the operator, but still this outcome must be regarded as a hazard.

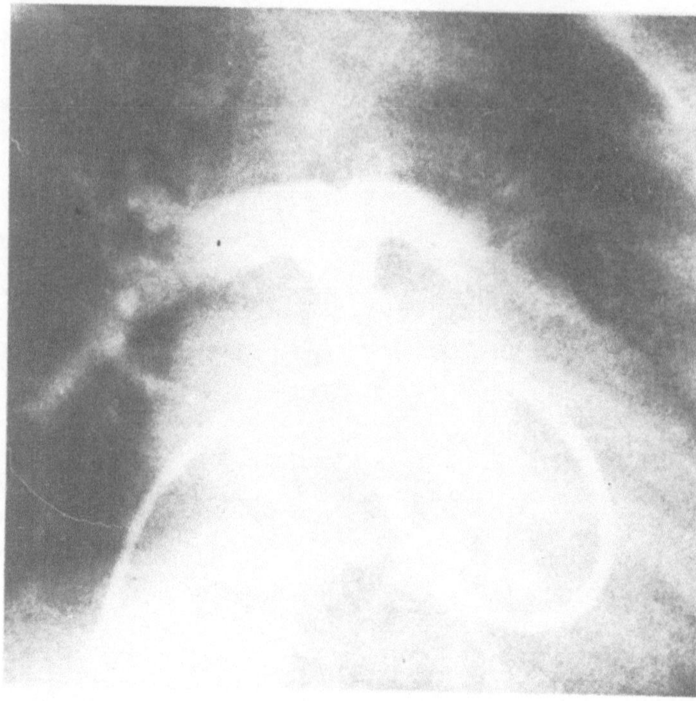

Figure 4 The complete approach. Entry into the pulmonary artery in a case of tricuspid atresia, ventricular septal defect, double outlet right ventricle with l-malposition and pulmonary stenosis. Catheter tip deflector technique

Embolic and thrombotic complications

Though these are the result of cardiac catheterization rather than the angiogram *per se*, they are a relevant hazard to the whole procedure. Catheter-induced embolus is an avoidable complication, and the risk of it is small. Emboli dislodged from the heart, notably fragments of calcified aortic valve, portions of left atrial thrombus and infective vegetations, occur in patients who can be identified as at-risk. In these cases, the need for catheterization has to be particularly clearly defined.

Thrombosis at the point of catheter insertion is an occasional problem; it used to be not uncommon after balloon septostomy in the neonate, but present-day catheter sheath techniques have rendered it infrequent. Spontaneous venous thrombus in severely cyanosed, polycythaemic cases is a sporadic and unpredictable complication, and usually occurs in the cerebral veins leading to significant neurological impairment. The precipitating cause is probably the dehydration consequent to patient preparation before the procedure, exacerbated by contrast media. Operator skill and experience – which shortens the procedure, and adequate hydration during the procedure mitigate against this hazard.

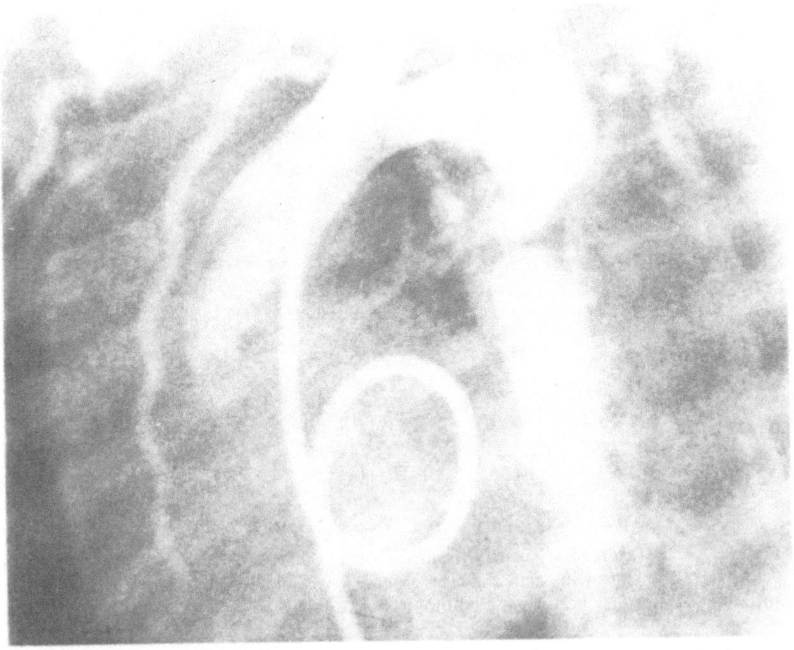

Figure 5 Transvenous aortography in coarctation of the aorta. The catheter is via a patent foramen ovale, mitral and aortic valves. Tip deflector technique

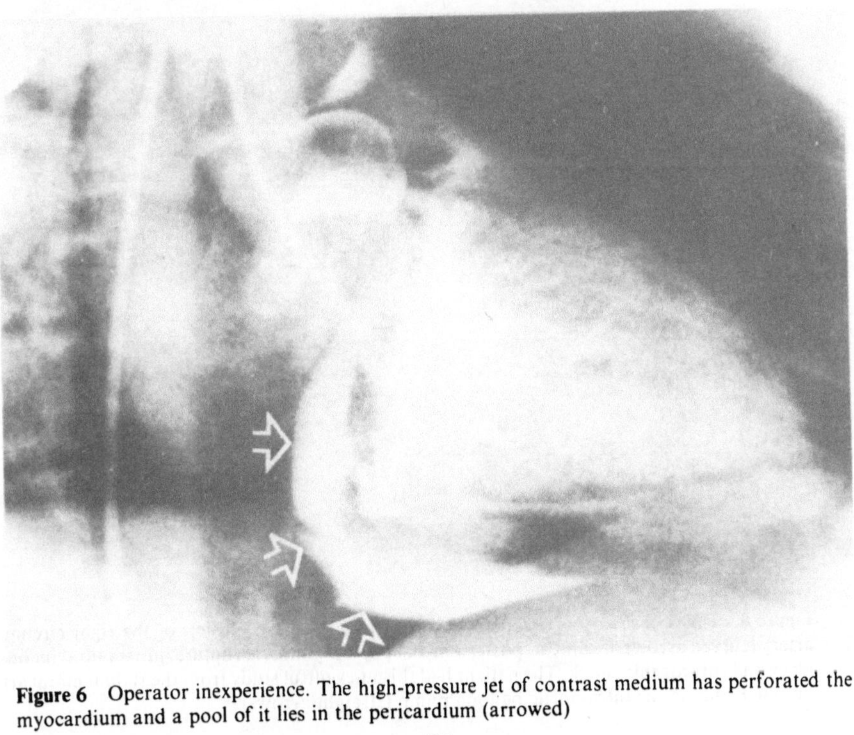

Figure 6 Operator inexperience. The high-pressure jet of contrast medium has perforated the myocardium and a pool of it lies in the pericardium (arrowed)

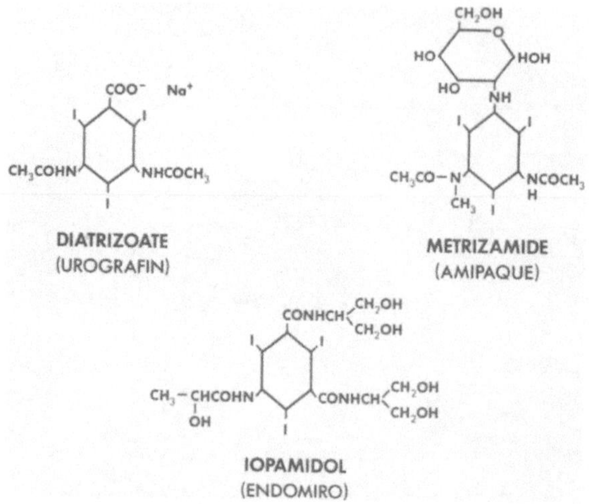

Figure 7 Contrast media. The routine media such as diatrizoate are fully ionized, hyperosmolar acids. Replacement of the acid chain by glucose gives metrizamide, a costly but safer medium. Iopamidol is another non-ionic medium, not yet available

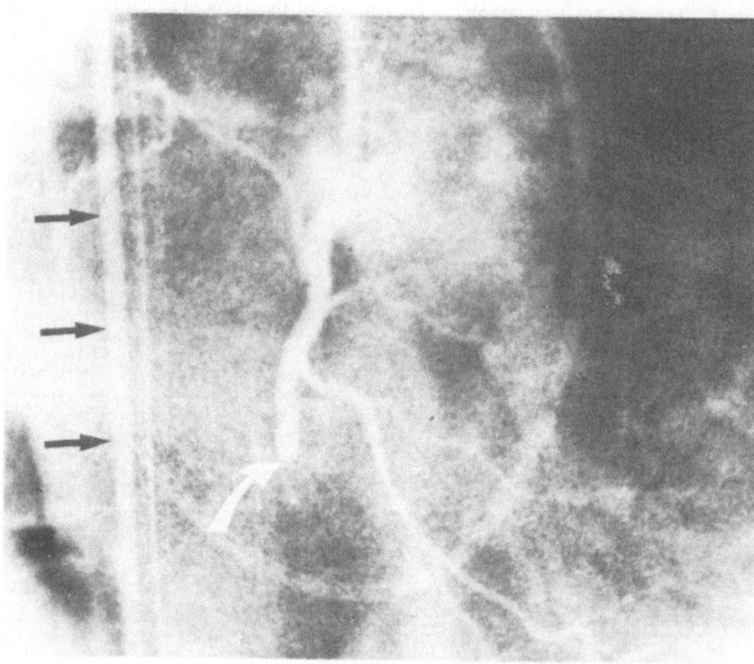

Figure 8 Right coronary arteriogram demonstrating acute occlusion of the right circumflex artery (curved arrow), leading to posteromedial papillary muscle rupture, gross mitral incompetence and cardiogenic shock. The patient had this uneventful study from the right femoral artery despite being on the intra-aortic balloon pump (straight arrows)

CONCLUSION

The hazards of angiocardiography are lessening in the face of increasing expertise and improved equipment, and the surgeon should expect a high standard of investigation and not hesitate at least to request that any doubt in anatomic interpretation be resolved.

References

1. Bargeron, L. M., Elliott, L. P., Soto, B., Bream, P. R. and Curry, G. C. (1977). Axial angiography in congenital heart disease: Section I. Concept, technical and anatomic considerations. *Circulation*, **56,** 1075
2. Elliott, L. P., Bargeron, L. M., Bream, P. R., Soto, B. and Curry, G. C. (1977). Axial cineangiography in congenital heart disease: Section II. Specific lesions. *Circulation*, **56,** 1084
3. Singh, S. P., Rigby, M. L. and Astley, R. (1978). Demonstration of pulmonary arteries by contrast injection into pulmonary vein. *Br. Heart J.*, **40,** 55
4. Albrechtsson, U. and Olsson, C. G. (1979). Thrombosis after phlebography; a comparison of two contrast media. *Cardiovasc. Radiol.*, **2,** 9
5. Almen, T., Hartel, M., Nylander, G. and Olivecrona, H. (1973). Effects of metrizamide on silver staining of aortic endothelium. *Acta Radiologica (Suppl. 335)*, 197
6. Gonsette, R. E. (1973). Biologic tolerance of the central nervous system to metrizamide. *Acta Radiologica (Suppl. 335)*, 25
7. Salveson, S. (1973). Acute toxicity tests of metrizamide. *Acta Radiologica (Suppl. 335)*, 5
8. Partridge, J. B., Scott, Olive, Fiddler, G. I., Williams, G. and Walker, J. K. (1980). Angiocardiography with metrizamide in the neonate and infant. *Clin. Radiol.* (In press)
9. Almen, T. (1973). In vitro aggregation of red blood cells following exposure to metrizamide and other agents. *Acta Radiologica (Suppl. 335)*, 223

10
The mechanisms and hazards of echocardiography

P. N. T. WELLS

INTRODUCTION

Ultrasound is a form of energy which consists of mechanical vibrations the frequencies of which are so high that they are above the range of human hearing. The lower frequency limit of the ultrasonic spectrum may generally be taken to be about 20 kHz. Most biomedical applications of ultrasound employ frequencies in the range 1–15 MHz.

Elementary outlines of the physics of ultrasound may be found in the literature cited in the Bibliography at the end of this chapter. The higher the frequency of the ultrasound, the shorter its wavelength. In any method of imaging, the wavelength is one of the factors which limits the resolution which can be obtained. At a frequency of 1 MHz, for example, the wavelength is about 1.5 mm in the soft tissues of the body. Consequently, in order to visualize structures with a resolution of around a millimetre or less, the frequency must be around 1.5 MHz or more. Although in principle the resolution could be improved simply by operating at a higher frequency, in practice the maximum frequency is limited by the attenuation of ultrasound in tissue. This is because the attenuation increases with the frequency.

PULSE–ECHO DIAGNOSTIC METHODS

An ultrasonic pulse is reflected when it strikes the boundary between two media of differing characteristic impedances (the characteristic impedance of a medium is equal to the product of its density and the speed of ultrasound), and the time delay that occurs between the transmission of the pulse and the reception of its echo depends on the propagation speed and the path length. The propagation speeds in different soft tissues are so closely similar (approximately equal to that in water, and around 1500 m/s), that a constant relationship between time and distance can usually be assumed. Ultrasound travels 10 mm in about 6.7 μs at this speed.

The ultrasonic pulse–echo method depends on the estimations of the ranges and directions of echo-producing targets within the tissue volume interrogated by the ultrasonic beam. Instruments range in complexity from the simple range-finding A-scope with hand-held probe, through the time-position recording system and the static two-dimensional B-scope, to real-time systems gathering data from two-dimensional planes within three-dimensional volumes.

The A-scope

The basic elements of the simplest type of pulse–echo system for medical diagnosis, called an 'A-scope', are illustrated in Figure 1. The rate-generator (or 'clock') simultaneously triggers the transmitter, the swept-gain generator (or 'time gain control', 'tgc', generator), and the timebase generator. The voltages which appear across the transducer in the probe are amplified by the receiver, and the output from the receiver is arranged to deflect the time-base line on the display. Thus, vertical deflections of the horizontal timebase occur at positions corresponding to echo-producing targets along the ultrasonic beam within the patient. Rapid repetition of the process (typically 1000 times per second) results in a flicker-free display.

Swept gain

A substantial improvement in the usefulness of the displayed information is obtained if the echo signals from deeper structures are amplified more than those which originate closer to the probe. This is because deeper echoes are more attenuated by the greater tissue path length; swept gain compensates for this. Ideally, swept gain should lead to similar deflection amplitudes on the display for similar surfaces, irrespective of their distances from the probe. In practice, however, accurate swept gain is difficult to achieve, for two main reasons. First, there is a variation in the attenuation rates of different tissues, so that compensating on the basis of 1 dB cm^{-1} MHz^{-1} is at best only a compromise. (Note that the decibel, abbreviated 'dB', is a logarithmic measure of relative ultrasonic signal strength. For example, an attenuation of 3 dB corresponds to a reduction of signal power by a factor of two.) Secondly, the energy in the ultrasonic pulse is distributed over quite a wide frequency spectrum, and the higher frequency components of the pulse are increasingly attenuated with increasing penetration, since the attenuation coefficient in soft tissues is roughly proportional to the frequency. This exacerbates the problem of applying accurate swept-gain compensation.

Resolution in pulse–echo systems

Within the limitations imposed by noise and by the maximum permissible transmitted power, the maximum useful dynamic range between the largest and the smallest echoes received in conventional medical diagnostic pulse–echo systems is about 100 dB (corresponding to an amplitude ratio of 100 000 to 1). This dynamic range is shared between the variations in echo

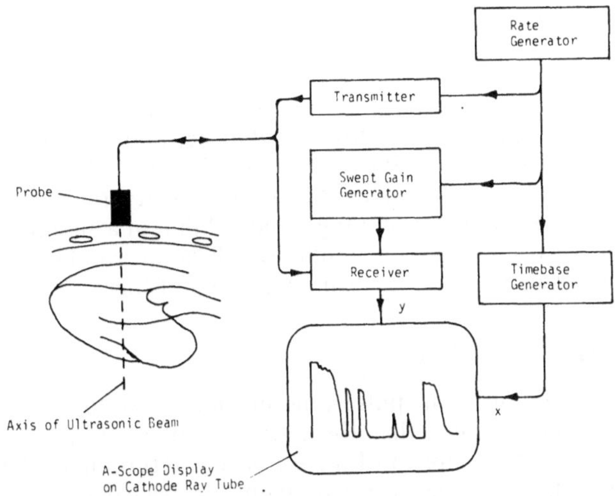

Figure 1 Basic elements of the A-scope. The probe contains a transducer which generates a short-duration ultrasonic pulse in response to excitation from the transmitter. This pulse is transmitted into the patient along the narrow ultrasonic beam. Echoes returning to the transducer produce electrical signals which are amplified by the receiver. The output from the receiver is connected to the vertical (y) deflection plates of the cathode-ray tube, and that from the time-base generator, to the horizontal (x) plates

amplitude at particular ranges, and the attenuation of echoes which increases with distance. In practice, at any particular range, an echo amplitude variation of about 30 dB (about 32 to 1) is the maximum which may usefully be employed, since the azimuthal resolution is unlikely to be acceptable with a larger dynamic range. Therefore, around 70 dB is available to provide swept-gain compensation for attenuation. An attenuation of 1 dB cm^{-1} MHz^{-1} corresponds to 0.15 dB per wavelength, or to 0.3 dB per wavelength of penetration (taking account of the go-and-return path). With 70 dB of swept gain, a penetration of 233 wavelengths would thus seem to be possible; 200 wavelengths is a more realistic figure.

The resolution of any imaging system may be defined in several different ways. The usual definition is that the resolution is equal to the reciprocal of the minimum distance (in range or in azimuth) between two point targets, at which separate registrations can just be distinguished on the display. An alternative definition, equivalent in concept but sometimes more convenient in practice, is that the resolution is equal to the reciprocal of the distance which appears on the display to be occupied by a point target in the field. Measurements based on this definition avoid problems which arise due to interference between waves scattered by two closely spaced point (or line) targets.

The resolution cell is the volume of material within which the interaction providing the data takes place. Except in simple and idealized situations, the dimensions of the resolution cell depend on the distance between the transducer and the target (that is, the range). At any particular range, the length of the resolution cell depends on the duration of the ultrasonic pulse (the shorter the pulse, the shorter the length, and the better the range resolution), and its width, on the diameter of the ultrasonic beam (the smaller the diameter, the better the resolution in azimuth and in elevation). In echocardiography, optimum resolution and penetration are obtained at frequencies of around 2–5 MHz. For example, at 2.5 MHz the maximum penetration is about 120 mm, and the resolution at a range of about 80 mm is typically around 0.6 mm in range, and 1.2 mm in azimuth and elevation. This value of resolution in azimuth and elevation would correspond to a focused ultrasonic beam over its limited depth of focus.

Multiple reflection artifacts

A serious limitation of the pulse–echo method is due to the multiple reflections, or reverberations, that the ultrasonic pulse may suffer during its propagation. For example, in Figure 1 echoes returning to the probe from within the patient are themselves partially re-reflected at the probe surface, and these pulses themselves act as if they were transmitted pulses, relatively small in amplitude and appropriately delayed in time. Echoes of these small pulses produce registrations, if they are large enough to be detected, at positions corresponding to twice (and higher multiples of) the distances at which the true echoes are registered. These 'multiple reflection' artifacts may often be quite easily recognized because of their regular spacings. Those due to gas and bone are generally inconveniently large, and they are a fundamental limitation in ultrasonic diagnosis. In echocardiography, common sources of multiple reflection artifacts are the ribs and lung.

The B-scope

The information obtained with a pulse–echo system is a combination of range and amplitude data which can simply be presented as an A-scan. The same information, however, may alternatively be displayed on a brightness-modulated timebase, in such a way that the brightness increases with echo amplitude; this type of display is called a B-scan. The B-scope is the basis of the time-position recording technique (the 'M-mode' recording technique which is the cornestone of echocardiography), and the two-dimensional scanner (which in its real-time form is becoming increasingly important in cardiological investigations).

Time-position (M-mode) recording

A time-position recording of structure position along the ultrasonic beam may be generated from a B-scan as shown in Figure 2. Most instruments based on this principle generate time and distance (i.e. ultrasonic timebase) markers on the recording to assist in interpretation.

A time-position recording is composed of many separate B-scan lines lying side-by-side. Conventionally, increasing distance into the patient is represented by more downward deflection on the recording, and earlier time, horizontally towards the left. The time required to form a single B-scan line

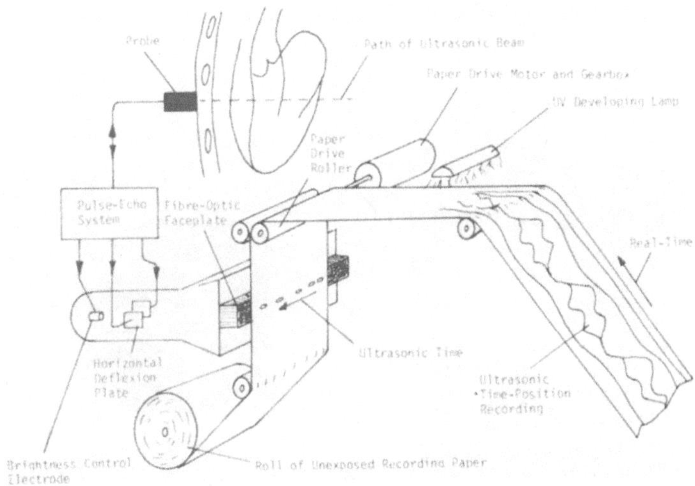

Figure 2 Time-position recording system using a continuous strip of photographic paper sensitive to ultraviolet light. The B-scan is displayed on a cathode-ray tube with a fibre-optic faceplate. This display is extremely bright, and a continuous image of the time-position trace is produced (and developed within a few seconds) as the paper is driven at constant speed past the cathode-ray tube

depends on the depth of penetration; for example, a time of 133 μs corresponds to a depth of 100 mm. Generally structures within the body do not move significant distances during so short a time, so that (provided that the pulse repetition rate is fast enough) the movements of structures such as heart valves may be studied.

Two-dimensional B-scanning

The production of an image of a cross-section through soft tissue structures of the body may be accomplished by relating the positions of registrations on the display to the positions of the corresponding echo-producing structures within a defined two-dimensional plane in the patient.

The first type of ultrasonic two-dimensional scanner to come into widespread clinical use was of the so-called 'static' variety. This type of scanner, illustrated in Figure 3, is still commonly used for the ultrasonic visualization of the pregnant uterus and its contents, and of the relatively static contents of the abdominal cavity. The image is built up on some kind of storage device, whilst the transducer is moved, often by hand and in contact with the skin, across the anatomical structures to be visualized.

In cardiological investigations, images of at least limited usefulness can be obtained by means of a static two-dimensional ultrasonic scanner, especially if the display is 'gated' from the electrocardiogram so that a cross-sectional picture at a particular phase in the cardiac cycle is built up over several cardiac cycles. A potentially much more useful type of instrument, however, has been developed: this is the so-called 'real-time' two-dimensional scanner. Real-time imaging systems have image frame rates which are

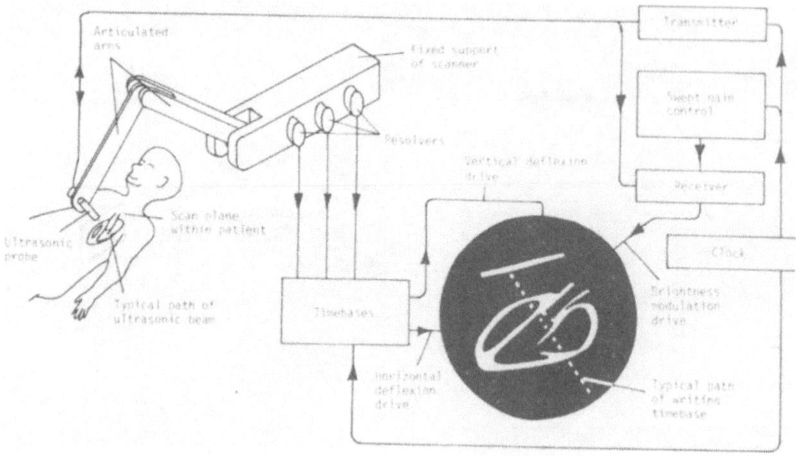

Figure 3 Block diagram showing the basic principles of the conventional 'static' two-dimensional B-scanner. The scanning arrangement shown is one of several different designs. The horizontal and vertical deflection circuits are driven by separate ultrasonic timebases, simultaneously triggered by the clock. The x and y coordinates of the start of the timebases which form the image are controlled by x and y resolvers in the scanner, and the relative velocities of the two timebases are determined by a third resolver which measures the direction of the ultrasonic beam across the patient. Thus the output from the video amplifier, arranged to z-modulate the display, produces registrations on the resultant timebase in positions corresponding to echo-producing targets within the patient. A two-dimensional image is built up by moving the probe so that the part of the anatomical cross-section which it is desired to visualize is scanned by a sufficient number of discrete ultrasonic lines. Gating from the ECG can be used to make a 'static' image of the heart

sufficiently fast to allow movement to be followed. The actual frame rate necessary to satisfy this definition depends on the circumstances of the particular clinical investigation. For example, if the movement to be followed is that of the heart, a frame rate of at least 40/s is necessary to avoid missing details of valve action.

Ultimately the frame rate is limited by the speed of ultrasound in tissue. If, for example, a penetration of 120 mm is required, the time which elapses between the transmission of the ultrasonic pulse and reception of the echo from the maximum range is equal to 167 μs (taking the speed to be 1500 m/s). The corresponding maximum pulse repetition rate is almost 6000/s (although in practice 2000–3000/s would still be more likely to be used). Thus the maximum theoretically achievable line rate is 6000/s; equal to the product of the number of lines per frame and the number of frames per second. Again, for example, at 40 frames/s, there could be up to 150 lines per frame.

Some of the many methods of rapid scanning to produce real-time images are illustrated in Figure 4. In the first technique, a conventional single-element transducer, or group of single-element transducers, is mechanically driven to form images in real-time but otherwise similar to those made by conventional 'static' two-dimensional scanners.

The principles of the electronically addressed linear array type of real-time scanner are illustrated in Figure 5. In the earliest linear array systems,

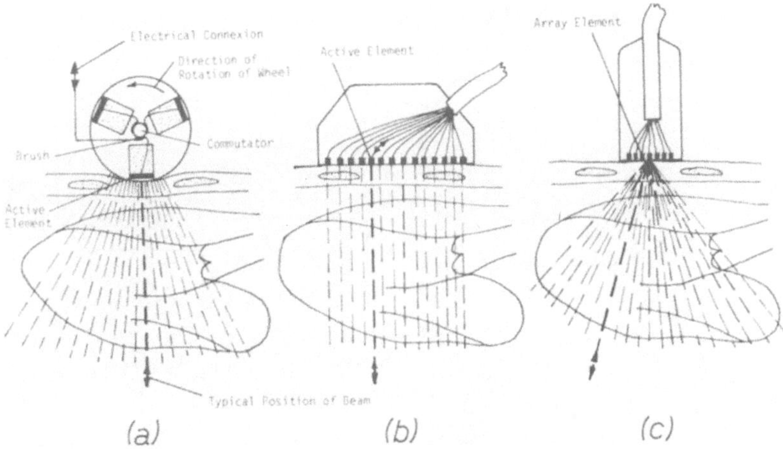

Figure 4 Methods of real-time scanning: (a) fast mechanical scanner – in this example, three single-element transducers are mounted on a wheel which rotates continuously, and as each transducer in turn comes into contact with the patient, it sweeps out a new frame made up of an image sector; (b) electronically scanned linear array transducer array – the transducer elements are addressed sequentially, to sweep out image frames with a rectangular format; (c) transducer array with electronic beam steering – delays are introduced into the separate signal paths associated with the individual elements in the array, to sweep out image frames with a sector format

the transducer elements were addressed one at a time. In this situation, a compromise is necessary. On the one hand, it is desirable to have a large number of lines in the image, and this requires a large number of transducers. On the other hand, it is desirable to have good resolution, which depends on having a non-divergent (or even focused) beam of ultrasound. Unfortunately, the beam divergence in the far field increases as the transducer is made more narrow. The difficulty can be circumvented by having an array of many narrow transducers (so that the objective of high line density can be achieved) operated in groups to ensure an adequate aperture (so that the resolution is acceptable). A common arrangement is to have 64 elements operated in groups of 4, stepped one element between lines, thus giving 61 lines of ultrasonic information.

The second type of electronically controlled real-time scanner makes use of the beam-steering capability of an array. Consider the array, consisting of four long, narrow elements, illustrated in Figure 6. The introduction of appropriate time delays in the signal paths allows the beam to be directed through any desired angle (within certain limitations), and also to be focused. Moreover, on reception the position of the focus may be swept continuously to coincide with the instantaneous position of the target, thus giving greatly improved resolution in azimuth, comparable with the resolution at the focal length of a fixed focus (i.e., lens) system. Of course, this technique is also valuable with linear array scanners. Typically, electronically steered arrays have around 20 elements, and the external dimensions of the probe are similar to those of a conventional single-element transducer probe.

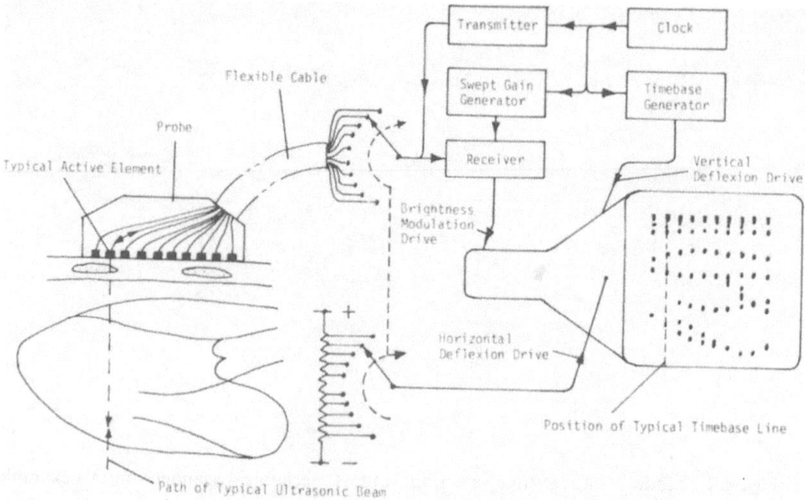

Figure 5 Linear array real-time scanning system. In this diagram, the probe contains 10 separate transducer elements (in a practical system, the number is usually between 20 and 128). The clock, typically operating at a rate of 2000/s, triggers the transmitter. In this simple example the transmitter pulse is applied, through a sequencing switch, to one of the transducer elements. (Again, in a practical system, this sequencing switch and the second switch operating synchronously with it are usually electronic and not mechanical.) Simultaneously, the clock triggers the timebase generator connected to the vertical deflection plates of the cathode-ray tube display. Echoes returning from within the patient are detected by the transducer element which emitted the original pulse, fed through the sequencing switch, and amplified (under swept-gain control, triggered by the clock), to brightness-modulate the display. Each element is rapidly addressed in sequence, and a two-dimensional image is built up by the second sequencing switch applying appropriate horizontal deflection voltages to the display

Of the two main types of real-time scanner, the electronically controlled system (either linear or steered array) has one particularly important advantage in cardiological investigations. This is the ability which it has to allow the selection of one (or more) scan-line positions for simultaneous M-mode recording (see the section on Time-position Recording) of the movement of a structure identified on the two-dimensional image. The best that can be done with mechanical scanners is first to identify the structure of interest on a two-dimensional scan, and then progressively to decrease the scan angle until there is a single stationary line passing through the structure whose motion it is desired to record.

The real-time image is at present invariably displayed on a cathode-ray tube during the scanning procedure. The scan format of a linear array system can be arranged to be TV-raster-compatible, permitting the convenient use of standard TV monitors, character generators and videotape-recorders. Where the scan format is not directly compatible with the TV raster, scan conversion can be accomplished either by viewing the initial ultrasonic scan display tube by a closed-circuit TV camera, or by an analogue or a digital 'scan converter'.

At any moment during scanning, the operator may see an image which merits detailed study. In this case, a 'frame freeze' capability is most useful. Basically there are two methods by which this may be provided. One method uses a conventional analogue scan converter, such as that commonly used as an image store in static scanners; but this does have the disadvantages that selective erasure of part of an image is difficult and time-consuming (in relation to the frame time of the image). These problems are avoided in the second method of frame freeze, which uses a digital image store.

In many clinical applications, it is important to be able to make measurements of distance from the ultrasonic images. It is not satisfactory to measure directly from the cathode-ray tube display, even when the image is stationary

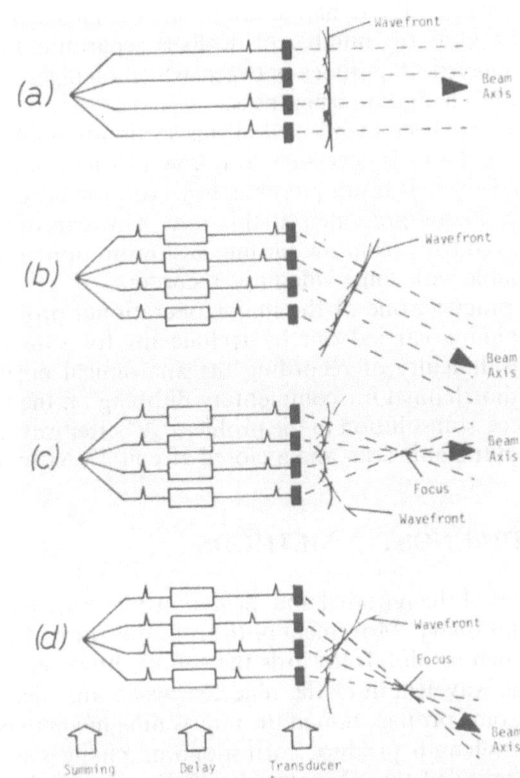

Figure 6 Principles of electronically steered array scanning. These diagrams illustrate the transmission of ultrasound by an array of four long, narrow elements; the same principles apply to the reception of ultrasound. The long axes of the elements are normal to the plane of the diagram, and viewed in this direction each element emits a cylindrical wavelet in response to electrical excitation: (a) when the elements are excited simultaneously (as indicated by the simultaneous 'blips' on the connecting wires), the wavelets combine to form a wavefront of which the corresponding beam travels directly away from the array; (b) when the elements are excited in sequence, the beam is deviated off the central axis; (c) when spherical time-grading is used, the beam is focused; (d) when the time-grading consists of combined linear and spherical distributions, the beam is both deviated and focused

for long enough to make this possible, because the image is distorted by non-linearities in the deflection system. Electronic calipers may be provided to eliminate this problem, and several arrangements have been devised: generally the choice depends on the personal preference of the operator.

Before the mid-1970s, ultrasonic two-dimensional scanners were generally designed to produce tissue maps with the emphasis on the display of organ boundaries. The best scans were considered to be those in which the anatomy was depicted by thin white lines on a black background, for which purpose a black-and-white display is ideal. Subsequently, it has become clear that the echo amplitude conveys useful diagnostic information, and that grey-scale displays are generally greatly superior to those limited to presenting black-and-white images. The grey-scale capability of a display system can be described in terms of the dynamic range of the image. The dynamic range may be expressed as the number of decibels separating the minimum and maximum displayed amplitudes between which changes in amplitude produce perceptible changes in brightness.

It has previously been mentioned in this section that an image frame rate of at least around 40/s is necessary to follow fast movements such as those of the cardiac valves. It is not possible, however, for the eye of the observer to follow movements presented at this rate. This can only be done if the images are played back from a recording in slow motion; and this is a facility which is available with some videotape recorders.

In clinical practice, one of the major operational problems in real-time ultrasonic scanning carried out by technicians for subsequent review by doctors is the difficulty of recording the anatomical position of the scan plane. An audio channel for commentary dubbing on the videotape is only a partially successful solution to the problem. A better way is simultaneously to record the ultrasonic scan and a closed-circuit TV view of the patient.

DOPPLER DIAGNOSTIC METHODS

The frequencies of the reflected and incident waves are equal if the reflecting boundary is stationary. Movement of the reflector (or scatterer, or ensemble of scatterers such as blood) towards the source, however, results in a compression of the wavelength of the reflected wave, and vice-versa. Since the speed of ultrasonic propagation in the intervening medium is constant, these changes in wavelength produce corresponding changes in frequency. The phenomenon is called the 'Doppler effect'. Quantitatively, a 2 MHz ultrasonic wave, for example, is shifted in frequency by about 260 Hz on reflection from a surface (or ensemble of scatterers) moving along the axis of the beam at a velocity of 100 mm s^{-1}. For practical purposes, the Doppler shift frequency may be taken to be proportional both to the ultrasonic frequency and to the reflector velocity.

Ultrasonic Doppler methods are nowadays both widely used and of established value in the study of moving structures in clinical diagnosis. In most applications, the Doppler shift in frequency of a continuous-wave ultrasonic beam reflected from a moving structure (or ensemble of scatterers) is used to provide information about the velocity of the structure (or ensemble), either for interpretation by ear, or for analysis by instrument. Two-dimensional Doppler scanning is becoming accepted. Pulsed Doppler systems, which combine the range-measuring capability of the pulse-echo method with the velocity-measuring capability of Doppler, are beginning to demonstrate their potential value in scanning and analysis.

The choice of the best ultrasonic frequency depends on the clinical application. A compromise is necessary to optimize the penetration, the variation of Doppler shift frequency for a given variation in target velocity, the sensitivity to small reflectors, and the size and shape of the ultrasonic field. In cardiology, the optimum frequency is generally 2–3 MHz, but in blood flow studies in superficial vessels it may be as high as 10 MHz.

The same restrictions and limitations (such as the necessity to maintain good ultrasonic coupling, and the inability to operate successfully through gas) which apply to ultrasonic pulse-echo methods, also apply to ultrasonic Doppler methods.

The reflection (backscattered) ultrasonic Doppler method is used in many types of instrument, simple and complex, for measuring the velocities of structures and flow within the heart and blood vessels. Usually the examination is transcutaneous.

Continuous-wave systems

The block diagram of a continuous-wave Doppler system is shown in Figure 7. The transmitter operates continuously, providing an output of

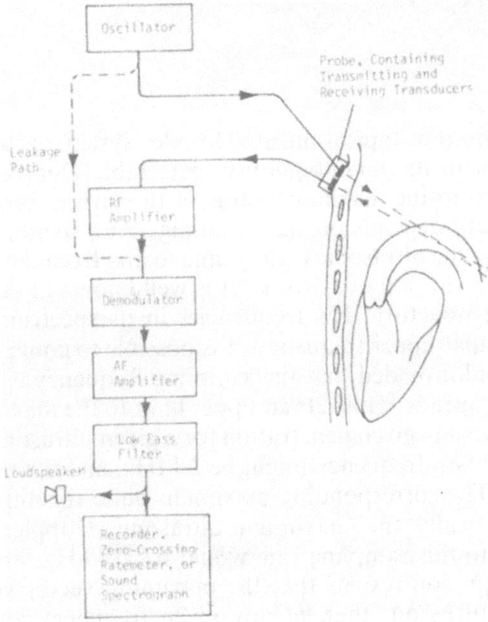

Figure 7 Block diagram of typical continuous-wave ultrasonic Doppler system: a blood flow velocity detector is shown here

constant amplitude and frequency. The ultrasonic probe contains separate transmitting and receiving transducers. (These are generally necessary, because it is important to minimize the direct transfer of energy from the transmitter to the radiofrequency amplifier, in order to avoid overloading the receiver.) The output from the radiofrequency amplifier consists of a mixture of signals, some of frequency equal to that of the transmitter (these are due to reflections from stationary structures in the ultrasonic field, and electrical leakage), and some of frequencies shifted by the Doppler effect (due to reflections from moving structures). These signals are all mixed in the demodulator, the output from which contains the difference frequencies between the transmitted ultrasonic wave and the Doppler-shifted received waves. The output from the demodulator is filtered to allow these difference frequencies to pass, whilst unwanted (higher) frequencies are stopped. The useful difference frequencies, which, as already explained, fall in the audible range, are amplified, and either an operator listens to them, or they are analysed electronically. In clinical applications, the Doppler-shifted signals do not consist of a single frequency, but they extend over a frequency spectrum (since the beam simultaneously interrogates structures moving at different velocities). For this reason, measurements of Doppler shift signals made by ratemeters, such as the zero-crossing frequency meter, need to be interpreted with caution. In most cardiological investigations with Doppler techniques, it is generally very much safer to subject the Doppler signals to frequency spectrum analysis; this may be done by on-line or off-line instruments.

Pulsed systems

A block diagram of a typical pulsed Doppler system is shown in Figure 8. The upper limit to the unambiguously detectable Doppler shift frequency (which is related to the maximum value of the target vector velocity which can be measured) depends on the sampling rate. The maximum sampling rate is limited by the ultrasonic transit time to and from the target of interest, and by the reverberation decay time. It is well known in information theory that if a signal waveform has frequencies in its spectrum extending from zero to a particular upper frequency, it is possible to convey all the information in the signal provided that the sampling frequency is at least twice the upper signal frequency. This sets an upper limit to the maximum measurable velocity vector at any given penetration for a given ultrasonic frequency. For example, the chosen frequency might be 2 MHz, and the necessary penetration, 200 mm. The corresponding maximum pulse repetition rate would be 3750/s. Theoretically the maximum ultrasonic Doppler shift frequency corresponding to this sampling rate would be 1875 Hz; and substitution in the Doppler equation reveals that the maximum vector velocity would be 720 mm/s[1]. It turns out that, at any given frequency and geometry, the product of the maximum vector velocity and the maximum target range is equal to a constant.

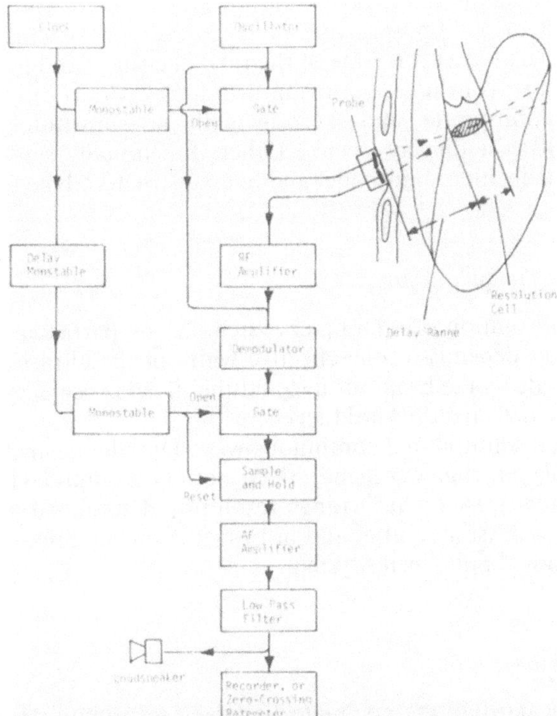

Figure 8 Block diagram of typical pulsed Doppler system. The pulse repetition rate is controlled by the clock, which triggers the monostable to open the gate to allow the transmitting transducer to be excited for a period corresponding to the width of the target volume which it is desired to study. Echoes returning from within the patient are amplified, and mixed in the demodulator with the signal from the oscillator (equal in frequency to that which was transmitted). The delay monostable triggers the monostable controlling the receiver gate, so that the gate opens to allow a voltage, which is in effect a sample corresponding to the Doppler shift due to motion in the target volume, to be stored in the sample-and-hold circuit. The sample-and-hold is reset immediately prior to being updated by a new sample resulting from the following ultrasonic pulse. The output from the sample-and-hold is thus a rectangular wave with a long 'mark' and a short 'space', the envelope of which is an audible signal representing the Doppler shifted information from the target volume

Directionally sensitive Doppler systems

Simple Doppler systems merely measure the magnitude of the frequency difference between the transmitted and received ultrasonic signals, and not the sign of the difference. This sign carries the information about the direction of the movement of the target, either towards or away from the probe. Directional information is vital in some diagnostic situations.

If the signal always consists, at any instant in time, of movement (or flow) in only one direction, a detector capable of switching a logic circuit to indicate whether the movement is in the forward or reverse direction would be satisfactory. (This is the method employed in many commercially manufactured systems.) Almost invariably, however, in practice the Doppler signal consists, at least for some of the time in each periodic cycle, of simultaneous signals from targets moving in opposite directions. Logic circuits are then inappropriate, and there is really no substitute for the sound spectrograph as a display device. Other directionally sensitive detection arrangements include single-sideband and superheterodyne techniques.

Resolution in Doppler systems

The lateral resolution of a Doppler system at any particular distance from the transducer depends on the effective width of the ultrasonic beam. This in turn depends on the beam profile, and the signal processing arrangements including the detector threshold level.

The range resolution of a continuous-wave Doppler is, in effect, such that any detectable target gives a signal; the penetration is limited by attenuation. Pulsed Doppler systems have range resolution determined by the effective length of the ultrasonic pulse, and in principle the situation resembles that in a conventional pulse–echo system.

Doppler imaging

In many clinical situations, adequate diagnostic information can be obtained with a hand-held Doppler probe. It is necessary, however, for the investigator to know the anatomy of the structures being studied in order to interpret the results.

In studies of the vascular system it is often useful to have a two-dimensional map showing the position of blood vessels. The ultrasonic Doppler-shifted signals from flowing blood are sufficiently characteristic to allow their presence to be detected by logic circuitry. This capability is exploited in the two-dimensional scanner shown in Figure 9. The probe is mounted on a two-dimensional coordinate measuring scanner, the resolvers of which provide data enabling computation of the x and y voltages that control the deflection circuits of a direct-view electronic storage tube. The probe is arranged so that the ultrasonic beam is at least slightly inclined to the direction of flow in the vessels to be visualized. This ensures that when the beam passes through moving blood the Doppler detector generates an output signal. This signal is filtered (to remove artifacts due to low-velocity movements such as those of the probe over the skin) and, provided that the output exceeds a preset threshold level, it switches on the electron beam of the display. A two-dimensional map showing those regions in which flow has been detected is constructed on the display by scanning the probe over the area of skin overlying the vessel. Since arteries and veins often lie close together, a directionally sensitive circuit is arranged to inhibit the display when the only flow detected is in the opposite direction to that in the vessel under study.

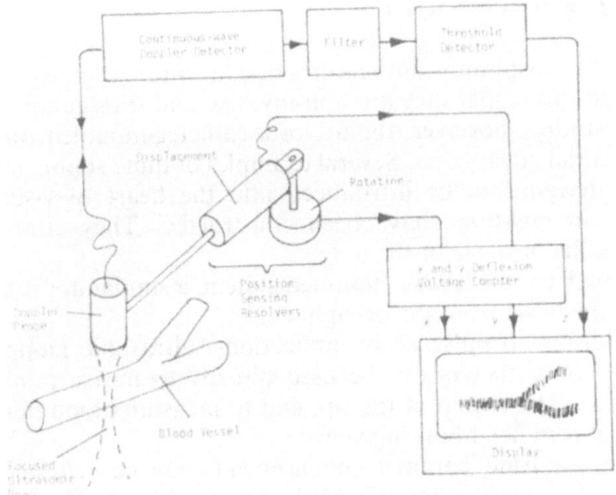

Figure 9 Continuous-wave Doppler system for two-dimensional visualization of blood vessel distribution

A two-dimensional scan of a blood vessel made with a continuous-wave Doppler instrument is a plan view, representing the projection of the blood vessel onto the skin surface along the line-of-sight of the ultrasonic beam. The same type of image can be obtained with a pulsed Doppler scanner range-gated to a constant depth (or even to a variable depth, under the control of the operator) within the blood vessel. Because the pulsed Doppler scanner is capable of measuring range (as well as velocity), and thus of displaying the depth of detected flow, cross-sectional and longitudinal images of the blood vessel lumen can also be produced. Typically a pulsed Doppler scanner has 32 serial gates, each representing flow in a 1 mm increment along the ultrasonic beam, and the system operates at 5 MHz and is directionally sensitive. Furthermore, in appropriate anatomical situations, it is possible to determine the orientation, lumen cross-sectional area, and flow velocity profile, by means of pulsed Doppler scanning, and thus to estimate the rate of blood-flow volume. With contemporary equipment, this estimation cannot be made in real-time, because several separate measurements have to be made. Moreover, the attainable resolution is such that the estimation becomes progressively less accurate as the diameter of the blood vessel becomes smaller.

Combined pulse–echo imaging and Doppler measurement

The combination of pulse-echo two-dimensional imaging of blood vessels (or of structures suspected of being blood vessels, or of the heart) with pulsed Doppler measurement of blood velocity in defined volume elements in the image is becoming established as a powerful technique. It may be expected to be further refined.

INVASIVE TECHNIQUES

One of the most important features of conventional ultrasonic cardiological investigations is that they are non-invasive and transcutaneous. For certain clinical studies, however, the use of a catheter-mounted transducer system has potential advantages. Several examples of quite sophisticated transducer arrays, designed to be introduced into the heart to visualize transverse sections in real-time, have been constructed. They afford a method of avoiding the obstacle of the lung.

Although not a catheter-mounted system, a similar approach may be used to scan the heart from the oesophagus.

In addition to pulse–echo applications, ultrasonic Doppler transducers mounted on catheters can be used directly to measure intraluminal flow velocities in the region of the tip, and to measure blood flow in arteries by scanning from neighbouring veins.

Ultrasonic echo contrast enhancement may be achieved by the introduction of a cloud of microbubbles into the blood. This can be done very easily, for example by injecting normal saline, or even by reinjecting blood, since the drop in pressure at the tip of the needle is sufficient to cause cavitation. Although the microbubbles have quite short lifetimes (in the order of 10 s), they act as strong scatterers. Blood carrying such microbubbles produces relatively high-amplitude echoes, in comparison with the echoes from within solid tissues, which are of medium amplitude, and from blood itself, which is, of course, practically anechoic in a pulse–echo examination.

POSSIBLE HAZARDS OF ULTRASONIC CARDIOLOGY

The fact that ultrasound can modify biological tissues has been known since early in this century, when the pioneers of 'sonar' (underwater 'sound navigation and ranging') noticed that small fish were killed by their transmitters. Much enthusiasm for the ultrasonic therapy as a cure-all was built up in the 1930s, but the unscientific basis of this work and its indifferent results drove the method into disrepute. Since around 1955, however, there has been steady progress in the understanding of the biological effects of ultrasound.

There are two distinct mechanisms by which ultrasound may produce biological effects. The first of these, the thermal mechanism due to heat produced by the absorption of ultrasound, may be discounted as a possible source of hazard in ultrasonic cardiological investigations, since the average ultrasonic power used is generally around only $10\ \mathrm{mW\ cm^{-2}}$. The corresponding heat can easily be dissipated by conduction, convection (including blood flow) and radiation, without any conceivably significant increase in temperature.

The second mechanism involves 'cavitation' which is the term used to describe the behaviour of gas-filled cavities in liquid media supporting ultrasonic waves. 'Transient' cavitation is the phenomenon in which voids suddenly grow from nuclei in the supporting liquid, and then collapse, under the influence of the changing pressure in the ultrasonic field. This whole process of growth and collapse occupies less time than the wave period. During the collapse of a bubble, a strong pressure pulse is set up in the liquid and high temperatures occur within the bubble. It is practically certain that the exposure conditions used in cardiological examinations are too low to cause transient cavitation.

The behaviour of a gas-filled bubble pre-existing in an ultrasonic field of intensity below that necessary to cause transient cavitation is known as 'stable' cavitation. A resonant system exists in which the surrounding liquid behaves as a mass set into vibration, the elasticity being provided by the gas in the bubble. A resonant air-filled bubble in water at atmospheric pressure has a diameter of about 0.7 μm at 1 MHz; it is roughly proportionately larger at lower frequencies, whereas at higher frequencies the effect of surface tension increasingly modifies this proportionately.

The biological effects of stable cavitation at low megahertz frequencies in liquids of low viscosity are quite well understood. Stable cavitation is effective at these frequencies if the specimen is rotated to neutralize unidirectional forces. At least about 1000 cycles of oscillation are necessary for stable cavitation to become effective at 1 MHz, and under these conditions DNA is degraded by intensities of a few watts per square centimetre. In solid tissues, however, it is clear that effects due to stable cavitation have much higher intensity thresholds, if indeed they occur at all.

Not all changes taking place in biological materials as a result of ultrasonic irradiation can be explained simply in terms of thermal or cavitational mechanisms. Some examples of these effects serve to demonstrate this. For instance, blood flow in small blood vessels may be arrested by irradiation with ultrasound of around 0.5 W cm^{-2} at 1 MHz. The phenomenon seems to be due to radiation forces in standing waves. Wound-healing may be accelerated, and this effect seems to be marked with 5 min irradiations, on alternate days, using 3.6 MHz with a pulse intensity of 0.5 W cm^{-2}, pulse duration 2 ms, duty cycle 0.2. Heat can almost certainly be excluded as a contributing factor under these conditions. As another example, there is evidence, although not statistically significant, that 5 h irradiation at 40 mW cm^{-2} with 2.25 MHz ultrasound may be teratogenic in the mouse.

One constructive way of approaching the question of the possibility that ultrasonic exposures used in diagnostic applications may be hazardous is to review the literature on the biological effects of ultrasound. A pair of zones can then be defined on a chart of intensity and time, such that in one zone the conditions have been shown to produce biological effects, and, in the other, they have not. The results of three literature surveys are shown in Figure 10. Once it has been recognized that a particular irradiation does not fall in the 'safe' region, many considerations need to be taken into account in assessing the 'hazard'. For example, it would probably be considered reasonable to assume that irradiation of the adult heart might be safer than irradiation, under the same conditions, of the early fetus.

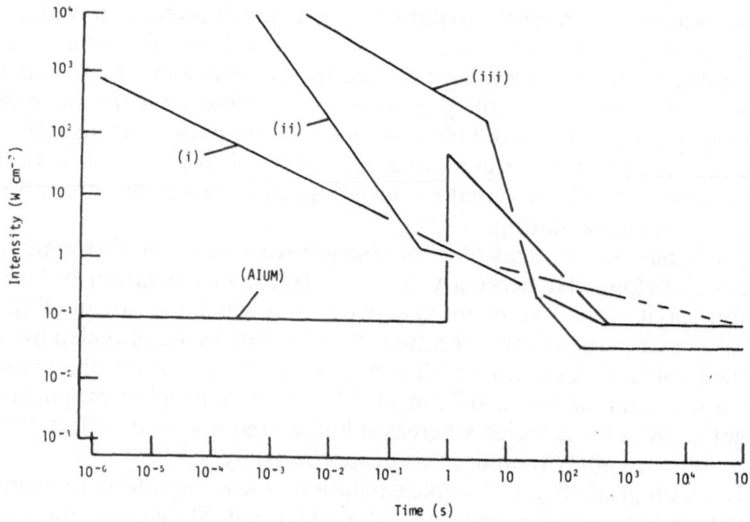

Figure 10 Three pairs of exposure zones, and the AIUM recommendations, showing 'safe' and 'potentially hazardous' conditions, as established from three independent literature surveys. Each line separates one pair of zones, the zone below the line being 'safe'. (i) and (ii): These refer to two separate surveys in which the intensity is the time average (TA) value, equal to the product of the on-intensity and the duty cycle, and the time is the total exposure, including intervals between pulses when appropriate; (iii): This line refers to a third survey in which the intensity is the on-intensity (generally the temporal peak, TP) and the time is the on-time. The AIUM conditions relate to SPTA exposures

In order to give guidance to practising clinicians, the American Institute of Ultrasound in Medicine (AUIM) has issued the following statement:

> In the low megahertz frequency range there have been, as of this date, no independently confirmed significant biological effects in mammalian tissues exposed to intensities (spatial peak, temporal average (SPTA) as measured in a free field of water) below 100 mW cm^{-2}. Furthermore, for ultrasonic exposure times (total time; this includes off-time as well as on-time for a repeated-pulse régime) less than 500 s and more than 1 s, such effects have not been demonstrated at higher intensities when the product of intensity and exposure time (as defined above) is less than 50 J cm^{-2}.

Whilst it would be wrong to be complacent, it is reassuring to observe that exposure conditions in contemporary routine cardiological investigations are well below the levels mentioned in the AIUM statement. The AIUM conditions are illustrated in Figure 11.

ECHOCARDIOGRAPHY'S CONTRIBUTION TO SAFER CARDIAC SURGERY

Ultrasonic measurement techniques could – and, indeed, in many situations, already do – contribute towards safer cardiac surgery in three distinct ways.

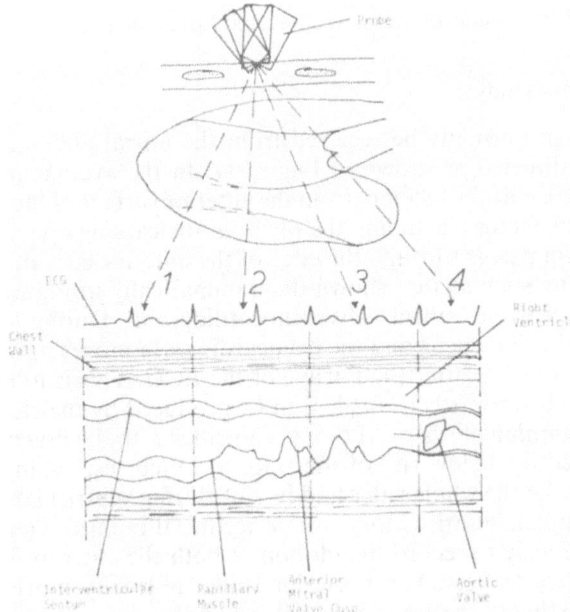

Figure 11 Longitudinal section of the heart shows the structures through which the ultrasonic beam passes as it is aimed in four successive directions through the organ as a time-position scan is made. The time-position scan obtained is shown diagrammatically at the bottom, with the traces from several structures labelled. Position 1 corresponds to the apex of the heart, 4 corresponds to the base of the heart, and 2 and 3 are in between. The time-position scan is shown in relation to a simultaneous recording from an electrocardiograph (ECG)

First, better preoperative definition of the nature and extent of disease could – and does – improve the planning of surgical strategy. Secondly, intraoperative imaging could reduce the incidence of technical failure, particularly in vascular reconstruction. Thirdly, postoperative monitoring of cardiac performance and blood flow could – and, again, already does – allow both the value of surgery to be assessed, and complications to be dealt with more expeditiously. Other chapters in this book deal with particular aspects in depth. In this chapter, an attempt is made superficially to review the whole impact – present and potential – of ultrasonic measurement on cardiac surgery.

The echocardiographer has to take account of anatomical constraints on ultrasonic access to the heart. Except for a small triangular area in the left parasternal region, the anterior of the heart is normally covered by lungs and pleura. The intercostal spaces in this area provide the most commonly used route to the heart in echocardiography. Occasionally, a suprasternal or subxiphoid route is used, and, even more rarely, the examination may be made from the oesophagus, or with a catheter-mounted transducer. These latter routes are not usually justifiable, however, except in patients precluded from the usual approach by emphysema or by previous surgery.

Heart valve studies

Echoes can normally be received from the mitral and aortic valves, if the probe is directed as shown in Figure 11. In the average normal adult, the anterior cusp lies 60–85 mm from the anterior surface of the chest, depending on various factors including the phase in the cardiac cycle. When the ultrasonic beam passes through the edge of the anterior cusp of the mitral valve, a recording such as that shown diagrammatically in Figure 12 is obtained. This is called the 'mitral valve echocardiogram'. During left atrial systole, the mitral valve opens and the echocardiogram moves upwards to point A, which occurs just after the P wave of the ECG. This is followed by a rapid deflection downwards through B to C, produced by the closing of the valve at the beginning of systole. Point C coincides with the first heart sound. This is followed by a slow rise of the trace to D, corresponding to the forward movement of the whole valve and its ring during ventricular systole. In order to be completely satisfactory from a technical point of view, it is necessary simultaneously to record the motion of both the anterior and the posterior mitral valve leaflets. The posterior leaflet normally moves with a similar pattern to that of the anterior leaflet, but in the opposite direction and with a

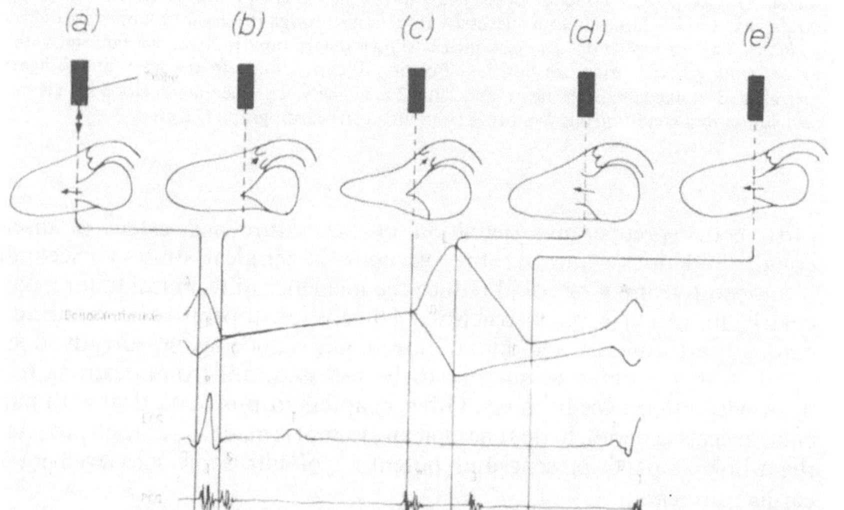

Figure 12 Normal mitral valve echocardiogram, showing the time-relationships to the electrocardiogram and the phonocardiogram. The arrows indicate the directions of blood flow in the diagrams of the left side of the heart. On the echocardiogram, increasing downward deflection of the trace corresponds to increasing depth of the anterior cusp of the valve (i.e. closing of the valve): (a) atrial systole; (b) early ventricular systole; (c) late ventricular systole; (d) ventricular diastole – rapid filling phase; (e) late ventricular diastole

smaller amplitude. The first component of the second heart sound, due to closure of the aortic valve, occurs 10–50 ms before point D. As the ventricle relaxes in diastole, the valve cusps swing wide open and the echocardiogram rises steeply upwards to point E. The ventricle fills rapidly with blood from the left atrium, and the anterior mitral valve cusp is forced backwards while the valve ring also moves in the same direction. During this phase, the echocardiogram transcribes a downward slope, sometimes called the 'diastolic slope', to point F. After point F, the trace may remain level during slow ventricular filling, particularly if the heart rate is slow. Occasionally a low amplitude rise may be seen shortly after point F, but usually the trace moves directly to the next A-wave. In sinus arrhythmia, which in the young is normal during respiratory inspiration, the A-wave disappears.

The mitral valve echocardiogram can be quantitated in terms of the diastolic slope (the slope of the E–F line) and the amplitude of its excursion (the distance C–E).

Mitral valve echocardiograms detected in various abnormalities are illustrated diagrammatically in Figure 13. In summary:

(i) *Mitral regurgitation*
The diastolic slope and amplitude are generally greater than in normals (see Figure 13a).

(ii) *Mitral stenosis*
The diastolic slope and amplitude are generally smaller than in normals (see Figure 13b).

(iii) *Combined mitral stenosis and regurgitation*
The shape of the echocardiogram depends on which lesion is dominant. If stenosis is dominant, the tracing resembles that in pure mitral stenosis. On the other hand, if regurgitation is dominant, the early diastolic slope is greater than that in pure stenosis, and a more gradual slope continues for the next phase of diastole (see Figure 13c).

(iv) *Mitral valve prolapse*
This condition is characterized by an abrupt posterior displacement of the anterior leaflet during systole (see Figure 13d).

(v) *Torn chordae*
In patients with torn anterior chordae, the anterior leaflet of the mitral valve moves erratically in diastole; the fluttering is much coarser than that seen in aortic regurgitation. With torn posterior chordae, the posterior mitral valve leaflet remains posterior throughout systole and returns anteriorly during ventricular diastole. Prolapse of the mitral valve, on the other hand, does not affect the posterior leaflet motion in early systole.

(vi) *Hypertrophic cardiomyopathy*
Whether or not there is obstruction, mitral valve echocardiography reveals that the normal gradual anterior systolic movement (C–D) is replaced by a

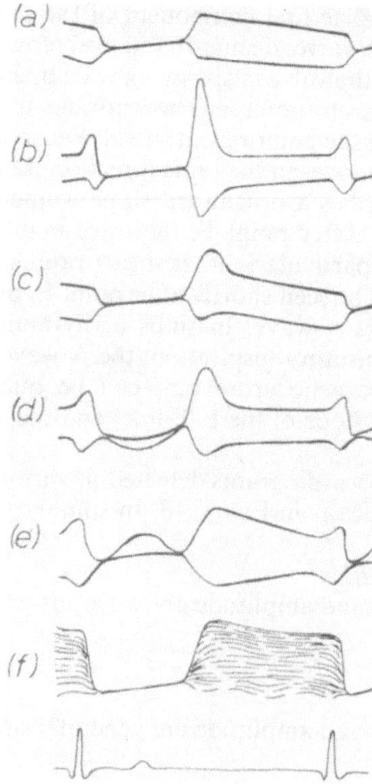

Figure 13 M-mode mitral valve echocardiograms in various abnormalities: (a) mitral regurgitation; (b) mitral stenosis; (c) combined mitral stenosis and regurgitation, with dominant regurgitation; (d) mitral valve prolapse; (e) idiopathic hypertrophic subaortic stenosis; (f) left atrial myxoma. The bottom trace is the electrocardiogram

more pronounced deflection which begins after the onset of ejection from the ventricle and continues to the end of systole. This is because the anterior mitral valve leaflet and the interventricular septum come into contact during systole in patients with hypertrophic obstructive cardiomyopathy (HOCM). Clinically it is often difficult to distinguish these patients from those with coronary artery disease. In addition there may be a reduced diastolic (E–F) slope due to the reduced rate of filling resulting from the low compliance of the ventricle. Even in the presence of fixed left ventricular outflow obstruction, abnormal systolic anterior movement of the anterior mitral valve leaflet may be found on retrospective examination of the echocardiograms of patients who subsequently proved to have HOCM (see Figure 13e).

(vii) *Left atrial myxoma*

This type of tumour may be diagnosed from its echocardiogram which is reminiscent in shape of that which occurs in mitral stenosis, and which is characterized by multiple echoes in the left atrium, particularly in diastole (see Figure 13f).

(viii) *Austin–Flint murmur*

In the presence of aortic regurgitation, an apical diastolic rumbling is often heard. In the presence of this (the Austin–Flint) murmur, it is not possible to determine, using conventional methods of diagnosis, whether or not the mitral valve is diseased. Echocardiography of the mitral valve can quickly resolve this problem.

(ix) *Prosthetic valves*

M-mode studies of mitral valve prostheses can often be clinically useful, although the results are not always definitive. The Starr–Edwards valve gives rise to a pattern which resembles that seen from a natural valve with mitral stenosis. The ball remains in the fully open position throughout diastole, and any movement which may be seen during this phase is that of the cage. There seems always to be some regurgitation at the beginning of systole. Malfunction of the prosthesis may be due to fibrous overgrowth causing the ball to stick, and this can usually be seen on the M-mode tracing. Malfunction of other types of prostheses usually also have characteristic M-mode tracings, but a difficulty in practice is that satisfactory recordings cannot often be obtained because of the orientation of the ultrasonic beam in relation to the valve movement.

In order to record the aortic valve echocardiogram, the position of the probe is first adjusted to receive echoes from the mitral valve, and the ultrasonic beam is then directed medially 10–15° towards the sternum and slightly upwards towards the right shoulder. Echoes are then detected (in around 80 % of normal patients) from the aortic valve ring, the right coronary cusp, and either the left coronary or posterior cusp. The normal aortic valve echocardiogram is seen within the aortic root as slender cusp echoes producing a box-like configuration during systole and a single, nearly central, line in diastole, as shown diagrammatically in Figure 14a. Figure 14b illustrates

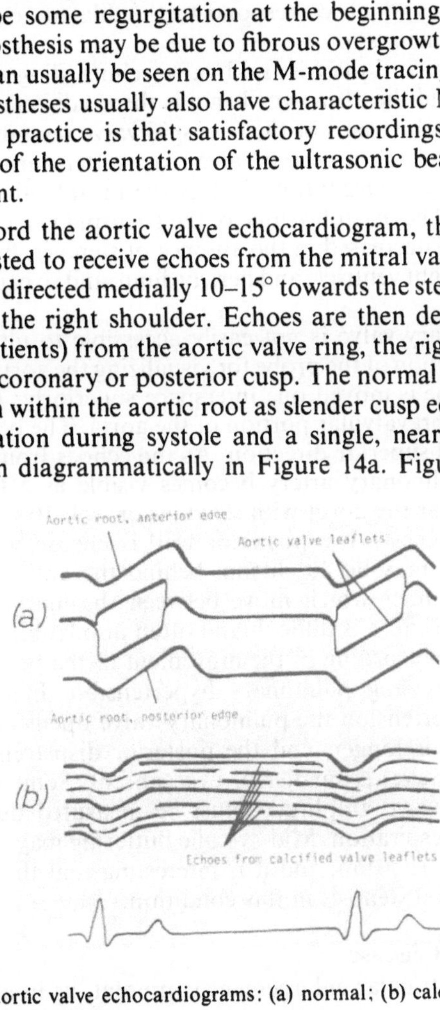

Figure 14 M-mode aortic valve echocardiograms: (a) normal; (b) calcified aortic valve. The bottom trace is the electrocardiogram

the increase in the density of the cusp echoes which correlates quite well with the assessment of valve calcification made at operation. Unfortunately the presence of these echoes makes it impossible to measure the movements of the cusps. Consequently, aortic echocardiography is not very helpful in grading the severity of aortic stenosis. In the rare absence of calcification, the expected reduction in the separation of the aortic valve cusps in stenosis is not seen if the valve is domed so that the orifice is displaced superiorly beyond the ultrasonic beam, as with a biscuspid aortic valve. In aortic regurgitation, however, the valve separation is generally greater than in the normal: if the separation is increased, regurgitation is almost certain to be present. False negative diagnoses are, however, occasionally made.

Dissecting aortic aneurysm may be diagnosed from the appearance on the echocardiogram of normal valve leaflets within two anterior and two posterior echoes which correspond to the dilated aortic root and the false lumen of the aneurysm.

In order to record the tricuspid valve echocardiogram, the aortic valve is first located, and the ultrasonic beam is then redirected medially and downwards. Echocardiograms of the tricuspid valve resemble those of the mitral valve. Moreover, the tricuspid valve may flutter during diastole in patients with pulmonary regurgitation, just as the mitral valve may do with aortic regurgitation. The diastolic slope of the tricuspid valve echocardiogram may be significantly decreased in the absence of stenosis, by restrictive processes involving the right ventricle and pericardium, and so caution in interpretation is necessary.

The pulmonary valve is not easily accessible to ultrasonic examination. Taking the position of the probe for visualizing the aortic valve as the starting point, the probe is moved one interspace superiorly: the beam then passes through the supravalvular portion of the aorta. The beam is then redirected in a lateral and superior direction. As the echoes from the aortic walls disappear, the pulmonary artery becomes visible as a transonic space lying superficially near the aorta with its anterior wall 10–20 mm from the inner surface of the chest. The posterior wall is characterized by a thick echo complex which may lie 20–40 mm behind the anterior echo. Valve cusps appear as thin lines which move between the margins of the pulmonary artery. The procedure is difficult and often impossible.

The M-mode recording of the movement of the pulmonary valve may be of value in assessing pulmonary hypertension. In comparison with the normal, in hypertension the pulmonary valve opens more rapidly, the pre-ejection period is longer, and the posterior displacement following atrial systole (the A-wave) is smaller or even absent. Some caution is necessary, because the A-wave amplitude must be measured during the inspiratory phase of quiet respiration. Mid-systolic fluttering may occur in patients with pulmonary hypertension, and it is interesting that the mitral valve motion may mimic mitral stenosis in this condition.

Congenital heart disease

When right ventricular enlargement is present, as in atrial septal defect or complete transposition of the great vessels, the septum is located more posteriorly than normal, and so is the position of the anterior cusp of the fully open mitral valve. Discontinuity in the echoes from the mitral valve and the aortic root indicates the presence of a double-outlet right ventricle. Congenital mitral valve disease is associated with abnormalities in the movement of the anterior cusp. If the absence of an interventricular septum is demonstrated by echocardiography, differential diagnosis becomes much easier because it excludes many conditions in which two atrioventricular valves and two ventricles are present.

In those patients in whom it is possible to obtain M-mode recordings of the pulmonary valve, both the C–D and E–F slopes are increased in the presence of increased pulmonary blood flow due to left-to-right shunt.

Measurements of left ventricular volume and function

The stroke volume can be estimated if the assumption is made that the ventricular volumes in diastole and systole are given by the cubes of the corresponding transverse 'diameters' measured by echocardiography. Access difficulties make the method inapplicable in a substantial proportion of patients, and its accuracy is further reduced in some cardiac abnormalities.

Echocardiographic diagnosis of hypertrophic cardiomyopathy may generally be made by the observation of abnormal mitral valve motion. These patients, however, represent only one subgroup of a cardiac disease in which the characteristic anatomical abnormality is asymmetric septal hypertrophy (ASH). In most patients with ASH, left ventricular outflow is unobstructed and cardiac dysfunction is presumably due to widespread left ventricular myocardial abnormality; a few patients exhibit HOCM. The interventricular septum is thickened in obstructive ASH. Moreover the thickening of the free wall behind the posterior mitral leaflet appears to regress after surgery for the relief of outflow obstruction.

In favourable circumstances, it is possible echographically to measure the thickness of the posterior left ventricular wall. This has been used to measure stress–strain relationships and to estimate pre-load and after-load.

The velocity of circumferential fibre shortening (VCF) may be measured from ultrasonic recordings of the posterior left ventricular wall during systole. Mean VCF is often depressed in patients with non-localized impaired left ventricular function.

Pericardial effusion

In normal individuals, the space between the two layers of pericardium investing the heart is a potential space only, and on echocardiography it is not possible to differentiate the echoes from the chest wall or the posterior pleura and the walls of the heart. If fluid develops in the pericardial space, however, it may separate the heart walls from the chest wall in front and the pleura behind, and these structures can then be identified on echocardiography as separate echoes, because the space where the intervening pericardial fluid has collected is echo-free.

The role of two-dimensional scanning in cardiology

In principle, two-dimensional scans (whether single-frame or real-time) are built up from the same information that is used to make M-mode recordings. Consequently, they do not contain new information but rather they present the information in a way (represented diagrammatically in Figure 15) which may be more meaningful to an observer. Thus, real-time two-dimensional scanning improves the accuracy of structure identification, because anatomical relationships are demonstrated. Real-time scanning can also improve the reliability in diagnosis of some mitral valve disorders, for example in the measurement of the valve orifice area in patients with rheumatic heart disease, in the sometimes tricky matter of determining the presence of mitral valve prolapse, and in the assessment of vegetations.

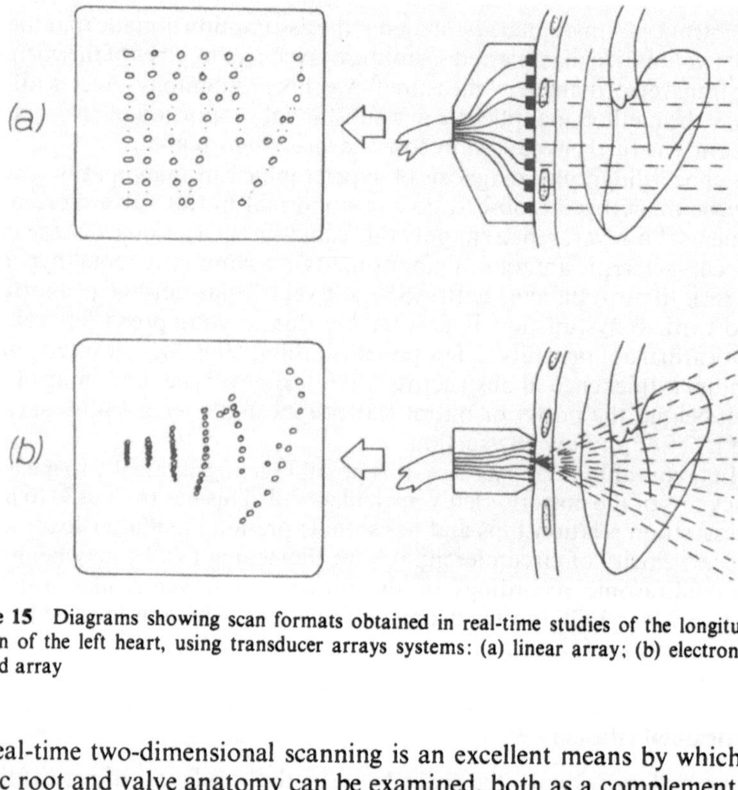

Figure 15 Diagrams showing scan formats obtained in real-time studies of the longitudinal section of the left heart, using transducer arrays systems: (a) linear array; (b) electronically steered array

Real-time two-dimensional scanning is an excellent means by which the aortic root and valve anatomy can be examined, both as a complement and a guide to M-mode recording of structure motion. It is particularly useful for the detection of small solitary calcific deposits, and for the assessment of aortic valve mobility in patients with heavy valvular calcification. Serial study of vegetation is useful, but two-dimensional real-time imaging of prosthetic valves does not seem to provide much additional information. There is substantial scope, however, for the use of the technique in patients with congenital aortic valve disease.

Some of the basic problems of assessing left ventricular function from M-mode recordings, which arise because the technique is limited to one spatial dimension, can be avoided by the use of real-time two-dimensional imaging. Dyskinesia is then generally quite easy to detect, if not to quantify. The anterior and posterior ventricular walls, and the interventricular septum, can all be visualized in suitable patients. The medial lateral walls of the left ventricle, which are difficult to study by M-mode echocardiography, are accessible by two-dimensional scanning. The examination can also be carried out during stress testing.

Real-time two-dimensional scanning is capable of detecting left ventricular clots, and aneurysm formation (which may be a complication in chronic coronary artery disease). Success in surgical removal of an aneurysm depends partly on the amount of remaining myocardium: and in this connection preoperative scanning may be very useful in assessing the part of the ventricle not involved in the aneurysm.

Potentially, a most useful application of real-time two-dimensional scanning is in the serial study of patients with acute myocardial infarction. It offers to be an excellent way of assessing changes in myocardial function, and of detecting complications such as clots, pericardial effusion, aneurysm formation, and disruption of the mitral valve apparatus.

Two-dimensional real-time scanning is generally superior to M-mode studies in the detection of right-sided heart abnormalities. This is because the wide field of view, particularly with sector scanners, results in easy spatial recognition of structures such as the right atrium, coronary sinus, the leaflets of the tricuspid valve, the right ventricle, the pulmonary valve leaflets, and the proximal pulmonary artery and its bifurcation. Abnormalities which are detectable include tricuspid valve disease, Ebstein's anomaly, atrial septal defect, vegetative endocarditis, and tumour.

Two-dimensional real-time studies of the right heart can be improved, in some cases, by contrast techniques. Suitable contrast is provided by rapid injection of 8–10 ml of normal saline into an antecubital vein. The method is helpful in the detection of tricuspid regurgitation, especially when bubbles appear in the inferior vena cava. The appearance of bubbles on the left side of the heart is a sensitive indication of right-to-left shunt.

A most important application of real-time two-dimensional scanning is in the evaluation of congenital heart disease in the paediatric patient. The examination should follow a rational procedure. The atrial situs should first be established, and then the ventricles should be located and identified. Next, the great arteries should be identified. The heart can then be examined in detail: the ventriculo-arterial connections should be visualized, and the possible presence of obstructive lesions and shunts should be considered. Many of these diagnoses are made easier by positive or negative contrast studies.

The role of Doppler techniques in cardiology

In the study of the heart, three main approaches with Doppler techniques have shown promise. Firstly, measurements of flow in the thoracic aorta reflect left heart function. These data can be obtained with a continuous-wave Doppler system operating at a frequency of around 2 MHz, by positioning the probe in the suprasternal notch. The orientation of the aortic arch is such that the ultrasonic beam can, when directed from the suprasternal notch, intersect the direction of blood flow tangentially. Other angles of attack occur, due to the curvature of the vessel, but the highest Doppler shift frequency corresponds to the highest velocity along the beam. The use of a real-time sound spectrograph to display directionally detected Doppler shift signals allows the operator to obtain optimal orientation, and to recognize flow signals from branch arteries which, since they serve the head and neck, are in the opposite direction to the flow in the aortic arch. The spectral display allows turbulence to be identified, and can be interpreted even if the signal-to-noise ratio is poor.

The clinical usefulness of transcutaneous aortovelography is still being assessed. The part of the aorta in which the flow velocity is monitored is close to the heart, so that information on left heart action is obtained. In any particular individual, instantaneous cardiac output is likely to be proportional to the measured velocity, provided that the systolic cross-sectional area of the aorta, the velocity flow profile, and the fraction of flow in the branches of the aortic arch, all remain constant. Preliminary observations bear out the validity of these assumptions, and therefore the method may be useful in critical-care situations. The waveform of the envelope of the frequency spectrum also seems to reflect the cardiac performance in other respects. Thus, it is possible to estimate indices of early systolic acceleration, peak velocity, and durations of acceleration and deceleration phases of the systolic period. Because of the difficulty of absolute measurement, in clinical practice it is likely that changes in these indices will prove to be more useful than their actual values. In addition, the frequency spectrum may reflect functional abnormalities in the heart and aorta, such as aortic regurgitation, coarctation of the aorta, and so on.

The second promising application of the Doppler effect in cardiology arises because the waveform of blood flow detected with a continuous-wave Doppler probe placed transcutaneously over the jugular vein depends on right heart function. The waveform is, for example, modified in tricuspid valve disease.

Thirdly, potentially valuable information can be obtained by measuring blood flow within the heart. Thus, the continuous-wave Doppler method can be used to measure the instantaneous maximum blood-flow velocity within the cardiac chambers, and especially in the region of the valves. Using present techniques, this is not easy to do because of the problems of structure identification in the absence of real-time two-dimensional imaging for guidance. Continuous-wave Doppler instruments do not suffer from the range-velocity limitation of pulsed systems, however, and the technique is a sensitive way of detecting regurgitation and turbulence. Generally, however, this disadvantage of pulsed Doppler is not a serious problem at least for qualitative diagnosis, and the great advantage of range selection deserves to be emphasized. The combination of pulsed Doppler flow measurement with real-time two-dimensional visualization is emerging as an extremely powerful diagnostic tool. The small size of the resolution cell allows turbulent volumes to be detected: in this way, murmurs can be identified which relate to the diastolic rumbles of mitral and tricuspid stenoses, mitral regurgitation, left ventricular outflow obstruction, aortic stenosis, aortic regurgitation, augmented right ventricular filling sound in atrial septal defects, pulmonary stenosis, pulmonary regurgitation, and high-velocity flow through the obstruction in coarctation of the aorta. The analyses generally depend on inspection of the frequency spectrum. In many respects, transcutaneous pulsed-Doppler studies could replace intracardiac phonocardiography.

Another area where Doppler ultrasound can provide data of value to the cardiac surgeon is in the study of blood flow in the periphery. For example, Doppler ultrasound is a sensitive method of detecting the presence or absence of the pulse in blood-pressure measurement. Again, in generalized arterial disease, the characteristics of the arteries in the leg may reflect the progress of atherosclerosis throughout the arterial system. Arterial disease may modify the shape of the blood-flow pressure pulse at the ankle. This may be determined non-invasively by using the ECG R-wave as a timing reference, and measuring the delays in the arrivals of different parts of the pressure wave beyond a cuff with decreasing pressures, at a Doppler probe positioned over the posterior tibial artery. Another approach to arterial characterization depends on measurements of the transit times of the arterial pulse past consecutive segments of artery, and from measurements of the pulsatility of the arterial pulse waveforms at the input and output sites of the arterial segments. Measurement of the pulsatility depends on obtaining the waveform of the maximum Doppler shift frequency, and this is usually done manually by tracing from the frequency spectrum, although reliable maximum frequency followers have been developed. This approach allows the collateral circulation to be graded into one of four classes, according to its status. Another promising method involves the concept of characterizing the arterial segment between the heart and measurement site (at the common femoral artery, for example) in terms of the Laplace transform of the blood flow velocity/time signal. Thus it is possible to obtain numerical indices of arterial stiffness, proximal lumen size, and distal peripheral impedance.

Two dimensional Doppler imaging of blood vessels gives further important data on localized peripheral arterial disease, and is a valuable guide for selecting sites for the monitoring of flow waveforms. The relatively inexpensive continuous-wave instruments are only capable of imaging the projection of the blood vessels; but pulsed Doppler systems can also make cross-sections and longitudinal sections, thus increasing the reliability of lesion detection.

Studies of venous flow are limited by the general absence, except in vessels close to the heart, of natural pulsation. Deep-vein thrombosis can sometimes be detected by changed flow characteristics in the superficial femoral vein, in response to squeezing the calf or foot. Doppler imaging has a valuable place in assessing the local site of deep-vein thrombosis.

These techniques of measuring and visualizing blood flow have an important role in monitoring patients in the postoperative period, in addition to their presently better accepted place in diagnosis and preoperative assessment.

Invasive techniques

Although invasive techniques are generally less attractive than non-invasive studies, they do have a place in clinical care. For example, atrial septal defects have been demonstrated in radial ultrasonic two-dimensional scans produced by rotating small transducers mounted at the tips of catheters introduced through the external jugular or the femoral veins into the right atrium. The method is neither convenient nor safe, and so it has not come into general clinical use. The potential value of scanning from the oesophagus has still to be determined, but it seems unlikely that this approach will have widespread application.

Doppler techniques also have a limited role in invasive studies. Thus, left ventricular blood ejection velocity has been measured by means of a Doppler transducer mounted at the tip of a catheter introduced via a brachial artery and aorta into the left ventricle. Characteristic and reproducible flow velocity waveforms have been obtained from various sites. Inflow tract blood velocity is characterized by a predominant diastolic wave related to left ventricular filling, succeeded by a smaller systolic component. Mid-cavity blood flow velocity is triphasic in nature. Outflow tract blood velocity is associated with a major systolic wave, resulting from left ventricular ejection.

Ultrasonic visualization and flow measurement methods have potentially invaluable, but as yet virtually untested, applications for the cardiac surgeon during operative procedures. For example, a small sterilizable, real-time scanner head and associated display could be used by the surgeon as a guide during the surgical approach, and as a method of assessing operative success or failure during the closing stages of intervention. Doppler methods of blood-flow detectors might be equally valuable in vascular reconstructive surgery.

Bibliography

Feigenbaum, H. (1972). *Echocardiography*. (Philadelphia: Lea & Febiger)

Lancée. C. E. (ed.) (1979). *Echocardiology*. (The Hague: Nijhoff)

Reneman, R. S. (ed.) (1974). *Cardiovascular Applications of Ultrasound*. (Amsterdam: North Holland)

Roelandt, J. (1977). *Practical Echocardiography*. (Forest Grove: Research Studies Press)

Ross, F. G. M. (1977). Ultrasonic investigation of the heart. In Wells, P. N. T. (ed.). *Ultrasonics in Clinical Diagnosis*, 2nd Edn., pp. 114–41. (Edinburgh: Churchill Livingstone)

Wells, P. N. T. (1977). *Biomedical Ultrasonics*. (London: Academic Press)

11
The importance of echocardiography in preoperative diagnosis

L. COTTER AND D. GIBSON

Although the diagnosis of valcular heart disease is nearly always apparent on clinical grounds, it is generally agreed that before surgery is undertaken confirmation by some independent method is desirable. Until recently this required cardiac catheterization. However, using M-mode echocardiography – a technique available in most district hospitals – it is possible to assess the anatomy and movement of all four valves. It is also possible to gain a comprehensive picture of left ventricular function, not only detecting how it has been altered by valve stenosis or regurgitation, but also allowing an assessment to be made of independent left ventricular disease. These echocardiographic methods of assessing left ventricular function are dealt with in Chapter 7, but their relevance in preoperative diagnosis can scarcely be overemphasized.

RHEUMATIC MITRAL VALVE DISEASE

The well-known echocardiographic features of rheumatic mitral valve disease are due to the pathological changes in the valve caused by rheumatic involvement, and the nature and severity of the haemodynamic disturbance. These lead to fibrosis and eventually calcification of the valve cusps, with consequent thickening of the cusp echoes and diminution of the diastolic closure rate. Fusion of the smaller posterior cusp to the dominant anterior cusp results in anterior movement of the posterior cusp in diastole in about 90 % of cases, and fibrosis of the subvalvar apparatus may cause diminution in the amplitude of cusp movement. These anatomical abnormalities lead to disturbances in the pattern of left ventricular filling.

The mobility and calcification of the mitral valve have been assessed echocardiographically by Nanda and his colleagues[1], allowing the feasibility of performing a conservative procedure on the mitral valve to be predicted. In 57 preoperative patients the mitral valve amplitude was measured from the closed position at the onset of systole to the fully open position in diastole. The mobility of valves with amplitudes of less than 20 mm was considered to be impaired, and severely impaired if less than 16 mm. Light calcification was considered to be present when tiered multiple linear echoes were present in diastole, and this calcification was considered heavy when thick conglomerate echoes were present (Figure 1). If thin single or duplicate valve echoes were obtained calcification was deemed absent (Figure 2). Using these criteria 18 of 19 patients with no echocardiographic evidence of calcium were correctly assessed and 23 of 28 patients considered to have a mobile valve were also correctly judged suitable for valvotomy.

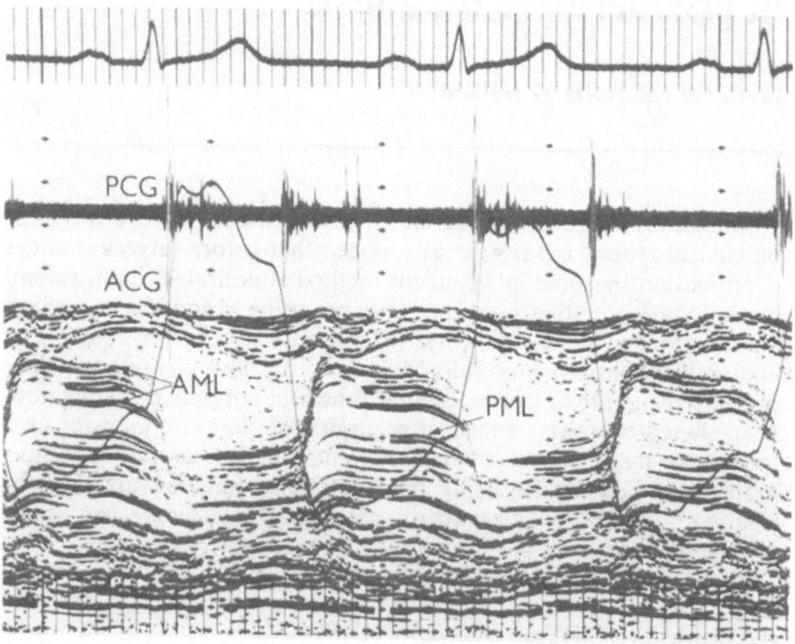

Figure 1 Echocardiogram of patient with calcific rheumatic mitral valve disease showing evidence of severely thickened and deformed anterior and posterior leaflets. (PCG = phonocardiogram, ACG = apex cardiogram, AML = anterior mitral leaflet, PML = posterior mitral leaflet). (Courtesy of the editor of the *British Heart Journal*)

Similar information may be obtained using the cross-sectional echocardiogram. The restriction of movement of the anterior cusp in rheumatic mitral stenosis causes an angular shape or 'knee' with the aortic root and thickened echoes fróm the fibrous or thickened cusps are seen (Figure 3). The cross-sectional technique is the best method for demonstrating disease of the subvalvar apparatus, and in rheumatic involvement fibrosis and thickening, sometimes with calcification, is easily appreciated. A number of studies have shown correlations between mitral valve area estimated by cross-sectional echograms and that estimated at cardiac catheterization. However, the velocity of ultrasound through fibrotic cusps is less than that through

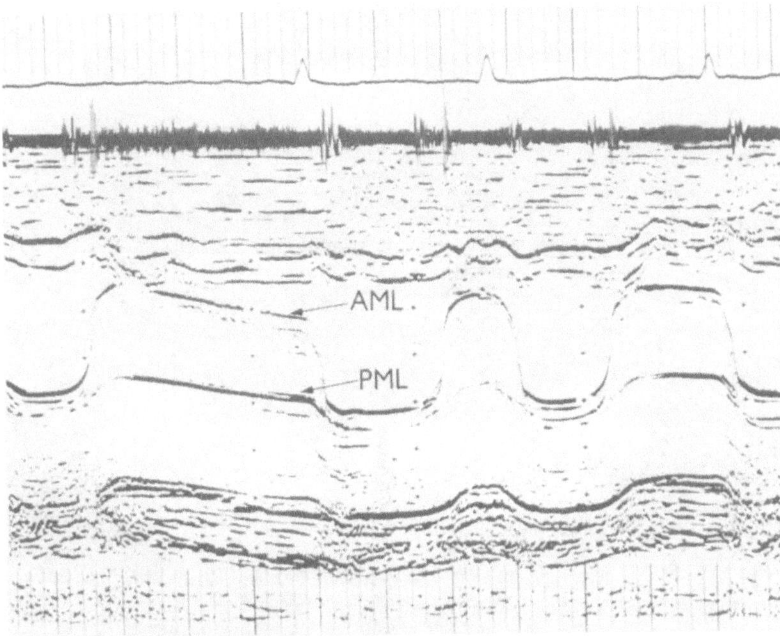

Figure 2 Echocardiogram of patient with rheumatic mitral stenosis without calcification and echocardiographically suitable for a valvotomy. (AML = anterior mitral leaflet, PML = posterior mitral leaflet). (Courtesy of the editor of the *British Heart Journal*)

blood. This increases the time taken for the reflected beam to return to the transducer, and as the instrument interprets this increase in time as an indication that the sound beam has travelled further, such changes in velocity in denser tissue may give an echogram much thicker than the actual structure represented. This problem is further compounded because in a calcified valve sound-waves may be reflected by a posterior part of the cusp causing internal reverberations, again interpreted as increased distance. When this is an increased distance between the anterior and posterior surfaces of a cusp, the echogram is much thicker than the cusp it represents and so the apparent valve area is too small. For these reasons only the position of the anterior surface of the valve is precisely located. Estimates of valve area made echocardiographically should thus be viewed as no more than semiquantitative.

Although the presence of rheumatic involvement and the degree of mobility and of calcification can be assessed fairly accurately echocardiographically, examination of the valve echocardiogram has proved an unsatisfactory means of detecting the functional effects of the valve disease. Indeed even differentiation between rhematic mitral stenosis and regurgitation cannot be made from the valve record. The EF slope, which is usually less than 35 mm/s in rheumatic mitral regurgitation and is also affected by left ventricular disorders with no obstruction of the mitral valve, is clearly of no use as a means of assessing functional severity[2].

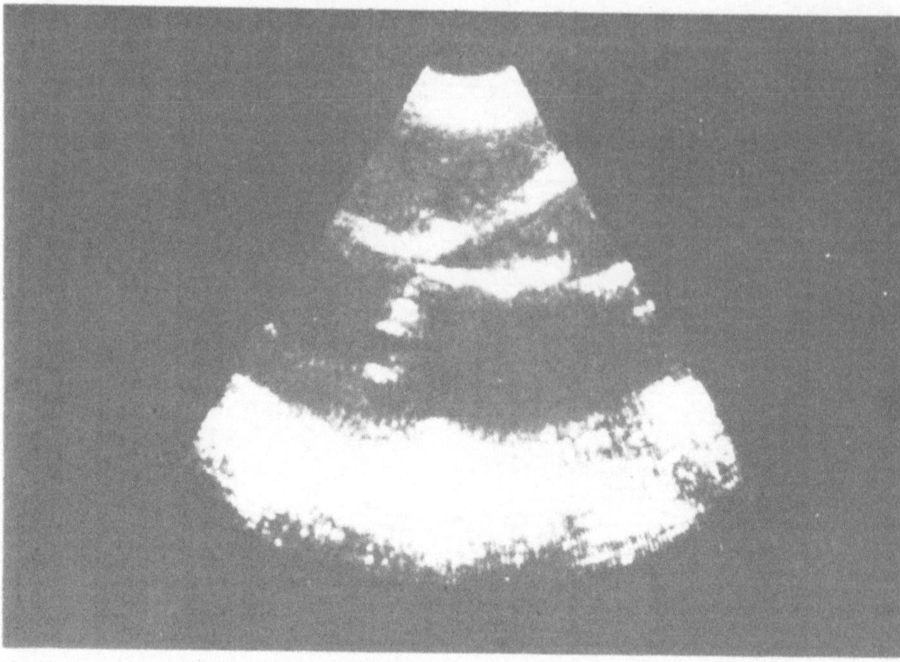

Figure 3 Cross sectional echocardiogram of patient with rheumatic mitral stenosis with thickened immobile cusps. (Courtesy of the editor of the *British Heart Journal*)

Identification and quantification of the functional disturbance caused by mitral valve disease depends on assessing the pattern of left ventricular filling. This can be performed by using a simple digitizing technique to derive instantaneous measurements of left ventricular dimension and its rate of change from a standard echocardiogram of the left ventricular cavity[3]. In normal subjects the initial accelerating phase of left ventricular filling lasts 0.11 ± 0.033 s (mean ± 1 SD). During this time the rate of change of left ventricular dimension rises progressively to reach a peak value of 11 ± 3.9 cm/s. This initial rapid filling phase is followed by progressive reduction in the rate of outward wall movement which declines to 20% of its peak value 0.21 ± 0.026 s after the onset of ventricular filling (Figure 4). In contrast in patients with pure mitral regurgitation the end diastolic dimension is large and its peak rate of increase (22.4 ± 5.9 cm/s) is approximately double the normal value. The normal pattern of left ventricular filling with respect to the duration of acceleration is, however, unchanged. In patients with mitral stenosis the pattern of left ventricular filling is markedly altered (Figure 5). The peak rate of increase in left ventricular dimension is greatly reduced (6.9 ± 2.5 cm/s) and this low rate is maintained throughout diastole with no rapid filling phase being identifiable. It is clear then that the haemodynamic disturbance is closely reflected in the pattern of dimension increase on the echocardiogram. Furthermore a reduction in peak rate of dimension increase always requires explanation. In the absence of rheumatic mitral valve disease it may be due to severe left ventricular hypertrophy as described in detail below, or less commonly to congenital mitral stenosis, supravalvar mitral diaphragm or cor triatriatrum.

However obvious the clinical picture may be, the diagnosis of rheumatic mitral valve disease should always be confirmed by echocardiography. Prospectively the clinical features of atrial myxomas are usually indistinguishable from those of mitral valve disease, and misdiagnosis even before cardiac catheterization can be disastrous – particularly if a trans-septal puncture is performed. Furthermore the two conditions can give precisely the same haemodynamic picture[4], while severe mitral stenosis can exist with no discernible gradient[5].

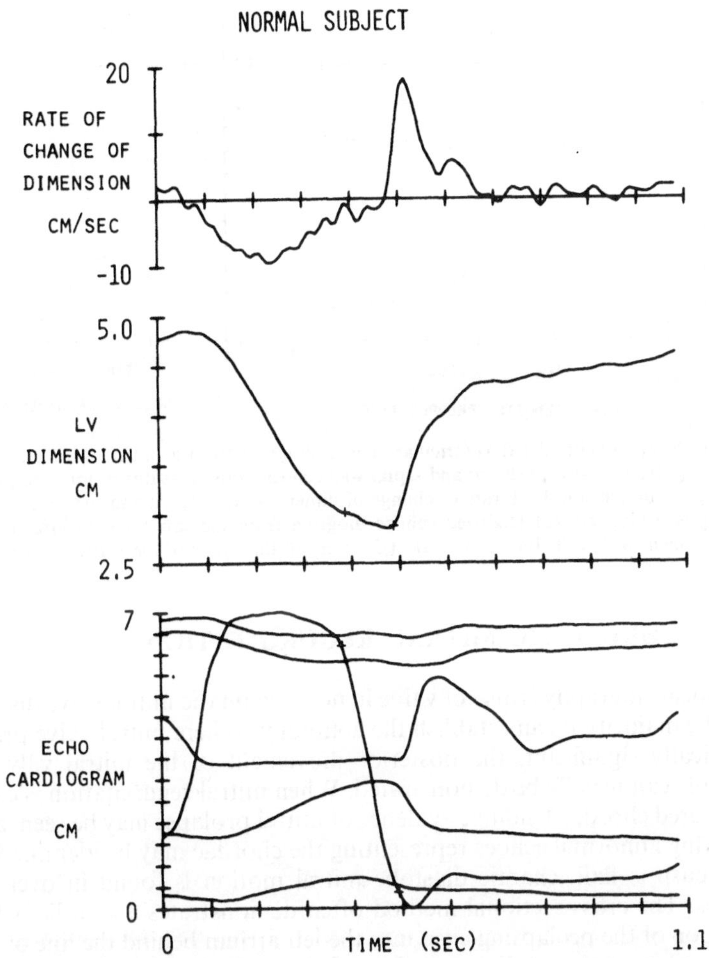

Figure 4 Digitized left ventricular echocardiogram from a normal subject, showing (from below) digitized data with superimposed apex cardiogram, left ventricular dimension, and (top) rate of change of dimension. The crosses represent the timing of aortic valve closure and mitral valve opening. (Courtesy of the editor of the *British Heart Journal*)

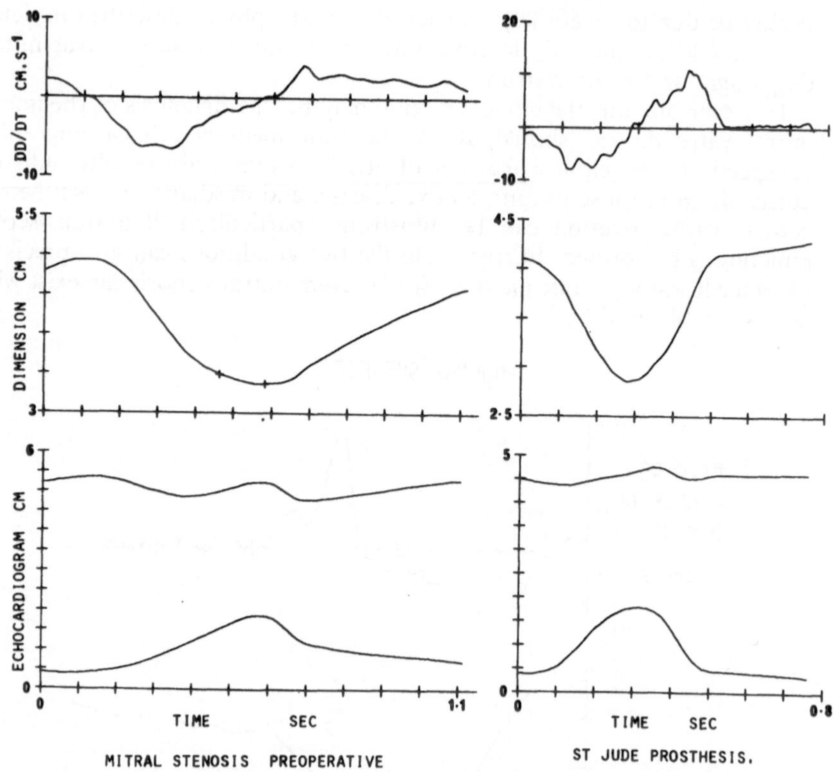

Figure 5 (a) Digitized left ventricular echocardiogram from a patient with mitral stenosis, showing (from below) posterior and septal wall echoes, transverse dimension, and (top) rate of change of dimension. Peak rate of change of dimension is reduced and the time to 20% peak filling is prolonged. (b) Digitized echocardiogram from the same patient after mitral valve replacement with a St. Jude prosthesis. (Courtesy of the editor of the *British Heart Journal*)

NON-RHEUMATIC MITRAL REGURGITATION

Echocardiography is also of value in non-rheumatic mitral valve disease, and in the majority it can establish the aetiology. Where mitral valve prolapse is clinically significant, the posterior movement of the mitral valve during systole can usually be demonstrated. When mitral regurgitation is caused by ruptured chordae tendinae evidence of mitral prolapse may be seen, and fast-moving abnormal echoes representing the chordae may be identified. Where the cusp is flail, chaotic diastolic mitral motion is found in over 90% of cases. The cross-sectional method often demonstrates a systolic 'whipping' motion of the prolapsing cusp into the left atrium behind the line of the A-V ring, abnormal systolic co-aption of the cusps and sometimes abnormal intra-atrial echoes[6].

Severe non-rheumatic mitral regurgitation, whether due to ruptured chordae, ruptured papillary muscles or severe mitral valve prolapse, causes left ventricular volume overload leading to exaggerated septal and posterior left ventricular wall movement with higher rates of dimension increase during diastole than those seen in rhematic mitral regurgitation.

Patients presenting with congestive cardiomyopathy with 'secondary' mitral regurgitation have generally been considered unsuitable candidates for mitral valve surgery. Seven such patients investigated haemodynamically and echocardiographically had low ejection fractions (less than 30%) and low peak velocities of 'circumferential fibre shortening' but had coordinate contraction patterns when assessed by M-mode echocardiography combined with apex cardiography (Figure 6). In view of this surprisingly coordinate pattern of contraction[7], surgical correction of the mitral regurgitation was recommended. Six of the seven patients benefited greatly[8]. Such patients often respond poorly to medical treatment and the possibility of surgical correction should be borne in mind when they are being assessed.

AORTIC STENOSIS

In valvar aortic stenosis, echocardiography is rarely as central to the correct diagnosis as it is in mitral valve disease. Nevertheless, in the majority of patients it has an important contribution to make. In older patients the aortic valve is calcified and appears on the M-mode echocardiogram as multiple linear echoes which may be conglomerate. The cross-sectional echogram also shows multiple dense echoes from a calcified valve but the same reservations as outlined above about estimation of valve area apply as in mitral disease, with even greater force. A normal aortic echogram in a middle-aged or elderly patient suspected of having aortic stenosis is incompatible with the diagnosis of a significant valvar aortic lesion. This is not so in young adults and children, in whom the ultrasonic beam may pass across the base of doming cusps giving a normal M-mode aortic echocardiogram even in the presence of severe valvar stenosis. In such patients it is usually possible to demonstrate the doming of the cusps with the cross-sectional technique, and to gain some idea of the size of the stenotic orifice.

Significant aortic stenosis causes left ventricular hypertrophy with little increase in left ventricular cavity size until left ventricular function deteriorates. This has allowed Bennett and his colleagues[9] to devise a formula for the calculation of the peak sytolic gradient across the aortic valve dependent upon the ratio between systolic wall thickness and systolic minor axis cavity dimension, assuming the persistence of normal peak wall stress. The significant correlation they obtained in patients with no cavity dilatation has been confirmed by others, but no surgical series relying on such calculations without cardiac catheterization has yet been reported.

Hypertrophic (obstructuve) cardiomyopathy (HCM) may be mis-diagnosed as valvar aortic stenosis and should be excluded by M-mode or 2D echocardiography. The characteristic feature of HCM is an asymmetrically hypertrophied akinetic septum, often with systolic anterior movement if the mitral valve apparatus. Severe left ventricular hypertrophy due to valvar stenosis or any other cause can mimic HCM[10] although concentric hypertrophy is less likely to be mistaken for HCM.

The aortic echocardiogram in subvalvar aortic stenosis – whether due to HCM, a discrete diaphragm, or a subaortic tunnel – may show early systolic closure of the aortic valve[11]. The extent and timing of this early systolic

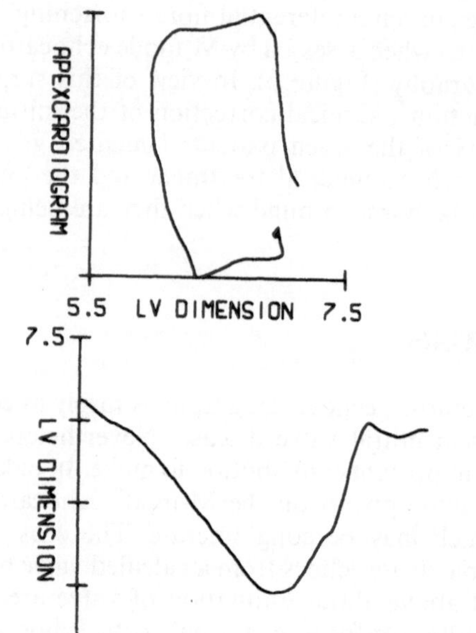

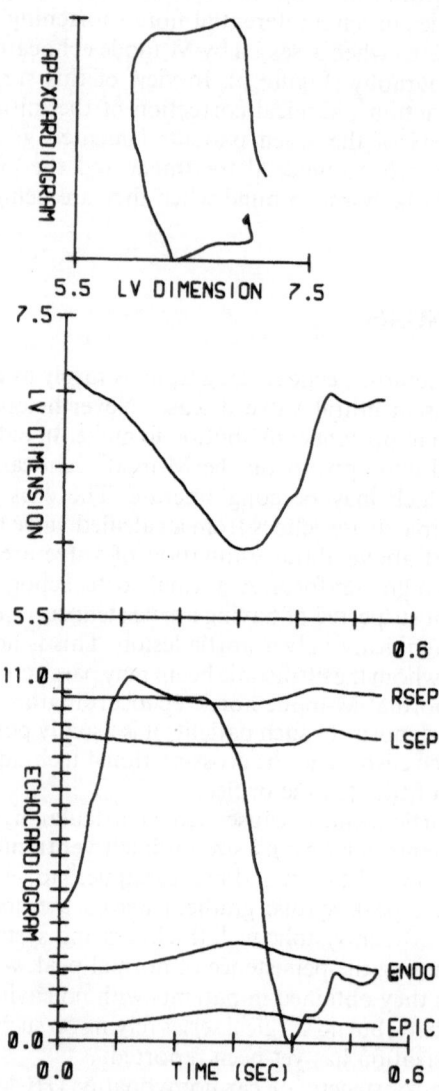

Figure 6 Computer output of digitized echo and apex cardiogram from a patient with congestive cardiomyopathy and 'secondary' mitral regurgitation showing from below echoes from posterior wall and septum and apex cardiogram, transverse dimension and the echo dimension–apex cardiogram loop which is approximately rectangular, indicating coordinate contraction (see also chapter 6). (Courtesy of the editor of the *British Heart Journal*)

closure has been suggested as an indication of the exact location and even severity of the subvalvar lesion. Unfortunately early aortic closure is a non-specific finding occurring in many different conditions[12], although if it does occur in the presence of left ventricular outflow tract obstruction, the possibility of a subvalvar lesion may be raised. In some cases of discrete subvalvar stenosis abnormal echoes have been identified in the left ventricular outflow tract using the M-mode, but the sensitivity and specificity of this finding requires further evaluation.

Since many cases of aortic stenosis have a rheumatic aetiology, concomitant mitral valve disease may be present even in the absence of diagnostic physical signs, so that all patients undergoing aortic valve surgery require mitral echocardiograms, particularly if cardiac catheterization is not to be performed. In this context it is essential to realize that disorders of diastolic function are found in left ventricular hypertrophy whether secondary or due to HCM. These abnormalities include significantly reduced peak rates of dimension increase, prolongation of the early diastolic period, and a reduced diastolic closure rate of the mitral valve[13]. This pattern can be distinguished from that due to rheumatic mitral valve disease most readily by the posterior movement of the posterior cusp during diastole, normal thickness of the cusp echo and normal or increased isovolumic relaxation time compared with short values seen in mitral valve disease, along with the presence of left ventricular hypertrophy.

These alterations may reflect the abnormal filling pattern occurring in both conditions, and can cause confusion if the evidence for rheumatic mitral valve disease is not examined critically.

AORTIC REGURGITATION

Direct ultrasonic examination of the aortic valve itself is not usually helpful in aortic regurgitation, except as described below in patients with suspected infective endocarditis. Apparent cusp separation in diastole is not a sign of aortic regurgitation, being often found in normal subjects. An eccentric line of coaption during diastole may suggest a bicuspid valve but gives no clue to the severity or even presence of aortic regurgitation. If the aortic valve is disorganized and calcified then multiple linear echoes are found, but in the younger patient with pure aortic regurgitation the aortic valve echocardiogram may be entirely normal. Early opening of the aortic valve is an unusual sign sometimes found in severe aortic regurgitation (Figure 7) signifying considerable elevation of the left ventricular end-diastolic pressure[14].

In aortic regurgitation the volume load on the left ventricle produces left ventricular dilatation, except in the early stage of an acute lesion. This may be extreme, with a minor axis cavity dimension as high as 9 cm. A vigorously moving free left ventricular wall and septum are found unless left ventricular disease is present. In the majority of patients the aortic regurgitant jet causes a high-frequency 'buzz' on the anterior mitral valve, and sometimes the interventricular septum. This may be associated with the rumbling mid-diastolic Austin Flint murmur, due to the partial closure of the mitral valve, which

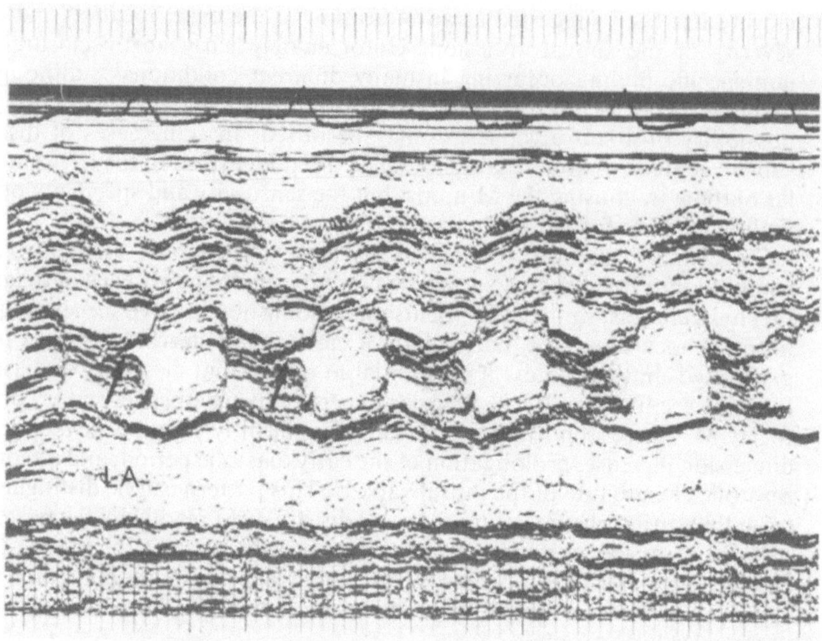

Figure 7 Echocardiogram of the aortic valve and root in a patient with severe aortic regurgitation due to infective endocariditis showing early opening of the aortic valve (arrowed). Thickened cusps with vegetations are also present and the anterior aortic root dimension is increased. (LA = left atrium). (Courtesy of the editor of the *British Heart Journal*)

requires the echocardiogram to distinguish it from concomitant mitral stenosis – this being a common practical differential diagnosis.

The correct timing of surgery in chronic aortic regurgitation is sometimes difficult. Attention is usually paid to clinical, electrocardiographic, and radiographic features. This can be usefully augmented by serial echocardiograms to identify increases in left ventricular cavity size which may influence the time at which surgery is performed.

In acute aortic regurgitation the left ventricular diastolic pressure may rise above the left atrial pressure well before ventricular systole, so that the echocardiogram may show premature closure of the mitral valve (Figure 8). This sign is an indication that the regurgitation is severe and that aortic valve surgery is essential as soon as is practicable.

MISCELLANEOUS CONDITIONS WHERE PREOPERATIVE ECHOCARDIOGRAPHY IS HELPFUL

Prosthetic valve dysfunction is increasingly common, the usual differential diagnosis resting between paraprosthetic valvar leak, prosthetic obstruction and poor left ventricular function. In the correct clinical context an echo-

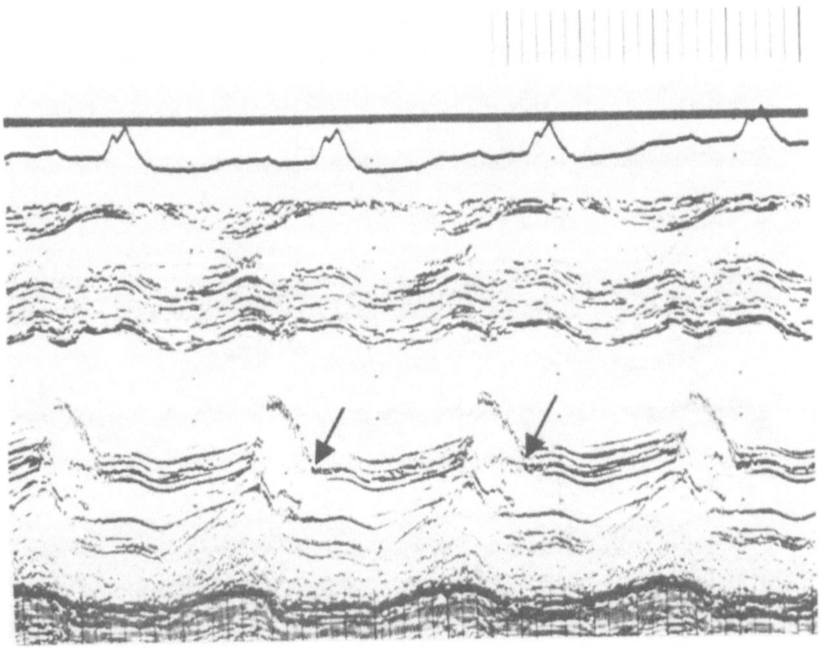

Figure 8 Echocardiogram of patient with acute severe aortic regurgitation showing closure of the mitral valve (arrowed) before the onset of ventricular systole. High frequency vibrations are present on the anterior cusp due to the aortic jet. (Courtesy of the editor of the *British Heart Journal*)

cardiogram which shows a vigorously moving septum and posterior left ventricular wall, usually with normal direction of septal movement, rules out the possibility of an obstructed prosthesis or poor left ventricular function as the cause of the patients' problems. This removes the need for cardiac catheterization in a high proportion of these severely ill patients.

The presence or absence of vegetations in infective endocarditis is rarely of paramount surgical importance, though they may in fact be identified by M-mode in at least a half of cases and nearly all by cross-sectional methods[15]. Also of practical significance is the identification of distorted aortic root anatomy by the demonstration of an abscess cavity (Figure 9) or even the line of dehiscence of an infected prosthetic valve (Figure 10).

CONCLUSION

Safe cardiac surgery requires preoperative diagnosis to be complete and exact. Echocardiography is an essential aid to a full diagnosis in virtually all cases of valvar heart disease in adults, and for some anatomical and functional details is the investigation of choice. In selected cases, when it is com-

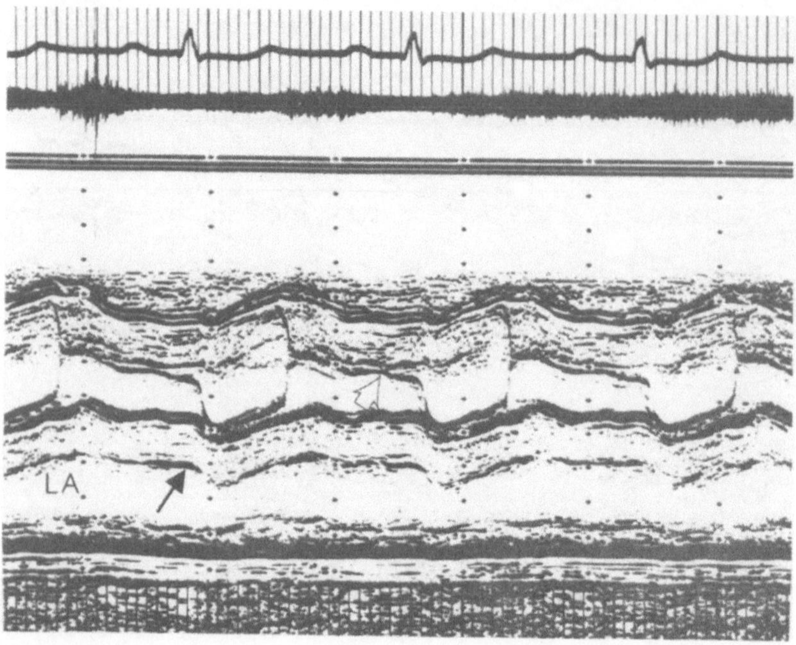

Figure 9 Echocardiogram of patient with infective endocarditis causing aortic regurgitation in whom an aortic root abscess cavity present, suspected due to the abnormal echoes in the left atrium (solid arrow). Early aortic valve opening is also present (open arrow). (Courtesy of the editor of the *British Heart Journal*)

bined with information from a careful history, examination, electrocardiogram, and chest X-ray, echocardiography may allow valve surgery to be performed without the need for preoperative cardiac catheterization.

References

1. Nanda, N. C., Gramiak, R., Shah, P. M. and DeWeese, J. (1975). Mitral commissurotomy versus replacement. Preoperative evaluation by echocardiography. *Cirvulation* **51**, 263
2. Cope, G. D., Kisslo, J. A., Johnson, M. L. and Behar, V. S. (1975). A reassessment of the echocardiogram in mitral stenosis. *Circulation*, **52**, 664
3. Gibson, D. G. and Brown, D. J. (1975). Measurement of peak rates of left ventricular wall movement in man. Comparison of echocardiography and angiocardiography. *Br. Heart J.*, **37**, 677
4. Sung, R. J., Ghahramani, A. R., Mallon, S. M., Richter, S. E., Sommer, L. S., Gottlieb, S. and Myzrburg, R. J. (1975). Haemodynamic features of prolapsing and nonprolapsing atrial myxoma. *Circulation*, **51**, 342
5. Traill, T. A., St John Sutton, M. G. and Gibson, D. G. (1979) Mitral stenosis with high left ventricular end-diastolic pressure. *Br. Heart J.* **41**, 405
6. Child, J. S., Skorton, D. J., Taylor, R. D., Krivokapich, J. K., Abbassi, A. S., Wong, M. and Shah, P. D. (1979) M-Mode and cross sectional echocardiographic features of flail posterior mitral leaflets. *Am. J. Cardiol.*, **44**, 1383

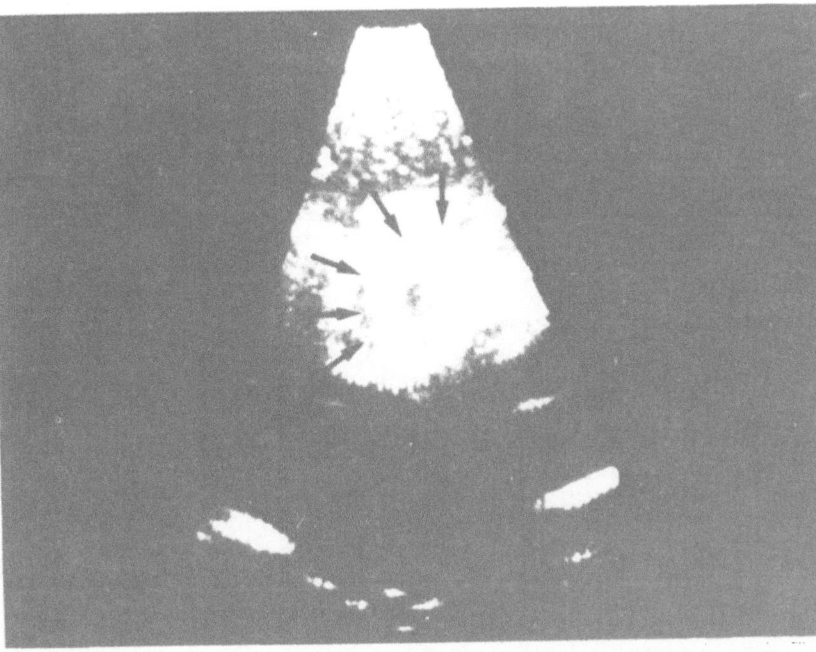

Figure 10 Cross sectional echocardiogram of a patient with an infected homograft prosthesis in the aortic position showing a distinct line of dehiscence. (Courtesy of the editor of the *British Heart Journal*)

7. Venco, A., St John Sutton, M. G., Gibson, D. G. and Brown, D. J. (1976). Non-invasive assessment of left ventricular function after correction of severe aortic regurgitation. *Br. Heart J.* **38,** 1324
8. Cotter, L., Gibson, D. G., Paneth, M. and Shiu, M. F. (1979). Surgery in congestive cardiomyopathy (abs.). *Circulation*, **59,** II, 220
9. Bennett, D. H., Evans, D. W. and Raj, M. V. J. (1975). Echocardiographic left ventricular dimensions in pressure and volume overload: their use in assessing aortic stenosis. *Br. Heart J.*, **37,** 971
10. Gibson, D. G., Traill, T. A., Hall, R. J. C. and Brown, D. J. (1979). Echocardiographic features of secondary left ventricular hypertrophy. *Br. Heart J.*, **41,** 54
11. Ten Cate, F. J., Van Drop, W. G., Hugenholtz, P. G. and Roelandt, J. (1979). Fixed subaortic stenosis: value of echocardiography for diagnosis and differentiation between various types. *Br. Heart J.*, **41,** 159
12. Wong, P., Cotter, L. and Gibson, D. G. (1980). Early systolic closure of the aortic valve. *Br. Heart J.* (In press)
13. Sanderson, J. E., Traill, T. A., St John Sutton, M. G., Brown, D. J., Gibson, D.G. and Goodwin, J. F. (1978). Left ventricular filling and relaxation in hypertrophic cardiomyopathy. *Br. Heart J.*, **40,** 596
14. Cohen, I. S., Wharton, T. P. and Neill, A. (1979). Pathophysiologic observations on premature opening of the aortic valve utilizing a technique for multiplane echocardiographic analysis. *Am. Heart J.*, **97,** 766
15. Wann, L. S., Dillon, J. C. and Weyman, A. E. (1976). Echocardiography in bacterial endocarditis. *N. Engl. J. Med.*, **295,** 135

12
The perioperative value of nuclear magnetic resonance

P. MANSFIELD

INTRODUCTION

Nuclear magnetic resonance (NMR) has long been used as an analytical tool by chemists and physicists in the study of inter- and intramolecular interactions in all phases of matter. The powerful analytical techniques developed and refined over many years are now finding increasing application in the biological and medical sciences[1].

More recently both in Britain and abroad intensive effort has been devoted to the development of new methods of imaging the interior of a living body by NMR[2-8]. The idea is to produce cross-sectional images related to the distribution of water, fat, or oil in biological structures. A number of techniques have been proposed and tried experimentally. All the methods, which are non-invasive, involve no ionizing radiation hazard and could therefore have some clinical value in medical diagnosis. Full descriptions of most of the imaging methods have been discussed and reviewed elsewhere[9-11].

NMR images of live human subjects have already been produced showing anatomical detail in finger cross-sections[12,13], hand, wrist and arm cross-sections[14,15], thoracic cross-sections[16,17] as well as abdomen[18] and head[19,20]. All the images to date have been representations of the proton spin distribution (hydrogen nucleus) in living tissue. In this paper, the potential of this new imaging modality will be emphasized, not only for the study of protons (^{1}H) but also for other naturally occurring nuclei, in particular, phosphorus (^{31}P). The exciting possibility of performing non-invasive, localized chemical analysis as well as imaging on cardiac muscle will also be discussed, and its perioperative value explored. However, before discussing details of the imaging technique and its applications, we shall briefly review the elements of nuclear magnetic resonance itself.

PRINCIPLES OF NMR[21]

Many naturally occurring high isotopic abundance elements exist with nuclei possessing a small magnetic moment. This magnetic moment arises because these nuclei possess an electric charge and behave like small spinning tops. Such nuclei are often referred to as spins, and their spin angular momentum or spin is denoted as I. Common biological examples are the nuclei of hydrogen, known as protons (^{1}H), and the magnetic nuclei of carbon (^{13}C), a low abundance species, and phosphorus (^{13}P).

Of course, protons are found in many different molecules both organic and inorganic. Water molecules, for example, each contain two protons. If, therefore, biological material containing water is placed in a strong magnetic field, a polarization of the nuclear spins results in a small measurable nuclear magnetization of the specimen. The strength of the magnetization varies from place to place in the specimen and depends on the density of protons present locally. This in turn depends on the local water concentration.

NMR imaging measures the local magnetization by utilizing a second important property of a proton in a magnetic field which arises from its spin. This is the Larmor precession which occurs when a spin is disturbed from alignment with the polarizing field. In addition to relaxing back to alignment with a time constant T_1 (the spin lattice relaxation time) individual spins perform a precessional motion, like the precession of a gyroscopic top when disturbed from the upright position. The precessional angular frequency or Larmor frequency is given by:

$$\omega_0 = \gamma B_0 \tag{1}$$

where B_0 is the magnitude of the magnetic field and γ a constant called the magnetogyric ratio. The Larmor frequency ($\omega_0/2\pi$) falls conveniently into the short radio waveband for magnetic fields of 1 kG or so. Table 1 lists a number of common nuclei, their isotopic abundance, spin, Larmor precessional frequency, and relative sensitivity for both constant magnetic field and constant frequency. In this comparison, protons head the list for sensitivity and since they occur in large numbers in biological material they are relatively easy to detect. Fluorine nuclei, though nearly as sensitive as protons, occur rarely in biological molecules and are therefore of less interest. All other nuclei in Table 1 compare rather poorly with proton sensitivity at constant field. However, if we consider the relative sensitivities at constant frequency, phosphorus begins to look an interesting possibility. However, we shall return to this point in a later section.

According to equation (1), if B_0 is spatially uniform, then all parts of a specimen residing in the magnetic field will have the same Larmor frequency. In practice, there are small spin–spin interactions present in all material, both solid and liquid, which cause the coherent precession predicted by equation (1) to dephase irreversibly with the spin–spin interaction time constant T_2. If the dephasing is caused by static inhomogeneities of the magnetic field, the resulting decay is reversible and can be recalled to form a spin echo[22]. However, the echo amplitude will decay with T_2, the lifetime of the transverse magnetization. Another important spin interaction is the isotropic chemical

Table 1 A number of common magnetic nuclei together with their respective Larmor frequencies in a magnetic field of 0.1 T (1000 G), and their isotopic abundance. Note the differences between sensitivities at constant magnetic field and at constant frequency relative to protons (^1H)

				Relative sensitivities for equal numbers of nuclei	
Nucleus	*Larmor frequency in 0.1 T field* (MHz)	*Isotopic abundance*	*Spin*	*Constant field*	*Constant frequency*
^1H	4.2577	100	1/2	1.00	1.00
^{19}F	4.0055	100	1/2	0.834	0.941
^{13}C	1.0705	1.108	1/2	1.59×10^{-2}	0.251
^{23}Na	1.1262	100	3/2	9.27×10^{-2}	1.67
^{31}P	1.7235	100	1/2	6.6×10^{-2}	0.405

shift δ[21]. This arises through a magnetic screening of the nucleus by the orbital electrons and results in the nucleus experiencing a slightly smaller effective field B_{eff} given by

$$B_{eff} = (1 - \delta)B_0 \tag{2}$$

The value of δ depends very much on the nucleus observed and its chemical environment, and can be related to the chemical bond structure. In hydrogen bonding, for example, δ is typically $1 - 2 \times 10^{-6}$. Phosphorus chemical shifts, on the other hand, exhibit a larger variation, typically $\sim 20 \times 10^{-6}$, depending on the bond character. As we shall see, these chemical shifts are characteristic of particular molecular constituents and can therefore form the basis of a non-destructive, non-invasive method of chemical analysis.

BIOLOGICAL TISSUE CHARACTERISTICS

Human biological tissue contains on average around 75% water which can readily be detected by NMR methods. Quite a large fraction of the water is contained within the cell cytoplasm but there is also a substantial amount of extracellular water in addition to the bulk fluids contained within the body. Different healthy body tissues contain different amounts of water and the variation in water content can be used to some extent to differentiate the various organs within the body. Figure 1 shows the water content of various human tissues. Many factors affect water content – for example, illness, nutrition, and age – and it is hoped that such detailed information on water distribution will be a valuable supplementary aid in diagnosis.

It has also been found experimentally that different normal tissues show differences in the important NMR parameter T_1. The T_1 differences are even more pronounced between normal and malignant tissue[23,24].

Other disease states, such as ischaemia following myocardial infarction, show a significant increase in water content in the infarcted area of around

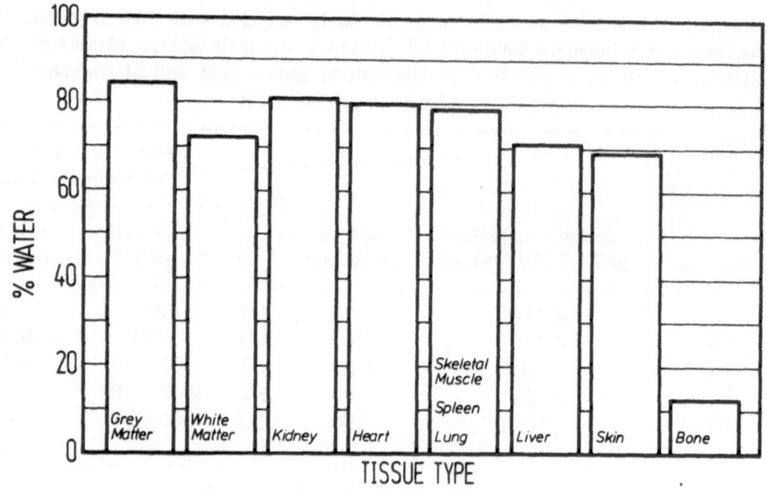

Figure 1 Water content of various human tissues

20 % over that of normal cardiac muscle[25]. It has been demonstrated that high water content and long T_1 values are quite well correlated[24] so that on this basis one might expect an elevation of T_1 in the ischaemic areas. From the tissue characteristics it is clear that an imaging method based on water content and/or T_1 can easily differentiate between the various tissue yielding cross-sectional images showing anatomical and pathological detail as reflected in the distribution of water throughout the body, and indeed this is the case experimentally, as we shall see later. It should be emphasized, however, that unique tissue typing does not seem possible at the present time on the basis of the two NMR parameters T_1 and density.

As already indicated in the section on principles, chemical shifts for protons are rather small and there seems little prospect of observing them with the magnetic field strengths currently used for whole-body NMR imaging; typically 0.1 T (1000 G). Furthermore, one requires exceptionally good uniformity of the static magnet over large volumes. To detect proton shifts, for example, would require a static field homogeneity of 1 part in 10^7. For phosphorus shifts, on the other hand, a static field homogeneity of 1 part in 10^6 would just suffice. However, there are other problems connected with experimental sensitivity, to which we shall refer later.

MEDICAL IMAGES BY LINE-SCANNING

If a linear magnetic field gradient is added to B_0 different parts of the specimen will experience different field strengths causing the localized spins to precess at different Larmor frequencies. By subjecting the specimen to suitable magnetic field gradients, therefore, spins from a specific region of the sample can be identified through their Larmor frequency, the received signal strength being proportional to the local spin concentration.

The precession of a nucleus when disturbed from magnetic alignment with the polarizing field is not unlike the ringing of a bell when struck. Using this analogy, we can visualize a thin layer of our specimen as represented by a collection of bells with pitches proportional to their position across the layer. A thin strip of material in the layer would thus be represented by a row of bells. A missing bell along the row corresponds to zero nuclear density at that point.

Line scanning in our analogy corresponds to simultaneously ringing all the bells in a row, recording the discordant din and then frequency-analysing it to determine which notes, and hence bells, are present and from their pitch where they are located. The process of frequency-analysing is often referred to as performing the Fourier transformation, after the French mathematician.

In line-scan imaging we imagine that a layer of undisturbed spin magnetization produced in the magnetic field B_0 is first prepared within a thin cross-sectional slice of thickness Δx through an extended specimen – Figure 2. A linear magnetic field gradient G_y is switched on and the spins within the shaded strip are selectively perturbed with a radio frequency pulse (in this case at a

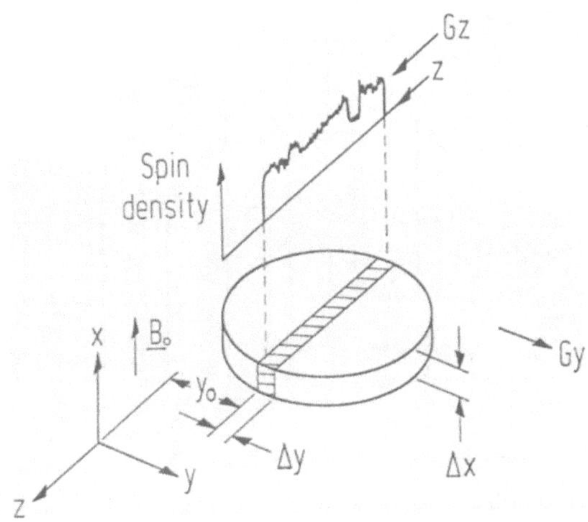

Figure 2 Sketch showing the principle of line-scan imaging

frequency of 4 MHz). The resultant transient signal from the spins is observed in the read gradient G_z and Fourier transformed to give the proton distribution along the strip.

By changing slightly the frequency of the pulse, successive strips may be irradiated and the spin density scanned line by line across the specimen. The digitized data are fed into a square array in a computer memory and later output to a television screen in picture form. Bright regions of the picture correspond to high mobile proton density. Darker regions correspond to lower proton density, the full range of mobile spin density being represented on a 16-level linear grey scale. In the colour pictures, each of the 16 signal levels is assigned a colour code. In this way, picture contrast between levels can be arbitrarily increased to accentuate particular detail if desired.

A single examination of the spin magnetization along a given strip usually does not produce a good enough signal/noise ratio for a recognizable and assignable picture. Picture enhancement may be performed by averaging the signal for a given strip. By this means the picture quality may be greatly improved at the expense of imaging time. For medical imaging one must settle for a compromise betwen imaging time and picture quality.

Figure 3 shows a typical four-coil magnet system and one possible patient disposition. The magnet used in our work was made by Oxford Instruments and produces a maximum field of 0.1 T at the centre. The magnet uniformity

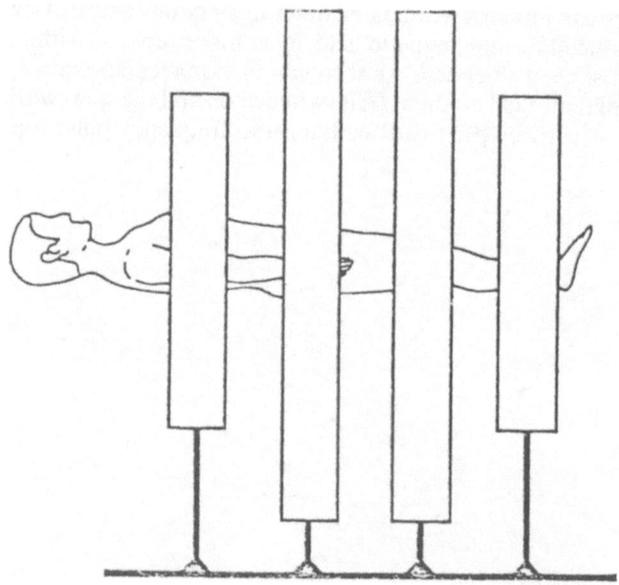

Figure 3 Sketch showing a side view of a whole-body electromagnet and the position of a patient

at present is a few parts in 10^5 but can be improved by fine coil movements and/or additional field shim coils.

An example of the many line-scan images that have been produced with our whole-body imaging system is shown in Figure 4. This is a cross-sectional image through the abdomen of P.M. at the L2–3 level[18]. The slice thickness in this case was about 4 cm and the image took 40 min to produce. The original data array was 90^2 points, corresponding to the largest array size that we could then display. The original data have been interpolated four times giving a 360^2 picture matrix. The tiled appearance is intentional and emphasizes the separate 90^2 picture sections which make up the whole. As well as the general outline of the body as seen from above, the picture shows some internal detail. The arrow indicates the posterior mid-line. The liver

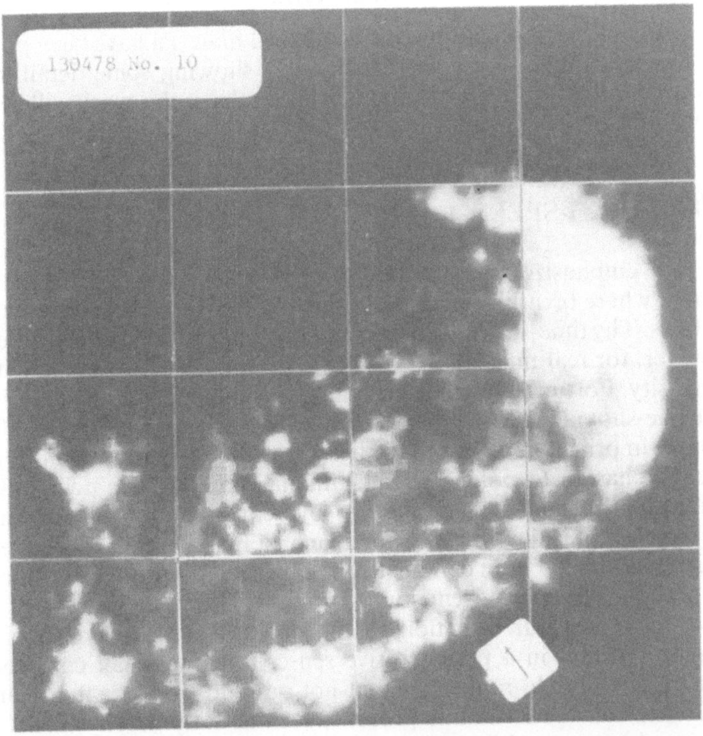

Figure 4 Cross-sectional NMR line-scan image through the abdomen of P.M. at the level of the second and third lumbar vertebrae. The slice thickness was about 4.0 cm. The imaging time was 40 min. The arrow indicates the midline posterior. The large bright zone to the right of the midline is the liver. See text for other details

shows as a bright well-defined zone to the right of the midline, the vertebral column is visible in the midline and the right kidney shows overlapping with the liver. Other recognizable features of this picture are the spleen on the left side, part of the pancreas, the circular outline of the aorta just anterior and to the left of the vertebral column, the gall bladder on the anterior lobe of the liver, and some gut. The anterior abdominal wall does not show in this picture. Loss of signal intensity is ascribed to wall movements during imaging. The unusual shape of the right kidney is no doubt due to motion. These motional artefacts emphasize the importance of speeding up the imaging process.

It is perhaps worth stressing here that line-scanning is one of several different methods of producing NMR images. For example, the so-called echo-planar imaging technique[26] is able to simultaneously examine and differentiate all picture points in a selected slice and is therefore a potentially very fast imaging method. Thus, whereas in line-scanning we can obtain images in several minutes, comparable quality pictures should be obtainable in seconds by echo-planar methods. Indeed, preliminary results obtained at 4.0 MHz on a small-scale probe assembly are extremely encouraging[27]. For example, averaged images of phantoms and biological material have been produced in 8 s, whereas single-shot complete pictures showing some detail have been produced in as short a time as 40 ms. The results of this work will be reported elsewhere[28].

ULTRA-HIGH-SPEED CARDIAC IMAGING

We have emphasized the importance of high-speed imaging in the previous section, where breathing and abdominal motions can introduce undesirable artefacts. The time-scale for this type of imaging could be of the order of 10 s. However, for real time studies of the heart, much shorter imaging times are a necessity. Fortunately, the echo-planar technique[26] is able to produce complete one-shot pictures in times of around 30 ms, and it would therefore seem feasible, in principle, to image the heart and even to study its motions in real time. We hasten to point out that this has not yet been achieved and the technical problems that have to be overcome should not be minimized. Nevertheless, it is theoretically possible on a human scale and, as referred to earlier, has already been demonstrated experimentally on a one-third human size scale[27]. The spin system studied comprised mobile protons.

We now turn our attention to the potential value of such high-speed imaging schemes in a perioperative sense. First, we shall consider proton imaging. We should remember that not only do we see water protons, but also other sources of mobile protons, such as fatty or oily tissue. Adipose tissue is characterized by high mobile proton density and short T_1 values[24], whereas blood, for example, though rich in mobile protons, possesses a somewhat longer T_1. Thus, T_1 discrimination enables one to locate fatty deposits. This point has been demonstrated in the case of yellow bone marrow in a live finger[13]. In the heart, of course, the blood is moving and it is expected, again on theoretical grounds, that blood flow will be measurable in NMR imaging.

From the clinical standpoint, valuable parameters necessary for a meaningful prognosis and therapy planning in heart disease are the ejection fraction, that is to say, the ratio of stroke volume at systole to left ventricular end-diastolic volume, and cardiac output. As well as directly measuring these parameters by three-dimensional imaging[10,26,30] studies of the ventricular wall movements should aid in locating and assessing the infarcted region. All this is within sight using present and projected proton imaging methods. In addition to the purely haemodynamic approach outlined, variations in water content and T_1 of the myocardium itself will supplement the diagnosis.

Although we have already indicated the possibility of observing other spin species we have so far concentrated on protons simply because they are easier to detect. The first generation of NMR imaging machines, therefore, have been designed specifically with this in mind. However, given magnets capable of producing sufficiently high fields, it will no doubt be possible to tune in on other nuclei listed in Table 1. In particular, we wish to consider in the next section the exciting possibilities of phosphorus imaging.

NMR IMAGING OF PHOSPHORUS

Phosphorus occurs naturally in biological tissue in membrane structures; for example, in the form of phospholipids and in many other tissues including muscle, where it occurs in the form of adenosine triphosphate (ATP) which provides the driving energy of the cell.

From Table 1 it would appear that all we have to do is raise the static field according to equation (2) to bring the ^{31}P nuclei into resonance at 4.0 MHz (say) and we can then expect a sensitivity comparable to that obtained from protons. The field increase required is only by a factor of 2.470. This would be true for equal numbers of phosphorus and hydrogen nuclei. Unfortunately, despite the 100% isotopic abundance, there is typically only one phosphorus nucleus per thousand protons in biological material, and so the actual relative sensitivity is more like 4×10^{-4}. On this basis, it might appear not worthwhile to contemplate phosphorus imaging at all. This might well be the case were it not for the fact that ^{31}P resonances contain extremely interesting and potentially useful medically diagnostic information[31]. To understand its importance, we must consider further the details of muscle metabolism.

ATP contains three phosphate groups, α, β and γ. The molecule is broken down by enzymes in the muscle to form adenosine diphosphate (ADP) and inorganic phosphate P_i. ADP contains only the α and β phosphate groups. However, ATP is regenerated under enzymic action from phosphocreatine (PCr) plus ADP yielding ATP and creatine (Cr). That is to say, the nett effect is to break down phosphocreatine to form creatine plus inorganic phosphate. This is summarized in equation (3)

$$PCr \rightarrow Cr + P_i + E \tag{3}$$

This process delivers the energy (E) required by the cell.

Because of the relatively large numbers of hydrogen atoms in these compounds and the surrounding protons, the high-resolution proton resonances of the reaction metabolites are extremely complicated and difficult to interpret. On the other hand, the small numbers of phosphorus nuclei yield relatively simple and interpretable ^{31}P resonances. This fact was first noticed only a few years ago and has been pioneered and exploited by a number of research groups both in Britain and elsewhere[32-35].

A typical ^{31}P resonance in normal muscle is sketched in Figure 5 and shows the α, β and γ ATP phosphate groups, the strong phosphocreatine line and the weaker inorganic and sugar phosphate resonances P_s. The different resonances are due to chemical shifts between the various metabolites. An important fact is that the chemical shift of the inorganic phosphorus resonance is dependent on the local pH value and thus provides a new way of measuring this parameter. For example, in ischaemia, lack of nutrient and oxygen resulting from an infarct causes the heart tissue to seek alternative supplies of ATP from glycolysis, the breakdown of glycogen. This process produces lactic acid as an end-product and so the localized pH increases producing a measurable shift of the P_i peak and an increase in the sugar phosphate P_s.

In addition to this effect, there is an even stronger intensity effect in ischae-

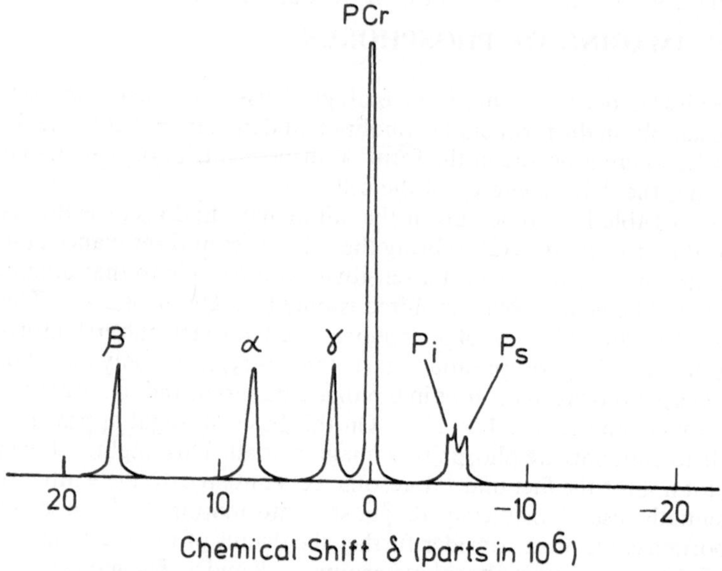

Figure 5 Sketch of a typical ^{31}P high-resolution NMR spectrum in muscle tissue. α, β and γ denote the three phosphorus peaks of ATP which are chemically shifted down-field from phosphocreatine (PCr) shown here centred with zero chemical shift. The small inorganic phosphate peak P_i, and the sugar phosphates P_s, are shifted slightly up-field. Note that the relative proportions of the various metabolites present are proportional to the areas under the respective absorption profiles

mia recently observed in simulated infarcts produced by ligation of the coronary arteries in both perfused beating hearts studies and in rat heart studies of anoxia performed *in vivo*[34–37]. It should be emphasized that none of these studies was performed by NMR imaging, but by invasive means in which the exposed heart or removed heart is enclosed in the NMR probe coil. Nevertheless, these important results indicate clearly that following ligation and the onset of ischaemia, the phosphocreatine peak drops while the P_i and P_S peaks increase. During this phase the ATP levels stay fairly constant. Finally, as glycogen reserves are used up the ATP levels drop. Similar results occur following respiratory arrest[37].

The implications of these exciting developments are clear. For we now have, at least in principle, a non-destructive and, if combined with NMR imaging, a non-invasive method of following the time course of the phosphorus metabolites in living cardiac tissue. In other words, chemical analysis relevant to the disease state of the heart can be performed *in vivo*.

As indicated at the beginning of this section, there are problems of signal sensitivity when considering human ^{31}P imaging. All the high-resolution work referred to above has been performed on very small specimens in very high magnetic fields corresponding to ^{31}P frequencies in the range 30–100 MHz. Quite apart from the cost of producing such high fields over large volumes, there is a limiting physical factor so far not discussed. This is radio frequency (r.f.) penetration of the specimen. Man, after all, is a conducting medium and above about 10 MHz it is virtually impossible to get significant penetration of the r.f. field[38]. For small animals and specimens the problem is ameliorated, but with man, even at 4.0 MHz the r.f. field penetration is not complete. In addition, troublesome r.f. phase shifts occur in both the transmitted pulse and received nuclear signal, resulting in additional picture artefacts. At 4.0 or 5.0 MHz these effects are tolerable. If we therefore settle for a ^{31}P imaging system operating at, say, 4.0 MHz and we wish to produce cross-sectional images through the thorax in the same time as that taken for a proton scan, it will be clear from our earlier discussion on signal sensitivity that the expected ^{31}P signal/noise ratio for the same picture resolution, or number of picture points, is simply 1/1000th of that obtained from the proton scan. This being so, we have a number of options available in order to bring the signal/noise ratios equal. The simplest is to signal-average, but this is costly on time which really we would like to keep to a minimum. If we also insist on examining the same slice thickness, the only variable left is the number of picture elements comprising the final picture. If we assume that the proton image comprises 128^2 picture elements, then the maximum number of picture elements allowable in the ^{31}P image is $(128/10\sqrt{10})^2 \simeq 4^2$. At first sight this might appear too coarse an image to be of any value. In spatial terms one picture element would correspond to an area of roughly 7^2 cm^2. Thus whole organs, like the heart or kidneys, could be arranged to fall into one or possibly two picture elements. The signals from whole organs thus isolated could then be made to yield their chemical information in the manner previously described.

In the course of producing this article a method of achieving non-invasive localized ^{31}P chemical analysis has been announced[39]. In this system, which is already commercially available with magnet access of 20 cm or 60 cm, the ^{31}P resonance is observed at a single sensitive point by profiling the static magnetic field. It is therefore not an imaging system *per se*. High-resolution spectra from live whole rats and localized liver regions demonstrate the virtual absence of the PCr peak in liver, a fact known from other work. The system operates at 32.5 MHz corresponding to a field of 1.89 T. This high field is produced using a superconductive magnet.

CONCLUSION

NMR imaging, although still under intensive development, has already demonstrated its potential for producing pictures showing morphological detail, and in some instances, the picture quality is close to that achievable by X-ray tomography. However, our feeling is that NMR imaging will find its true role in physiological applications. Of these, the most likely initial application will be proton studies of blood supply in situations where speed is not too important. As imaging speeds increase proton studies of the heart will become possible. Finally, with higher magnetic fields and larger magnets, *in vivo* chemical analysis will be possible studying phosphorus and possibly carbon and sodium.

Acknowledgments

The whole-body proton image referred to in this article was produced with support from the Medical Research Council, to whom we are grateful. Current work is continuing with support from both MRC and DHSS. The imaging project is, of course, a group effort. The group comprises Professor R. E. Coupland, Dr P. G. Morris, Dr I. L. Pykett, Mr R. J. Ordidge, Mr V. Bangert and Mr R. R. Rzedzian, whose help is gratefully acknowledged.

References

1. James, T. L. (1975). *Nuclear Magnetic Resonance in Biochemistry*. (London: Academic Press)
2. Lauterbur, P. C. (1973). Image formation by induced local interactions; examples employing nuclear magnetic resonance. *Nature* (*London*), **242,** 190
3. Garroway, A. N., Grannell, P. K. and Mansfield, P. (1974). Image formation in NMR by a selective irradiative process, *J. Phys., C.*, **7,** L457
4. Hinshaw, W. S. (1974). Spin mapping: the application of moving gradients to NMR. *Phys. Lett.*, **48A,** 87
5. Damadian, R., Minkoff, L., Goldsmith, M., Stanford, M. and Koutcher, J. (1976), *Science,* **194,** 1430
6. Hutchison, J. M. S., Mallard, J. R. and Goll, C. C. (1974). *In vivo* imaging of body structures using proton resonance. In Allen, P. S., Andrew, E. R. and Bates, C. A. (eds.). *Proceedings of the* 18*th Ampere Congress, Nottingham*. Volume 2, p. 435. (Amsterdam: North Holland)
7. Crooks, L. E., Grover, T. P., Kaufman, L. and Singer, J. R. (1978). Tomographic imaging with nuclear magnetic resonance. *Invest. Radiol.*, **13,** 63
8. Hoult, D. I. (1979). Rotating frame zeugmatography. *J. Mag. Reson.*, **33,** 183.
9. Mansfield, P. (1976). Proton spin imaging by NMR. *Contemp. Phys.*, **17,** 553
10. Brunner, P. and Ernst, R. R. (1979). Sensitivity and performance time in NMR imaging. *J. Mag. Reson.*, **33,** 83
11. Mansfield, P. and Morris, P. G. (1981). In Waugh, J. S. (ed.). *Advances in Magnetic Resonance* (London: Academic Press) (To be published)
12. Mansfield, P. and Maudsley, A. A. (1976). Planar and line scan spin imaging by NMR. In Brunner, H., Hausser, K. H. and Schweitzer, D. (eds.). *Proceedings of of the* 19*th Ampere Congress, Heidelberg*, p. 247 (Heidelberg/Geneva: Groupement Ampere)
13. Mansfield, P. and Maudsley, A. A. (1977). Medical imaging by NMR. *Br. J. Radiol.*, **50,** 188
14. Hinshaw, W. S., Bottomley, P. A. and Holland, G. N. (1977). Radiographic thin-section image of the human wrist by nuclear magnetic resonance. *Nature* (*London*), **270,** 722
15. Hinshaw, W. S., Andrew, E. R., Bottomley, P. A., Holland, G. N., Moore, W. S. and Worthington, B. S. (1979). An *in vivo* study of the fore-arm and hand by thin section NMR imaging. *Br. J. Radiol.*, **52,** 36
16. Damadian, R., Goldsmith, M. and Minkoff, L. (1977). NMR in cancer: XVI. Fonar image of the live human body. *Physiol. Chem. Phys.*, **9,** 97
17. Mallard, J., Hutchison, J. M. S., Edelstein, W. A., Ling, C. R., Foster, M. A. and Johnson, G. (1980). *In vivo* n.m.r. imaging in medicine; the Aberdeen approach, both physical and biological. *Phil. Trans. R. Soc.* (*London*), **B289,** 519
18. Mansfield, P., Pykett, I. L., Morris, P. G. and Coupland, R. E. (1978). Human whole body line-scan imaging by NMR. *Br. J. Radiol.*, **51,** 921

19. Clow, H. (1978). Unpublished work, presented at the British Institute of Radiology, November 1978. (See also *New Scientist*, 23 November 1978, p. 588)
20. Holland, G. N., Moore, W. S. and Hawkes, R. C. (1980). NMR tomography of the brain. *J. Comput.-Assist. Tomogr.*, **4,** 1
21. For introductory texts to NMR see Andrew, E. R. (1956). *Nuclear Magnetic Resonance* (Cambridge: Cambridge University Press); Slichter, C. P., (1978) *Principles of Magnetic Resonance* (Berlin/Heidelberg: Springer-Verlag); and Farrar, T. C. and Becker, E. D., (1971). *Pulse and Fourier Transform NMR* (London: Academic Press)
22. Hahn, E. L. (1950). Spin echoes. *Phys. Rev.*, **80,** 580
23. Damadian, R. (1971). Tumour detection by nuclear magnetic resonance. *Science, N.Y.*, **171,** 1151
24. Kiricuta, I. C. and Simplaceanu, V. (1975). Tissue water content and nuclear magnetic resonance in normal and tumorous tissue. *Cancer Res.*, **35,** 1164
25. Damadian, R. and Lauterbur, P. C., private communications. See also Lauterbur, P. C., Frank, J. A. and Jacobson, M. J. (1976). *Digest of the 4th International Conference on Medical Physics.* Abstract 33.9; Lauterbur, P. C. (1976). Feasibility of NMR zeugmatographic imaging of the heart and lungs. Engineering Foundation Conference on *Comparative Productivity of Techniques for non-invasive Medical Diagnosis.* New England College, Henniker, N.Y., 15–20 August; and also Frank, J. A., Feiler, M. A., House, W. V., Lauterbur, P. C. and Jacobson, M. J. (1976). Measurement of proton nuclear magnetic longitudinal relaxation times and water content in infarcted canine myocardium and induced pulmonary injury. *Clin. Res.*, **24,** 217A
26. Mansfield, P. and Pykett, I. L. (1978). Biological and medical imaging by NMR. *J. Mag. Reson.*, **29,** 355
27. Mansfield, P., Morris, P. G., Ordidge, R. J., Pykett, I. L., Bangert, V. and Coupland, R. E. (1980). Human whole body imaging and the detection of breast tumours by NMR. *Phil. Trans. R. Soc.* (*London*), **B289,** 503
28. Mansfield, P. and Ordidge, R. J. (to be published)
29. Lauterbur, P. C. and Lai, C.-M. (1977). Feasibility study of nuclear magnetic resonance zeugmatography for use in detecting arteriosclerosis. *Proceedings of the NHLBI Division of Heart and Vascular Diseases, Devices and Technology Branch Annual Contractors Meeting*, p. 158
30. Lai, C.-M. and Lauterbur, P. C. (1980). True three-dimensional image reconstruction by nuclear magnetic resonance. *Phys. Med. Biol.* (In press)
31. Gadian, D. G. (1977). Nuclear magnetic resonance in living tissue. *Contemp. Phys.*, **18,** 351
32. Hoult, D. I., Busby, S. J. W., Gadian, D. G., Radda, G. K., Richards, R. E. and Seeley, P. J. (1974). Observation of tissue metabolites using ^{31}P nuclear magnetic resonance. *Nature*, **252,** 285
33. Burt, C. T., Glonek, T. and Bárány, M. (1976). Phosphorus-31 magnetic resonance detection of unexpected phosphodiesters in muscle. *Biochemistry, N.Y.*, **15,** 4850
34. Garlick, P. B., Radda, G. K. and Seeley, P. J. (1979). Studies of acidosis in the ischaemic heart by phosphorus nuclear magnetic resonance. *Biochem. J.* **184,** 547
35. Hollis, D. P., Nunnally, R. L., Jacobus, W. E. and Taylor, G. J. (1978). Detection of regional ischaemia in perfused beating hearts by phosphorus nuclear magnetic resonance. *Biochem. Biophys. Res. Comm.*, **75,** 1086
36. Hollis, D. P. and Nunnally, R. L. (1980). Recent ^{31}P NMR studies of myocardium. *Phil. Trans. R. Soc.* (*London*), **B289,** 437
37. Ackerman, J. J. H., Bore, P. J., Gadian, D. G., Grove, T. H. and Radda, G. K. (1980). NMR studies of metabolism in perfused organs. *Phil. Trans. R. Soc.* (*London*), **B289,** 425

38. Bottomley, P. A. and Andrew, E. R. (1980). RF magnetic field penetration, phase shift and power dissipation in biological tissue; implications for NMR imaging. *Phys. Med. Biol.*, **23**, 630

39. Gordon, R. E., Hanley, P. E., Shaw, D., Gadian, D. G., Radda, G. K., Styles, P. and Chan, L. (1980). Localization of metabolites in animals using ^{31}P topical magnetic resonance. *Nature* (*London*) (In press)

13
Computed tomography of the heart

J. J. K. BEST

INTRODUCTION

Computed tomography is a radiographic method for visualizing the distribution of X-ray attenuation in the body. The method has acquired many names since it was introduced into clinical radiological practice in 1971, 'computerized axial tomography' or 'computer-assisted tomography' (CAT) and 'computed tomography' or 'computerized tomography' (CT) are terms in common use. The term 'computed tomography', CT, is generally used in radiology and will be used in this paper.

CT may be thought of as a method of X-raying transverse sections of the body which are typically 10 mm thick. The method employs the same physical properties of the tissues of the body as conventional X-ray techniques. A narrow fan of X-rays is created by collimating the output of an X-ray tube, and the X-rays are directed at the slice of the patient being investigated. The fan beam of X-rays passing through the body is attenuated by interaction with the body tissues. The amount of absorption depends on the physical density and atomic composition of the body and the energy of the X-ray beam. For the same X-ray energy a more dense material will attenuate the beam more than a less dense material. In order to measure the attenuation in conventional radiography a photographic film is used; for CT the radiographic film is replaced by sensitive scintillation or ionization detectors. The X-ray tube and dectectors are mounted on a gantry or frame which is mechanically rotated round the patient. The system allows measurements of the attenuation of X-rays to be made at different angles of rotation around the periphery of the patient and these measurements are referred to as projections (Figures 1 and 2). If sufficient projections are obtained a mathematical reconstruction of the X-ray absorption in the tissues of the slice of the patient through which the X-rays have passed may be reconstructed using a computer. It would be impractical to attempt the resolution of a conventional X-ray picture because of the very large number of measurements and calculations necessary. The computation process is reduced by calculating the absorption values for a two-dimensional matrix of imaginary boxes

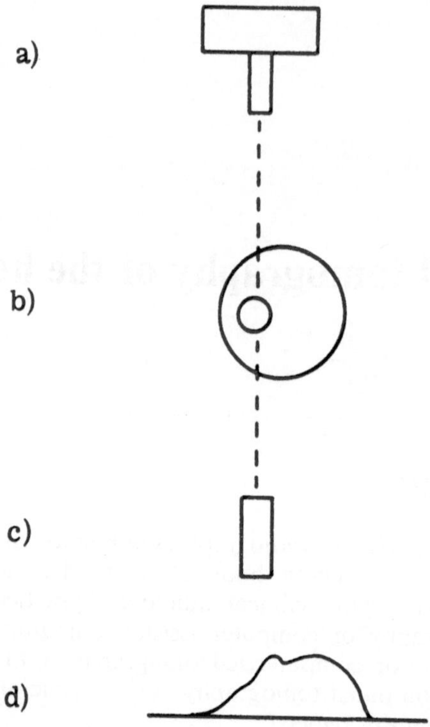

Figure 1 Schematic diagram of a very simple pencil-beam CT scanner: (a) X-ray tube; (b) body; (c) detector; (d) projection of X-ray attenuation data made during a single transverse

of tissue typically measuring 1 mm × 1 mm × the depth of the slice thickness–these are frequently referred to as 'voxels'. The thickness of the slice is dictated by the width of the X-ray beam. The values for the absorption of each 'voxel' are related to the attenuation coefficients for the tissues in the 'voxels' and are termed CT numbers or Hounsfield numbers (after Godfrey Hounsfield, the inventor of CT and joint winner of the Nobel Prize for Medicine, 1979). The computer displays these numbers as a two-dimensional array of figures called 'pixels'. The numerical values for the pixels may be presented as printed numbers but more usually are displayed as a picture of shades of grey on a television monitor. This display may be photographed to provide a permanent record, hard copy.

CT OF THE HEART

Changes in the size and shape of the heart during the cardiac cycle, together with an assessment of blood flow to the different regions of the heart, are the parameters of cardiac function that may be measured by an imaging technique. As the shape of the heart is dependent upon the myocardial anatomy and the mechanical properties of the heart, it may be argued that the dynamic

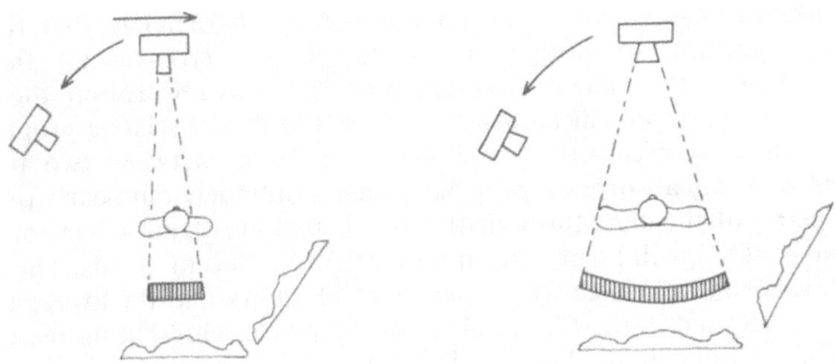

Figure 2 There are two types of CT scanner, the rotate–translate and the rotate-only; both produce projection data of X-ray attenuation from angles around the patient

changes recorded by an imaging technique may closely reflect the inter-relationship of the basic components of cardiac function. This premise is supported by the use of the left ventricular volume and ejection fraction as useful indices of cardiac function in clinical practice.

Conventional radiographic methods for measuring these indices employ projectional geometry, and it was the absence of this drawback in computed tomography – together with a demonstration of its very high sensitivity to small changes in tissue composition, leading to its successful application in radiology – which led a number of workers to investigate the possibility that CT scanning would be a useful technique for investigation of the heart[1–4]. Both normal and infarcted hearts were investigated in these experiments, and the general conclusions were that X-ray attenuation of the blood within the chambers of the heart, the myocardium, and infarcted myocardium were almost identical; but that after injection of iodinated contrast medium sufficient differences existed to distinguish between normal myocardium and ischaemic or infarcted muscle. It appears from a review of this work that a precision of measurement of the attenuation in the order of 0.5 % (difference between water and air being 100 %) is required[5]. In the presence of intravenous contrast a precision in the order of 1 % is required. More recent work using rapid sequential scanning[6] suggests that intravenous contrast given by a bolus may increase the myocardial density by 5 %.

PROBLEMS INHERENT IN CT SCANNING OF THE HEART

'Partial volume effect'

Commerical CT scanners currently available scan only one slice at a time. The picture produced represents the grey-scale analogue of numerical values for the pixels calculated by the computer. The pixel represents the voxel in the slice of tissue scanned, and whilst the linear resolution – that is the resolution of the plane of the scan, typically 1 mm × 1 mm – has the dimensions of the pixel, the third dimension of the voxel is the thickness of the slice, typically 10 mm. If the tissue occupying the voxel is of one histological type, the number generated by the computer may characterize that tissue. If, however, tissues of more than one histological type occupy the voxel, although each type may have a characteristic X-ray absorption, the number generated will represent an average influenced by the relative proportion of the tissues occupying the voxel. If the interface between two tissues of different X-ray absorption properties passes obliquely but nearly parallel to the plane of the slice through the voxel, this averaging effect, or 'partial volume effect', will be present in a number of adjacent voxels. The number of voxels will be related to the degree of obliquity and the averaging effect will be reflected in the CT numbers of the pixels representing these voxels, making it difficult to distinguish the boundary between the tissues. The 'partial volume effect' influence in the pixel numbers reflects the dimensions of the voxel; it is most marked when the interface is nearly parallel to the plane of the slice and is least marked when it is normal to the plane of the slice (Figure 3a,b).

When the particular problem of CT of the heart is considered, the principal interfaces in the thorax are the lung/myocardium and the myocardium/blood interfaces. Inspection of the anatomy of the heart shows that these interfaces have a wide range of obliquities. Thus, the precision of the delineation of the myocardium as affected by the partial volume effect will vary. This variation is made smaller as the slice thickness is reduced, and does not exist if the voxel is a cube. This will be the case when the linear resolution and the slice thickness are the same.

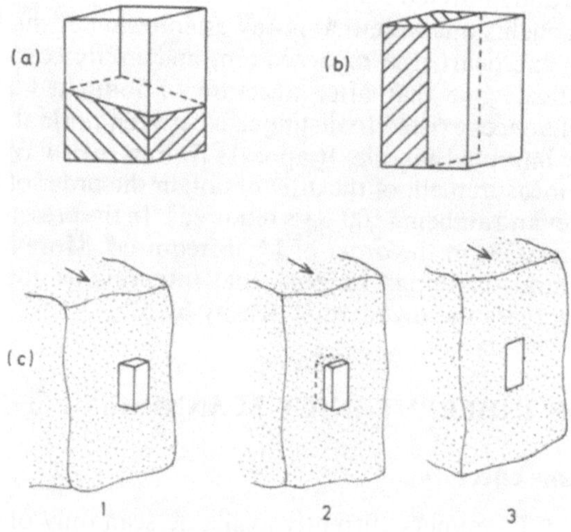

Figure 3 (a) A block of tissue representing the volume of reconstruction occupied by two types of tissue with an oblique interface. The dimensions of the reconstructed block of tissue are typically 1 mm × 1 mm × 10 mm. (b) Two types of tissue with an interface aligned with the long axis of the block of tissue. The partial volume effect will be small in this situation. (c) The effects of movement. Assume the tissue represents heart muscle and the interface is between heart and lung. During the period of the scan the value of reconstruction will be occupied by heart and then by lung, and the calculated attenuation will represent an average value.

Motion

Motion during the scan will also cause an averaging effect if a tissue interface moves through a voxel during scanning (Figure 3c). The time taken to make a scan – the temporal resolution – must therefore be sufficiently short so that motion greater than the spatial resolution does not occur during the scan. If one considers the left ventricular wall motion during the cardiac cycle and considers the motion apparent during short intervals of decreasing duration, motion is observed with 300 ms intervals during systole and the filling phase in diastole, but if the interval is decreased to 10 ms movement of the order of only 1 mm occurs at any time during the cardiac cycle (Figure 4). Thus, a temporal resolution of 10 ms is required if the heart is to be imaged during systole with a spatial resolution of 1 mm, but the scan time may be longer during diastole[7].

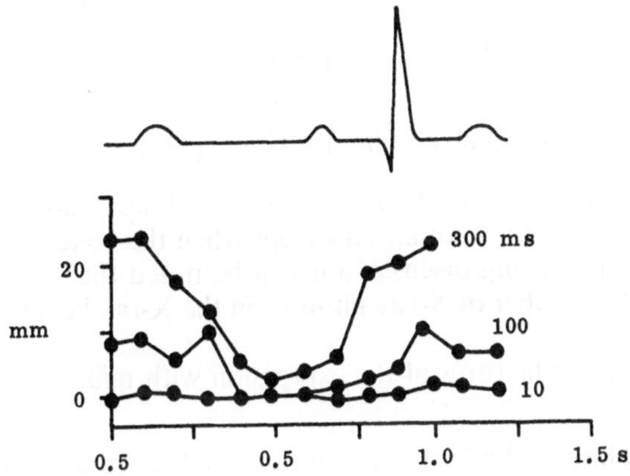

Figure 4 Graphs of left ventricular wall movement throughout the cardiac cycle representing apparent motion when viewed during intervals of 300, 100 and 10 ms (after Ritman[7])

Radiation dose to the patient

The sensitivity of a CT scanner enabling it to distinguish between different tissues may be considered under two general headings:

Spatial resolution
The dimensions of the voxel: the linear resolution in the plane of the scan × the thickness of the scan.

Accuracy of the measurement of X-ray attenuation: density discrimination
This is the ability to distinguish between tissues or materials or nearly similar X-ray absorbing properties.

X-ray attenuation is a random process and consequently the number of X-ray photons making up the X-ray beam which emerge from the patient and are detected are subject to fluctuation. The statistics of the process are such that the greater the number of photons detected, the more X-rays, the more precise the calculated attenuation values become. The precision of the measurements of spatial resolution and attenuation is dependent on the number of photons detected. This in turn is dependent upon the efficiency of the CT scanner detectors and the number of X-ray photons emerging from the patient. To increase the number of emerging photons means increasing the number of photons entering the patient, and this in turn means increasing the radiation dose to the patient. The radiation dose is the energy transferred to the patient during the process of attenuation of the X-ray beam.

The relation between the radiation dose, the spatial resolution and density discrimination has been derived[8–10], and has the following form:

$$D = \frac{1}{(\text{density discrimination})^2 \times a^3 \times t}$$

Where D is the radiation dose to the patient, a is the pixel size and t the slice thickness.

This expression may be crudely approximated to

$$D = \frac{1}{(\text{density discrimination})^2 \times (\text{spatial resolution})^4}$$

Spatial resolution = pixel size × slice thickness, so the term (spatial resolution)^4 is an approximation except when the voxel is a cube.

From the preceding discussion it will be noted that the radiation dose is related to the number of X-ray photons in the X-ray beam, the output of the X-ray tube.

The important features of the expression with relation to CT scanning of the heart are:

(a) Doubling of the spatial resolution, that is reducing the volume of the voxel by eight times, requires that the tube output and dose be increased sixteen times. If the slice thickness is maintained and the pixel size halved, the radiation dose will be increased by only eight times.
(b) Doubling the precision of the measurement of X-ray attenuation, density discrimination, requires an increase in dose by a factor of four.
(c) Whilst there is no expression for time in the equation, it is implicit in that radiation dose = the tube output × time. Thus the limiting factor of how short a scan-time can be achieved for a particular radiation dose is the X-ray tube output. That is, in how short a time can the number of photons required for a particular resolution and density discrimination be delivered by the X-ray tube.

THE IDEAL HEART CT SCANNER

The ideal heart-imaging system should be able to visualize the entire heart throughout the cardiac cycle with sufficient spatial resolution to resolve the anatomical detail necessary to make clinical decisions. It should not need the use of large volumes of iodinated contrast agents which may themselves alter the performance of the heart because of their pharmacological properties. The subject has been discussed in considerable depth by Ritman[7]. Ritman has assessed the imaging requirements in the following terms:

(a) Resolution of the major branches of the coronary arteries (2–3 mm diameter) opacified during coronary vessel arteriography.

(b) Localization and quantitation of transmural infarcts of moderate size (0.05 kg) to a precision of 5%.

(c) An estimate of left ventricular regional wall thickness and total muscle mass to a precision of 5%.

These requirements may be translated into specifications for an ideal CT scanner:

(a) Spatial resolution: 1 mm × 1 mm × 1 mm
(pixel: 1 mm × 1 mm; slice thickness 1 mm)

(b) Temporal resolution:
0.01 s during systole
0.1 s during diastole

(c) Density discrimination less than 0.5%.

(d) Ability to scan the whole heart during a single cardiac cycle.

These ideal specifications may be considered in terms of the general relationship. The patient dose varies inversely as (spatial resolution)^4 × (density discrimination)^2. This has been quantified by Pullan and Best[5] in terms of the performance of a commercial CT scanner, and the tube output necessary and dose to the patient appear impracticably large. If, however, the specifications are made less exacting the problem may be overcome. Two compromises are currently being employed to allow CT scanning of the heart. These are described in the following two sections.

THE DYNAMIC SPATIAL RECONSTRUCTOR

A multidisciplinary group at the Mayo Clinic and Foundation are developing a purpose-built CT scanner to image the heart[7,11–14]. The compromise they have chosen is to maintain the spatial and temporal resolution together with the facility to measure the whole heart during a single cardiac cycle, but to relax the density discrimination to 5%. This implies that they will require iodinated contrast to detect the myocardium and ischaemic areas within the myocardium. The technical solution they have used to overcome the limitations of X-ray tube output is to employ 28 X-ray tubes viewed by image-intensifiers with TV chains rotated around the patient. The line output of the TV chain is used as the projectional data. Whilst this latter system is less sensitive than the detectors used in conventional scanners it allows the whole heart to be imaged during one scan.

'GATING' CONVENTIONAL CT SCANNERS

Conventional scanners employ slice thicknesses considerably greater than the ideal 1 mm. Thus, by relaxing the spatial resolution in this way, a compromise is partially achieved. But even the latest CT scanners have scan times (1–2 s) considerably longer than the cardiac cycle and therefore the scans show considerable motion degradation. The effect of movement may be minimized by collecting projectional data at set intervals during the cardiac cycle triggered by an ECG (it will be remembered that projections are measurements of X-ray attenuation made at many angles around the periphery of the patient).

A number of gating methods have been proposed. The most difficult type of CT machine to gate is the translate–rotate type of CT scanner because the fan of rays which are measured at any one time see only a fraction of the scan field and the detector and X-ray tube have therefore to be at the position of the traverse during the period of the cardiac cycle for which the projectional data are to be collected. A method which has been used is illustrated in Figure 5. The rotate-only type of scanner allows much more freedom in the design of gating methods:

(a) the scanner can either be synchronized to the cardiac motion so that a full set of projections (covering one complete cardiac cycle) is gathered with the heart in one position; or
(b) projectional data can be gathered asynchronously (i.e. not in any predetermined position in the cardiac cycle), together with an ECG record, and the data subsequently allotted to particular intervals in the cardiac cycle after the scan is mechanically completed.

The two basic schemes for this purpose are illustrated in Figure 5, and it can be seen that the method which synchronizes both tube output and data gathering will lead to a lower radiation dose. Good gated pictures have been obtained by workers using rotate-only machines, notably the work of Berninger *et al.*[15]. It must be remembered, however, that several complete rotations must be made to collect the projectional data required to reconstruct an image, because only during one rotation-only part of the projection can data be gathered. This is because the ECG gated interval is shorter than the scan time. Additionally, the process will have to be repeated several times to scan the whole heart, thus there may be a limit to the technique due to the radiation dose incurred by the patient. Additionally, it should be remembered that iodinated contrast has to be given throughout the examination period to allow discrimination between the heart chambers and the myocardium; therefore there may be a second limit to using this technique due to the total amount of intravenous contrast needed during the study.

The two methods described represent the fundamentally different approaches. The first, a purpose-built machine employing unique technical solutions; the second the marrying of an established method, gating used in nuclear medicine, to conventional CT scanners. A third approach is technically feasible and has been proposed[5]. A machine of the rotate-only type – with three or

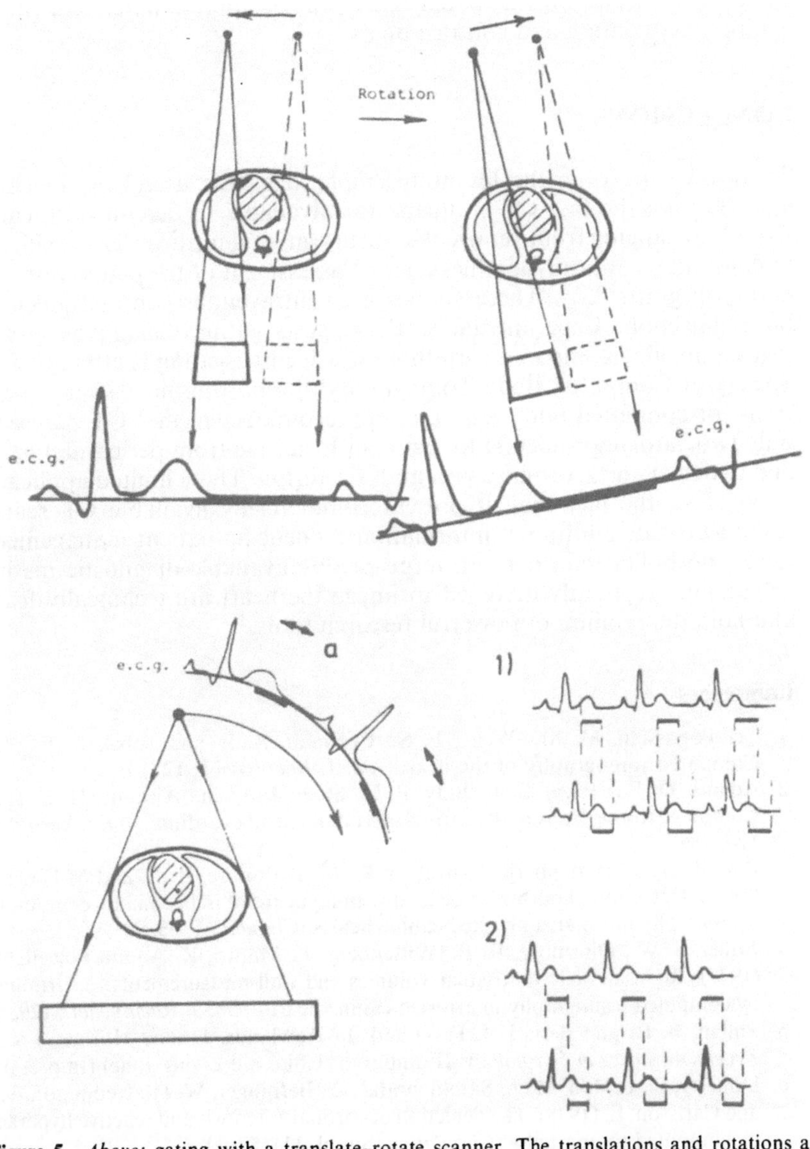

Figure 5 *Above*: gating with a translate–rotate scanner. The translations and rotations are synchronized to the heart rate such that the detectors and X-ray beam traverse the heart during diastole. *Below*: gating with a rotate-only scanner; 1 the data can be collected asynchronously leading to the overlapping of collection so that data are gathered more than once. 2 Alternatively the data can be gathered synchronously so that only the required transmission data measurements are made (after Pullan and Best[5])

four sets of detectors and the facility to record an ECG and sort the projection data into suitable time intervals – could be capable of producing clinically useful heart scans with a spatial resolution of approximately 0.4 cm with acceptable radiation and contrast doses.

CONCLUSIONS

There are reports in the literature emphasizing the usefulness of cardiac studies using the fast CT scanners now available to demonstrate cardiac pathology ranging from ventricular aneurysms and intracardiac calcification to congenital cardiomyopathies and the assessment of the patency of aorta-coronary grafts[16–18]. These studies used intravenous contrast given as a bolus injection. Experimental work suggests gating techniques give improved imaging compared with those in which no gating is attempted. The Society of Computed Body Tomography[19], reporting in 1979 new indications for computed body tomography, recommended that CT be used for only two cardiac problems: to distinguish cardiac from pericardial masses, and to detect aortacoronary vein graft occlusion. These limited applications may reflect the fact that at present commercially available CT scanners cannot provide additional information influencing patient management at lower morbidity than current, more readily available diagnostic methods. CT scanners specially designed to image the heart are technically feasible and hold the promise of powerful research tools.

References

1. Ter Pogossian, M. M., Weiss, E. S., Coleman, R. E. and Sobel, B. E. (1976). Computed tomography of the heart. *Am. J. Roentgenol.*, **127**, 79
2. Adams, D. F., Hessel, S. J., Judy, P. F., Stein, J. A. and Abrams, H. L. (1976). Computed tomography of the normal and infarcted myocardium. *Am. J. Roentgenol.*, **126**, 786
3. Powell, W. J., Wittenberg, J., Maturi, R. A., Dinsmore, R. E. and Miller, S. W. (1977). Detection of edema associated with myocardial ischaemia by computerized tomography in isolated arrested canine hearts. *Circulation*, **55**, 99
4. Miller, S. W., Dinsmore, R. E., Wittenberg, J., Maturi, R. A. and Powell, W. J. (1977). Right and left ventricular volumes and wall measurements: determination by computed tomography in arrested canine hearts. *Am. J. Roentgenol.*, **129**, 257
5. Pullan, B. R. and Best, J. J. K. (1980). In Rowlands, D. and Horner, J. (eds.). *Recent Advances in Cardiology*. (Edinburgh: Churchill Livingstone) (In press)
6. Doherty, P., Lipton, M. J., Skioldebrand, C., Berninger, W. H., Redington, R. W. and Carlsson, E. (1978). The detection of coronary stenosis and reactive hyperaemia by computed tomography. *Circulation* (Suppl. 11), **58**, 11
7. Ritman, E. L. (1977). Quantitative transaxial imaging of the heart. *Eur. J. Cardiol.*, **5**, 203
8. Brooks, R. A. and Di Chiro, G. (1976a). Principles of computer assisted tomography (CAT) in radiographic and radioisotope imaging. *Phys. Med. Biol.*, **21**, 689
9. Pullan, B. R., Rutherford, R. A. and Isherwood, I. (1976). Computerised transaxial tomography. In *Medical Images: Formation, perception and Measurement*, pp. 20–38. (London: The Institute of Physics/Wiley)

10. Tretiak, O. J. (1978). Noise limitations in X-ray computed tomography. *J. Comput. Assist. Tomogr.*, **2,** 477
11. Ritman, E. L., Robb, R. A., Johnson, S. A., Chevalier, P. A., Gilbert, B. K., Greenleaf, J. F., Sturm, R. E. and Wood, E. H. (1978). Quantitative imaging of the structure and function of the heart, lungs, and circulation. *Mayo Clin. Proc.*, **53,** 3
12. Ritman, E. L., Kinsey, J. H., Robb, R. A., Harris, L. D. and Gilbert, B. K. (1980). Physics and technical considerations in the design of the D.S.R.: a high temporal resolution volume scanner. *Am. J. Roentgenol.*, **134,** 369
13. Robb, R. A. and Ritman, E. L. (1979). High speed synchronous volume computed tomography of the heart. *Radiology*, **133,** 655
14. Wood, E. H. (1977). New vistas for the study of structural and functional dynamics of the heart, lungs and circulation by non-invasive numerical tomographic vivisection. *Circulation*, **56,** 506
15. Berninger, W. H., Redington, R. W., Doherty, P., Lipton, M. J. and Carlsson, E. (1979). Gated cardiac scanning: canine studies. *J. Comput. Assist. Tomogr.*, **3,** 155
16. Guthaner, D. F., Wexler, L. and Harell, G. (1979). C.T. demonstration of cardiac structures. *Am. J. Roentgenol.*, **133,** 75
17. Guthaner, D. F., Brody, W. R., Ricci, M., Oyer, P. E. and Wexler, L. (1980). The use of computed tomography in the diagnosis of coronary artery bypass graft patency. *Cardiovasc. Intervent. Radiol.*, **3,** 3
18. Vasile, N., Ferrane, J., Le Cudonnec, B., Casasoprana, A. and Vernant, P. (1979). On the computer tomographic diagnostic evaluation of certain congenital cardiopathies in children and adolescents. Preliminary report. *Electromedica*, **4,** 157
19. The Society for Computed Body Tomography (1979). New indications for computed body tomography – special report. *Am. J. Roentgenol.*, **133,** 115

14
Nuclear imaging techniques in cardiology and cardiac surgery

Part 1 Static imaging and myocardial blood flow

D. S. DYMOND

INTRODUCTION

The 'nuclear cardiologist' has taken his place alongside the 'electrophysiologist' and the 'echocardiographer', as a specialist within a specialty. Unlike electrophysiology or echocardiography, nuclear cardiology has evolved from the successful liaison between the disciplines of cardiology and nuclear medicine, and the ready application of the unique properties of radionuclides to the study of heart disease. Despite the rapid advances in imaging techniques, the limitations of currently available imaging devices and radionuclides do impose restrictions on the quantity and quality of information that can be gained from a nuclear test. The purpose of this chapter is to review the state of the art at present and to outline how radionuclide tests can be applied to patients undergoing cardiac surgery. The advantages and limitations of these tests will be discussed, as well as some aims for the future.

WHAT IS A RADIOISOTOPE?

At the present time there are known to be 105 distinct chemical elements, each of which exists in a number of forms known as isotopes. Isotopes of an element possess the same number of charged particles, or protons, in the nucleus, but differ in the number of uncharged particles, or neutrons. The combined number of protons and neutrons in the nucleus is the 'mass number' used to identify a given isotope. For example, thallium-201 is the radioisotope of thallium with 201 protons and neutrons in the atomic nucleus.

Many isotopes are radioactive, emitting radiation as they decay spontaneously from an unstable to a more stable configuration. Instability is itself brought about by a surplus or a deficiency of neutrons. Only very few of the known radioisotopes are stable and most are created artificially in cyclotrons or reactors. Some, such as technetium-99m, do not occur naturally in any form and are made synthetically.

Emission of radioactivity is a nuclear process and there are three types of radiation:

(1) alpha radiation, in which a particle consisting of two protons and two neutrons is ejected from the nucleus;
(2) beta, in which an electron is emitted;
(3) gamma, in which an electrically neutral photon or gamma ray is emitted.

Radiation from internally deposited alpha- and beta-emitting agents is easily absorbed in tissue and is poorly detected externally. In addition their absorption leads to a high radiation dose to the patient. Some agents, such as ^{43}K, formerly used in myocardial perfusion scintigraphy[1] are exclusive beta-emitters. Almost all nuclear medicine investigations today employ gamma-emitting radionuclides, since most gamma rays will escape from the body and can be detected, as well as being less harmful.

Any radioisotope or radionuclide has a characteristic physical property known as a half-life, which is the time taken for half the atoms present originally to decay. Thus after one half-life, the amount of radioactivity present (measured in Becquerels, Bq, which is one disintegration per second) will be one-half of the initial value. In the body the actual half-life is shorter than *in vitro* as the rate of disappearance of radioactivity depends on the rate of metabolism or excretion of the radionuclide as well as on its physical half-life. *In vivo* the time for radioactivity to fall by half is known as the biological half-life. Radionuclides with short half-lives are used where possible to reduce the radiation dose to the patient.

A radioisotope can be administered either in its unbound form, or bound to a chemical which localizes in a particular organ or organs. Thus unbound technetium-99m as pertechnetate may be used for first-pass radionuclide ventriculography (next chapter), and technetium bound to pyrophosphate is used for imaging infarcted myocardium.

The energy of radiation, usually expressed in kiloelectron volts (keV) also dictates the clinical usefulness of an agent. Medium-energy isotopes such as technetium-99m with an energy of 140 keV are more suitable for imaging with currently available gamma cameras than the high-energy agents which produce distorted images.

IMAGING EQUIPMENT

The invention of the scintillation camera, or gamma camera, by Hal Anger in 1958[2] was a major breakthrough in the detection of emitted radiation. For the first time an image of tracer distribution as a function of time within an organ was possible, following intravenous administration of that tracer. Prior to this, passage of radioactivity through an organ could only be seen in the form of curves with no anatomical detail. The gamma camera detector itself is a large single crystal of thallium-activated sodium iodide, some 50 cm in diameter and 1 cm thick. Since gamma rays cannot be focused, the field of view of the instrument is defined by a collimator, a block of lead with many (up to 60000) holes drilled through it placed in front of the crystal. Gamma photons passing through the collimator interact with the crystal which gives out a flash of light. The light is collected by an array of photomultiplier tubes mounted on the back of the crystal which yield electrical signals used to calculate the point in the crystal at which the gamma photon was incident. For each photon detected, a dot is displayed momentarily at the corresponding position on an oscilloscope display. The image, typically formed from 300000 to 500000 dots, is obtained by taking a continuous-exposure photograph of the display on either polaroid or X-ray film. The image information can be digitized and analysed by computer, so that regional count rates can be quantified, image enhancement may be performed and data can be manipulated arithmetically. Many gamma cameras available today come with dedicated digital computers.

IMAGING OF THE ACUTELY INFARCTED MYOCARDIUM

The idea of producing images of the infarcted myocardium was attractive to investigators as long ago as 1960, and several imaging agents were used with limited success[3-5]. With the expansion of coronary-care units interest has again been shown in radioisotopic methods for diagnosing acute myocardial infarction. There are two main ways of imaging infarction. Firstly, by administration of a radionuclide which accumulates only in infarcted tissue, not in healthy myocardium; and secondly by means of radionuclides which localize only in healthy muscle, not ischaemic or necrotic tissue.

'Cold spot' scanning

In the latter method, infarcted myocardium is visualized in the image as an area of decreased or absent tracer uptake in the region of the infarct, the so-called 'cold spot' image. Agents such as caesium-129 (ref. 6) and rubidium-81 (ref. 7) have been replaced by the newer potassium analogue, thallium-201 There is little doubt that thallium scintigraphy performed at rest has a high sensitivity for the detection and localization of transmural myocardial infarction manifest by electrocardiographic Q waves[8 10], regardless of whether the infarct is new or old. Defects in thallium uptake occur in the first few hours after the event[8] and the use of thallium scintigraphy as an early test for acute infarction has been suggested. However, as thallium is distributed in the myocardium in proportion to myocardial perfusion, the presence of a defect does not necessarily indicate infarction but possibly ischaemia. The presence of a defect also does not solely imply a recent ischaemic event, as prior myocardial infarction will also produce a permanent perfusion defect on the image. Another major disadvantage of the technique is that smaller defects such as those due to subendocardial infarction will be inconsistently detected. Mueller *et al.*[11] have previously defined a range of perfusion defects in dogs that may be identified, and they concluded that a perfusion decrease of 40% compared to normal myocardium was necessary, or an equivalent of 6 g of myocardium should be ischaemic, to allow consistent identification of abnormalities. It is quite probable that in man the scintigrams will be even less sensitive, due to the lower relative dose of thallium administered, and the difference in chest configuration which necessitates a greater distance between camera and left ventricle. There is therefore little place for the resting thallium scan in the diagnosis of acute myocardial infarction, although if prior myocardial infarction can be excluded, the method may be of value in helping to decide whether or not a patient's chest pain is due to ischamia early after the onset of symptoms.

Infarct-avid agents

Techniques involving radionuclides which accumulate only in acutely infarcted myocardium have grown in popularity over the last 5 years since the demonstration that organic phosphates labelled with technetium-99m localize in acutely necrotic myocardial cells[12,13]. The radionuclides have been used in clinical nuclear medicine for many years as bone-scanning agents[14], because of their high affinity for calcium. The mechanism of phosphate localization in the infarct is still not clear. It has been postulated that in the mitochrondria of necrotic cells calcium ions localize in a crystalline structure like hydroxyapatite[15], and that the phosphate moiety binds with the calcium[16]. Phagocytosis of technetium-99m by leukocytes migrating towards the infarct has been suggested as an alternative mechanism, although the animal experiments of Coleman *et al.*[17] refute this.

Whatever the precise mechanism, it is clear that the agents concentrate selectively in acutely necrotic myocardium irrespective of the cause of that necrosis. The most widely used of the agents has been technetium-99m–stannous pyrophosphate. Clinical experience has shown that scintigrams are not usually positive until 12 h after the infarction and the optimal imaging time is between 24 and 72 h after the pain. There is considerable temporal variation in the evolutionary patterns of the scintigraphic abnormalities and a negative scan 12–24 h after suspected infarction should be repeated 48–72 h after the event before being firmly classed as negative. The imaging protocol demands that scanning should be performed 2 h after intravenous administration of 10–15 mCi of the tracer, the time lapse being necessary for clearance of the tracer from the blood pool. Images performed earlier than 2 h after the injection of the isotope may be contaminated by the persistence of the isotope within the cardiac blood pool, and the image may be misinterpreted. Images performed later than 2 h may be difficult to interpret because of increasing activity in bony structures. Scans are usually performed in the antero-posterior, left anterior oblique and left lateral projection. The conventional method for grading scans is on a scale of 0–4, as described by Parkey *et al.*[12]. Figure 1 is an example of the five grades of scan with grades 0 and 1 considered

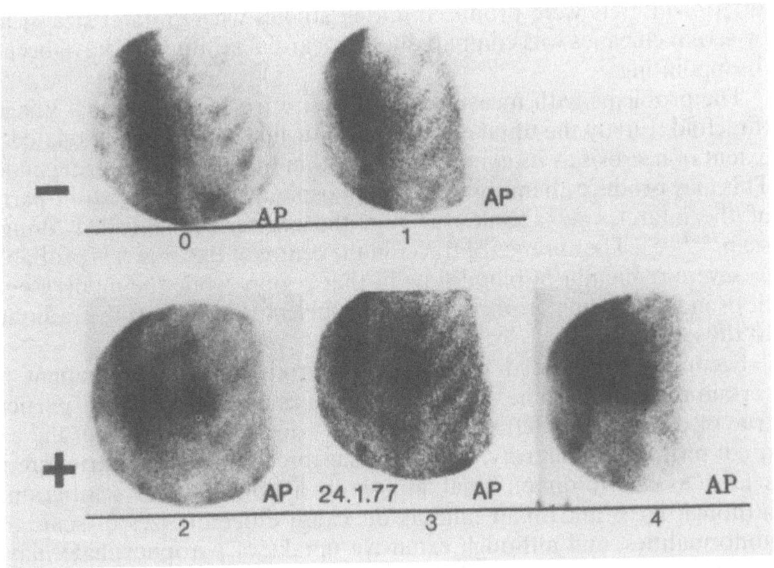

Figure 1 Examples of the five grades of pyrophosphate scan. Grades 0 and 1 are negative, grade 0 showing no myocardial uptake and grade 1 showing questionable uptake. Grades 2–4 are positive, with increasing densities of tracer uptake in the myocardium. All scans are anteroposterior (Reproduced from *Postgrad. Med. J.*[20] by permission of the publisher)

negative and grades 2–4 positive. The 2–4 grades represent increasing density of scan. Sternal and rib uptake is seen in each case. Infarct scintigrams should be interpreted by experienced observers familiar with the evolutionary patterns of scintigraphic abnormalities.

Transmural infarction

Acute transmural infarction can be detected and localized with this technique in more than 90% of cases[18-20], provided that imaging is carried out neither too early nor too late. The latest after an infarct that a positive scan may be obtained is uncertain, although in general scans tend to become negative at about 7 days[12] after the event. If detection of an infarct is all that is required by an investigator, there is little to be gained by carrying out a scintigram if the electrocardiogram and cardiac enzymes show typical evolutionary changes. Measurements of cardiac isoenzyme levels such as MB–CPK, if carried out at the appropriate time, are as sensitive as the infarct scintigram for the detection of acute infarction[17] but the scan is particularly valuable where the electrocardiogram contains prior abnormalities such as left bundle branch block[21] or ventricular paced complexes.

Sizing transmural infarction

Experimental studies in dogs have shown that the size of a scintigraphic abnormality does correlate with the size of the infarct[22-24], but in all cases anterior infarcts were produced. Other studies where infarct size measured by serum enzymes was compared to myocardial scintigrams have been more disappointing[25].

The problems with measuring infarct size from conventional images are threefold. Firstly the uptake of the radionuclide is not directly related to the extent of necrosis as its concentration within the infarct is flow dependent[26]. This may produce an image with pyrophosphate uptake only at the periphery of the infarct, and absent tracer in the centre, the so-called 'doughnut' scan[16,20,27]. The absence of tracer in the centre of the infarct is probably due to severe reduction of blood flow in that region, while the moderate reductions in flow at the periphery are still sufficient to transport the radionuclide to those areas.

Secondly, the limited resolution of current imaging equipment makes certain regions of the heart difficult to image accurately. This is particularly true of the posterior left ventricular wall which is farthest from the camera in all projections. Thirdly, the heart is a three-dimensional structure represented as a two-dimensional image on a conventional scintigram, and although large and small infarcts do cause different sizes of scintigraphic abnormalities, and although extensive uptake of pyrophosphate may have prognostic significance (see below), it is unlikely that an *accurate* size of an infarct can be obtained with pyrophosphate scans *in vivo*. The measurement of infarct size will be further discussed later in this chapter under the section on three-dimensional imaging.

Prognostic significance of pyrophosphate scans

Apart from the purely diagnostic value of the phosphate scans, several workers have attempted to glean information of prognostic value from the data. This has become increasingly investigated as active therapy to limit infarct size has developed[28]. Holman *et al.*[29] have recently reported that patients with large areas of pyrophosphate uptake have a greater incidence of complications both in hospital and after discharge. Complications described were cardiogenic shock, ventricular tachycardia, extension of infarction, unstable angina and sudden death. Rude *et al.*[27] have also recently reported the relationship between the 'doughnut' appearance and the incidence of left ventricular failure: 67% of patients with a doughnut pattern developed left ventricular failure, compared to 35% of patients with similar locations of infarcts but homogeneous radionuclide uptake. A persistently positive scintigram weeks or months following the acute infarct, in the absence of suspected re-infarction, suggests that the infarction was large and that the patient is at risk from developing cardiac failure[30].

Subendocardial infarction

Non-transmural, or subendocardial infarction is difficult to diagnose from electrocardiograms alone given the non-specific nature of ST segment and T wave changes and the difficulty in differentiating between acute ischaemia and infarction without Q waves electrocardiographically. The only evolution of the abnormal pattern is for depressed ST segments to return to baseline and the T waves to become upright over a period of days to weeks after the event. Occasionally no evolutionary changes occur. Cardiac enzymes are relied upon to substantiate the diagnosis but the levels may be equivocal. Pyrophosphate scintigraphy has been reported as highly successful by some workers in the detection of infarction[20,31] but others have found results disappointing[32]. The pattern of uptake usually differs from that found in transmural infarction inasmuch as it is not always possible to locate the infarction, rather the pattern of uptake of pyrophosphate is more diffuse and less intense. The problem here is that the diffuse pattern of uptake is not specific for subendocardial infarction, occurring in a wide variety of conditions from left ventricular aneurysms to calcified heart valves. In a comprehensive review of the current status of the pyrophosphate scan, Marcus and Kerber discuss the problems of lack of specificity of this pattern[33] and also of the localized pattern.

Unstable angina

Several reports have appeared of a high incidence of positive scans in patients with the unstable angina syndrome[19,20,32,34]. The incidence of positive scans ranges from 35 % to 100 % of cases, and the diffuse pattern of uptake is seen similar to that in non-transmural infarction. The question arose as to whether such patients have in fact sustained small areas of necrosis undetectable by other means, or whether ischaemic, non-necrotic cells take up the radionuclide. The current body of evidence would suggest that a positive scan indicates necrosis, not ischaemia[16,17,33]. It thus appears that unstable angina and non-transmural infarction may in fact be a confluent syndrome of necrosis with the difference being the presence or absence of abnormal cardiac enzymes. Unstable angina is often recognized as a medical emergency and many patients are treated by myocardial revascularization either as an emergency or after a 'cooling off' period of bed rest and medical therapy. It is not currently known whether the presence or absence of a positive pyrophosphate scan has prognostic significance in the outcome or risks of surgery in these patients, and investigation in this area is clearly necessary.

Perioperative infarction

The incidence of perioperative myocardial infarction following coronary artery saphenous vein bypass grafting has been an elusive statistic, primarily because of the difficulty in making the diagnosis. Chest pain, electrocardiographic changes and enzyme elevations may all result from the surgical procedure itself. Most data have been gathered from inspection of postoperative electrocardiograms and based on these the incidence of perioperative infarction has been reported as between 7 % and 40 %[35-37]. Only new Q waves are of value in the postoperative electrocardiogram, and conventional serum enzymes are of no value. Although the isoenzyme MB–CPK has been reported as reflecting only myocardial damage following bypass surgery[38], other reports contradict this belief[20,39,40]. The technetium-99m pyrophosphate scan is of major value in diagnosing perioperative infarction[21,39-41], provided two precautions are taken. Firstly, a preoperative scintigram should be available for comparison because some patients will have preoperative positive scintigrams[41] especially those with unstable angina. Secondly, because MB–CPK may be elevated in uncomplicated cardiac surgery, and electrocardiographic abnormalities may be non-specific, a postoperative scintigram could conceivably be positive for other reasons apart from perioperative infarction, for example repeated intraoperative defibrillations[33]. Thus the scans should, as always, be interpreted in the light of the entire clinical picture. Platt *et al.*[41] have compared two different operative techniques for myocardial revascularization and the perioperative infarction rate for each technique. Patients in whom the left ventricle was routinely vented, and in whom no aortic cross-clamping was used but haemostasis achieved with silastic tapes around the coronary arteries, had an infarction rate of 31 % scintigraphically. Another group of patients, who had no venting, aortic cross-clamping and left atrial pressure monitoring, had a 14 % infarction rate. Although the results of that particular study are not conclusive, the point is well made that modifications of surgical technique may well be shown to be beneficial or otherwise by use of the radionuclide technique. Figures 2 and 3 illustrate how the scintigram can help in a situation where the electrocardiogram may not. Figures 2a and 2b are pre- and postoperative electrocardiograms from a patient undergoing revascularization who was hypotensive postoperatively. The preoperative trace shows some inferior S–T segment and T wave changes, and the postoperative trace generalized non-specific changes of the S–T segments and T waves. Figures 3a and 3b are anteroposterior pyrophosphate scans taken pre- and postoperatively. It is evident that whereas no uptake in the myocardium was seen prior to surgery, the postoperative scan shows marked accumulation over the heart, indicating perioperative infarction.

One of the major advances in the application of scintigraphy to acutely ill, immobile patients has been the development of mobile gamma cameras enabling imaging to be carried out at the bedside[20]. Whereas most patients with infarcts in the non-surgical environment will be able to be moved to a nuclear medicine department 3 or 4 days after the event, this may not be so for surgical patients attached to a substantial amount of monitoring equipment. Figure 4 shows an example of a portable gamma camera in use on a ward.

Summary

Table 1 summarizes the current role of the pyrophosphate scan in clinical practice. In the majority of patients admitted to a coronary care unit, conventional electrocardiographic and enzyme testing will suffice to make a diagnosis. In the situations listed in Table 1 the scan may be helpful. The future of infarct imaging with phosphates will probably depend on its potential as a screening test, now that agents are available which can provide positive scans within the first few hours of infarction[42]. Work on agents which are independent of blood flow for delivery to the infarct, such as cardiac myosin specific antibodies[43] or neutrally charged liposomes[44],

Table 1 Defined role of the phosphate scan

History not available or unreliable
Infarcts 3 to 10 days old
Equivocal or unreliable enzymes
ECG conduction defects or ventricular paced complexes
Perioperative infarction
Myocardial contusion
Right ventricular infarcts

(or labelled white blood cells) has been promising. The role of three-dimensional imaging will be discussed later.

ASSESSMENT OF MYOCARDIAL PERFUSION

In the clinical and investigative study of coronary artery disease, an assessment of blood flow and perfusion to individual myocardial zones is very important. In the clinical setting, the use of non-invasive radioisotope techniques has enabled the visualization of areas of underperfused myocardium at rest and exercise, and perfusion scintigraphy now plays a significant part in the assessment of patients with chest pain, the physiological assessment of abnormal coronary anatomy, and the effects of surgical interventions on myocardial perfusion. The invasive methods employing intracoronary injection of radiotracers or the continuous infusion into the aortic sinuses, are less widely applicable but nevertheless important.

NON-INVASIVE MYOCARDIAL PERFUSION SCANNING

In the past, intravenously administered radionuclides such as potassium-43 (ref. 1), caesium-129 (ref. 6) and rubidium-81 (ref. 7) have been used to identify areas of infarcted myocardium and zones of transient ischaemia. Readers of articles on perfusion scintigraphy will be aware that these agents have largely been superseded by thallium-201 as the most widely used radiopharmaceutical for imaging the myocardium. Thallium is an analogue of potassium, and is distributed in myocardial cells in exchange with intracellular potassium. The principle of Sapirstein[45] dictates that regional concentration of tracer within an organ after intravenous injection of that tracer is directly proportional to regional blood flow.

Thallium-201

Thallium-201 is a monovalent cation which decays with the emission of abundant X-rays of low energy and few photons of medium energy. The energy spectrum of thallium is less than optimal but it may effectively be imaged with a gamma camera. It is superior as an imaging agent to ^{43}potassium, as it does not produce harmful beta radiation and in comparison to

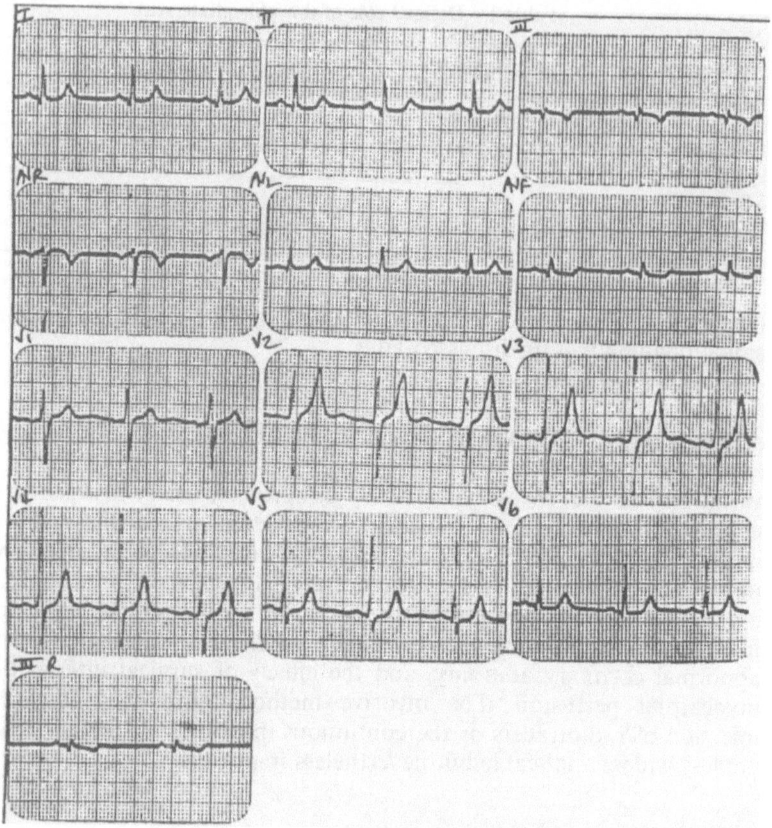

Figure 2 (a) Preoperative ECG of a patient undergoing saphenous vein graft surgery. There are inferior ST segment and T wave changes. (b) Postoperative ECG of the same patient. There are generalized ST segment and T wave changes of a non-specific nature (Reproduced from *Postgrad. Med. J.*[20] by permission of the publisher)

other potassium analogues it has a higher myocardial extraction efficiency than caesium, and appears to concentrate to a greater degree in the myocardium and less in the liver than rubidium[46]. This is advantageous in imaging the inferior regions of the left ventricle. Between 2 and 5% of the administered dose concentrates initially in the myocardium, the actual concentration depending on the rate of turnover in the myocardial cells. The half-life of thallium-201 is 73 h. This gives it an adequate shelf-life, and means that it is not necessary for it to be produced by an on-site cyclotron like many short half-life radioisotopes. It does mean that a long time (up to a week) is required between sequential studies in the same patient. The myocardial half-life is longer than that of potassium, and myocardial imaging may be performed up to 1 h after intravenous administration and still reflect myocardial perfusion at the time of injection[47]. The problem of redistribution will be discussed below.

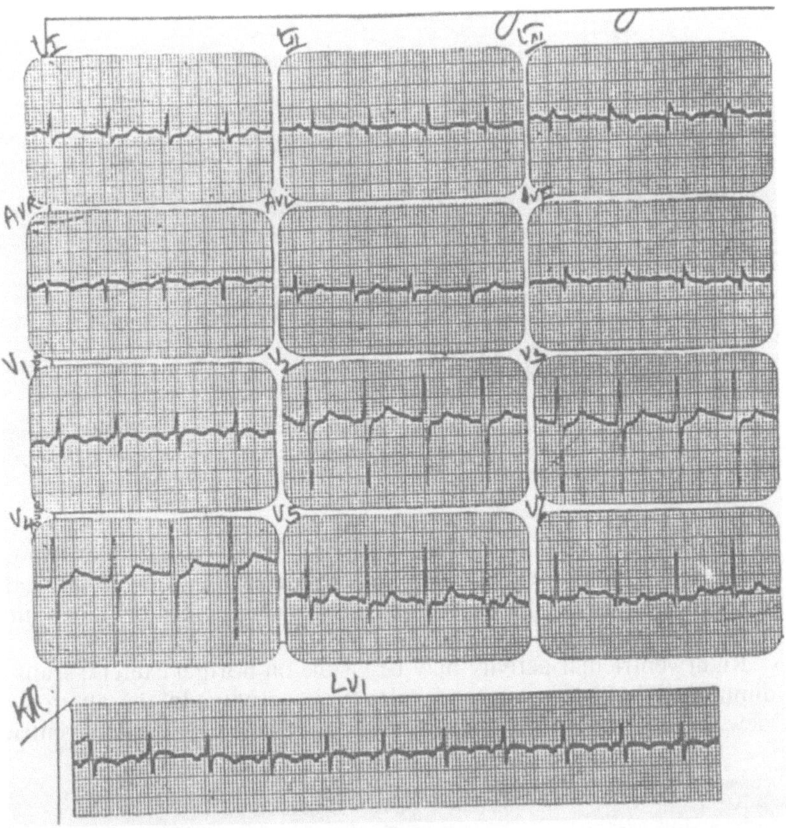

Factors influencing thallium distribution in the heart

The distribution of thallium-201 after injection is dependent both on coronary blood flow and cellular extraction. Under conditions of normal blood flow and of coronary occlusion regional thallium distribution correlates extremely well with radioactive microsphere distribution as an indicator of blood flow[46]. The extraction efficiency of thallium by the heart is 85–90 %[48] and is dependent on an intact sodium–potassium–ATPase system in the cell membranes. Hypoxia may reduce cellular extraction[48] and drugs such as porpranolol and digitalis may also reduce its extraction[49].

The normal image

The normal thallium-201 scintigram shows a relatively homogeneous image representing left ventricular tracer distribution in the shape of a horseshoe surrounding the left ventricular cavity which itself is nearly devoid of tracer. In a resting image, right ventricular activity is not usually seen, as the right ventricular myocardium is thinner and has a lower blood supply. Similarly

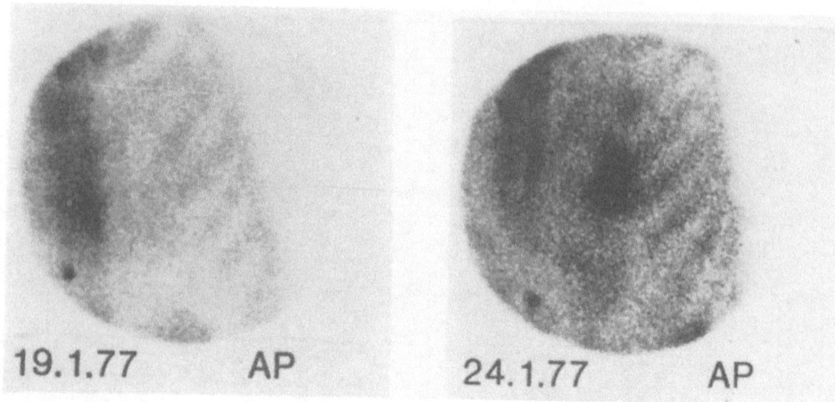

Figure 3 (a) Preoperative technetium-99m pyrophosphate scan in same patient. No myocardial uptake is seen. (b) Postoperative scan shows intense tracer accumulation in the myocardium (Reproduced from *Postgrad. Med. J.*[20] by permission of the publisher)

atria are rarely seen. The right ventricle may be well seen on the resting scintigrams of patients with pulmonary hypertension, and measured right ventricular free wall thickness is a more sensitive index of right ventricular hypertrophy than the electrocardiogram[50].

Right ventricular activity may be visible on normal exercise scans due to diminished lung, hepatic, and splanchnic activity. In the anteroposterior view, the anterolateral, apical and inferior walls of the left ventricle are

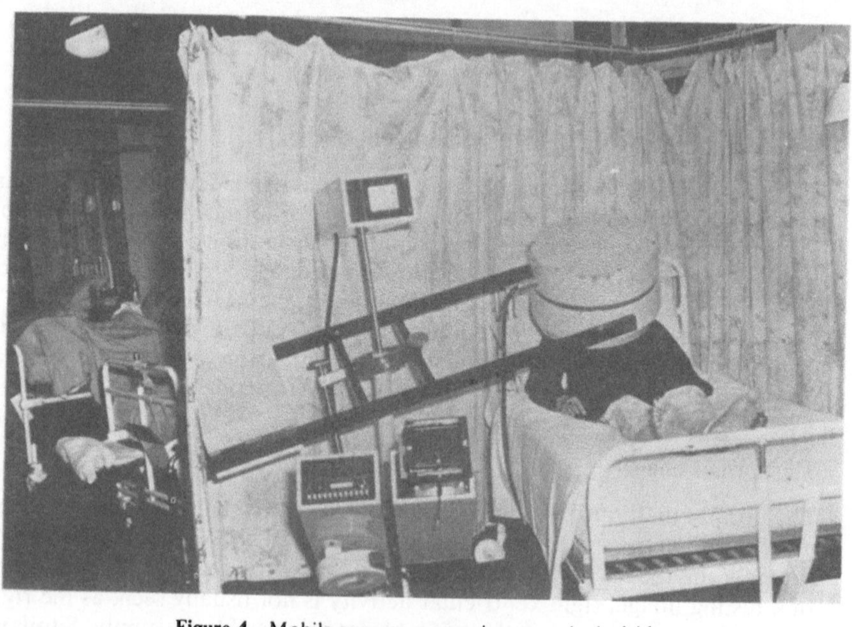

Figure 4 Mobile gamma camera in use at the bedside

visualized. The apex may appear to contain less activity than the rest of the ventricle due to anatomic thinning in that region. In the 45° left anterior oblique, the septum, apex, and posterolateral segments are seen and in the left lateral view the anterior wall, apex, inferior, and posterior walls are identified. Figure 5 shows in diagrammatic form the appearances of the left ventricle in the various views and their scintigraphic counterparts. Most centres image thallium distribution in four projections, a 30° or 55° left anterior oblique view being added to the above three. It is extremely important to obtain multiple projections of a perfusion scintigram to obtain as

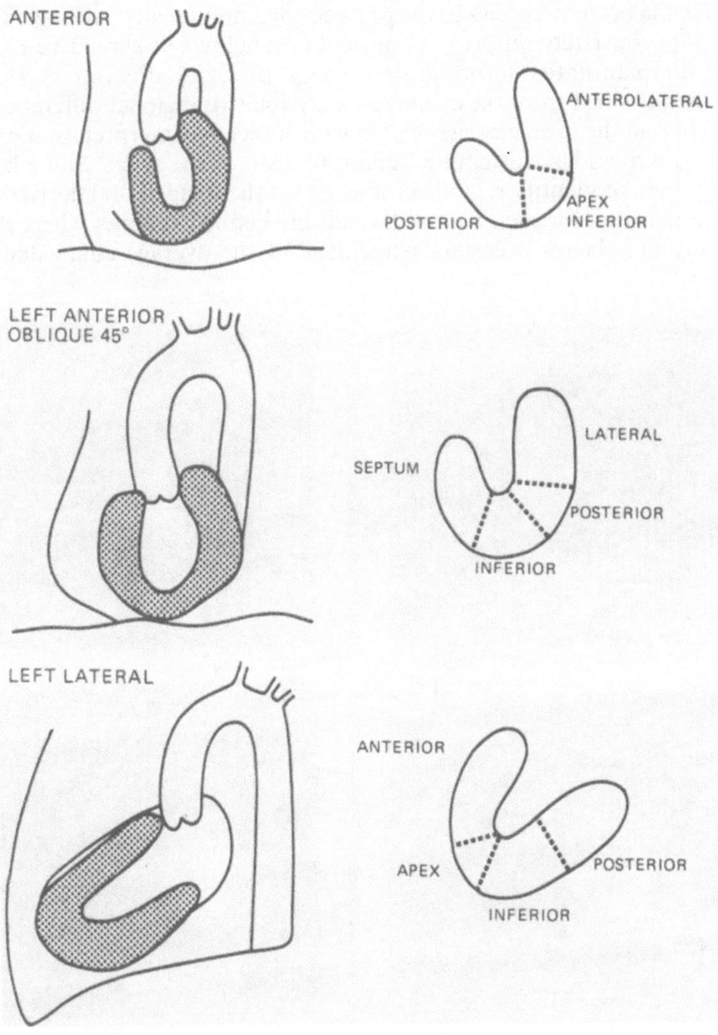

Figure 5 Diagrams of the different views utilized in perfusion scintigraphy. The different zones of the left ventricle imaged in each projection are shown

much segmental information as possible. Figure 6 is an example of a normal perfusion scintigram in anteroposterior, 30° and 50° left anterior oblique, and left lateral projections. Homogeneous thallium distribution is apparent in all cases.

Like many images in nuclear medicine, interpretation is based on pattern recognition by trained observers, and as such the observer of a scintigram can only interpret what his or her eye sees. The recognition of a perfusion defect on a thallium scan is dependent upon the perception of one or more areas of the image that appear to contain less radioactivity than another area. In other words, it is relative differences that make an image appear abnormal. This has great relevance in clinical practice, as situations where global ischaemia occur may lead to the presence of a homogeneous image which can be inappropriately reported as normal (see below). It should be recognized that no quantitative information on total or regional coronary blood flow can be obtained from these images: only relative regional differences.

To avoid the problems associated with subjective interpretation of images, several writers have attempted quantification of the scans. Some have used computers to identify regions of interest on the images, and derived average count densities for each region. Defects are defined as zones where the count density falls below a certain percentage of the average count density[51,52]

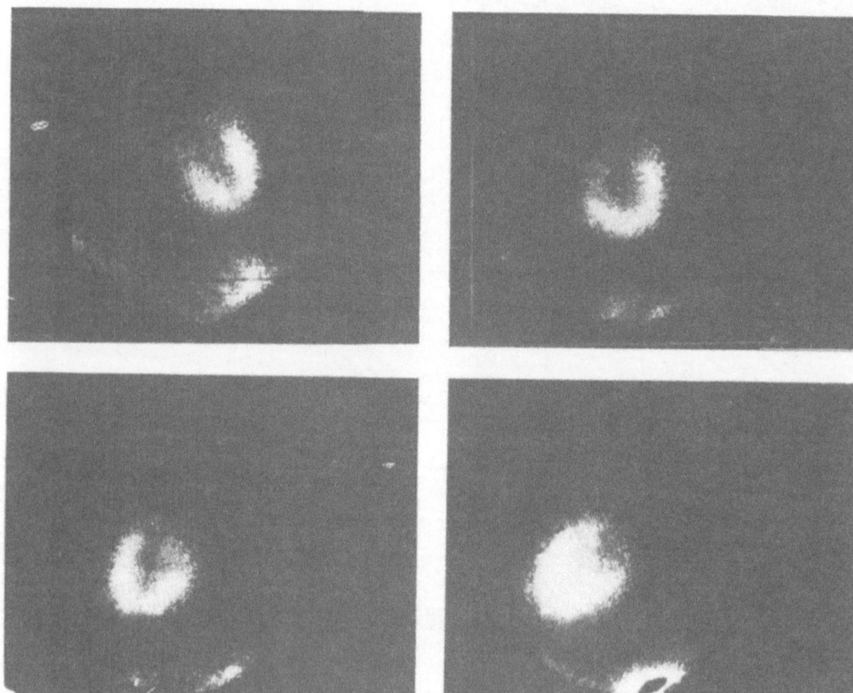

Figure 6 Examples of normal thallium-201 scans in anteroposterior, 30° and 50° left anterior obliques and left lateral projections. Homogeneity of tracer distribution is apparent in all cases

although there is no firm agreement on what count levels should be deemed abnormal. Others[53] have obtained count profiles from digitized images by dividing the myocardium into seven areas or cells with an electronic light pen. A range of normal counts per cell may then be obtained, and the differences between the counts in one cell and the average for the whole image may be quantified. Defects can be objectively defined therefore.

Figure 7 shows a normal anteroposterior and left anterior oblique scan with computer-generated 70% isocount contours superimposed, to illustrate how quantification may be achieved. There are several objections to the methods used for quantification of these images. Most revolve around the problems of the contribution of background non-cardiac radioactivity, and

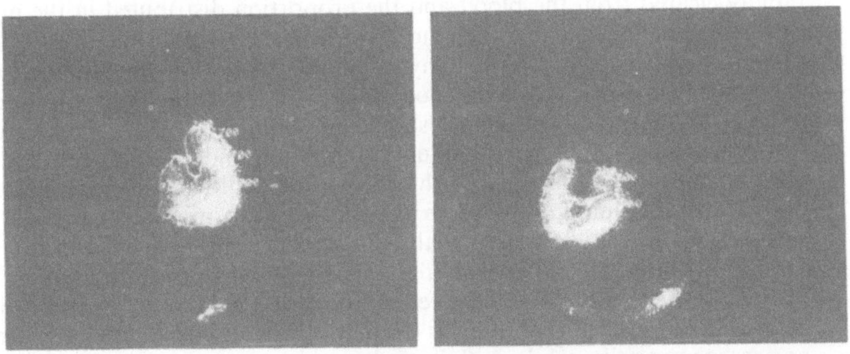

(a) (b)

Figure 7 Normal anteroposterior (a) and left oblique (b) thallium-201 scans with the 70% isocount contour superimposed. This is one of the methods used to quantify tracer distribution

the problems associated with the representation of a three-dimensional structure like the heart as a two-dimensional image. Counts emitted from the posterior left ventricle are overlain by more anterior counts, and the posterior counts are subjected to more attenuation of their energy than anterior counts as the distance from source to detector is longer. At best our attempts to quantify thallium scintigrams are crude, and some experienced workers rely wholly on visual interpretation of unprocessed data[54]. Three-dimensional imaging, discussed later, may offer a better way of quantifying thallium scans.

EXERCISE SCINTIGRAPHY IN OBSTRUCTIVE CORONARY ARTERY DISEASE

When patients with angina pectoris without myocardial infarction are imaged at rest, regional perfusion is usually normal. Viable areas of myocardium subtended by stenotic coronary arteries usually receive adequate perfusion either anterogradely or retrogradely, in the non-ischaemic state. In experimental animals, even coronary stenoses of 85% of luminal diameter failed to disturb resting coronary blood flow and regional distribution of flow[5]. However the ability to augment coronary flow in response to circulatory stress becomes increasingly poor with increasing coronary stenosis. Imaging the myocardium under stress produces an image with perfusion defects in the distribution of a coronary stenosis, whereas the corresponding rest image may be entirely normal[1,51,52,54].

A typical protocol for exercise scintigraphy involves exercising the patients on a treadmill or a bicycle ergometer until they are limited by angina, dyspnoea, fatigue, or the appearance of cardiac arrhythmias. Some workers use the attainment of 85% of the maximum predicted heart rate as the end-point: 1.5–2.0 mCi of thallium-201 are injected intravenously at the peak of exercise tolerance and the patients are encouraged to continue exercise for a further 60 s. The imaging may be carried out immediately as the thallium is very rapidly cleared from the blood and the proportion distributed in the myocardium remains virtually unchanged for at least 1 h after administration. Therefore the image reflects the physiological status at the time of injection, and imaging is carried out over about 45–60 min, while the patient is at rest. At least 200000 counts per image should be obtained.

Mechanisms of abnormal thallium distribution under stress probably involve quantitative differences in the amount of thallium being delivered to normal myocardium compared to that delivered to myocardium distal to stenoses, as well as decreased thallium extraction by ischaemic muscle[48]. Four hours later, the patients are re-imaged without further tracer administration, as the thallium will have redistributed in the myocardium over that period[56,57]. This redistribution is accomplished by loss of thallium from non-ischaemic cells, while initially ischaemic areas accumulate additional Thallium from the blood[58]. There is some experimental evidence that redistribution of thallium commences as early as 10 min after tracer injection[59], and delay in commencing imaging after the termination of exercise has been claimed to decrease the sensitivity of the technique for detecting transient ischaemia.

Most studies evaluating rest and exercise scintigraphy have demonstrated a sensitivity of 75–80% in detecting significant coronary artery disease[51,54,60–62]. A comprehensive review of the experience of all workers in this field is beyond the scope of this chapter, and the results in terms of specificity, predictive value for extent of coronary disease and localization of coronary disease are conflicting. Ritchie *et al.*[54], in a multicentre trial found the thallium scan more sensitive than the exercise electrocardiogram in identifying coronary disease, but concluded that combining the two tests further enhanced sensitivity.

Bailey *et al.*[60] concluded that the increased sensitivity of perfusion scanning compared to S–T segment depression in the electrocardiogram was due to the presence of patients with baseline electrocardiographic abnormalities and those who failed to achieve 85% of predicted maximum heart rate. The perfusion scan was particularly useful in patients with single-vessel disease. Botvinick and co-workers[61] also found the test useful in clarifying false-positive exercise tests. It is evident that the sensitivities and specificities of the scintigram will vary according to the criteria that are demanded for the diagnosis of 'significant' coronary artery disease. Botvinick *et al.*[61] demanded

75 % or more stenosis, while Ritchie *et al.*[54] utilized a 50 % luminal narrowing as significant. Reported differences in sensitivity and specificity may well be partly due to this. The higher sensitivities obtained by Murray *et al.*[62] were attributed to the semiquantitative analysis of the scans as opposed to their subjective interpretations. Figure 8a–d is an example of rest and exercise thallium scans in a patient with severe disease in circumflex and right coronary arteries. An inferior defect is apparent on exercise in the anterior–posterior scan (Figure 8a), and extensive posterolateral and apical tracer reduction is seen on the left oblique scan (8b). Resting images appear normal (Figures 8c and d).

The relation of thallium scintigrams to extent of coronary disease

It would be attractive to cardiologists if thallium scintigraphy could not only detect coronary disease but also quantify the extent of disease. It is well recognized that extent of coronary disease as judged arteriographically is closely related to patients' prognosis[63,64]. The published studies on the

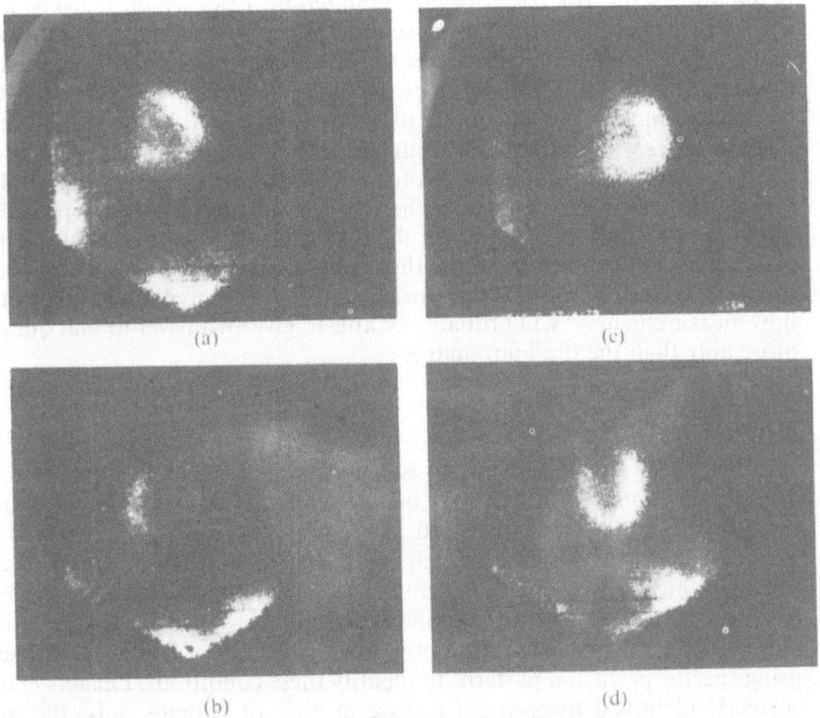

Figure 8 Exercise (a) and (b) and rest Thallium-201 scans from a patient with extensive disease in circumflex and right coronary arteries. The anteroposterior exercise scan (upper left) shows an inferior defect and the left oblique exercise scan shows tracer deficits apically and posterolaterally. The resting images (8c and d) obtained 4 hours later are normal.

ability of thallium scintigraphy to determine the extent of coronary disease give conflicting results. Several workers have concluded that although the scan may be sensitive for detecting coronary disease, it is of only limited value in quantifying the extent of disease[51,52,61,62,65,66]. Others[67] found excellent correlations between thallium scintigraphic appearances and extent of disease. The weight of evidence is against the reliability of predicting the extent of disease. In a review by McKillop *et al.*[52] the discrepancy between anatomic coronary arteriographic data and physiological perfusion scanning was attributed to the images reflecting relative, rather than absolute, reductions in myocardial blood flow. Images underestimate the extent of the abnormality either: (a) because performance is limited by ischaemia in the territory of the most abnormal vessel; or (b) more likely because the relatively greater reduction in myocardial blood flow in the territory of the most abnormal vessels causes the other areas to be interpreted as normal, despite reduction of flow in absolute terms.

Collateral vessels

Another factor which may be relevant in explaining the inaccuracies of prediction is the role of coronary collaterals. Frick *et al.*[68] using intracoronary injection of the inert gas xenon-133 found that in some patients the presence of angiographically demonstrated collateral vessels protected the myocardium from developing stress-induced hypoperfusion distal to a coronary stenosis. Not all collaterals exerted this effect, however. Two more recent studies with thallium have suggested a significant correlation between good collaterals and complete protection from ischaemia[69,70]. The role of scintigraphy in determining whether or not collateral-induced protection diminishes the necessity to revascularize a given area of heart muscle is as yet undefined. One must reiterate that only relative perfusion is indicated by the scintigram, not absolute perfusion, and quantitative myocardial blood flow measurements[68] will probably be able to give an answer to that question more ably than the thallium image.

Triple-vessel disease

In cases where global myocardial ischaemia occurs, such as in triple-vessel disease, left main stem or coronary ostial stenosis, a homogeneous image may in theory result[47,53]. As discussed in the lst section, it is unlikely that the scan can accurately predict which patients will have three-vessel disease angiographically, although abnormal scans usually occur and the presence of coronary disease may be identified. Dash *et al.*[71] found a low sensitivity (43 %) for the accurate detection of left main stenosis or triple-vessel disease using specific perfusion patterns to identify these conditions. Lenaers *et al.*[51] correctly identified three-vessel disease in 32 % of patients only, the other 68 % having patterns which suggested less extensive disease. Leppo *et al.*[72] found evidence of ischaemia in only 70 % of patients with triple-vessel disease and positive exercise electrocardiograms. This relatively low sensitivity in this particular patient group had been previously reported by Rouleau *et al.*[73], and one must conclude that thallium stress testing cannot always be relied upon to exclude *severe* coronary artery disease.

Angina at rest

Thallium scintigraphy has been shown to be of value in demonstrating the presence of myocardial ischaemia not only on exercise but also at rest. Patients with rest chest pain due to coronary spasm ('variant' angina) have been shown to develop transient ischaemia[74,75]. Although it is difficult to predict the onset of pain in this condition, the technique of perfusion scintigraphy offers a potential for proving that spontaneous chest pain has an ischaemic basis.

Wackers *et al.*[76] studied a group of patients with unstable angina in the pain-free period and found 39 % incidence of positive scans: 76 % of patients with a complicated course (who were refractory to medical treatment or who developed acute infarction) had thallium defects, compared to only 32 % of those with an uncomplicated course. The technique thus may allow recognition of a very high-risk subgroup within an already high-risk group of patients.

The assessment of coronary artery vein graft surgery

The decision whether or not to graft a particular area of myocardium is often difficult. The questions to be answered are:

(1) Is an area of myocardium viable enough to warrant revascularization, or is it dead?
(2) Is a given angiographically demonstrated stenosis contributing to angina pectoris.

The first question may be readily answered, as the demonstration that an area of myocardium fails to take up thallium at rest or on exercise nearly always indicates infarcted myocardium with little or no viable tissue. Revascularization of that area is not likely to be profitable. There are exceptions to that rule, as has been discussed under the section on unstable angina, where resting perfusion defects may indicate severe continuing ischaemia. The question as to whether a stenosis is significant is not so easy. In single-vessel disease, one can relate stenosis to tracer deficit easily enough, but in multivessel disease, when relative hypofusion will only be apparent in the most ischaemic zones, such a 'cause and effect' conclusion cannot be drawn. This problem has been previously discussed at length.

Following surgery, as many as 20 % of patients may require re-investigation to evaluate recurrent or persistent chest pain, which often is non-cardiac in origin or musculoskeletal. Relief of pain after revascularization is positively related to graft patency[35] but there remains the possibility that the closure of grafts does not necessarily cause pain[77]. Exercise stress-testing may be unreliable, as significant increases in the pressure-rate double product have been reported after surgery, even in the presence of total graft occlusions[78].

Several studies have shown the value of exercise thallium-201 scintigraphy for the detection of impairment in regional perfusion following surgery and in the non-invasive demonstration of graft closure[53,54,72,79,80]. One study[80] has suggested a modification of surgical technique, based on the scintigraphic findings of relative ischaemia in the distribution of angiographically normal diagonal branches of the left anterior descending artery when grafts to the main anterior descending artery were patent. It is proposed that large diagonal arteries should receive independent grafts even though they appear unobstructed. Figure 9 is an example of rest and exercise perfusion scans in a patient with recurrent symptoms 1 year after a saphenous vein graft to his right coronary artery. It is evident that an infero-apical defect is present on exercise. Figure 9c shows a severe stenosis in the graft. An uncontroversial use of this test is in the assessment and follow-up of grafted patients.

Anomalous coronary arteries

Congenital anomalies of the coronary arteries are among the rarest of cardiac conditions that may have practical significance. A variety of syndromes, from angina pectoris to sudden death, may be associated with abnormal origin of one or more coronary arteries[81]. Thallium-201 perfusion scintigraphy has been applied to the diagnosis of anomalous left coronary artery in the young[82] and in the serial assessment of myocardial perfusion in cases where the left coronary artery arises from the pulmonary artery[83]. Recently, we have described the presence of an exercise-induced anterior perfusion defect in a patient with congenital atresia of the left main coronary artery, and the abolition of that defect after coronary artery surgery[84]. Figure 10(a) and (b) shows exercise and rest scans from this patient, with a frame from the coronary arteriogram showing complete retrograde filling of the left coronary system from the right coronary injection (Figure 10c). Although contact with such conditions is unusual, a rational basis for the use of coronary surgery has been demonstrated by perfusion scintigraphy. The role of dynamiccardiac imaging in this context is discussed in the next chapter.

Non-coronary conditions

Thallium scintigraphy has been carried out in patients with mitral valve prolapse and chest pain[85]. It has been found superior to the exercise electrocardiogram in diagnosing associated coronary disease, as the cardiogram had a 53 % false-positive rate. Scintigraphy was uniformly negative in patients with angiographically normal arteries who had anginal chest pain, and uniformly positive in those with coronary disease. It is possible that small zones of ischaemia are present that are outside the resolution of the scan[11], or that hypoxia occurs independently of perfusion.

Nevertheless the reliability of thallium scintigraphy in this condition in excluding surgical coronary artery disease is attractive, as chest pain is so common a symptom. Thallium-201 has been used to differentiate non-coronary congestive cardiomyopathy from ischaemic myopathies, by the appearance of uniform uptake or focal defects respectively[86]. Hypertrophic cardiomyopathy demonstrates an increase in the thickness of the intraventricular septum relative to the free wall seen on the scan, and it has been claimed that in the obstructive case the posterolateral wall is thicker than in the non-obstructive case[87]. Infiltrative disease such as sarcoidosis, which may produce cardiac dysfunction, has been associated with focal decreases of

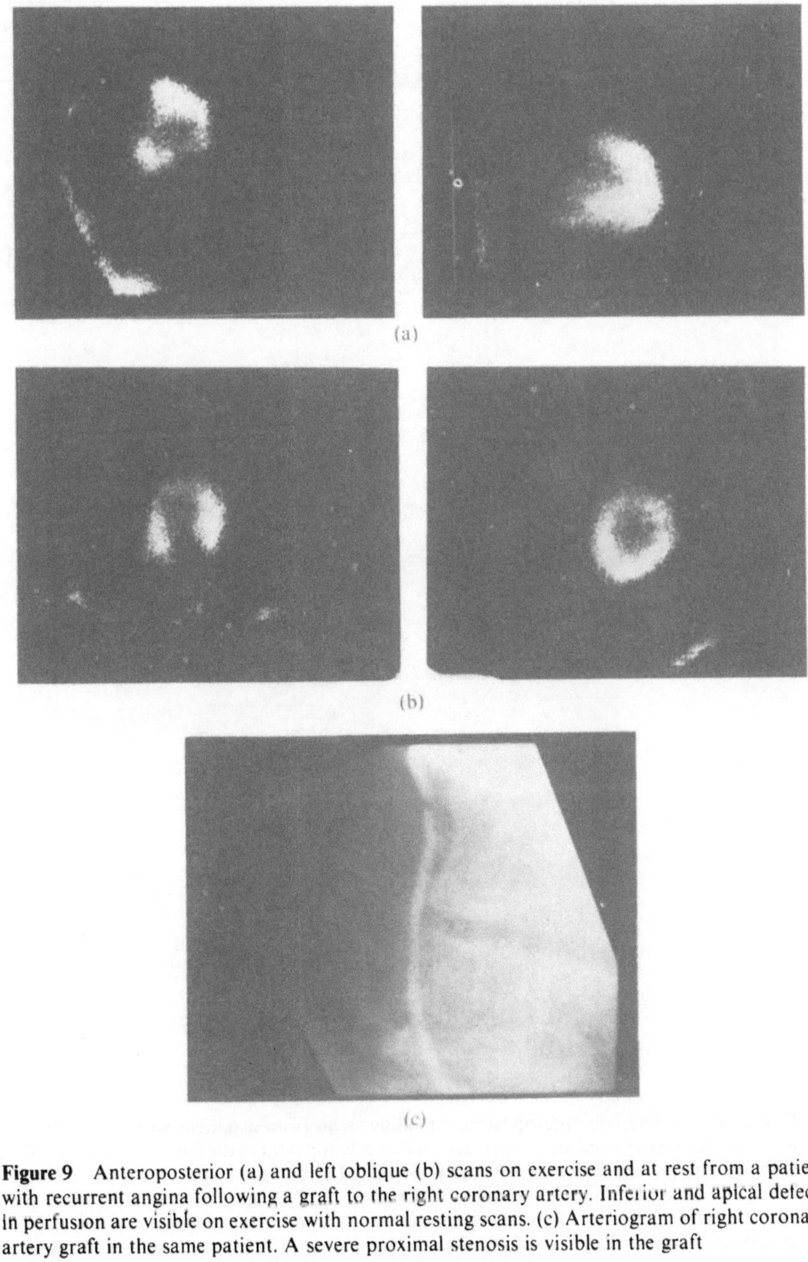

Figure 9 Anteroposterior (a) and left oblique (b) scans on exercise and at rest from a patient with recurrent angina following a graft to the right coronary artery. Inferior and apical defects in perfusion are visible on exercise with normal resting scans. (c) Arteriogram of right coronary artery graft in the same patient. A severe proximal stenosis is visible in the graft

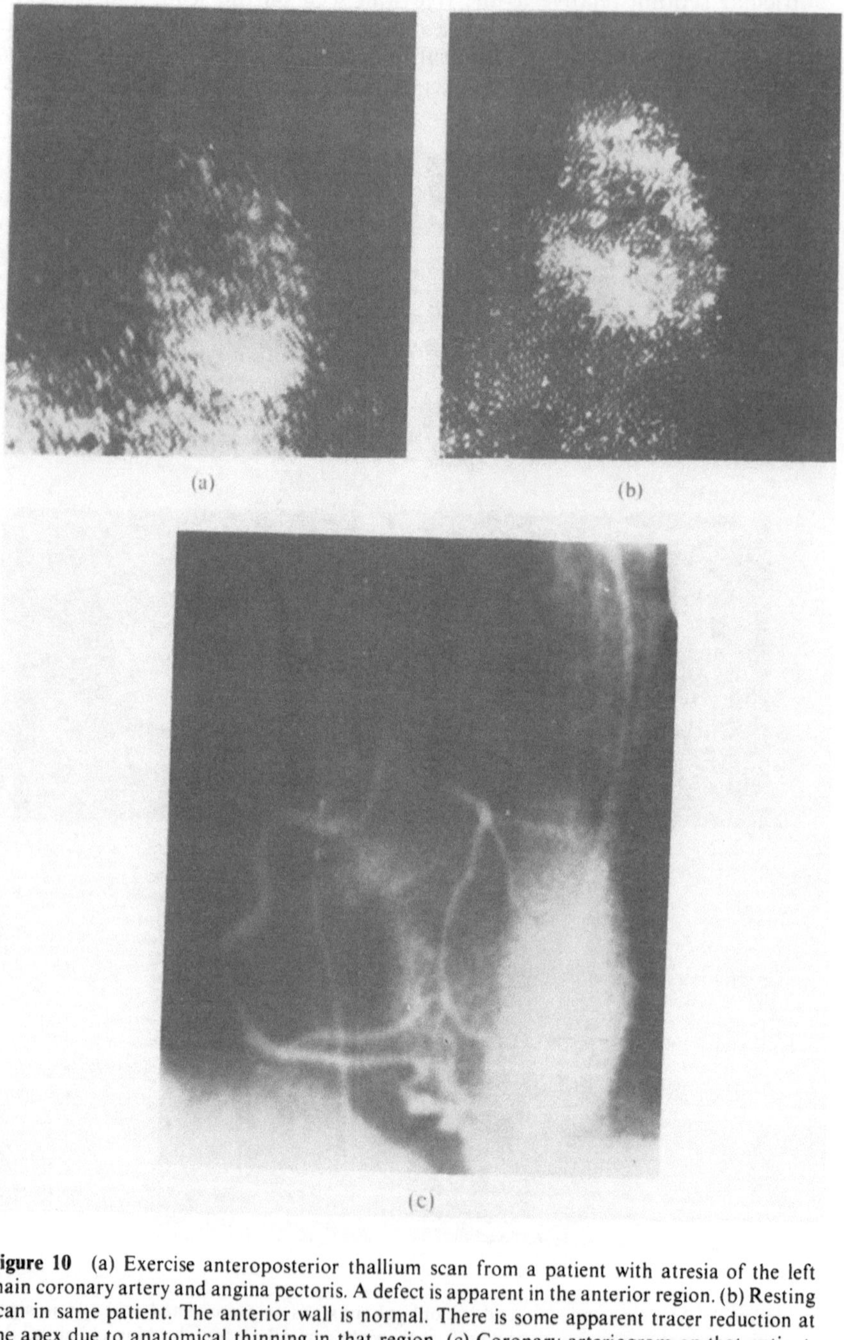

Figure 10 (a) Exercise anteroposterior thallium scan from a patient with atresia of the left main coronary artery and angina pectoris. A defect is apparent in the anterior region. (b) Resting scan in same patient. The anterior wall is normal. There is some apparent tracer reduction at the apex due to anatomical thinning in that region. (c) Coronary arteriogram on that patient, showing total retrograde filling of left coronary system from right coronary. No atheromatous lesions are present. (Reprinted from *British Heart Journal*[84], by permission of the publisher.)

thallium uptake but the appearances are not specific, and cannot exclude coronary disease[88]. Patients with the tetralogy of Fallot have been discriminated from those with a single ventricle by the appearance of the septum on the scintigram[89]. The role of thallium in the diagnosis of right ventricular hypertrophy[50] has been previously discussed.

SUMMARY

It is evident that thallium scintigraphy has many uses and many limitations. Tables 2 and 3 summarize the current indications for thallium scintigraphy and the limitations as gleaned from the now considerable experience with thallium-201. It is very tempting to employ stress perfusion scintigraphy as the first-line test for patients with chest pain. This may be reasonable in a situation such as pain after coronary bypass surgery, but is probably naive in many situations. In an articulate review by Turner *et al.*[90] it was shown that the test is inappropriate in a population with a high prevalence of coronary disease. In these cases, the post-test probability of disease does not significantly diminish even when the scintigram is normal. Turner *et al.* also con-

Table 2 Indication for thallium scintigraphy

Non-invasive detection of coronary disease (75–80 % sensitivity)
Identification of the false-positive exercise test
Improved sensitivity for detection of single-vessel coronary disease[60,61] (73 % for scan *vs.* 48 % for ECG)
Assessment of chest pain following vein graft surgery
Assessment of chest pain with mitral valve prolapse
Assessment of effect of coronary collaterals on myocardial ischaemia
Functional significance of coronary anomalies
Assessment of myocardial viability prior to revascularization
Non-coronary disease – single ventricle *vs.* Fallot's or right ventricular hypertrophy

Table 3 Limitations of thallium scintigraphy

Long half-life makes sequential studies impractical
Poor energy spectrum
No differentiation between old and recent infarction
Lesions less than 2.5 cm size not detected[11]
Posterior infarcts less well detected than anterior
Subendocardial infarcts or ischaemia not detected
Possibility of normal scans in triple-vessel disease or ostial stenosis
Extent of coronary disease not reliably detected
False negatives in single vessel disease especially of circumflex[62] artery
Previous infarction reduces sensitivity of detecting other lesions
Quantification very limited

cluded that in a patient population without prior infarctions the sensitivity of stress perfusion scintigraphy is not as high as in the population with prior infarction. It was pointed out in this article that in patients with 'atypical chest pain', of whom 30–50% will turn out to have significant coronary artery disease, the probability of disease being present is still high even in the presence of normal scans. Decisions on whether coronary arteriography should be performed cannot therefore be reliably made on the basis of thallium scans in patients with typical or atypical angina[90]. In a similar Bayesian approach to analysis of thallium scintigraphy, Murray *et al.*[91] concluded that thallium scanning is an inappropriate test in a low-prevalence population and thus as a screening test is not useful. Its major usefulness as a discriminating test lies in a population with a probability for coronary disease of 30–70%.

FUTURE POSSIBILITIES FOR PERFUSION SCANNING

If the limitations in thallium-201 scintigraphy as widely performed are accepted, there is obviously room for advancements in techniques for assessing myocardial perfusion. One possible approach to improve the quality of thallium images is the use of electrocardiographically 'gated' images, so that imaging is performed only at preset time intervals in the cardiac cycle, for example, the 50 ms associated with end-diastole. In this way, artefact produced by cardiac motion is eliminated. This approach has been shown to produce higher-resolution images in which perfusion defects are more readily apparent[92]. However, collecting so few counts per cardiac cycle means that the imaging time required to produce 300000 counts is vastly prolonged, and thus the applications of this technique to stress scintigraphy where multiple views are required is limited.

There are two other possible approaches to non-invasive perfusion scanning:

(1) Conventional imaging with newer radiopharmaceuticals.
(2) Three-dimensional imaging with conventional radionuclides or short half-life positron emitting agents.

Conventional imaging

As long ago as 1962 the uptake of radiolabelled fatty acids by the heart was demonstrated[93]. The techniques seemed satisfactory for experimental animal imaging, but the labelling method used seemed to alter the biological behaviour of the fatty acid and decrease myocardial extraction efficiency. Iodine-123 emits an almost pure 159 keV gamma photon in abundance, and the energy is ideal for use with a gamma camera. The half-life is short (13 h) so sequential studies can be more easily performed than with thallium. Fatty acids are an important energy source for the heart and are extracted efficiently by the myocardium. If they could be labelled with iodine-123, then a physiological radiopharmaceutical with ideal energy is produced, and limited studies on myocardial metabolism are possible. Labelling of hexadecanoic acid by radioiodine exchange with bromine has been found to produce a compound which retains the myocardial extraction efficiency of non-iodinated long-chain fatty acids[94]. Problems in the use of this type of agent include the fact that as the acids are rapidly metabolized the iodine label is released into the iodine pool which raises the non-myocardial background radioactivity[95].

Some very early clinical experience with iodine-123-labelled heptadecanoic acid suggests that the elimination of tracer, which is dependent on intact metabolic pathways, is abnormal in ischaemic and infarcted areas of heart muscle[96]. Detection of impaired myocardial metabolism in the presence of normal coronary arteries has also been postulated[97]. It remains to be seen whether these promising agents will displace thallium as the radiopharmaceuticals of choice for perfusion scanning, but their physiological nature and excellent physical properties will doubtless be an incentive for further research in this field.

The use of short half-life radionuclides which emit positrons will be discussed in more detail below, but basically they emit high-energy photons which are by no means ideal for use with an ordinary gamma camera. Walsh *et al.*[98] have described the use of one of these agents, nitrogen-13, administered as labelled ammonia, in the non-invasive assessment of myocardial perfusion in patients, with the imaging being performed with a mobile gamma camera. They found that a specially constructed tungsten collimator was necessary to produce satisfactory images, and concluded that the technique was a valid and sensitive method for the assessment of regional myocardial perfusion, and for the rapid sequential imaging of patients at short intervals. The limitations that are imposed on the widespread use of this technique are those of radionuclide production, which requires an on-site cyclotron (see below).

THREE-DIMENSIONAL IMAGING

The use of the gamma camera for cardiac imaging is limited by the following basic handicaps, some of which have been mentioned above.

(1) The image of a three-dimensional object is represented in two dimensions, and the activity overlying and underlying the region of interest are superimposed, introducing artefacts and 'noise' and decreasing image contrast[99], especially in the inferior myocardium.
(2) The field of view and resolution of a gamma camera vary greatly with depth, which complicates quantification of images.
(3) The attenuation of gamma radiation in tissues between the area of interest and the detector introduces a variable which allows only a qualitative relationship between the image and tracer distribution in the heart[99]. Corrections cannot be made for depth or attenuation.

The development of emission computerized axial tomography (ECAT) goes some way to overcoming these obstacles. This is a technique that provides transaxial sectional images of organs that contain gamma-emitting isotopes. The concepts are identical to those applied to the transmission scanner, such as the EMI scanner, but the distribution of *emitted* radionuclide, rather than attenuation of *transmitted* X-rays, is imaged. ECAT provides an image that is less encumbered by activity in surrounding structures and the problems due to varying depth can be overcome partially or totally, depending on the radiopharmaceutical used.

Figure 11 is a diagrammatic representation of the normal myocardial image and thorax in cross-section, with the horseshoe-shaped left ventricle in black.

There are two approaches to emission tomography.

(1) Single-photon emission tomography using conventional radiopharmaceuticals.
(2) Positron-emission tomography, or annihilation coincidence detection.

Single-photon tomography

Single-photon ECAT has been found superior to conventional imaging in the central nervous system[100]. Single-photon transaxial scanners have now become available for use in thoracic and abdominal imaging. They involve an assembly of scanning detectors which rotate around the patient at various degree increments and at each position a scan is performed[101,102]. Reconstruction of the image is undertaken by a computer and the image is viewed after data collection. The study of patients with thallium-201 has been described[101,102] and areas of infarction have been seen as areas of reduced

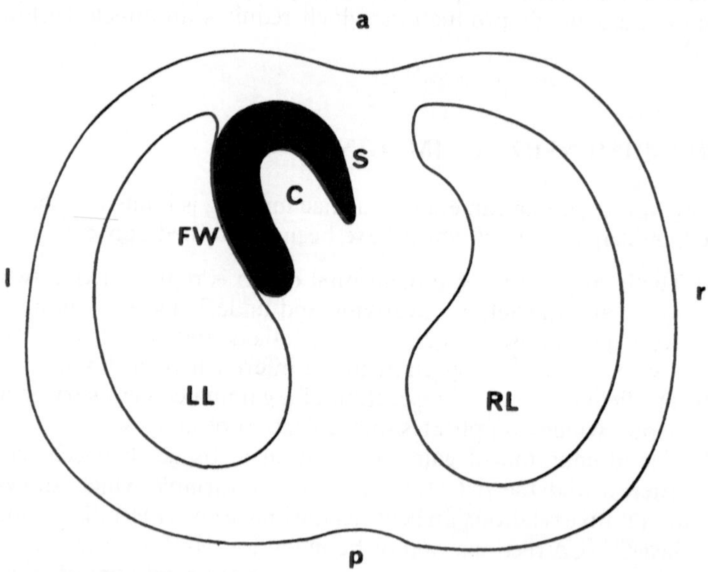

Figure 11 Diagrammatic representation of the thorax in cross-section. The horseshoe-shaped image of the left ventricle is shown in black. FW = free wall of left ventricle, S = septum, C = ventricular cavity, LL = left lung, RL = right lung, l = left, r = right, a = anterior, p = posterior.

tracer uptake in the ECAT images that correlate well with sites of reduced tracer uptake on the conventional images. Figure 12 is an example of conventional and ECAT images in a patient with anterior infarction. The use of this technique to image the heart at rest and on exercise has been described[101] and initial results suggest that it is feasible provided imaging can be carried out before redistribution of the thallium occurs. If both conventional and ECAT imaging are required then exercise scans may be logistically difficult as more than 1 h will be required to obtain multiple views and multiple sections. Approximate corrections for depth attenuation effects are possible with single-photon tomography[101] either from a set of approximate correction factors obtained from the initial reconstructed image, or from transmission measurements made prior to emission scanning[103]. One possible

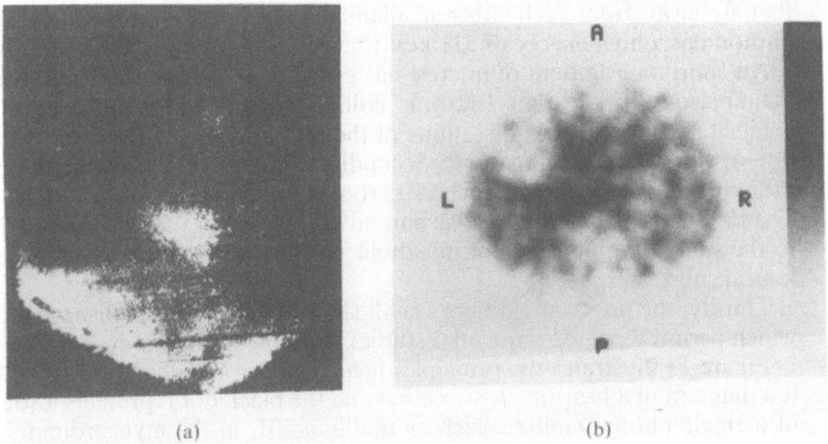

Figure 12 Conventional (a) and ECAT (b) images from a patient with anterior infarction. Anterior and apical defects in thallium-201 uptake are seen on the conventional scan. The sectional image shows a large defect of free wall, apex and septum

use of this technique is in the more accurate quantification of myocardial infarct size. Keyes *et al.*[104] have used computed tomography to image the distribution of technetium-99m pyrophosphate in experimental infarcts in dogs. The volume of the infarcts was assessed by measuring the number of picture elements representing infarction in all sections of the reconstructed image, and a weight was obtained by multiplying this by average myocardial density. The correlations with actual infarct weight were good, although the size of large infarcts was underestimated *in vivo*.

It remains to be seen whether these techniques will eventually contribute anything to our diagnostic capabilities. Although the use of conventional isotopes is attractive, the cost of the imaging equipment is considerable and most departments would be wary of purchasing dedicated ECAT devices whose clinical usefulness may be limited. The cost benefits of single-photon tomography may be heightened by the use of the seven-pinhole collimator gamma camera attachment[105]. Longitudinal tomographs obtained with thallium-201 by this technique have a 95% sensitivity for detecting significant coronary stenosis[106]. This technique has the disadvantage of producing distorted images that may limit measurements of infarct size. Also a wide normal variation in regional count density was found, so subjective interpretation of images should be performed cautiously.

Position tomography

What is a positron?

In positron (positive electron) emission, a photon in a nucleus changes into a positive electron and a neutron. The ejected positron combines with an electron and the reaction between positively and negatively charged particles is called an annihilation reaction. The energy associated with the masses of the two particles is 1022 keV which is divided equally between two photons that fly away from each other in diametrically opposite directions. Each photon has a high energy of 511 keV ($\frac{1}{2} \times 1022$ keV).

An enormous amount of interest has grown in positron imaging for three main reasons. Firstly, the 'electronic' collimation and better scatter rejection is facilitated by the 180° directions of the photons, so positron cameras do not require lead collimators. Secondly, among the positron-emitting radionuclides are elements such as carbon-11, oxygen-15, and nitrogen-13. The production of isotopes of carbon, nitrogen, and oxygen provides access to the study of a multitude of metabolic pathways by radiolabelled physiological substrates.

Thirdly, the positron-emitters are all short half-life radiopharmaceuticals which permit repeated sequential studies with low radiation dosages.

Figure 13 illustrates the principles behind positron detection. Figure 13a is a diagram of a heart in cross-section and the black dot represents a source of a single photon emitter, such as thallium-201, in the myocardium. The path length for the photon within the body depends upon the point of origin within the organ. Photons from the front of the heart have less distance to travel than those from the back of the heart, if the detector is placed anteriorly. If the detector is posterior, the situation is reversed. Thus, the degree of scatter and attenuation of photons depends on their point of origin. Since the point of origin is unknown, only approximate attenuation corrections can be made.

Figure 13b illustrates the situation with positron emitters. The annihilation reaction results in the emission of two photons at an angle of 180° to each other. By placing detectors on opposite sides of the source, it is possible to detect the two events simultaneously. When the simultaneous detection occurs, the origin of the annihilation reaction can be said to have taken place along a line between the two detectors[107]. If banks of detectors are placed around the isotope source then when one of the annihilation photons strikes one detector, its opposite *must* strike a crystal at 180° for the event to be recorded as valid. The electronic timing circuits are usually set to accept avents as coincident from the same annihilation reaction if they reach opposite detectors within 20 ns or less[107]. This 'electronic collimation' imposes a large burden on the coincidence circuiting which must discriminate valid

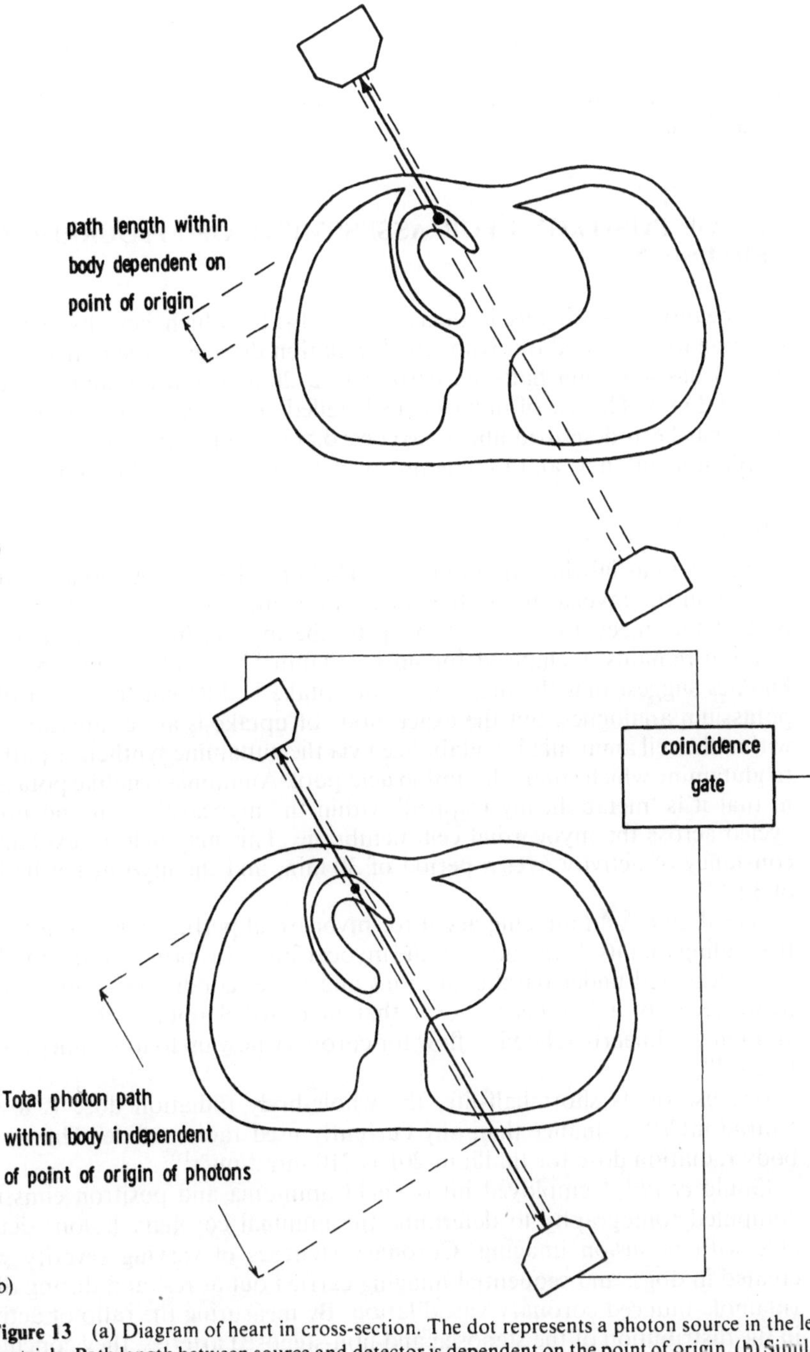

(a)

(b)

Figure 13 (a) Diagram of heart in cross-section. The dot represents a photon source in the left ventricle. Path length between source and detector is dependent on the point of origin. (b) Similar diagram showing that with positron-emitting agents, the path length between the photon source and the two detectors is the same regardless of the point of origin of the photons events from scattered ones. A constant count rate is possible regardless of the position of the source of radioactivity within the field of view of the paired detectors. In such a system, it is possible to make an accurate correction for attenuation effects, thereby significantly improving the quality of data obtained.

USE OF POSITRONS FOR ASSESSMENT OF MYOCARDIAL PERFUSION

The beauty of positrons is their short half-life, which permits sequential imaging to be carried out with small radiation dosage to the patient. Nitrogen-13 has a 10 min half-life, carbon-11 a 20 min half-life and oxygen-15 one of 2 min. The use of nitrogen-13-labelled ammonia with a gamma camera[98] has been described above. Myocardial imaging with positron emitters is still in its infancy, and to date nitrogen-13 and carbon-13 have been tried.

Nitrogen-13

Nitrogen-13 as labelled ammonia ($^{13}NH4^{+}$) has been shown to accumulate rapidly in the myocardium after intravenous injection[108]. Two to four per cent of the injected dose is taken up by the myocardium and in man this fraction remains unchanged for up to 30 min[108]. Its blood-disappearance kinetics suggest that the mechanism of uptake is different from that of the potassium analogues, but the exact mode of uptake is as yet unclear. Once within the cell ammonia is metabolized via the glutamine synthetase pathway to glutamine which enters the amino acid pool. Ammonia is unlike potassium in that it is 'metabolically trapped' within the myocardial cell and not recycled across the myocardial cell membrane. This may help to explain the constancy of activity over a period of 30 min, and the myocardial half-life of 3 h[109].

Its validity as an imaging agent for myocardial perfusion is confirmed by the finding that its distribution in the myocardium was proportional to blood flow measured under basal conditions and under conditions of low flow[98]. More recently it has been shown that myocardial uptake of nitrogen-13 ammonia is linearly related to flow for coronary flow up to four times resting levels[110].

Because of its short half-life, the whole-body radiation dose is low at 5 mrad/mCi[108], smaller than any currently used radionuclide. The whole-body radiation dose for thallium-201 is 210 mrad/mCi[107].

Gould *et al.*[111] employed nitrogen-13 ammonia and positron emission-computed tomography to determine the minimal coronary lesions detectable with perfusion imaging. Coronary stenoses of varying severity were created in dogs, and sequential imaging carried out at rest and during dipyridamole-induced coronary vasodilation. By measuring the ratio of activity in the distribution of the stenosed and non-stenosed arteries, they concluded that perfusion defects occurred with luminal narrowings of 47 % or greater. Although these experimental data cannot be extrapolated with certainty to exercise-induced or drug-induced angina in humans, the possibility of producing high-quality images in rapid succession before and after an intervention requires further evaluation in the future.

Walsh *et al.*[98] performed sequential studies on patients in the acute phase of myocardial infarction or unstable angina, and found a good correlation between sequential changes in regional myocardial perfusion and the clinical status of the patient, which may be helpful in the assessment of prognosis in such patients.

Carbon-11

Carbon-11 can be incorporated into fatty acids for access to metabolic pathways of carbohydrates and lipids. Decreased extraction of [^{11}C]palmitate has been observed in isolated perfused hearts subjected to ischaemia for 30 min, even though extraction remained normal for a period of 1 min despite low blood flow. Decreased extraction appears to be a characteristic of the metabolic alterations induced by ischaemia rather than simply reduction of perfusion and poor delivery of radionuclide to the myocardium[112]. The rate of metabolism of incorporated substrates has been determined in animal hearts by external detection[113]. Selective alterations in determinants of cardiac work produced increases in the rate of clearance of intracellular counts, and potassium cardioplegia drastically reduced clearance. Although the experience in humans has largely been confined to the detection of previous myocardial infarction[114], the possible applications of positron emission tomography to the assessment of *in vivo* regional metabolism are enormous. One can at this stage only speculate on the questions that might be answered. The syndrome of angina or infarction with angiographically normal coronary arteries demands a deeper investigation into regional myocardial metabolism, and labelled substrates may provide an insight into poorly understood pathophysiological processes.

Despite the potential of positron imaging, the techniques are handicapped by the awesome cost of the positron cameras and the necessity for on-site cyclotrons for radionuclide productions. It seems unlikely that these constraints will ever allow widespread application of positron tomography, and their use will probably remain confined to a few fortunate centres.

INVASIVE ASSESSMENT OF MYOCARDIAL PERFUSION

In contrast to the technique of myocardial perfusion scanning with agents such as thallium-201 which demand no more than a venepuncture, invasive techniques must be carried out at the time of cardiac catheterization. They involve either the injection of tracer directly into the coronary arteries, or into the aortic sinuses. The techniques are:

(1) The injection of labelled biodegradable particles into the coronary arteries. Either microspheres or macroaggregates (MAA) are used.
(2) The infusion of the ultra-short half-life krypton-81m into the aortic sinuses.

Microspheres and macroaggregates (MAA)

Myocardial imaging with isotopically tagged non-diffusible particles injected directly into the coronary circulation was shown to be feasible in humans in 1970[115]. Prior to this lung scanning with albumin MAA labelled with iodine-131 had been routinely used for some years. When MAA are injected intravenously their pulmonary distribution is in proportion to regional pulmonary blood flow, and imaging is carried out after the particles have 'micro-embolized' in the pulmonary capillaries. Unlike potassium analogues and metabolic markers, these agents have no affinity for the myocardium.

The potential hazards of producing a myocardial capillary block are self-evident. Grames *et al.*[116] reported the experience of particle injection in 800 cases undergoing coronary angiography. They found that the incidence of minor dysrhythmias was similar to that produced by contrast medium and only two patients showed significant dysrhythmias. No patient had sequelae after the procedures. Workers concluded that if the size and number of particles were adequately controlled then the technique was safe[116,117]. Methods for preparing MAA generally yield particles of 10–80 microns (μm) in size with 90% being 20–40 μm[118]. The particles can be labelled with technetium-99m, indium-113m, or iodine-131. The two former radionuclides are generally used nowadays. The wide variation in particle size of MAA prompted the introduction of human albumin microspheres (HAM). These have a more uniform particle size which makes quality control easier and the microspheres are adaptable to the kit method which offers long-term storage and rapid labelling with technetium-99 or indium-113. Higher specific activity is achievable which reduces the number of particles needed for injection.

The primary advantages of this approach are the improved resolution that results from the higher target to background ratio than one achieves with intravenous administration of a tracer. Also, the ability to label the HAM with two different radionuclides means that the evaluation of perfusion of the territory supplied by each coronary may be imaged separately. Thus, technetium-99m microspheres may be injected into the left coronary artery, and indium-113m microspheres into the right. Imaging is performed either in the catheter laboratory with a mobile gamma camera or after the patient has been transferred to the nuclear medicine department.

If imaging is performed in the resting state, coronary artery stenoses of 70% or more are generally associated with recognizable regional hypoperfusion, especially when collateral vessels are scarce, when multiple vessels are involved, or where there is substantial scarring of the myocardium[119]. In a large series reported by Jansen *et al.*[120], 25% of patients had both normal coronary arteries and normal perfusion, 9% had normal arteries but abnormal perfusion, and 16% had abnormalities of both. Abnormal arteries and normal perfusion were found in 50%. It would be expected, as with resting thallium scintigraphy, that resting defects represent previously infarcted tissue and in fact HAM scintigraphy has proved compatible with left ventricular angiography in nearly all cases. The microsphere technique also appears to be more sensitive in predicting scar tissue than non-invasive perfusion scintigraphy with potassium analogues[119]. The group with normal arteries and abnormal perfusion was the smallest group in Jansen's series, but a flow defect due to selective injection or streaming accounted for one-third of the abnormalities in this group, and the remainder had myopathic ventricles. The implication in the large group with normal perfusion and abnormal arteries is that the capillary bed is intact and bypass grafting is worthwhile. The converse holds for the group with abnormal perfusion and abnormal arteries, where a highly abnormal capillary bed is suggested and bypass grafting would be a futile exercise.

Resting HAM scintigraphy can therefore offer fairly unique data on the state of capillary beds distal to a stenosed or occluded artery. It provides no information on metabolism and quantitative measurement of blood flow, but is a valuable adjunct to the evaluation of the patient considered for coronary surgery.

If a different isotope is utilized for each coronary artery, then studies on microsphere distribution after an intervention are not possible. If, however, only one coronary artery is studied then the two isotopes may be used to study perfusion at rest and after an intervention. Gould *et al.*[121] studied regional flow distribution in experimental animals subjected to circumflex artery stenoses of varying severity. Iodine-131-labelled particles were injected at rest, and technetium-99m-labelled particles after the intracoronary injection of Hypaque contrast medium. Myocardium supplied by the normal left anterior descending artery responded normally with an increase in perfusion due to Hypaque-induced hyperaemia, but the circumflex territory could not. Pharmacologically induced hyperaemia thus unmasked regional perfusion abnormalities.

Ritchie *et al.*[122] extended this technique to humans and found that the dual isotope technique helped to ascertain the haemodynamic importance of a stenosis of questionable significance anatomically.

Overall, in all 10 patients with no, or insignificant, coronary disease, (<50% stenosis) images were normal at rest and during hyperaemia. Of 39 patients with significant (>50%) stenosis, 37 demonstrated perfusion abnormalities, 14 of which were only seen during the contrast-induced hyperaemia. However, the absence of a perfusion defect does not prove the absence of a significant coronary stenosis. Balanced lesions in anterior descending and circumflex vessels will impair flow in both, and defects of perfusion may not be seen[123]. This situation is analogous to the 'normal' thallium-201 image in global ischaemia, which has been previously discussed.

Postoperative studies

Direct injection of particles into saphenous vein grafts was carried out by Hamilton *et al.*[124] to assess the clinical utility of the technique. Normally functioning grafts presented characteristic scintigraphic patterns. Right coronary grafts had a 'ball and tail' pattern, with the tail representing right ventricular myocardium and the ball the inferior left ventricle. Collateral flow through the graft to myocardium may also be visualized, and collateral flow was more frequently seen by scintigraphy than by angiography (53% versus 18% of cases).

It was suggested that the demonstration of collateral flow through the grafts to other areas of myocardium is an indication of good graft function. MAA or HAM perfusion scintigraphy was judged a poor indicator of the amount of graft flow, however. The application of the dual-isotope technique to graft and native circulation was of value only when the grafted native vessels remained patent. In these circumstances the distribution of flow often differed from the arteriographic appearances. The technique may possibly offer a way of assessing perfusion in patients who do badly after revascularization, as well as in assessing significance of graft stenosis. The current role of this method in assessing grafted vessels is still uncertain.

SUMMARY

The HAM technique is safe and applicable to all centres with imaging facilities. The advantages of high-resolution images are partly offset by the disadvantages of the invasive nature of the technique, the possibility of artefacts being produced by streaming and superselective intracoronary injection, and the limitations imposed upon segmental studies. It is questionable whether the benefits of high-resolution images are outweighed by these limitations above, especially as high-resolution non-invasive perfusion scanning with newer radiopharmaceuticals appears possible[98].

KRYPTON-81m

Krypton-81m is an inert, freely diffusing metastable breakdown product of rubidium-81, that is produced by a cyclotron. It has an ultra-short half-life of 13 s and thus is totally unsuitable for non-invasive perfusion scanning. If it is introduced directly into the coronary circulation, however, as a continuous infusion, a scintigraphic image is constantly maintained as the new generation of krypton replaces the amount lost by decay. The isotope emits a single 190 keV gamma ray that is well suited to gamma camera detection. Krypton-81m is available in the form of a portable generator-delivery system based on the spontaneous decay of rubidium-81m. The eluted solution contains dissolved krypton-81m gas, which is chemically and biologically inert. In experimental animals, the agent has been introduced directly into the coronary circulation by a Teflon catheter threaded into various branches of the left coronary artery, and images of myocardial perfusion obtained[125]. In man, krypton-81m has been infused continuously into the aortic sinuses using a specially constructed looped cardiac catheter[126]. A constant-infusion pump and timed collections from each loop were used to ascertain that equal volumes were delivered to each sinus. High-quality myocardial images free of background activity may be obtained. The technique has been used to image myocardial perfusion under the stress of atrial pacing in patients with coronary artery disease[126]. Studies have demonstrated that maldistribution of regional counts occurs before the onset of ECG changes or angina.

Krypton-81m scintigraphy has also been used to assess saphenous vein graft function at the time of surgery[127]. Myocardial flow per unit volume was measured from the krypton-81m washout curves when grafts were inserted into the left anterior descending coronary artery in patients with a history and ECG evidence of previous anterior infarction. Low flow through the grafts was recorded. This technique thus offers a way of assessing perfusion through individual grafts before the chest is closed.

The advantages of krypton-81m perfusion scanning are that a continuous image of perfusion may be obtained due to the ultra-short half-life of the agent, with high spatial resolution and low background counts. The disadvantages are the invasive nature of the technique, the need for a special catheter, the prolongation of catheterization time, and the need for a mobile gamma camera to image in the catheter laboratory or operating theatre. The method is obviously not widely applicable.

MEASUREMENT OF MYOCARDIAL BLOOD FLOW WITH SPECIAL REFERENCE TO XENON-133

Quantification of myocardial blood flow by radioactive tracers has been attempted by many groups. Knoebel *et al.*[128] used a coincidence counting system and a single bolus injection of the positron-emitting rubidium-84. The technique was based on the Sapirstein[45] principle that the fractional uptake of rubidium-84 by the heart equalled the fraction of cardiac output received by the heart. Washout curves following the intracoronary injection of nitrous oxide[129] or xenon-133 (ref. 130) have also been used. When there are spatial differences in regional blood flow as a result of coronary arterial obstructions, the single curves obtained by an external detector over the left ventricle or by coronary sinus sampling contain a family of curves with inhomogeneous exponential washouts[131]. Areas of regional underperfusion may therefore be obscured as prolonged times for the washout from these zones are required. The problem with xenon-133 is that apart from the inhomogeneity of regional washout, the gas diffuses rapidly into the fat in the epicardium and washes out slowly from zones with a high epicardial fat content. Regional differences in xenon-133 washout may be partly related to varying amounts of epicardial fat[130]. If attempts are made to overcome this by using the mean washout time from the monoexponential that fits only the initial part of the curve, then the errors due to the obscuring of underperfused areas will appear. A modification of the technique has been to produce multiple xenon-133 washout curves by recording from different regions of the heart using a multicrystal scintillation camera[131,132]. With the aid of a computer, rate constants of regional tracer clearance from the myocardium are calculated by monoexponential analysis of the data recorded by each crystal. The pattern of regional flow can be superimposed upon a tracing of the coronary arteriogram. The method has been utilized to produce perfusion patterns in patients with coronary disease and ventricular aneurysms[132], and in the demonstration of abnormal perfusion under the stress of atrial pacing[131].

It has been possible to separate clearly territories perfused by normal vessels from those distal to significant stenosis. The advantages of xenon-133 as a tracer include the negligible recirculation, as 95% of the gas is exhaled during the first passage through the pulmonary circulation. Disadvantages include its expense, the low count rates associated with high resolution collimation, and xenon's low energy and its differing solubilities in fat, muscle, and scar tissue.

Krypton-81m (ref. 127) washout rates may be able to provide more accurate quantification of myocardial blood flow in the future, but it is difficult to foresee such measurements being available with the more widely applicable techniques for perfusion scanning.

References

1. Zaret, B. L., Strauss, H. W., Martin, N. D., Wells, H. P. Jnr. and Flamm, M. D. (1973). Non-invasive regional myocardial perfusion with radioactive potassium: study of patients at rest, with exercise and during angina pectoris. *N. Engl. J. Med.*, **288,** 809
2. Anger, H. O. (1958). Scintillation camera. *Rev. Sci. Instrum.*, **29,** 27
3. Dreyfuss, F., Ben-Porath, M. and Menczel, J. (1960). Radioiodine uptake by the infarcted heart. *Am. J. Cardiol.*, **6,** 237
4. Carr, E. T., Bierwaltes, W. H., Patno, M. E., Bartlett, J. E. and Wegst, A. V. (1962). The detecting of experimental myocardial infarcts by photoscanning. *Am. Heart J.*, **64,** 650
5. Malek, P., Kolc, J. and Zastava, V. L. (1963). Fluorescence of tetracycline analogues fixed in myocardial infarction. *Cardiology*, **42,** 303
6. Romhilt, D. W., Adolph, R. J., Sodd, V. J., Levenson, N. I., August, L. S., Nishiyama, H. and Berke, R. A. (1973). Cesium^{129} myocardial scintigraphy to detect myocardial infarction. *Circulation*, **48,** 1242
7. Martin, N. D., Zaret, B. L., McGowan, R. L., Wells, H. P. and Flamm, M. D. (1974). Rubidium^{81}, a new myocardial scanning agent; non-invasive regional myocardial perfusion scans at rest and exercise and comparison with potassium 43. *Radiology*, **3,** 651
8. Wackers, F. J. Th., v.d. Shoot, J. B., Sokole, E. B., Samson, G., v. Niftrik, G. J. C., Lie, K. I., Durrer, D. and Wellens, H. J. J. (1975). Non-invasive visualisation of acute myocardial infarction in man with Thallium 201. *Br. Heart J.*, **37,** 741
9. Hamilton, G. W., Trobaugh, G. B., Ritchie, J. L., Williams, D. L., Weaver, W. D. and Gould, K. L. (1977). Myocardial imaging with intravenously injected Thallium-201 in patients with suspected coronary artery disease: analysis of technique and correlation with electrocardiographic, coronary anatomic and ventriculographic findings. *Am. J. Cardiol.*, **39,** 347
10. Pabst, H. W., Hör, G., Lichte, H., Sebening, H. and Kreigel, H. (1976). Experience with ^{201}Thallium in detection of myocardial infarction. *Eur. J. Nucl. Med.*, **1,** 19
11. Mueller, T. M., Marcus, M. L., Ehrhardt, J. C., Chaudhuri, T. and Abboud, F. M. (1976). Limitations of Thallium-201 myocardial perfusion scintigrams. *Circulation*, **54,** 640
12. Parkey, R. W., Bonte, F. J., Meyer, S. L., Atkins, J. M., Curry, G. L., Stokeley, E. M. and Willerson, J. T. (1974). A new method for radionuclide imaging of acute myocardial infarction in humans. *Circulation*, **50,** 540

13. McLaughlin, P., Coates, G., Wood, D., Cradduck, T. and Morch, D. (1975). Detection of acute myocardial infarction by Technetium-99m polyphosphate. *Am. J. Cardiol.*, **35**, 390
14. Subramanian, G., Mcafee, J. G., Bell, E. G., Blair, R. J., O'Mara, R. E. and Ralston, P. H. (1972). 99m Tc-labelled polyphosphate as a skeletal imaging agent. *Radiology* **102,** 71
15. D'Agostino, A. N. and Chiga, M. (1970). Mitochondrial mineralization in human myocardium. *Am. J. Clin. Pathol.*, **53,** 820
16. Buja, L. M., Parkey, R. W., Dees, J. H., Stokely, E. M., Harris, R. A., Bonte, F. J. and Willerson, J. T. (1975). Morphologic correlates of technetium-99m stannous pyrophosphate imaging of acute myocardial infarcts in dogs. *Circulation*, **52,** 596
17. Coleman, R. E., Klein, M. S., Ahmed, S. A., Weiss, E. S., Bucholz, W. M. and Sobel, B. E. (1977). Mechanisms contributing to myocardial accumulation of Technetium 99m stannous pyrophosphate after coronary arterial occlusion. *Am. J. Cardiol.*, **39,** 55
18. Berman, D. S., Amsterdam, E. A., Salel, A. F., Denardo, G. L., Baily, G. J. and Mason, D. T. (1975). Diagnostic accuracy of Tc-99m-pyrophosphate scintigraphy in the detection of acute myocardial infarction. *Circulation*, **51/52** (Suppl. 2), 53
19. Lessem, J., Johannson, B. W., Nosslin, B. and Thorell, J. (1977). Clinical analysis of myocardial scintigraphy with 99m-Tc-pyrophosphate. In *Medical Radionuclide Imaging, Proceedings of Symposium, Los Angeles*, **II**, 231 (Vienna: IAEA)
20. Dymond, D. S., Jarritt, P. H., Britton, K. E., Langley, D. and Spurrell, R. A. J. (1978). Positive myocardial scintigraphy at the bedside – evaluation using a portable gamma camera. *Postgrad. Med. J.*, **54,** 641
21. Klein, M. S., Coleman, R. E., Weldon, C. S., Sobel, B. E. and Roberts, R. (1976). Concordance of electrocardiographic and scintigraphic criteria of myocardial injury after cardiac surgery. *J. Thorac. Cardiovasc. Surg.*, **71,** 934
22. Stokely, E. M., Buja, L. M., Lewis, S. E., Parkey, R. W., Bonte, F. J., Harris, R. A. Jr. and Willerson, J. T. (1975). Measurement of acute myocardial infarcts in dogs with ^{99m} Tc-stannous pyrophosphate scintigrams, *J. Nucl. Med.*, **17,** 1
23. Botvinick, E. H., Shames, D., Lappin, H., Tyberg, J. V., Townsend, R. and Parmley, W. W. (1975). Noninvasive quantitation of myocardial infarction with technetium 99m pyrophosphate. *Circulation*, **52,** 909
24. Zaret, B. L., Lange, R. C. and Lee, J. C. (1977). Comparative assessment of infarct size with quantitative Thallium-201 and Technetium-99m pyrophosphate dual myocardial imaging in the dog. *Am. J. Cardiol.*, **39,** 309
25. Willerson, J. T., Parkey, R. W., Harris, R. A. Jr, Bonte, F. J., Stokely, E. M. and Buja, L. M. (1975). Sizing acute myocardial infarction utilizing technetium stannous pyrophosphate myocardial scintigrams in dogs and man. *Clin. Res.*, **23,** 214A
26. Bruno, F. P., Cobb, F. R., Rivas, F. and Goodrich, J. K. (1976). Evaluation of 99m technetium stannous pyrophosphate as an imaging agent in acute myocardial infarction. *Circulation*, **54,** 71
27. Rude, R. E., Parkey, R. W., Bonte, F. J., Lewis, S. E., Twieg, D., Buja, L. M. and Willerson, J. T. (1979). Clinical implications of the Technetium-99m stannous pyrophosphate myocardial scintigraphic 'doughnut' pattern in patients with acute myocardial infarcts. *Circulation*, **59,** 721
28. Maroko, P. R. and Braunwald, E. (1973). Modification of myocardial infarction size after coronary occlusion. *Ann. Intern. Med.*, **79,** 720
29. Holman, B. L., Chisholm, R. J. and Braunwald, E. (1978). The prognostic implications of acute myocardial infarct scintigraphy with 99m-Tc-pyrophosphate. *Circulation*, **57,** 320

30. Olson, H. G., Lyons, K. P., Aronow, W. S., Brown, W. T. and Greenfield, R. S. (1977). Follow-up technetium ^{99m} stannous pyrophosphate myocardial scintigrams after acute myocardial infarction. *Circulation*, **56**, 181
31. Willerson, J. T., Parkey, R. W., Bonte, F. J., Meyer, S. L. and Stokely, E. M. (1975). Acute subendocardial myocardial infarction in patients. Its detection by Technetium 99m stannous pyrophosphate myocardial scintigrams. *Circulation*, **51**, 436
32. Walsh, W., Lessem, J., Fill, H., Harper, P. V. and Resnekov, L. (1976). Value of 99m Tc pyrophosphate myocardial scintigraphy in patients with suspected myocardial infarction. *Am. J. Cardiol.*, **37**, 180
33. Marcus, M. L. and Kerber, R. E. (1977). Present status of the 99m Technetium pyrophosphate infarct scintigram. *Circulation*, **56**, 335
34. Donsky, M. S., Curry, G. C., Parkey, R. W., Bonte, F. J., Platt, M. R. and Willerson, J. T. (1976). Unstable angina pectoris: clinical angiographic and scintigraphic observations. *Br. Heart J.*, **38**, 257
35. Alderman, E. L., Matlof, H. J., Wexler, L., Shumway, N. E. and Harrison, D. C. (1973). Results of direct coronary artery surgery for the treatment of angina pectoris. *N. Engl. J. Med.*, **288**, 535
36. Brewer, D. L., Bilbro, R. H. and Bartel, A. G. (1973). Myocardial infarction as a complication of coronary by-pass surgery. *Circulation*, **47**, 58
37. Espinoza, J., Lipski, J., Litwak, R., Donoso, E. and Dack, S. (1974). New Q waves after coronary artery by-pass surgery for angina pectoris. *Am. J. Cardiol.*, **33**, 221
38. Dixon, S. H., Limbird, L. E., Roe, C. R., Wagner, G. S., Oldham, H. W. and Sabiston, D. C. (1973). Recognition of post-operative acute myocardial infarction: application of isoenzyme techniques. *Circulation*, **47/48** (Suppl. III), 137
39. Coleman, R. E., Klein, M. S., Roberts, R. and Sobel, B. E. (1976). Improved detection of myocardial infarction with Technetium-99m stannous pyrophosphate and serum MB creatine phosphokinase. *Am. J. Cardiol.*, **37**, 732
40. Righetti, A., O'Rourke, R. A., Schelbert, H., Henning, H., Hardarson, T., Daily, P. O., Ashburn, W. and Ross, J., Jr. (1977). Usefulness of pre-operative and post-operative Tc-99m-(Sn)-pyrophosphate scans in patients with ischemic and valvular heart disease. *Am. J. Cardiol.*, **39**, 43
41. Platt, M. R., Mills, L. J., Parkey, R. W., Willerson, J. T., Bonte, F. J., Shapiro, W. and Sugg, W. L. (1976). Peri-operative myocardial infarction diagnosed by Technetium ^{99m} stannous pyrophosphate myocardial scintigrams. *Circulation*, **54** (Suppl. III), III-24
42. Ell, P. J., Langford, R., Pearce, P., Lui, D., Elliott, A. T., Woolf, N. and Williams, E. S. (1978). 99m Tc-imidodiphosphonate: a superior radiopharmaceutical for in vivo positive myocardial infarct imaging. *Br. Heart J.*, **40**, 226
43. Beller, G. A., Lehaw, B. A., Haber, E. and Smith, T. W. (1977). Localization of radiolabelled cardiac myosin-specific antibody in myocardial infarcts. Comparison with technetium 99m stannous pyrophosphate. *Circulation*, **55**, 74
44. Caride, V. J. and Zaret, B. L. (1977). Liposome accumulation in regions of acute myocardial infarction. Effect of surface charge. *Clin. Res.*, **25**, 211A
45. Sapirstein, L. A. (1956). Fractionation of cardiac output in rats with isotopic potassium. *Circ. Res.*, **4**, 689
46. Strauss, H. W., Harrison, K., Langan, J. K., Lebowitz, E. and Pitt, B. (1975). Thallium 201 for myocardial imaging. Relation of Thallium 201 to regional myocardial perfusion. *Circulation*, **51**, 641
47. Corne, R. A., Gotsman, M. S. and Atlan, H. (1979). Radionuclide assessment of regional myocardial perfusion with thallium-201. *Am. Heart J.*, **97**, 112
48. Weich, H. F., Strauss, H. W. and Pitt, B. (1977). The extraction of thallium-201 by the myocardium. *Circulation*, **56**, 188

49. Costin, J. C. and Zaret, B. L. (1976). Effect of propranolol and digitalis upon radioactive thallium and potassium uptake in myocardial and skeletal muscle. *J. Nucl. Med.*, **17,** 535
50. Cohen, H. A., Baird, M. G., Rouleau, J. R., Fuhrmann, C. F., Bailey, I. K., Summer, W. R., Strauss, H. W. and Pitt, B. (1976). Thallium-201 myocardial imaging in patients with pulmonary hypertension. *Circulation*, **54,** 790
51. Lenaers, A., Block, P., van Thiel, E., Lebedelle, M., Becquevort, P., Erbsmann, F. and Ermans, A. M. (1977). Segmental analysis of Tl-201 stress myocardial scintigraphy. *J. Nucl. Med.*, **18,** 509
52. McKillop, J. H., Murray, R. G., Turner, J. G., Bessent, R. G., Lorimer, A. R. and Greig, W. R. (1979). Can the extent of coronary artery disease be predicted from Thallium-201 myocardial images? *J. Nucl. Med.*, **20,** 715
53. Wainwright, R. J. (1977). Radioisotopes in cardiology. In Besser, G. M. (Ed.) *Advanced Medicine*, **13,** pp. 462–87 (Tunbridge Wells: Pitman Medical)
54. Ritchie, J. L., Zaret, B. L., Strauss, H. W., Pitt, B., Berman, D. S., Schelbert, H. R. Ashburn, W. L., Berger, H. J. and Hamilton, G. W. (1978). Myocardial imaging with Thallium-201: a multicenter study in patients with angina pectoris or acute myocardial infarction. *Am. J. Cardiol.*, **42,** 345
55. Gould, K. L., Lipscomb, K. and Hamilton, G. W. (1974). A physiological basis for assessing critical coronary stenosis: instantaneous flow response and regional distribution during coronary hyperaemia and measures of coronary flow reserve. *Am. J. Cardiol.*, **33,** 87
56. Pohost, G. M., Zir, L. M., Moore, R. H., McKusick, K. A., Guiney, T. E. and Beller, G. A. (1977). Differentiation of transiently ischaemic from infarcted myocardium by serial imaging after a single dose of Thallium 201. *Circulation*, **55,** 294
57. Blood, D. K., McCarthy, D. M., Sciacca, R. R. and Cannon, P. J. (1978). Comparison of single-dose and double-dose Thallium-201 myocardial perfusion scintigraphy for the detection of coronary artery disease and prior myocardial infarction. *Circulation*, **58,** 777
58. Beller, G. A. and Pohost, G. M. (1978). Time-course and mechanism of resolution of thallium-201 defects after transient myocardial ischaemia. *Am. J. Cardiol.*, **41,** 379
59. Schwartz, J. S., Ponto, R., Carlyle, P., Forstrom, L. and Cohn, J. N. (1978). Early redistribution of Thallium-201 after temporary ischaemia. *Circulation*, **57,** 332
60. Bailey, I. K., Griffith, L. S., Rouleau, J., Strauss, H. W. and Pitt, B. (1977). Thallium-201 myocardial perfusion imaging at rest and during exercise. Comparative sensitivity to electrocardiography in coronary artery disease. *Circulation*, **55,** 79
61. Botvinick, E., Taradash, M. R., Shames, D. M. and Parmley, W. W. (1978). Thallium-201 myocardial perfusion scintigraphy for the clinical clarification of normal, abnormal and equivocal electrocardiographic stress tests. *Am. J. Cardiol.*, **41,** 43
62. Murray, R. G., McKillop, J. H., Bessent, R. G., Turner, J. G., Lorimer, A. R., Hutton, I., Greig, W. R. and Lawrie, T. D. V. (1979). Evaluation of thallium-201 exercise scintigraphy in coronary heart disease. *Br. Heart J.*, **41,** 568
63. Bruschke, A. V., Proudfit, W. L. and Sones, F. M. (1973). Progress study of 590 consecutive nonsurgical cases of coronary disease followed 5–9 years. 1. Arteriographic correlations. *Circulation*, **47,** 1147
64. Humphries, J. O., Kuller, L., Ross, R. S., Friesinger, G. C. and Page, E. E. (1974). Natural history of ischaemic heart disease in relation to arteriographic findings *Circulation*, **49,** 489
65. Rehn, T., Griffith, L., Achuff, S., Bulkley, B., Pond, M. and Becher, L. (1978).

Rest and stress thallium-201 imaging in left main coronary disease: sensitive but not specific. *Am. J. Cardiol.*, **41**, 413
66. Massie, B., Dash, H., Botvinick, E., Brundage, B. and Shames, D. (1978). Identification of high risk coronary disease by myocardial perfusion scintigraphy during exercise testing. *Am. J. Cardiol.*, **41**, 413
67. Wainwright, R. J., Maisey, M. N. and Sowton, E. (1978). Segmental quantitative thallium scintigraphy in diagnosis of coronary artery disease – correlation with coronary arteriography and exercise stress testing. *Br. Heart J.*, **40**, 447
68. Frick, M. H., Valle, M., Korhola, O., Riihimäki, E. and Wiljasolo, M. (1976). Analysis of coronary collaterals in ischaemic heart disease by angiography during pacing induced ischaemia. *Br. Heart J.*, **38**, 189
69. Rigo, P., Becker, L. C., Griffith, L. S. C., Alderson, P. O., Bailey, I. K., Pitt, B., Burow, R. D. and Wagner, H. N. (1979). Influence of coronary collateral vessels on the results of Thallium-201 myocardial stress imaging. *Am. J. Cardiol.*, **44**, 452
70. Wainwright, R. J., Maisey, M. N., Edwards, A. C. and Sowton, E. (1980). Functional significance of coronary collateral circulation during dynamic exercise evaluated by thallium-201 myocardial scintigraphy. *Br. Heart J.*, **43**, 47
71. Dash, H., Massey, B. M., Botvinick, E. and Brundage, B. H. (1979). The non-invasive identification of left main and three-vessel coronary artery disease by myocardial stress perfusion scintigraphy and treadmill exercise electrocardiography. *Circulation*, **60**, 276
72. Leppo, J., Yipintsoi, T., Blankstein, R., Bontemps, R., Freeman, L. M., Zohman, L. and Scheuer, J. (1979). Thallium-201 myocardial scintigraphy in patients with triple vessel disease and ischaemic exercise stress tests. *Circulation*, **59**, 714
73. Rouleau, J., Griffith, L., Strauss, H. W. and Pitt, B. (1975). Detection of diffuse coronary artery disease by quantification of thallium 201 myocardial images. *Circulation*, **52** (Suppl. II), II-111
74. Maseri, A., Parodi, O., Severi, S. and Pesola, A. (1976). Transient transmural reduction of myocardial blood flow, demonstrated by Thallium-201, as a cause of variant angina. *Circulation*, **54**, 280
75. McLaughlin, P. R., Doherty, P. W., Martin, R. P., Goris, M. L. and Harrison, D. C. (1977). Myocardial imaging in a patient with reproducible variant angina. *Am. J. Cardiol.*, **39**, 126
76. Wackers, F. J. Th., Lie, K. I., Liem, K. L., Sokole, E. B., Samson, G., Van Der Schoot, J. B. and Durrer, D. (1978). Thallium-201 scintigraphy in unstable angina pectoris. *Circulation*, **57**, 738
77. Di Luzio, V., Roy, P. R. and Sowton, E. (1974). Angina in patients with occluded aorto-coronary vein grafts. *Br. Heart J.*, **36**, 139
78. Block, T., Murray, J. and English, M. (1977). Improvement in exercise performance after unsuccessful myocardial revascularisation. *Am. J. Cardiol.*, **40**, 673
79. Robinson, P. S., Williams, B. T., Webb-Peploe, M. M., Crowther, A. and Coltart, D. J. (1979). Thallium-201 myocardial imaging in the assessment of results of aorto-coronary bypass surgery. *Br. Heart J.* **42**, 455
80. Wainwright, R. J., Brennand-Roper, D. A., Maisey, M. N. and Sowton, E. (1980). Exercise Thallium-201 myocardial scintigraphy in the follow-up of aorto-coronary bypass graft surgery. *Br. Heart J.*, **43**, 56
81. Kimbiris, D., Iskandrian, A. S., Segal, B. L. and Bemis, C. E. (1978). Anomalous aortic origin of coronary arteries. *Circulation*, **58**, 606
82. Ferrer, P. L., Gottlieb, S., Garcin, O. L. and Miale, A. (1977). Non-invasive diagnosis of anomalous left coronary artery in the young with Thallium-201 myocardial imaging. *Paed. Res.*, **11**, 389
83. Finley, J. P., Howman-Giles, R., Gilday, D. L., Olley, P. M. and Rowe, R. D. (1978). Thallium-201 myocardial imaging in anomalous left coronary artery

arising from the pulmonary artery. Applications before and after medical Nnd surgical treatment. *Am. J. Cardiol.*, **42,** 675

84. Dymond, D., Camm, J., Stone, D., Rees, S., Rees, G. and Spurrell, R. (1980). Dual isotope stress testing in congenital atresia of the left coronary ostium: applications before and after surgical treatment. *Br. Heart J.*, **43,** 270
85. Massie, B., Botvinick, E. H., Shames, D., Taradash, M., Werner, J. and Schiller, J. (1978). Myocardial perfusion scintigraphy in patients with mitral valve prolapse: its advantages over stress electrocardiography in diagnosing associated coronary artery disease and its implications for the aetiology of chest pain. *Circulation*, **57,** 19
86. Bulkley, B. H., Hutchins, G. M., Bailey, I., Strauss, H. W. and Pitt, B. (1977). Thallium-201 imaging and gated cardiac blood pool scans in patients with ischaemic and idiopathic congestive cardiomyopathy. A clinical and pathologic study. *Circulation*, **55,** 753
87. Bulkley, B. H., Rouleau, J., Strauss, H. W. and Pitt, B. (1975). Idiopathic hypertrophic subaortic stenosis: detection by thallium-201 myocardial perfusion scanning. *N. Engl. J. Med.*, **293,** 1113
88. Bulkley, B. H., Rouleau, J. R., Whitaker, J. Q., Strauss, H. W. and Pitt, B. (1977). The use of 201 thallium for myocardial perfusion imaging in sarcoid heart disease. *Chest*, **72,** 27
89. Strauss, H. W. and Pitt, B. (1977). Thallium-201 as a myocardial imaging agent. *Sem. Nucl. Med.*, **7,** 49
90. Turner, D. A., Battle, W. E., Deshmukh, H., Colandrea, M. A., Snyder, G. J., Fordham, E. W. and Messer, J. V. (1978). The predictive value of myocardial perfusion scintigraphy after stress in patients without previous myocardial infarction. *J. Nucl. Med.*, **19,** 249
91. Murray, R. G., McKillop, J. H., Bessent, R. G., Hutton, I., Lorimer, A. R. and Lawrie, T. D. V. (1980). Bayesian analysis of stress thallium-201 scintigraphy. *Br. Heart J.*, **43,** 110
92. Hamilton, G. W., Narahara, K. A., Trobaugh, G. B., Ritchie, J. L. and Williams, D. L. (1978). Thallium-201 myocardial imaging: characterisation of the ECG-synchronized images. *J. Nucl. Med.*, **19,** 1103
93. Evans, J. R., Gunton, R. W. and Beanlands, D. S. (1962). Use of radio-iodinated fatty acid (RIFA) for photoscans of the heart. *Circulation*, **26,** 714
94. Poe, N. D., Robinson, G. D. and Macdonald, B. S. (1975). Myocardial extraction of labelled long chain fatty acid analogs. *Proc. Soc. Exp. Biol. Med.*, **148,** 215
95. Poe, N. D., Robinson, G. D., Graham, L. S. and Macdonald, N. S. (1976). Experimental basis for myocardial imaging with 123-I labelled hexadecanoic acid. *J. Nucl. Med.*, **17,** 1077
96. Freundlieb, Chr., Höck. A., Vyska, K., Feinendegen, L. E., Machulla, H. J. and Stöcklin, G. (1979). Quantitative assessment of myocardial energy metabolism by use of ω-I-123-heptadecanoic acid. *Abstracts of the European Society of Cardiology Workshop use of isotopes* Tours, 21–22 May, p. 78
97. Lösse, B., Höck, A., Rafflenbeul, D., Vushka, K., Krönert, H., Freundlieb, Chr. and Feinendegen, L. E. (1979). Comparative myocardial scintigraphy with 123-I-heptadecanoic acid and 201-thallium. *Abstracts of the European Society of Cardiology Workshop use of isotopes* Tours, 21–22 May, p. 79
98. Walsh, W. F., Harper, P. V., Resnekov, L. and Fill, H. (1976). Non-invasive evaluation of regional myocardial perfusion in 112 patients using a mobile scintillation camera and intravenous Nitrogen-13 labelled ammonia. *Circulation*, **54,** 266
99. Ter-Pogossian, M. M. (1976). Limitations of present radionuclide methods in the

evaluation of myocardial ischaemia and infarction. *Circulation*, **53** (Suppl. I), I-119

100. Kuhl, D. E. and Sanders, T. P. (1971). Characterizing brain lesions with use of transverse section scanning. *Radiology*, **98,** 317
101. Dymond, D. S., Stone, D. L., Elliott, A. T., Britton, K. E. and Spurrell, R. A. J. (1979). Cardiac emission tomography in patients using 201-Thallium. A new technique for perfusion scintigraphy. *Clin. Cardiol.*, **2,** 192
102. Holman, B. L., Hill, T. C., Wynne, J., Lovett, R. D., Zimmerman, R. E. and Smith, E. M. (1979). Single-photon transaxial computed tomography of the heart in normal subjects and in patients with infarction. *J. Nucl. Med.*, **20,** 736
103. Cho, Z. H., Cohen, M. B., Singh, M., Eriksson, L., Chan, J., Macdonald, N. and Spolter, L. (1977). Performance and evaluation of the circular ring transverse axial positron camera (CRTAPC). In: *Medical Radionuclide Imaging*, Vol. I, p. 269 (Vienna: IAEA)
104. Keyes, J. W., Leonard, P. F., Brody, S. L., Svetkoff, D. J., Rogers, L. and Lucchesi, B. R. (1978). Myocardial infarct quantification in the dog by single photon emission computed tomography. *Circulation*, **58,** 227
105. Vogel, R. A., Kirch, D., Lefree, M. and Steel, P. (1978). A new method of multiplanar emission tomography using a sevenpinhole collimator and an Anger scintillation camera. *J. Nucl. Med.*, **19,** 648
106. Vogel, R. A., Kirch, D. L., Lefree, M. I. and Steele, P. (1978). Quantitative analysis of standard and tomographic myocardial perfusion scintigraphy. *Circulation*, **58** (Suppl. IV), II-9
107. Budinger, T. F. and Rollo, F. D. (1977). Physics and instrumentation. *Prog. Cardiovasc.* Dis., **20,** 19
108. Harper, P. V., Lathrop, K. A., Krizek, H., Lembares, N., Stark, V. and Hoffer, P. B. (1972). Clinical feasibility of myocardial imaging with $^{13}NH_3$. *J. Nucl. Med.*, **13,** 278
109. Phelps, M. E., Hoffman, E. J., Coleman, R. E., Welch, M. J., Raichie, M. E., Weiss, E. S., Sobel, B. E. and Ter-Pogossian, M. M. (1976). Tomographic images of blood pool and perfusion in brain and heart. *J. Nucl. Med.*, **17,** 603
110. Schelbert, H. R., Phelps, M. E., Hoffman, E. J., Huang, S. C., Selin, C. E. and Kuhl, D. E. (1979). Regional myocardial perfusion assessed with N-13 labelled ammonia and positron emission computerised axial tomography. *Am. J. Cardiol.*, **43,** 209
111. Gould, K. L., Schelbert, H. R., Phelps, M. E. and Hoffman, E. J. (1979). Non-invasive assessment of coronary stenosis with myocardial perfusion imaging during pharmacologic coronary vasodilatation. Detection of 47 per cent diameter coronary stenosis with intravenous Nitrogen-13 ammonia and emission-computed tomography in intact dogs. *Am. J. Cardiol.*, **43,** 200
112. Weiss, E. S. Hoffman, E. J., Phelps, M. E., Welch, M. J., Henry, P. D., Ter-Pogossian, M. M. and Sobel, B. E. (1976). External detection and visualization of myocardial ischaemia with ^{11}C-substrates in vitro and in vivo. *Circ. Res.*, **39,** 24
113. Klein, M. S., Goldstein, R. A., Welch, M. J. and Sobel, B. E. (1978). External quantification of myocardial metabolism with ^{11}C-labelled fatty acids. *Am. J. Cardiol.*, **41,** 378
114. Sobel, B. E., Weiss, E. S., Welch, M. J., Siegel, B. A. and Ter-Pogossian, M. M. (1977). Detection of remote myocardial infarction in patients with positron emission transaxial tomography and intravenous ^{11}C-palmitate. *Circulation*, **55,** 853
115. Endo, M., Yamazaki, T., Konno, S., Hiratsuka, H., Akimoto, T., Tanaka, T. and Sakakibara, S. (1970). The direct diagnosis of human myocardial ischaemia using ^{131}I-MAA via the selective coronary catheter. *Am. Heart J.*, **80,** 498

116. Grames, G. M., Jansen, C., Gander, M. P., Wieland, B. S. and Judkins, M. P. (1974). Safety of the direct coronary injection of radiolabelled particles. *J. Nucl. Med.*, **15,** 2
117. Ashburn, W. L., Braunwald, E., Simon, A., Peterson, K. and Gauit, J. (1971). Myocardial perfusion imaging with radioactive-labelled particles injected directly into the coronary circulation of patients with coronary artery disease. *Circulation*, **44,** 851
118. Hamilton, G. W., Ritchie, J. L., Allen, D. R., Lapin, E. and Murray, J. A. (1975). Myocardial perfusion imaging with ^{99} Tc or ^{113} In macroaggregated albumin: correlation of the perfusion image with clinical, angiographic, surgical and histologic findings. *Am. Heart J.*, **89,** 708
119. Holman, B. L. (1976). Radionuclide methods in the evaluation of myocardial ischaemia and infarction. *Circulation*, **53** (Suppl. I), I-112
120. Jansen, C., Grames, G. M. and Judkins, M. P. (1974). Myocardial blood flow in man – albumin microsphere technique. In Strauss, H. W., Pitt, B. and James, A. E. (Eds.). *Cardiovascular Nuclear Medicine*, pp. 211 25 (Saint Louis: C V. Mosby)
121. Gould, K. L., Lipscomb, K. and Hamilton, G. W. (1974). Physiologic basis for assessing critical coronary stenosis. Instantaneous flow response and regional distribution during coronary hyperaemia as measures of coronary flow reserve. *Am. J. Cardiol.*, **33,** 87
122. Ritchie, J. L., Hamilton, G. W., Gould, K. L., Allen, D., Kennedy, J. W. and Hammermeister, K. E. (1975). Myocardial imaging with Indium-113m- and Technetium-99m-macroaggregated albumin. New procedure for identification of stress induced regional ischaemia. *Am. J. Cardiol.*, **35,** 380
123. Gould, K. L., Hamilton, G. W., Lipscomb, K. and Kennedy, J. W. (1974). A method for assessing stress-induced regional malperfusion during coronary arteriography: experimental validation and clinical application. *Am. J. Cardiol.*, **34,** 557
124. Hamilton, G. W., English, M. T., Ritchie, J. L. and Allen, D. R. (1977). Myocardial perfusion imaging with MAA following coronary artery surgery. In Serafino, A. N., Gilson, A. J. and Smoak, W. M. (Eds.). *Nuclear Cardiology – Principles and Methods*, pp. 111–22 (New York: Plenum)
125. Kaplan, E., Mayron, L. W., Friedman, A. M., Gindler, J. E., Frazin, L., Moran, J. M. Loeb, H. and Gunner, R. M. (1976). Definition of myocardial perfusion by continuous infusion of Krypton-81m. *Am. J. Cardiol.*, **37,** 878
126. Selwyn, A. P., Steiner, R., Kivisaari, A., Fox, K. and Forse, G. (1979). Krypton-81m in the physiologic assessment of coronary arterial stenosis in man. *Am. J. Cardiol.*, **43,** 547
127. Selwyn, A. P., Sapsford, R., Forse, G., Fox, K. and Myers, M. (1979). Assessment of coronary venous bypass graft function using Krypton-81m. *Am. J. Cardiol.*, **43,** 554
128. Knoebel, S. B., McHenry, P. L., Stein, L. and Sonel, A. (1967). Myocardial blood flow in man as measured by a coincidence counting system and a single bolus of ^{84}RbCl. *Circulation*, **36,** 187
129. Eckenhoff, J. E., Hafkenschiel, J. H., Harmel, M. H., Goodale, W. T., Lubin, M., Bing, R. J. and Kety, S. S. (1968). Measurement of coronary blood flow by the nitrous oxide method. *Am. J. Physiol.*, **152,** 356
130. Maseri, A., Mancini, P., L'Abbate, A. and Magini, G. (1971). Method for regional dynamic study of myocardial blood flow in man. *J. Nucl. Biol. Med.*, **15,** 54
131. Schmidt, D. H., Weiss, M. B., Casarella, W. J., Fowler, D. L., Sciacca, R. R. and Cannon, P. J. (1976). Regional myocardial perfusion during atrial pacing in patients with coronary artery disease. *Circulation*, **53,** 807

132. Cannon, P. J., Sciacca, R. R., Fowler, D. L., Weiss, M. B., Schmidt, D. H. and Casarella, W. J. (1975). Measurement of regional myocardial blood flow in man: description and critique of the method using Xenon-133 and a scintillation camera. *Am. J. Cardiol.*, **36**, 683

15
Nuclear imaging techniques in cardiology and cardiac surgery
Part 2 Dynamic imaging

D. S. DYMOND

INTRODUCTION

In the first of these 2 chapters on the subject of nuclear imaging, the techniques that have been described for infarct scanning and perfusion scanning produce images that are static. In other words, an image produced over a few minutes shows no appreciable change in tracer distribution over the imaging period. The dynamic imaging techniques to be described in this chapter differ, in that tracer distribution changes rapidly with time within a region of interest.

HISTORICAL REVIEW OF DYNAMIC IMAGING

As long ago as 1927, Blumgart and Weiss[1] injected solutions of Radium C intravenously in patients, and recorded the arrival in the other arm with an imaging device called a cloud chamber. They found that the mean arm-to-arm circulation time was prolonged in patients with heart disease. In the early 1940s, a Geiger–Müller tube was used to measure the time for intravenously injected sodium-24 to travel from injection site to a distant point in the circulation[2]. The effects of various drugs on circulatory dynamics were measured in this way[3]. In 1948 Prinzmetal and co-workers[4] recorded graphically the appearance and concentration of sodium-24 over the heart following intravenous injection. Filling and emptying of both sides of the heart was demonstrated, and the term 'radiocardiography' was coined for this technique. The method was too imprecise to provide data on the nature and severity of cardiac disease. Over the next 20 years, most of the efforts in the field of radiocardiography were directed towards overcoming the limitations of external counting. Quantitative radiocardiography[5] has been used in the measurement of mean pulmonary circulation time, pulmonary blood volume, and cardiac output.

The graphic recordings lent themselves to the detection of intracardiac shunts. Iodine-131-labelled renografin was used to detect right-to-left shunts by recording its early appearance over the femoral artery[6] and left-to-right shunts were detected by recording the early arrival of an intracardiac injection of krypton-85 in expired air[7], or by continuous sampling from the right side of the heart after phosphorus-32-labelled erythrocytes were injected into the pulmonary artery[8].

The development of devices that provided anatomical information as well as data in curve format was a major advance. Imaging of the cardiac blood pool was first used clinically for the detection of pericardial effusions, using radioiodinated human serum albumin and a rectilinear scanner[9]. After the arrival of the Anger camera radionuclide angiocardiograms were obtained in 1965[10], the passage of a radioactive bolus being followed through the heart and great vessels. In 1969, temporal resolution of one-sixtieth of a second was achieved on such angiocardiograms by the use of a stop-action video-recorder[11]. Throughout the 1970s, improvements in imaging devices and computer technology have led to the quantification of nuclear angiograms and their wide usage in clinical practice.

BASIC PRINCIPLES OF MODERN DYNAMIC IMAGING

The instrument capabilities which influenced the accuracy of dynamic studies included all performance characteristics pertinent to static studies, such as collimator design, accurate event positioning, and field uniformity. The greatest limitation for quantitative dynamic studies was without doubt the low count-rates achieved with available imaging devices, and the earliest instruments for cardiac dynamics achieved a count-rate of less than 30000 counts per second[12]. Count-rates of a high level are needed to resolve the rapidly occurring events of the cardiac cycle. Low count-rates themselves are not a problem when static images are required, as the imaging time can be prolonged to obtain enough counts. In dynamic imaging low count-rates limit the statistical accuracy of the dynamic function measurements. The ability of a camera system to resolve the rapid events of the cardiac cycle depends on three components:

(a) temporal (or framing rate);
(b) statistical (or information density);
(c) spatial.

These three components are not mutually independent[13], and an attempt to improve the temporal resolution by faster framing rates, without a concomitant increase in count-rates may degrade the final image by reducing the information density. Rapid framing rates are necessary in cardiac studies to achieve definition of each phase of the cardiac cycle, and 20 frames per second will provide this[13]. At longer framing intervals a frame designated as end-diastole may already include early systolic elements. Rapid framing rates will have minimal clinical usefulness if there are not an adequate number of counts in each frame to provide a satisfactory signal to noise ratio. The noise per unit area of an image is dependent on the square root of the number of counts in that image and hence on the square root of the data density[14]. An image with only 100 counts per matrix element will have a statistical error of 10 %, but an image with one million counts per matrix element will have an error of only 0.1 %. If counts are so low that changes in counts between diastole and systole are within statistical errors then measurements of ejection fraction based on count changes will be inaccurate[13]. The limitations in count rates and the consequences are at least partly responsible for the development of two different methods for dynamic cardiac imaging, namely:

(a) first pass radionuclide angiography;
(b) equilibrium gated blood pool imaging.

The former involves the imaging of the first transit only of an injected bolus of radionuclide through the individual cardiac chambers and lungs. The second method involves the injection of a non-diffusible indicator into the blood stream, and imaging is carried out over several minutes after the tracer has equilibrated in the cardiac blood pool. Temporal resolution of the different phases of the cardiac cycle is achieved by electrocardiographic gating devices which permit imaging only at certain phases of the cardiac cycle. The gating devices may be triggered by the 'R' wave of the electrocardiogram and have delay controls and record controls. At its simplest, imaging is carried out only at the extremes of the cardiac cycle by having the gate open during the immediate 40 ms associated with end-systole and 60 ms associated with end-diastole[15].

Imaging may take several minutes, and data from several hundred cardiac cycles are summed to achieve enough counts for a statistically accurate image. Advances in computer techniques have allowed extension of this method into multiple gated acquisition studies (MUGA) when the cardiac cycle may be gated into up to 28 segments[16]. 200000 counts per frame over the heart may be achieved in 12–16 min.

ADVANTAGES AND DISADVANTAGES OF FIRST PASS AND GATED STUDIES

A full list of the differing technical prerequisites and advantages and disadvantages of each technique are shown in Table 1. The major advantages of the first pass technique are:

(a) the ability to perform right anterior oblique studies due to temporal separation of the ventricles;
(b) the short data-acquisition time, which permits studies to be peformed at the end-point of a stress test;
(c) low background counts in other chambers;
(d) no ECG gating is necessary.

Table 1 Advantages and disadvantages of first pass and gated studies

	First pass	*Gated*
Isotope	Technetium-99m as pertechnetate. Separate injection for each study. Small bolus necessary	Technetium-99m bound to human serum albumin or red cells. Repeat studies possible from one injection of indicator
Camera	High count-rate capabilities and high temporal resolution needed for adequate statistics. Wall motion may not be possible with ordinary camera. Multi-crystal camera ideal	Conventional camera and computer only needed
Projection	RAO possible	LAO preferred due to spatial separation of ventricles
Time	50 s only for data acquisition	Up to 5 min
Background	Low outside chamber of interest	High background at equilibrium
Selection of end-diastole and end-systole	Achieved by count density only. ECG unnecessary	ECG gating required, and assumptions made about relation of electrical to mechanical events that may be altered in cardiac disease
Right ventricular contribution	Very important. Studies not possible if RV function poor, or tricuspid insufficiency present. Pulmonary artery injection required in such cases	Independent of RV function, provided LAO is used
Arrhythmia	Representative cycle of little value in presence of atrial fibrillation or multiple ectopic beats. Limited data available means it is difficult to reject cardiac cycles	Beats may be rejected if fall outside selected cycle length
Stress testing	Dynamic exercise possible. True end-point studies obtainable. Exercise can be terminated at moment of injection	Dynamic studies of dubious technical validity due to motion artefacts, and long data-acquisition time. Non-dynamic stress tests preferable, e.g. isometric, cold-pressor
Intervention studies	Dual study possible. Two or three data points only with currently available radionuclides	Multiple data points possible over 4 h

The major disadvantages are:

(a) the limited number of cardiac cycles available to accumulate an image of sufficient data density;

(b) the dependence on adequate right ventricular function to eject the bolus as a compact unit prior to entry into the left ventricle;

(c) the difficulties in obtaining reliable data if the patient is in atrial fibrillation or has multiple premature beats;
(d) each study requires a separate injection of radionuclide.

The major advantages of gated scanning are:

(1) multiple studies can be obtained from a single injection of tracer, allowing the effects of an intervention to be studied over a period of hours;
(2) data collection time can be as long as is desired, and data density is therefore satisfactory;
(3) premature beats or beats with excessively short or long cycle lengths can be rejected.

The major disadvantages of gated scanning are:

(1) the necessity to perform left anterior oblique studies to provide spatial separation between right and left ventricles. This projection is not the optimum for studying ventricular wall motion[17];
(2) high background counts in other cardiac chambers;
(3) assumptions about relation of electrical events to mechanical ones;
(4) long data-acquisition time hinders end-point stress studies.

There is little doubt that the count-rate limitations of single-crystal gamma cameras restrict their ability to provide accurate information on wall motion when first pass studies are performed. A different concept in imaging devices is that of a multi-crystal gamma camera[12,13] which has higher count-rate capabilities than any other available imaging system and is able to perform fast dynamic cardiac studies by the first pass technique[12,13,18-20]; it is therefore able to overcome the constraints imposed by collecting data from a few cardiac cycles only.

RADIATION DOSAGES

The radiation dosages received by patients undergoing radionuclide angiography are small. Patients receiving a total of 20 mCi of technetium-99m will be exposed to less than 400 mrad, compared to 3900 mrad for cardiac catheterization and angiography[21].

MEASUREMENTS OF VENTRICULAR FUNCTION BY RADIONUCLIDE VENTRICULOGRAPHY

Equilibrium gated blood pool scans are able to provide information on left ventricular ejection fraction, regional wall motion and indices of ejection, such as ejection rate. First pass angiograms can in addition provide information on transit times, cardiac output, and left-to-right shunts (see below). In clinical practice ejection fraction and regional wall motion are the most useful parameters and can be obtained from either technique.

EJECTION FRACTION

The earliest attempt to measure left ventricular ejection fraction by radioisotopic methods was made in 1962, when a radioactive tracer was introduced directly into the left ventricle and a precordial detector was used to record the dilution of the tracer to estimate ejection fraction[22]. The technique produced highly inaccurate estimates, attributed to the incomplete mixing of tracer with blood caused by a direct ventricular injection. In 1971, Strauss and co-workers[23] described the measurement of left ventricular ejection fraction from end-systolic and end-diastolic images of gated studies. Ejection fraction was measured by the application of geometric-area–length formulae to the scintigraphic outlines in the same way as to contrast angiograms.

In 1972 a new method for estimating ejection fraction was described, which exploited the relationship of counts within a chamber to the volume of that chamber at any one time, assuming complete mixing had occurred[24]. With ECG gating devices, good correlations were found between this 'count-volume' ejection fraction and contrast angiographic values[25]. Since then, many reports have appeared of good correlation between radionuclide ejection fractions and contrast angiographic values both from first pass studies[18–20,26,27], or gated scans[16,23,28]. The formula in all cases for calculation of ejection fraction is:

$$\text{Ejection fraction} = \frac{\text{End-diastolic counts minus end-systolic counts}}{\text{End-diastolic counts minus background counts}}$$

The main differences in all the methods described relate to the various methods by which background corrections are made in the application of the above formula. A full review of all the techniques for background correction is beyond the scope of this chapter but suffice it to say that good correlations seem to be produced with contrast angiographic values for most methods, despite the valid criticisms that may often be made about some of the assumptions used.

At St Bartholomew's Hospital, the method for calculation of ejection fraction is as follows:

(1) From the initial first pass radionuclide angiocardiogram a frame from the left ventricular phase is chosen and a region of interest entered using a magnetic pen. Figure 1 is an example of such a region of interest.

(2) A high-frequency time–activity curve (Figure 2) is generated to display the change of counts with time occurring in that region. The flat portion of the top curve in Figure 2 contains the spatial and temporal data of the washout of activity from lungs and left atrium. The peaks and troughs of the curves represent the end-diastolic and end-systolic phases of the individual cardiac cycles involved in the first pass. The numbers above the curves are the frame numbers and the counts per frame. Thus frame 1100 contains 852 counts, etc.

(3) The frame numbers of the peaks and troughs are fed into the computer and summed. Background correction is made by choosing the lowest point on the plateau, pre-ventricular phase (frame 1126 of Figure 2, with 542 counts), and background counts are subtracted dynamically from the peak and trough counts, as background changes temporally as the activity enters and leaves the left ventricle.

Such background corrections have produced excellent correlates with contrast angiography in anterior[18] and right anterior oblique[20] projections. It is open to debate whether or not radionuclide or contrast angiographic measurements of ejection fraction are the more accurate. The geometric formulae applied to contrast angiograms assume that the left ventricle conforms to a predetermined shape. Whereas this may be a reasonable assumption in normal hearts, diseased hearts may deviate from the prolate spheroid model and hence geometric measurements may be less valid. Radionuclide measurements make no geometric assumptions and therefore may be more accurate. Radionuclide measurements are extremely reproducible[29,30] and the techniques are therefore suitable for intervention studies (see below).

Given the importance of left ventricular ejection fraction as one of the most useful indices of left ventricular function in terms of its relationship to patients' clinical status, the results of surgery and eventual prognosis[31,32], then radionuclide ventriculography has an important role to play in the assessment of cardiac patients.

REGIONAL WALL MOTION

Whereas left ventricular ejection fraction is a useful index of global function, it is just as important to have information about regional ventricular performance. The cardiac literature has contained an abundant number of reports which show radionuclide techniques to be capable of providing accurate information on wall motion[13,15,18–20,27]. The first pass technique, by permitting right anterior oblique studies to be carried out, has a major advantage over gated scanning, as the left anterior oblique is not the projection of choice for studying wall motion. Pierson *et al.*[33] have found that anterior segments of ventricle may be poorly visualized when gated scanning is used. Problems of defining the edge of the ventricle are more difficult to solve from radionuclide angiograms than from contrast studies. In the latter, where contrast is injected directly into the left ventricle, high-contrast images are produced. In radionuclide studies, an image is seen of counts within a cavity but the edge of that cavity is not defined. Several methods exist of identifying the position of the ventricular wall. Among the most widely used are (a) the isocount contour technique[18,20], whereby a count band is enhanced around the ventricular image, and (b) first or second derivative method[27], from a profile across the matrix containing the image.

Figure 3a and 3b are images of the left ventricle at end-diastole and end-systole from a right oblique first pass angiogram. The colour display shows

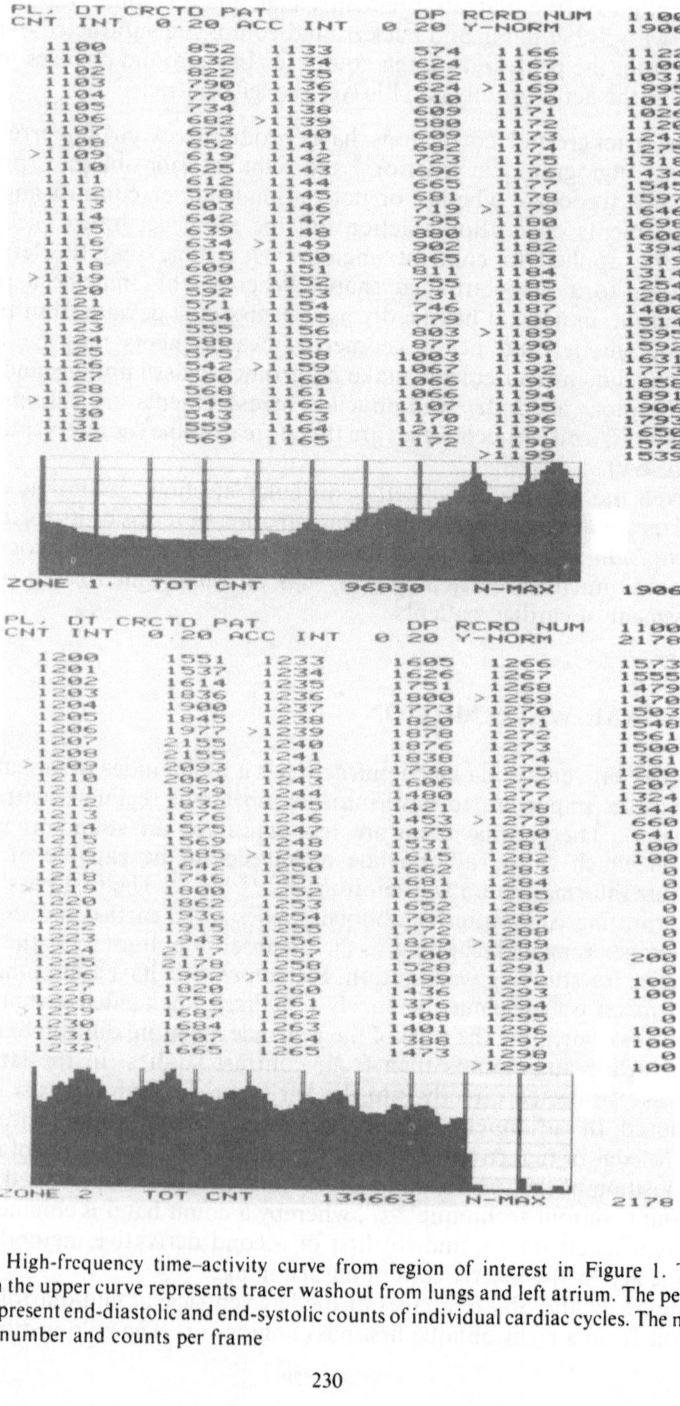

Figure 2 High-frequency time–activity curve from region of interest in Figure 1. The flat portion on the upper curve represents tracer washout from lungs and left atrium. The peaks and troughs represent end-diastolic and end-systolic counts of individual cardiac cycles. The numbers are frame number and counts per frame

the distribution of activity in 16 colours, with yellow representing the maximum number of counts per cell in the image. Decreasing activity is shown by a different colour for every 6.25% decrement in count density scaling down from red to dark green. In Figure 3a the maximum count density is in the left ventricle and in Figure 3b the most dense counts are seen in the aortic root. The isocount contours of each image may be produced and superimposed. Figure 4 shows the two contours superimposed to provide an image from which regional wall motion may be assessed. The end-diastolic perimeter is in white, the end-systolic perimeter in yellow. Uniform wall motion is apparent throughout the left ventricle. The assessment of normality and abnormality can be made either visually, which depends upon subjective interpretation of either a cine-display or of a static image such as Figure 4, or objectively. Objective quantification of wall motion has been carried out by the application of a hemiaxial model to the ventricular perimeter, and percentage shortening for each axis may be measured. This has been validated against contrast angiograms[19]. Such an objective approach has proved useful in detecting stress-induced abnormalities of regional ventricular function, as will be discussed later.

Regional Ejection Fraction

Another approach to the assessment of regional function is that of the regional ejection fraction. This method does not demand structural resolution sufficient to define the edges of the ventricles, but instead relies only on the relative stroke volume counts of each region, compared to end-diastolic counts[34-36]. The regional ejection fraction can be displayed as an image which represents in 16 colour shades the relative contribution of each zone to ejection fraction. Figure 5 is an example of a normal regional ejection fraction image. The homogeneity of function is apparent from the yellow colour throughout the image. This image has been found valuable in the demonstration of asynergy at rest[34] and under stress[35,36] (see below).

Like ejection fraction, regional wall motion has been found to be reproducible from radionuclide studies[30].

TRANSIT TIMES

Since the development of quantitative radiocardiography[5] there has been wide interest in the study of the transit of blood through the central circulation. Chamber-to-chamber transit times index the efficiency of blood flow and appear to provide data that relate to haemodynamic variables[37]. This is evident in the work of Steele *et al.*[38] who described the relationship of a shortened pulmonary transit time to the presence of a pulmonary embolus, and in the work of other groups who have defined the relationship of a prolonged pulmonary curve to the presence of left-to-right shunting[39]. This will be discussed in more detail later. Transit time measurements can be obtained from recordings of a single probe over the heart[38] or by generation of time–activity curves from imaging equipment. The latter method involves entering a region of interest of both right and left ventricles of a radionuclide angiogram. Figure 6 is an example of a time–activity curve from those regions of interest spanning a period of 20 s. The twin peaks are right and left ventricular phases respectively, and the trough in between is the pulmonary phase. Mean right-to-left transit times are calculated from the difference in mean right and mean left transit times[40]. The individual transit times are obtained by a curve-analysis computer programme which searches for the peaks in the curve and 'strips' one peak from the other. A semi-logarithmic extrapolation is applied to each component curve, assuming a mono-exponential washout of tracer from each chamber. Mean chamber transit times can then be calculated by the formula:

$$\text{Mean transit time} = \Sigma_i(\text{sum of counts at time } i \times \text{time } i) \div \text{sum of total counts (ref. 37).}$$

Although transit time measurements have been used in clinical diagnosis, as discussed above, the values are far less useful than first appeared because many factors affect the measurements in the same way as cardiac output may be influenced. In conjunction with other measurements such as ventricular images, ejection fraction and chamber volumes, they are of more use. For example, the presence of a large end-diastolic volume, a high stroke volume and a prolonged chamber transit time might indicate valvular regurgitation.

VOLUMES

Calculation of ventricular volumes from radionuclide angiogram depends on application of geometric formulae to the radionuclide perimeters (Figure 4c). In 1969 the measurement of ventricular volumes was described from first pass studies recorded in synchrony with the electrocardiogram[41] Several end-diastolic and end-systolic frames were summed and the edges of the projected images defined. Since then several studies have reported good correlation with contrast angiographic volumes in various projections[23,42,43].

Errors in the choice of the ventricular edge for the images almost certainly contributed to the underestimation of volumes by the isotope method in one study[42]. Using the isocount edge-enhancement technique described above, the tendency is for the radionuclide studies to overestimate volumes[20], especially when large volumes are present. Nevertheless the correlations are good, as shown in Figure 7. Recently we have described the use of right and left anterior oblique radionuclide venticulograms[44] to provide volumes from a biplane geometric formula. Biplane volumes may be more accurate than single-plane values[17,44].

INDICES OF CONTRACTILITY

Left ventricular contractility can be quantified from cineventriculograms by relating the instantaneous velocity of fibre shortening of the minor axis to maximal wall tension during ejection[45]. Mean circumferential fibre shorten-

PL. DT CRCTD PAT RCRD NUM 4221
CNT INT 0.05 ACC INT 0.20 Y-NORM 6220

3601	76	3733	5022	3865	1379
3605	252	3737	4920	3869	1365
3609	265	3741	4745	3873	1419
3613	404	3745	4515	>3877	1478
3617	922	3749	4354	3881	1495
3621	2155	3753	4053	3885	1533
3625	3647	>3757	3826	3889	1550
3629	5180	3761	3581	3893	1544
3633	5842	3765	3434	3897	1491
>3637	6220	3769	3271	3901	1466
3641	5764	3773	3117	.3905	1486
3645	5530	3777	2928	3909	1507
3649	4840	3781	2703	3913	1578
3653	4530	3785	2520	>3917	1615
3657	3912	3789	2436	3921	1668
3661	3539	3793	2299	3925	1657
3665	3108	>3797	2236	3929	1600
3669	2834	3801	2095	3933	1652
3673	2674	3805	2072	3937	1738
>3677	2597	3809	1987	3941	1836
3681	2590	3813	1903	3945	1789
3685	2568	3817	1849	3949	1763
3689	2614	3821	1775	3953	1760
3693	2900	3825	1725	>3957	1780
3697	3081	3829	1634	3961	1834
3701	3464	3833	1640	3965	1834
3705	3774	>3837	1548	3969	1853
3709	4204	3841	1514	3973	1884
3713	4395	3845	1506	3977	1872
>3717	4670	3849	1499	3981	1862
3721	4952	3853	1457	3985	1801
3725	5065	3857	1442	3989	1900
3729	5108	3861	1404	3993	1968
				>3997	2002

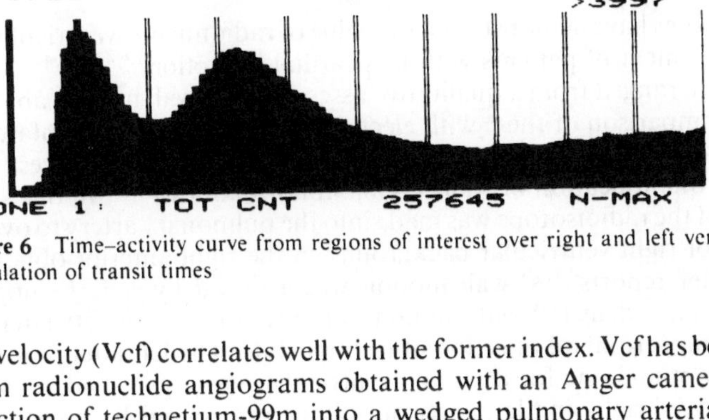

ZONE 1: TOT CNT 257645 N-MAX 6220

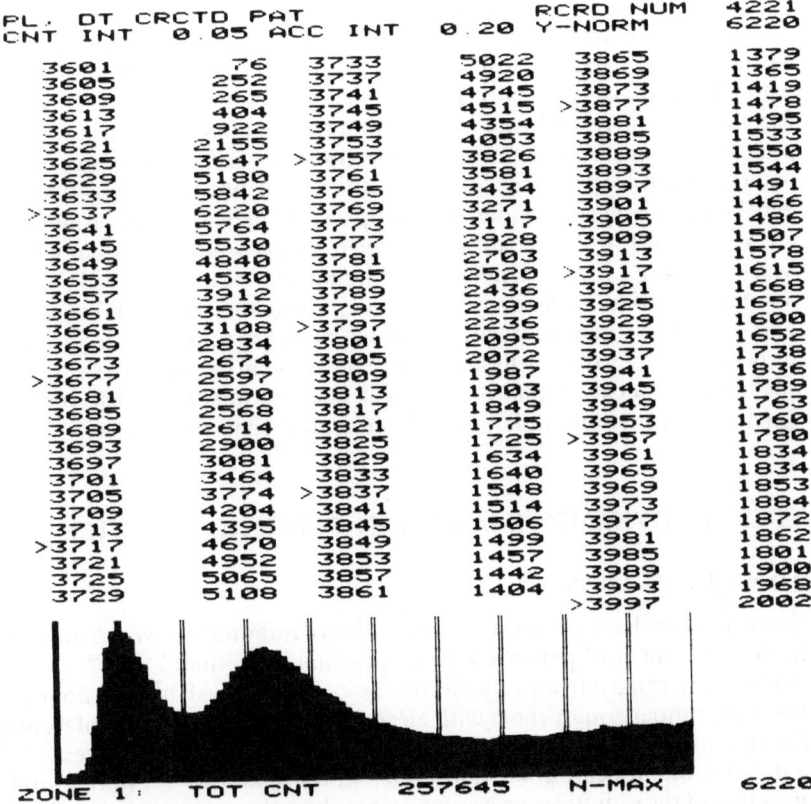

Figure 6 Time–activity curve from regions of interest over right and left ventricles, used for calculation of transit times

ing velocity (Vcf) correlates well with the former index. Vcf has been measured from radionuclide angiograms obtained with an Anger camera, following injection of technetium-99m into a wedged pulmonary arterial catheter[46]. A region of interest and time–activity curve were constructed over the minor axis of the ventricle. Vcf was calculated in circumferences per second, from the formula:

$$\text{Mean Vcf (radionuclide)} = \frac{\sqrt{C_{ED}} - \sqrt{C_{ES}}}{ET} \times \frac{1}{\sqrt{C_{ED}}}$$

where $\sqrt{C_{ED}}$ and $\sqrt{C_{ES}}$ are the square roots of the count-rates at end-diastole and end-systole respectively and ET is the ejection time.

Systolic ejection rate was measured in the same study. Values for Vcf and ejection rate correlated very closely with contrast angiographic values. Contractility indices also correlated well with measurements of ejection fraction. In another study[18], left ventricular ejection rate was measured from the representative cardiac cycle obtained by summing the individual cardiac cycles from a first pass angiogram. With a weighted least-squares analysis and a desk-top computer, a straight line was fitted to the high-frequency ejection phase data. The slope of this line represented the change in counts with time. This was normalized to the average counts over the ejection phase. Ejection rate correlated well with ejection fraction but not with end-diastolic pressure or stroke volume index. Ejection rate increased dramatically in patients when isoprenaline was infused[18] and it has been suggested that it may be a more sensitive index of inotropic state than is ejection fraction. The problems of fitting a slope to high-frequency data will be apparent when fast heart rates are present. Under these circumstances there are very few data points per cardiac cycle, and the errors in fitting the slope will be increased. These problems may be partly overcome by more rapid framing rates than 20 per second, as these will allow more data points per cycle. In the radionuclide assessment of pharmacological interventions upon left ventricular function, contractility indices may have a promising role to play.

USES OF DYNAMIC IMAGING IN CLINICAL PRACTICE

Myocardial infarction

Several studies have demonstrated the value of radionuclide ventriculography in the assessment of patients with myocardial infarction[13,43,44,47–50]. Such studies have ranged from a qualitative assessment of wall motion abnormalities and comparison of these with electrocardiographic sites of infarction[13], through assessments of ejection fraction from time–activity curves[47–49] to a detailed quantification of wall motion abnormalities[44,50]. In one study[47], injection of the radioisotope was made into the pulmonary artery to overcome problems of right ventricular background in the right anterior oblique, and in two other reports[48,49] wall motion was assessed by radarkymography. Kostuk *et al.*[43] detected wall motion abnormalities in the left lateral projection using peripheral injection of radionuclide. The left lateral projection is not the optimal one for assessing ventricular asynergy[17] and studies that have employed right and left anterior oblique projections have been carried out[44,50].

Both these studies measured ejection fraction, wall motion abnormalities, and chamber volumes. In one study[44] the use of biplane projection was advocated especially when multiple areas of infarction were present. Single-plane right or left obliques appeared equally able to detect akinesis in isolated anterior or postero-inferior infarction but each single projection had a substantial failure rate in multiple infarctions. The combined projections successfully demonstrated abnormalities in all areas. Figure 8 is an example of right and left anterior oblique ventriculograms from a patient with lateral and posterior myocardial infarction. The right oblique image (left hand) shows an akinetic segment anteriorly, but normal inferior function. The left oblique image shows akinesis of posterolateral wall.

The relationship between the extent of akinesis and left ventricular ejection fraction was also investigated[44]. For mean percentage akinesis from both obliques, akinesis from single-plane right oblique, and akinesis from single-plane left oblique, there was a definite inverse relationship with ejection fraction. The correlations are shown in Figure 9(a–c). Whereas mean percentage akinesis and percentage akinesis from right oblique studies showed equally good negative correlation with ejection fraction, the left oblique akinetic percentage was less well related to ejection fraction. The left oblique alone may give a false impression of the amount of akinesis, possibly due to the fact that in that projection the view is from the apex of the left ventricle rather than perpendicular to the long axis. The same study found that multiple infarctions led to a greater percentage akinesis and greater depression of ejection fraction than did anterior infarctions, which in turn led to more akinesis than inferior infarctions. These findings are in agreement with contrast angiographic data[51] and support the concept that more myocardial damage occurs after anterior than inferior infarction, as suggested by enzyme kinetic studies[52]. Rigo and co-workers[50] found that left ventricular end-diastolic volume was increased in patients with infarction only when left ventricular filling pressure was increased and cardiac index reduced, findings which relate to patients' prognosis[53]. Measurements of volume may therefore

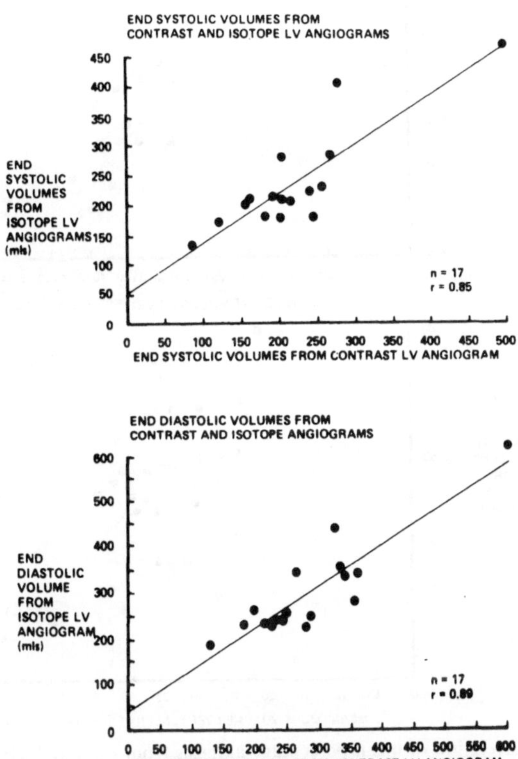

Figure 7 Correlations for end-systolic (above) and end-diastolic volumes between contrast and radionuclide angiograms. (Reproduced from *Br. Heart J.*[20] by permission of the publisher)

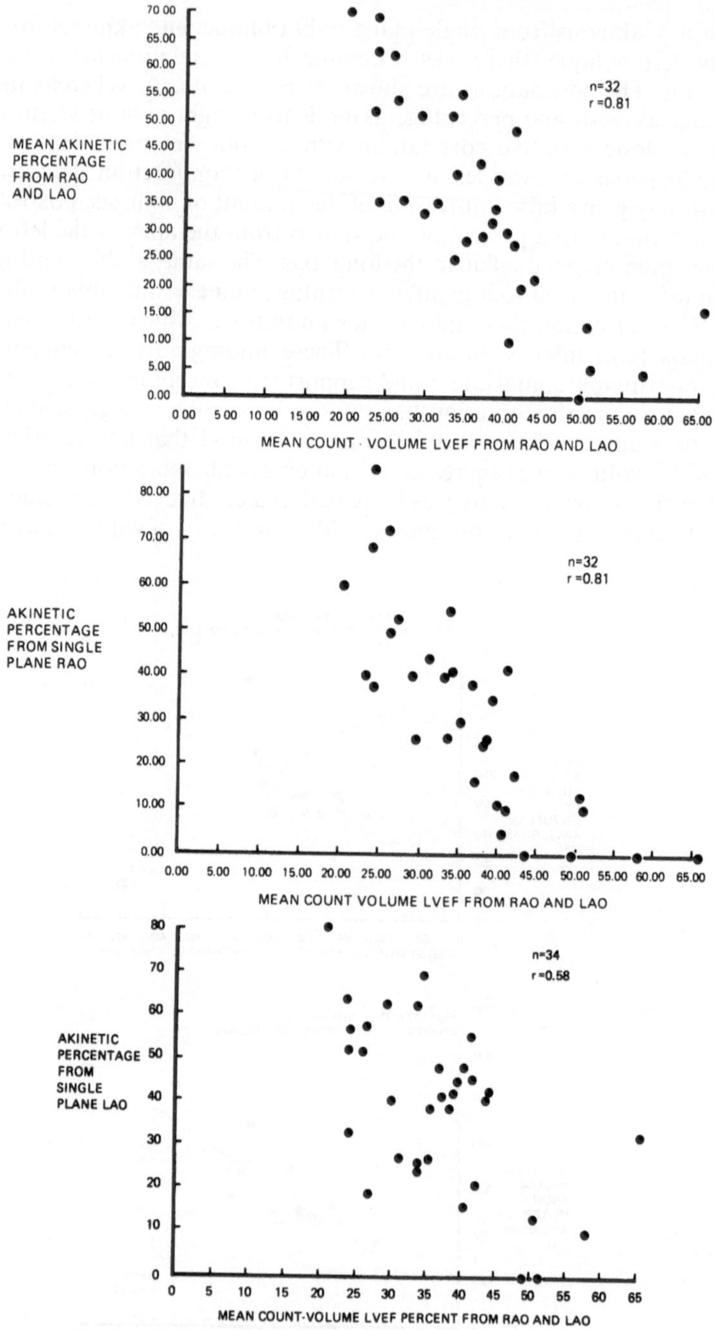

Figure 9 (a) Correlation of mean percentage akinesis from right and left obliques with mean ejection fraction from two obliques. (b) Correlation of percentage akinesis from single-plane right-oblique study with mean ejection fraction. (c) Correlation of percentage akinesis from left oblique study with mean ejection fraction (Reproduced from *Br. Heart J.* [44] by permission of the publisher)

provide prognostic information in such patients, and radionuclide ventriculography appears to be superior to single-beam echocardiography in this respect, the latter frequently overestimating ventricular performance[48]. The radionuclide ventriculogram thus appears to be capable of providing information on infarct size by measurements of akinetic percentages, as well as providing data on prognosis. The problems of measuring infarct size *in vivo* by other radioisotope methods have been discussed in detail in the preceding chapters. If dynamic imaging were performed at the bedside of acutely ill patients, effects on left ventricular function of interventions designed to reduce infarct size could be assessed. This appears to be a promising possibility for the future.

DETECTION OF LEFT VENTRICULAR ANEURYSMS

The development of left ventricular failure or congestive cardiac failure following infarction may be the result of a localized left ventricular aneurysm or of global ventricular dysfunction[54]. The differentiation between these derangements of ventricular function is crucial in the assessment of patients with such symptoms after infarction, as those with hypokinetic ventricles are rarely aided by surgical resection. Cardiac catheterization and contrast angiography has been successfully used to diagnose ventricular aneurysms, but the non-invasive radionuclide ventriculogram now has an important part to play in such diagnosis.

Gated blood pool scans have been reported as successful in detecting left ventricular aneurysms[55,56]. In the first of these studies[55], left ventricular ejection fraction was calculated from a geometric formula, not from time–activity curves, and in the second study[56] no quantitative data on wall motion were presented, although the technique appeared qualitatively reliable in the detection of such aneurysms. First pass angiography successfully differentiated between aneurysms and diffuse hypokinesis in 18 patients with recurrent symptoms after infarction[20]. In this study, ejection fraction and ventricular volumes correlated well with the contrast angiographic measurements. The extent of wall motion defect produced by ventricular aneurysms has been expressed as a percentage of the total end-diastolic circumference of the ventricle, and two studies have shown excellent correlations between this simple index of aneurysm size from radionuclide and contrast studies[20,55].

Radionuclide ventriculography can be recommended as a screening test in the pre-catheterization phase of investigation of patients with symptoms following myocardial infarction.

SELECTION OF PATIENTS FOR ANEURYSMECTOMY

Just as important as the differentiation between global and segmental ventricular dysfunction is the demonstration that patients with ventricular aneurysms have sufficiently good residual function to permit surgical intervention. This was recognized as long ago as 1968, when Key *et al.*[57] commented on the necessity for 'good left ventricular deep constrictor activity' to increase the likelihood of a successful operation. Such observations have been superseded by methods for quantification of contractile segment function. Ejection fraction of the contractile segment of ventricle (EFCS) has been found to be related to the results of aneurysmectomy[58]. Recently, we have described the measurement of EFCS from radionuclide ventriculograms and the correlation with contrast angiographic measurements[59]. Changes in EFCS occurred on exercise, and after administration of the vasodilator drug isosorbide dinitrate. The changes in EFCS appear to be independent of coronary artery status. If the function of the contractile segment does prove to be of importance in determining the results of aneurysmectomy, then radionuclide ventriculography can provide unique angiographic data to aid in the selection of patients for surgery. The demonstration that isosorbide dinitrate can improve exercise function in some patients with aneurysms allows logical identification of patients likely to benefit from nitrate therapy when operation is not contemplated or contraindicated.

ASSESSMENT OF VENTRICULAR FUNCTION FOLLOWING ANEURYSMECTOMY

The postoperative assessment of patients who have undergone left ventricular aneurysmectomy has often been limited to a subjective evaluation of symptoms[60] or, more recently, to a study of changes in resting haemodynamics[61]. Data on the results of aneurysmectomy indicate that the operation may not lead to improvements in symptoms or in haemodynamic measurements[60,61].

The ease of repetition, and the non-invasive nature of radionuclide ventriculography make the technique ideal for the study of the effects of surgery on left ventricular function.

Recently, we have investigated the effects of aneurysmectomy on left ventricular function at rest and on exercise, in 12 patients[62]. Resting ejection fraction improved significantly after surgery, from a mean of 26.6% to 33.3%, although it remained abnormal in all cases. End-diastolic volume fell from a mean of 344 ml before surgery to a mean of 232 ml postoperatively. In parallel with this improvement was a reduction in left ventricular filling pressure. Symptomatically dyspnoea improved in seven patients by one New York Heart Association (NYHA) clinical class, and five remained unchanged.

Exercise ejection fraction failed to improve over preoperative levels and although exercise filling pressure did show an improvement over the levels preoperatively, the improvement was only marginal, and filling pressure remained abnormally elevated in all cases.

Postoperative resting ejection fraction showed a significant relation to NYHA clinical class, but exercise ejection fraction, and rest and exercise filling pressure, did not (Figure 10). These results confirm the findings that ejection fraction is one of the most useful indices of left ventricular function in relation to patients' clinical status[31]. Similarly, resting preoperative EFCS

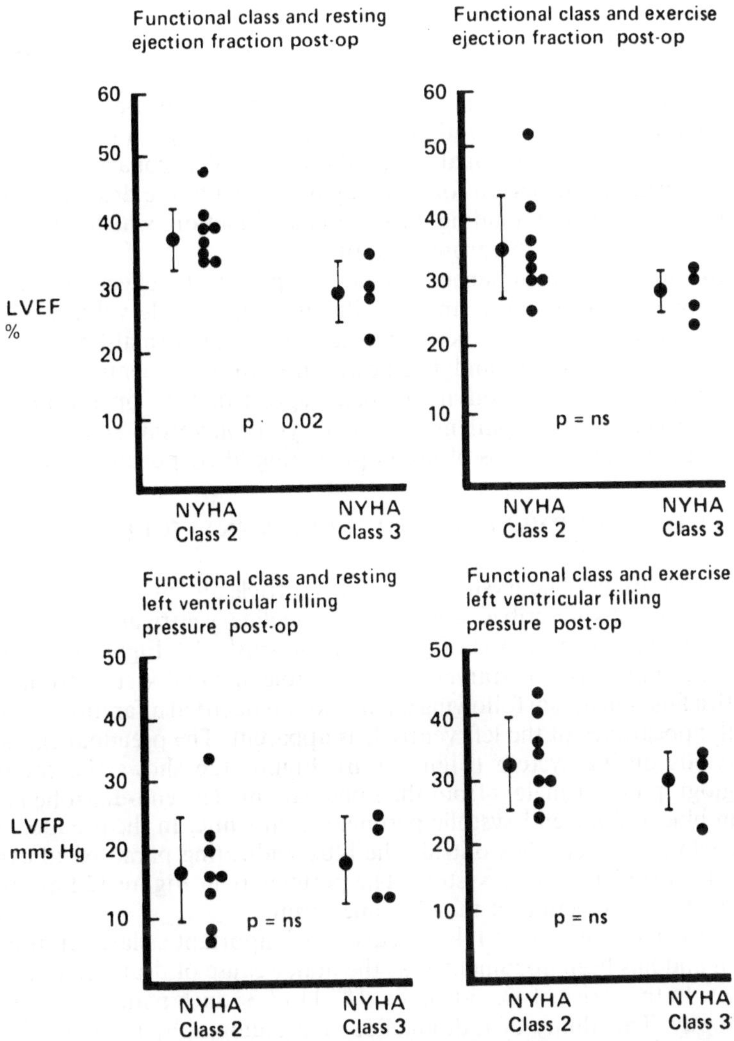

Figure 10 Relation of postoperative NYHA clinical class to rest and exercise ejection fraction, and rest and exercise ventricular filling pressure postoperatively

related to postoperative clinical class, but exercise EFCS did not. This finding does confirm the idea that EFCS is of major importance in predicting the result of aneurysmectomy.

A striking finding in this study[62] was the poor postoperative ventricular performance of patients with single-vessel coronary disease, in whom perfusion of the non-aneurysmal area of ventricle was normal. These patients showed a variable response in ejection fraction to exercise, and all showed a marked rise in filling pressure. Figure 11 is an example of rest and exercise postoperative ventriculographic perimeters for a patient with single-vessel disease. The resting study shows an akinetic segment anteriorly but the exercise study shows the ventricle to have taken on a diffusely hypokinetic appearance.

The influence of coronary disease on survival post-aneurysmectomy is debatable[63,64], but the radionuclide and haemodynamic findings suggest that in terms of functional result the extent of coronary disease may be unimportant. The reason for this may be related to the deleterious effects of chronic volume overloading on ventricular function, which may be irreversible and unrelated to coronary status[65].

In summary, aneurysmectomy does appear to be effective in improving resting ejection fraction, and in reducing end-diastole volume and resting filling pressure. Exercise performance remains abnormal however in terms of both angiographic and haemodynamic measurements. The combined radionuclide and haemodynamic data suggest that the operation may be of most benefit to those patients in whom symptoms from an aneurysm occur at rest, and that EFCS is of use in predicting likely postoperative status.

PSEUDOANEURYSM OF THE LEFT VENTRICLE

False, or 'pseudoaneurysms' of the left ventricle are much less common than the aneurysms described above. Radionuclide ventriculography has been successful in the detection of pseudoaneurysms[66-68]. Figure 12(a and b) are contrast angiographic frames at end-diastole and end-systole from a patient with a false aneurysm following an inferior myocardial infarction. The 'dumbbell' appearance of the left ventricle is apparent. The pseudoaneurysmal sac expands during systole (Figure 12b). Figure 12c shows the radionuclide angiographic perimeters from the same patient. The end-diastolic perimeter is in blue and the end-systolic perimeter is in white. In the pseudoaneurysm the white perimeter lies outside the blue, indicating paradoxical expansion of the aneurysm during systole. The perimeters in Figure 12d are from the patient after resection of the false aneurysm.

The early diagnosis of false aneurysm is important as late rupture is common and has been documented as the major cause of death in non-operated cases. In the series of Davidson *et al.*[69] 11 of 36 such patients succumbed in this way. The ability of radionuclide ventriculography to detect these false aneurysms provides a rational basis for its use in the evaluation of patients with cardiomegaly following infarction.

THE EFFECTS OF DRUGS ON VENTRICULAR FUNCTION

The increasing use of radionuclide ventriculography in clinical and research environments has led to the investigation of the effect of pharmacological interventions on left ventricular function.

Nitroglycerine

Resting ventricular function has been investigated before and after this drug.

In the first of these studies[70], equilibrium gated blood pool scanning after nitroglycerine showed improvement in the inward motion of ventricular segments that were hypokinetic originally. The conclusion was drawn that abnormal segments that improve after the drug were ischaemic, not infarcted, and were worthy of revascularization. In another study[71] first pass radionuclide ventriculography before and after nitroglycerine was advocated as a method to aid in the decision whether or not to revascularize dyssynergic segments of myocardium. Salel *et al.*[72] found that in patients with electrocardiographic evidence of infarction the post-nitroglycerine images showed significantly less decrease in end-systolic volumes than those of patients with no infarction. The changes in end-diastolic volumes after nitroglycerine were not significantly different between the two groups. Similarly patients with previous infarction showed less improvement in regional wall motion abnormalities compared to patients without infarction. This study also used post-nitroglycerine images to predict the effect of revascularization, and confirmed findings from invasive investigations that the demonstration of reversible dyssynergy allows prediction of successful revascularization[73].

This technique thus does provide a non-invasive method to aid in the decision whether or not to revascularize an area of myocardium.

Exercise function has been studied by exercise radionuclide ventriculography before and after nitroglycerine. Borer *et al.*[74] demonstrated that in patients with coronary artery disease, nitroglycerine reversed exercise-induced wall motion abnormalities and falls in ejection fraction when the drug was administered before exercise. Such changes occurred in patients without angina as well as those with angina. Exercise ejection fraction did not improve in normal subjects, and therefore the beneficial effects of the drug may be directly related to its sparing effect on myocardial oxygen demand[74]. The improvement in exercise function by isosorbide dinitrate in patients with ventricular aneurysms[59] has been discussed earlier.

Propranolol

Marshall *et al.*[75] studied the effects of incremental dosages of oral propranolol on ejection fraction, ejection rate and wall motion in 22 patients with coronary disease. All patients had stable angina pectoris, and all improved symptomatically on the drug. All showed a fall in heart rate and achieved therapeutic serum levels of propranolol. No significant changes in ejection fraction, ejection rate or wall motion occurred. The absence of deleterious effects of the drug on ventricular performance in the basal resting state was attributed to the low level of adrenergic support at rest. This appeared to be the case even in patients with reduced ejection fractions before the drug. The lack of depression of ventricular function at rest by propranolol was confirmed in another study[76]. Exercise ventricular function improved on propranolol in patients with coronary disease, however[76]. Although ejection fraction, not regional wall motion, was measured in the latter study, two points were of major importance. Firstly, exercise after propranolol in coronary patients may lead to improvements in ventricular function compared to before treatment, possibly due to reductions in exercise heart rate–blood pressure

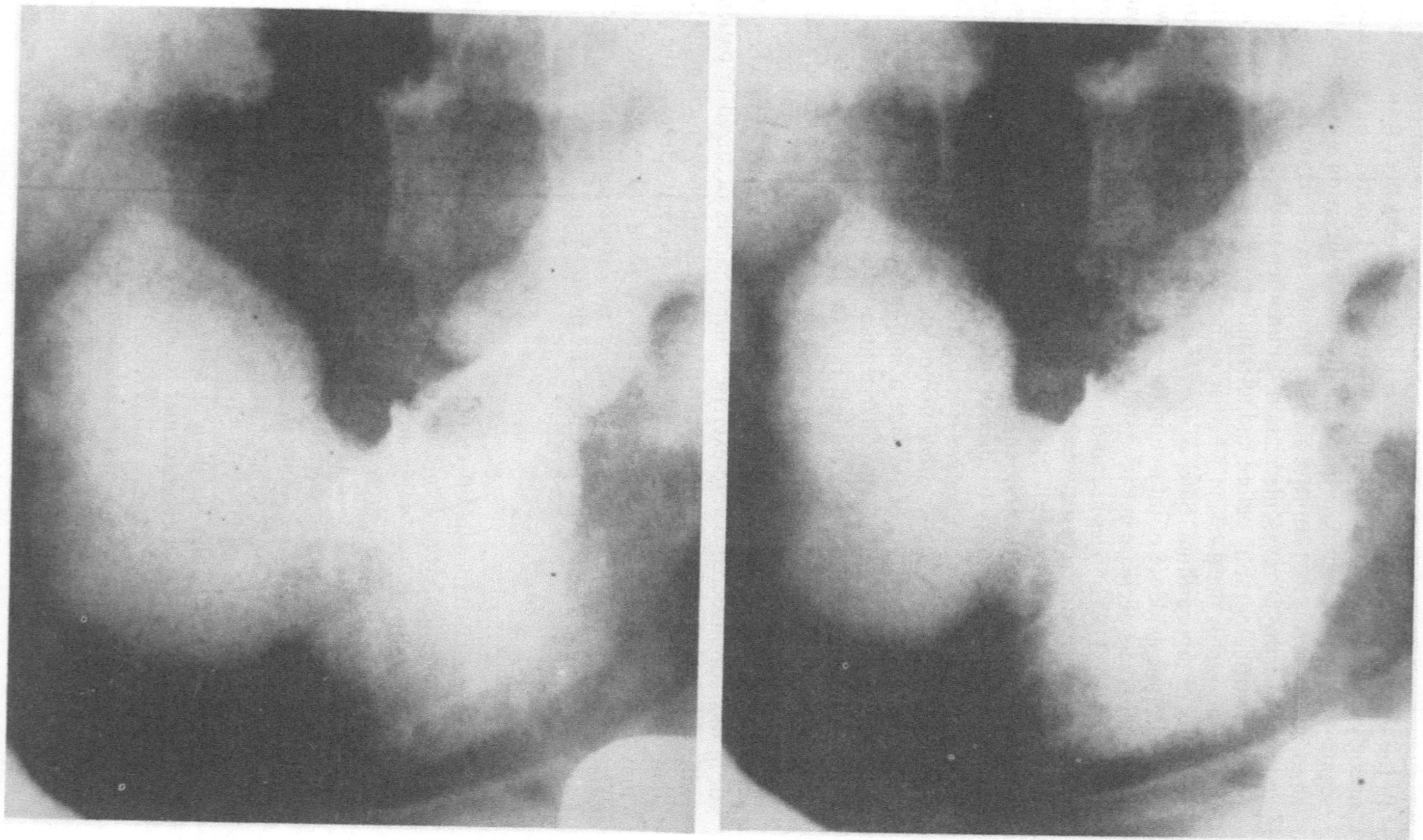

Figure 12 Contrast angiographic frames at end-diastole (a) and at end-systole (b) from a patient with a false aneurysm

product, increases in diastolic time per minute or redistributions of coronary flow. Secondly, when radionuclide ventriculography is performed under stress for diagnostic purposes (see below) a normal response while the patient is on propranolol does not exclude coronary artery disease.

CARDIOTOXIC DRUGS

A recent report has described the use of radionuclide ventriculography to study ventricular function sequentially in a group of patients receiving the cardiotoxic drug Doxorubicin for cancer chemotherapy[77]. A deterioration in measured ventricular function occurred before clinical manifestations of cardiac failure and the technique has been advocated as a method of judging the right time to stop chemotherapy and to avoid cardiac failure.

STRESS RADIONUCLIDE VENTRICULOGRAPHY IN THE DETECTION OF CORONARY ARTERY DISEASE

The detection of changes in ventricular function under situations of circulatory stress has proved feasible with radionuclide ventriculography. In coronary artery disease ventricular function may be normal at rest in the absence of previous infarction, even when coronary artery stenoses are extensive and severe. Ventricular wall motion is very sensitive to ischaemia and global and segmental function change when ischaemia is induced. Using gated blood pool scanning, Borer *et al.*[78] imaged coronary patients during dynamic bicycle exercise, data-collection beginning before the onset of angina and being continued for at least 2 min until fatigue or angina developed. The reasons why imaging was performed for that length of time have been discussed at the beginning of this chapter. Falls in ejection fraction occurred and new areas of regional dysfunction developed. Normal subjects did not show this response.

To validate changes induced by stress, a study was carried out to compare the changes in contrast angiography and first pass radionuclide ventriculography when incremental atrial pacing was carried out in patients with coronary disease[79]. The results of this study showed that falls in ejection fraction and regional dysfunction that occurred at angina were equally well seen on both techniques. Moreover, pacing-induced wall motion abnormalities could be related to anatomical coronary stenoses.

Several studies have shown the value of exercise first pass ventriculography in the evaluation of coronary disease[35,80,81]. The advantages of the first pass technique are that dynamic exercise studies can be performed at the true end-point of exercise as imaging time is short; also the right anterior oblique view may be used (Table 1). One study employed upright bicycle exercise[80] and another supine bicycle exercise[81]. Both studies showed falls in ejection fraction and the development of new wall motion abnormalities on exercise, and both used computer-generated ventricular perimeters at end-diastole and end systolc to assess wall motion. Quantification of wall motion may be made by the use of a hemiaxial model which has been validated against coronary arteriography[19]. Our policy at St Bartholomew's Hospital is to measure the percentage shortening of each hemiaxis on the radionuclide ventriculogram[79,81]. A normal range of shortening was defined from a series of radionuclide ventroculograms of patients with normal hearts. Abnormal wall motion was thus objectively defined as a percentage shortening of less than 2 standard deviations from the mean percentage shortening of each axis. With this approach, regional wall motion abnormalities were successfully demonstrated.

The regional ejection fraction image described earlier has also been used to identify changes occurring under stress[35,82]. Regional ejection fraction was found to be superior to wall motion analysis in the detection of regional dysfunction. Sensitivities for such detection were 67 % by wall motion and 91 % by regional ejection fractions. Specificity was high for both. These studies utilized isometric handgrip exercise, thus indicating that dynamic exercise is not necessary to demonstrate abnormalities. This is especially useful when equilibrium gated imaging is used, as the problems of motion artefact during dynamic imaging are avoided. In fact, the detection of coronary disease by the cold-pressor test has been recently described[83]. Here the patient's arm is immersed in iced water, and imaging is carried out through the peak haemodynamic response. The exact pathophysiological mechanisms involved in the production of global and regional abnormalities by this method are unclear, but may be related to vasospasm.

Figure 13 shows examples of regional ejection fraction images at rest (left hand) and on dynamic exercise. If the resting image is compared to the normal regional ejection fraction image shown in Figure 5, it is apparent that inferior and anterior function is normal, as manifest by the yellow and red colours. The apex is abnormal, and the blue colour indicates a severely hypokinetic segment. On exercise, the abnormality of regional function has extended to the entire inferior wall (black) but the anterior wall remains normal. This patient had a previous apical infarction and a 90 % stenosis of the right coronary artery. The important clinical implications of these findings are that radionuclide ventriculography may be used in the non-invasive assessment of patients with chest pain, and as a screening test in asymptomatic patients. The significance of a given stenosis may also be evaluated, as the demonstration of dysfunction distal to a stenosis of dubious severity would be a logical basis on to which to graft that vessel.

As discussed in the chapter on static imaging, the value of stress tests in screening does depend on which populations have the tests applied. The same cautions apply to radionuclide ventriculography as they do to thallium-201 scintigraphy in that decision-making is rarely aided by such screening tests in populations with a high prevalence for that disease.

ASSESSMENT OF THE SEVERITY OF CORONARY DISEASE

In a study of regional ejection fractions with handgrip exercise[82], it was found that patients with double- or triple-vessel disease developed more widespread

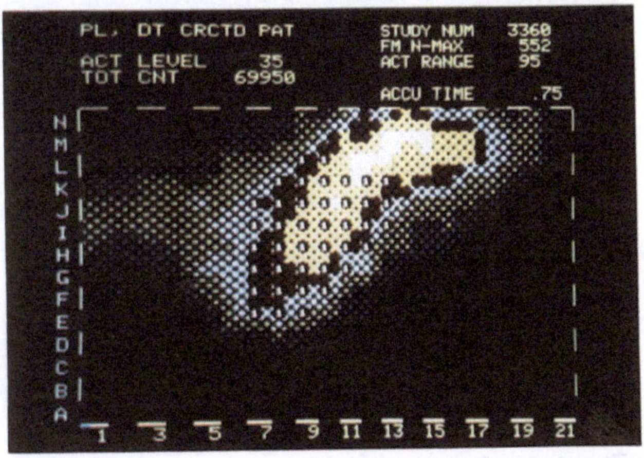

Figure 1 A frame from the left ventricular phase of the radionuclide angiogram, with region of interest entered (1's). The apex of the left ventricle is to the lower left

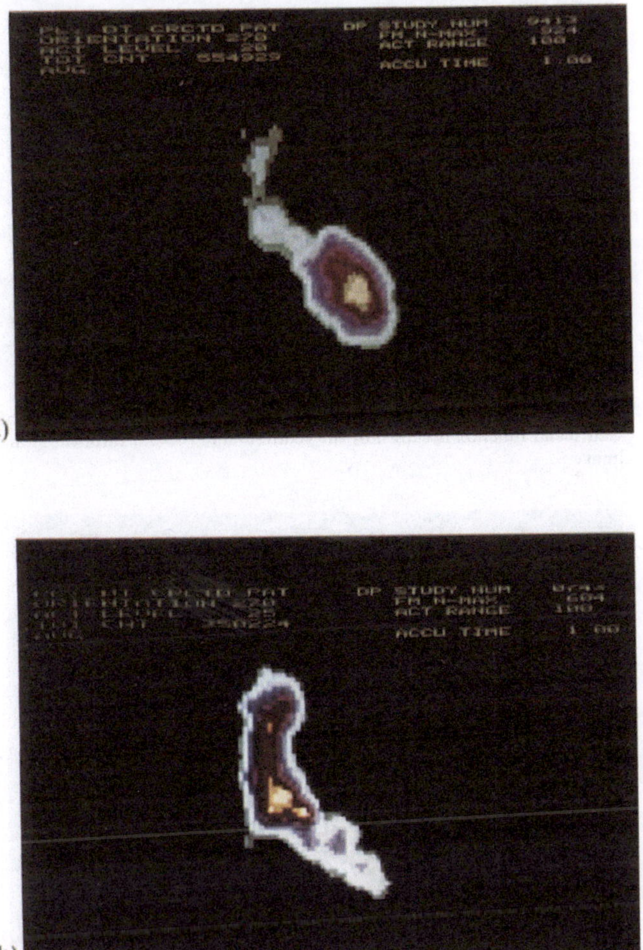

(a)

(b)

Figure 3 Radionuclide images of the left ventricle at end-diastole (a) and end-systole (b). The maximum density of counts is represented by yellow, which is apparent in the ventricle in Figure 3a, and in the aortic root in Figure 3b.

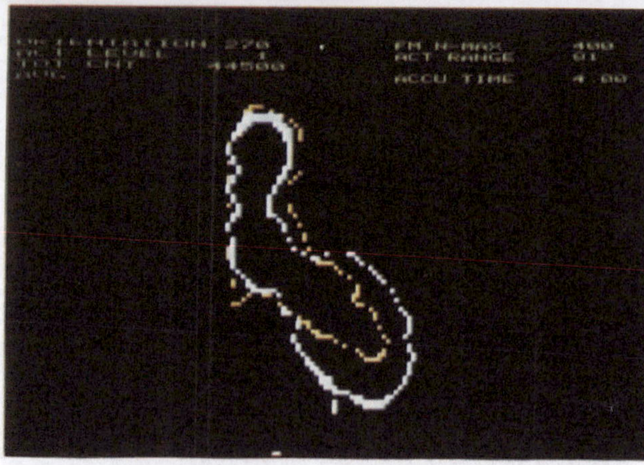

Figure 4 Superimposed end-diastolic (white) and end-systolic (yellow) perimeters from the images in Figure 3

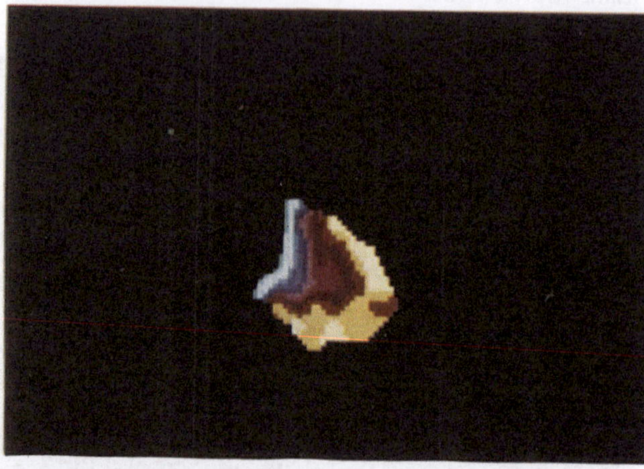

Figure 5 Normal regional ejection fraction image. The homogeneity of ventricular function is shown by the yellow and red colour throughout the image

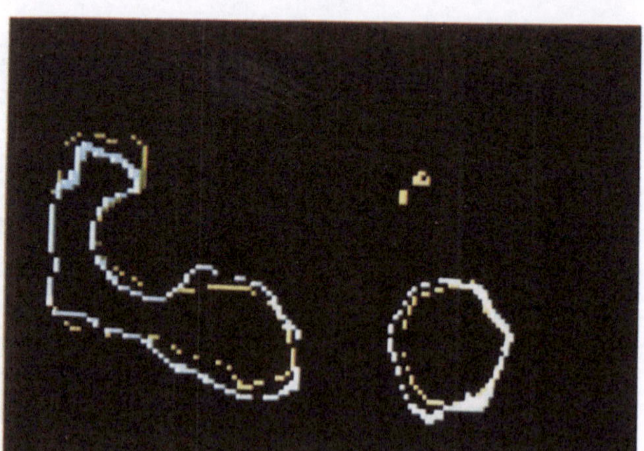

Figure 8 Right and left anterior oblique ventriculograms from a patient with anterior and posterolateral myocardial infarction. Right anterior oblique (left hand) shows anterior akinesis; left oblique image shows posterolateral akinesis. End-diastolic perimeter = blue; end-systolic = yellow (Reproduced from *Br. Heart J.*[44] by permission of the publisher)

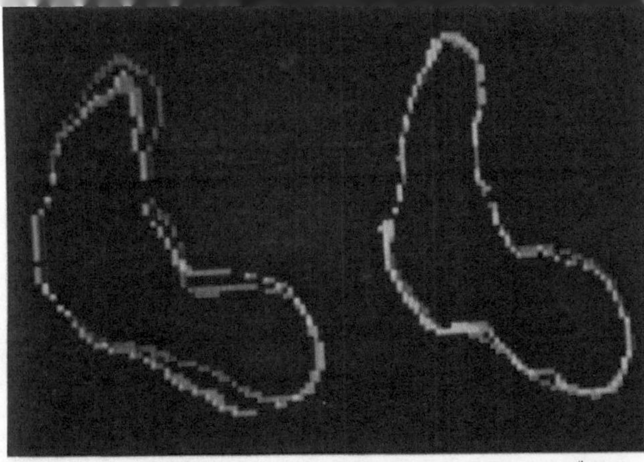

Figure 11 Rest (left-hand image) and exercise ventricular perimeters from a patient with single-vessel disease, post-aneurysmectomy. The resting study shows an area of akinesis anteriorly, but on exercise the ventricle appears diffusely hypokinetic

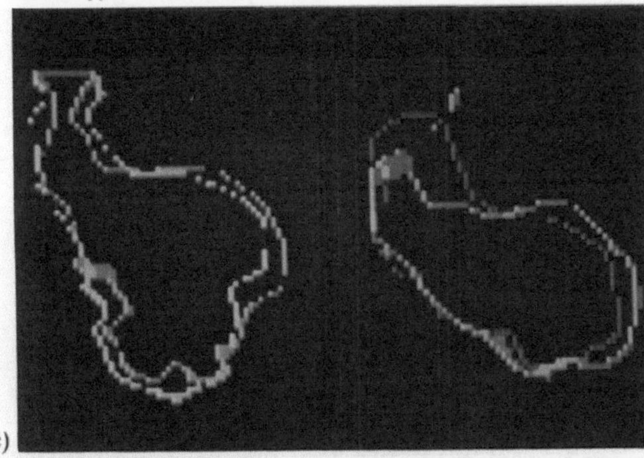

(c) (d)

Figure 12 See text for Figures 12a and b. (c) Superimposed radionuclide perimeters from same patient. End-systolic perimeter in white; end-diastolic in blue. (d) Postoperative perimeters, end-systole now in brown, showing absence of aneurysm (Reproduced from *J. Nucl. Med.*[67] by permission of the publisher)

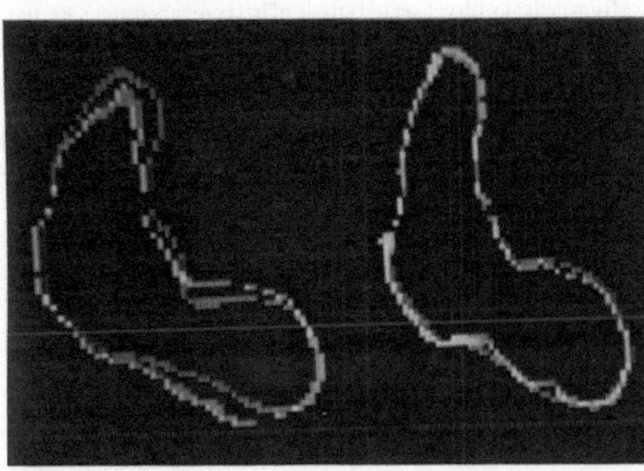

Figure 13 Rest (left hand) and exercise regional ejection fraction images from a patient with an apical infarction and a severe stenosis of right coronary artery. On exercise the abnormality of regional function has extended to whole of inferior wall (purple and black). The anterior wall (red and yellow) remains normal. End-diastolic perimeter is added in each case

(a)

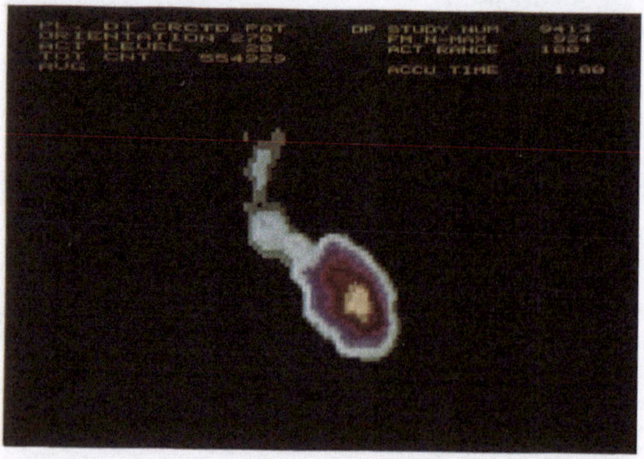

(b)

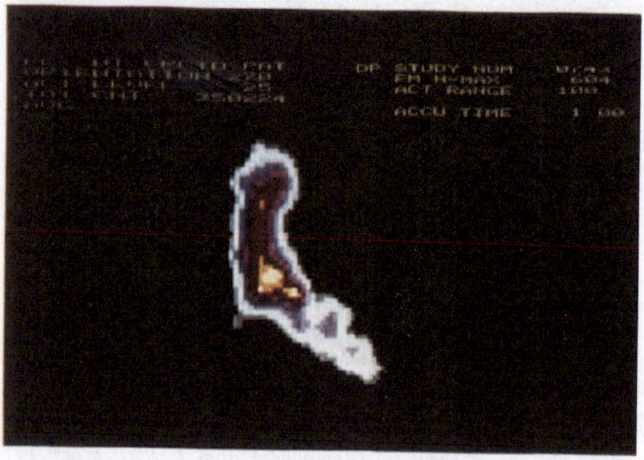

Figure 14 (a) Rest (left hand) and exercise regional ejection fraction images from patient with congenital atresia of left coronary ostium. Resting image is normal, exercise image shows anterior wall dysfunction (blue and black) (b) Rest (left hand) and exercise regional ejection fractions from same patient postoperatively. Normal pattern at rest, and on exercise (Reproduced from *Br. Heart J.*[36] by permission of the publisher)

abnormalities than those with single-vessel disease. In the study with supine bicycle exercise, Stone *et al.*[81] found that patients with triple-vessel disease showed a significantly greater fall in ejection fraction than those with less extensive disease, although both groups developed a fall in ejection fraction on exercise. No patient with triple-vessel disease showed a rise in ejection fraction on exercise. The combination of regional wall motion data and ejection fraction improved detection of coronary disease, and the findings of multiple abnormal areas coupled with large falls in ejection fraction suggest triple-vessel disease or left main stem stenosis. With the weight of evidence presented in the static imaging chapter suggesting that thallium scintigraphy is limited in this respect, then dynamic imaging under stress may be the method of choice for selection of patients with high-risk coronary disease.

ANOMALOUS CORONARY ARTERIES

Dynamic imaging has been applied to the study of atresia of the left coronary ostium[36], (see Figure 10 – previous chapter). Figure 14a shows the rest and exercise regional ejection fraction images from such a patient. A fall in anterior regional ejection fraction is apparent on exercise. The physiological significance of such anomalies may be effectively evaluated by imaging techniques.

EFFECTS OF REVASCULARIZATION SURGERY

The efficacy of coronary artery vein graft surgery has been shown by dynamic imaging before and after surgery. Improvement in resting function has been demonstrated in cases where preoperatively resting function was abnormal[70,72]. The reversal of both exercise-induced wall motion abnormalities and falls in ejection fraction has been described following surgery[84,85] while resting function may not change significantly[85]. Patients with recurrent angina and unsuccessful revascularization do not show such favourable improvements[85]. In anomalous coronary arteries, surgery also may lead to abolition of exercise-induced abnormalities[36]. Figure 14b shows rest and exercise regional ejection fractions from the same patient shown in Figure 14a. Exercise function is normal now.

ASSESSMENT OF VALVULAR HEART DISEASE

The quantification of valvular disease has been problematic. Contrast cineangiography, the standard by which valvar regurgitation is judged, is often unreliable for assessing the degree of regurgitation. Catheter position, the presence of ectopic beats, atrial and ventricular size and compliance are all variables that can influence the appearances of a contrast angiogram. In 1972 it was suggested by Morch *et al.*[86] that a left ventricular infusion of xenon-133 be used, and sampling carried out from left atrium, aorta and brachial artery, which permitted the measurements of relative concentrations at steady state. The invasive nature of the technique, and the necessity for many arterial catheters, limited its value. A computerized radionuclide angiocardiographic method for quantification of valvar regurgitation on right or left sides of the heart was described by Kirch *et al.*[87] The flow model used depended on the labelling of the atrium proximal to the regurgitant valve by a discrete bolus injection of radioisotope. The bolus was injected into the superior vena cava for right-sides studies, and into the pulmonary arterial wedge position for left-sided investigation. Time–activity curves of atrium and ventricle were generated, and data manipulated mathematically to produce quantitative information on total and forward stroke volumes. Comparison with contrast angiography produced high correlation coefficients for all measured volumes.

A different approach recently described by Rigo *et al.*[88] compared right and left ventricular stroke volume indices measured by the cyclical change in counts in each ventricle. In a group of controls the ratio was near unity. In patients with aortic or mitral regurgitation the left-to-right-sided index was increased. In the presence of simultaneous right ventricular volume overload the ratio could not grade left-sided valvar insufficiency. The technique may not yet be sophisticated enough to detect mild degrees of regurgitation and the data suggest that the regurgitant volume must be approximately 30% of the stroke volume before it will be detected. Technical improvements, such as the use of a slanting-hole collimator, may improve this.

The role of radionuclide ventriculography in the assessment of patients with valve disease has been extended by Borer *et al.*[89] who have attempted to unmask ventricular dysfunction on exercise as a guide to the timing of operative intervention. Symptomatic and asymptomatic patients with aortic valve regurgitation were exercised. Both groups contained a substantial proportion of patients who showed a deterioration in ejection fraction on exercise. Such dysfunction was not related to the size of the left ventricle or arterial pressure. It was weakly related to the presence of a raised resting left ventricular end-diastolic pressure. The possibility of being able to predict the onset of ventricular dysfunction before the onset of symptoms is an attractive one, and may lead to more logical timing of valve replacement.

The quantification of valvar stenosis has not yet been successfully achieved, and scintigraphic patterns in these conditions are as yet qualitative only[90].

DETECTION AND QUANTIFICATION OF SHUNTS

Non-invasive methods of shunt detection and quantification have been described for some years, although the methods do not seem to have become widely applied in the clinical environment. Radionuclide pulmonary dilution curves obtained after intravenous injection of tracer are sensitive for the qualitative demonstration of left-to-right shunts and are easily performed on an outpatient basis[91]. The detection of right-to-left shunts has been based on the principle that certain tracers are completely removed from the circulation by the lungs after administration, for example, the gases Xenon and Krypton, or the particulate microspheres[92]. A detector placed over a systemic arterial bed would detect significant activity after intravenous administration only in the presence of shunting. Quantification of right-to-left shunts is difficult, and the invasive nature of arterial sampling in the determination of tracer concentration offers no great advantages over oximetric methods employed in the catheter laboratory. Another method for quantification of right-to-left shunting evaluates the right-to-left-sided transit curves. A normal curve has equal areas under right- and left-sided peaks (Figure 6 is an example of such a curve). In right-to-left shunting the initial upslope and initial sharp down-slope of the right ventricular curve remains but there is little or no secondary left ventricular curve. The slope of the curve depends upon the magnitude and location of the shunt[92], but again quantification is difficult and many assumptions and subjective decisions are made.

Another simple method for purely qualitative evaluation of right-to-left shunts is the lung scan. When the kidneys are seen on a routine lung perfusion scan, then a shunt of greater than 15% is probably present[93].

Quantification of left-to-right shunts by the transit curve method suffers from the effect of the pulmonary capillary bed on the length of the bolus. Often it is not possible to record two discrete peaks when a detector is placed over the lungs[92]. Maltz and Treves[94] described a computerized analysis of pulmonary time–activity curves using a least-squares fit to a gamma variate. A region of interest over the lungs was generated which was free from extra-pulmonary contamination. The curve fitted with the gamma variate was subtracted from the remainder of the original data to obtain a second histogram which was again fitted to the gamma function. The areas of the two gamma-fitted histograms were measured, and the ratio represented the pulmonary : systemic flow ratio. The results were excellent when compared to oximetric values for a range of shunts from 1.2 : 1 to 3 : 1. The application of this technique to a variety of clinical problems has been described[95]. Atrial and ventricular septal defects may be quantified, and patent ductus arteriosus may be differentiated from intracardiac shunts by the demonstration of a different pulmonary : systemic flow ratio for each lung, as pulmonary blood flow is asymmetric and usually favours the left lung in this condition.

Residual shunts following surgical correction may be detected[95]. Drawbacks of the method include the necessity for a small discrete bolus of isotope to avoid distorted time–activity curves, and quality control of the bolus is imperative. The technique may not be able to detect shunts of less than 1.2 : 1 because of statistical fluctuations, although at this low level of shunt surgical intervention may not be contemplated.

The knowledge of exact anatomical detail is important in congenital heart disease, and radiotracer methods for quantification of shunts may provide data complementary to that obtained at cardiac catheterization, but will probably not replace it.

OTHER CONGENITAL HEART DISEASE

Radionuclide angiocardiography can detect changes in flow patterns due to Fallot's tetralogy, transposition of the great vessels, single-ventricle, pulmonary atresia and truncus arteriosus[96,97]. Radionuclide angiograms performed in both anterior and left oblique projections in infants have been described as useful in this respect[96].

STUDIES OF RIGHT VENTRICULAR FUNCTION

Recently the right ventricle has become increasingly investigated by radionuclide techniques. The relative paucity of data on right ventricular function has stemmed from the fact that its geometry is complicated, which makes calculation of volumes and ejection fraction from contrast angiograms difficult, although there are geometrical formulae for such calculations[98]. Also it has been generally assumed that right ventricular damage does not lead to cardiac decompensation[99]. More recently, haemodynamic syndromes of right ventricular infarction accompanying left ventricular infarction have been described[100], and such right ventricular infarction has been recognized from post-mortem examinations as more common than previously thought[101]. There are now an increasing number of reports indicating the possibility of calculating right ventricular ejection fraction from geometry-independent time–activity curves, both from first pass studies[102,103], and from equilibrium imaging[104]. The method described by Berger *et al.*[102] corrected right-ventricular time–activity curves by subtracting a right atrial time–activity curve from the ventricular one. Right ventricular ejection fraction was sensitive to changes in inotropic state produced by isoprenaline, was abnormal in patients with cardiomyopathy, and was lower in patients with cor pulmonale than in patients with obstructive airways disease without cor pulmonale. In another study the corrected right-ventricular curve was obtained by subtraction of a curve generated from a region of interest over a semi-annular region away from the right ventricle[103]. In patients with anterior or lateral infarction, right ventricular ejection fraction was normal but left ventricular ejection fraction was reduced. In patients with inferior infarction right ventricular ejection fraction was reduced, more so in patients with increased uptake of technetium-99m-pyrophosphate in the right ventricle. These findings concur with morphological studies[101]. Sharpe *et al.*[105] found that patients with pyrophosphate accumulation in the right ventricle exhibited akinesis of the right ventricular free wall on gated scintigraphy but those without pyrophosphate accumulation in the right ventricle did not. In a group of patients with coronary artery disease, resting right ventricular ejection fraction was not reduced in the presence of right coronary artery disease[104]. Steele *et al.*[106], using a collimated probe, found that a depressed right ventricular ejection fraction returned promptly to normal in patients with acute inferior infarction, but left ventricular ejection fraction did not improve so much. The value of a technique that can accurately measure right ventricular ejection fraction should be high, as the presence of a low right ventricular ejection fraction in patients with low cardiac output states following infarction would help to identify patients who would benefit from aggressive volume-loading therapy[100]. In addition right and left ventricular function can be evaluated from the same radionuclide angiocardiogram.

The potential use of exercise ventriculography in determining right ventricular function under stress is also under investigation[107].

ASSESSMENT OF CARDIAC TRANSPLANTATION

With the apparently successful use of cardiac transplantation on both sides of the Atlantic Ocean, ways of assessing the function of the transplanted heart are continuously being sought. Radionuclide transit curves have been shown to be of value in sequential studies of the function of the heart[38] and the response to inotropic agents. Scintiphotographic images before and after transplantation have also been obtained[90]. Whether or not tracer techniques will prove sensitive enough to detect rejection of a heart in the early stages remains to be seen.

CARDIOPLEGIA

The radionuclide ventriculogram has been useful in showing the beneficial effects of potassium cardioplegia in left ventricular function post-cardiopulmonary bypass[108].

MISCELLANEOUS

Scintigraphic techniques have been used in the demonstration of asymmetric septal hypertrophy in hypertrophic obstructive cardiomyopathy[70] in the visualization of intraventricular thrombi[90] and in the detection of left atrial myxomas[109].

In conclusion, dynamic cardiac imaging has developed into a highly useful technique in clinical and research media. The development of newer radiopharmaceuticals with shorter half-lives[110] will doubtless aid in the extension of these techniques in adults and children, without the constraints of excessive radiation dosages.

References

1. Blumgart, H. L. and Weiss, S. (1927). Studies on the velocity of blood flow. II. The velocity of blood in normal resting individuals and a critique of the method used. *J. Clin. Inv.*, **4,** 15
2. Hubbard, J. P., Preston, W. W. and Ross, R. A. (1942). The velocity of the blood flow in infants and young children determined by radioactive sodium. *J. Clin. Inv.*, **21,** 613
3. Mufson, I., Quimby, E. H. and Smith, B. C. (1948). Use of radioactive sodium as a guide to the efficacy of drugs used in the treatment of diseases of the peripheral vascular system. Preliminary Report. *Am. J. Med.*, **4,** 73
4. Prinzmetal, M., Corday, E., Bergman, H. C., Schwartz, L. and Spritzler, R. J. (1948). Radiocardiography: a new method for studying the blood flow through the chambers of the heart in human beings. *Science*, **108,** 340

5. Donato, L. (1973). Basic concepts of radiocardiography. *Sem. Nucl. Med.*, **3,** 111
6. Greenspan, R. H., Lester, R. G., Marvin, J. F. and Amplatz, K. (1959). Isotope circulation studies in congenital heart disease. *J. Am. Med. Assoc.*, **169,** 667
7. Braunwald, E., Long, R. T. L. and Morrow, A. G. (1959). Injections of radioactive Krypton (Kr 85) in the detection and localization of cardiac shunts. *J. Clin. Inv.*, **38,** 990
8. Weitzman, D. and McAlister, J. (1958). Tracer method for localizing left to right cardiac shunts. *Lancet*, **2,** 1356
9. Rejali, A. M., MacIntyre, W. J. and Friedell, H. L. (1968). A radioisotope method of visualization of blood pools. *Am. J. Roentgenol.*, **79,** 129
10. Anger, H. O., Van Dyke, D. C., Gottschalk, A., Yano, Y. and Schaer, L. R. (1965). The scintillation camera in diagnosis and research. *Nucleonics*, **23,** 57
11. Mason, D. T., Ashburn, W. L., Harbert, J. C., Cohen, L. S. and Braunwald, E. (1969). Rapid sequential visualization of the heart and great vessels in man using the wide-field Anger scintillation camera. Radioisotope angiography following the injection of Technetium-99m. *Circulation*, **39,** 19
12. Jones, R. H., Grenier, R. P. and Sabiston, D. C. Jr. (1972). Description of a new high count rate gamma camera system. *Medical Radioisotope Scintigraphy*, **I,** 299 (Vienna: IAEA)
13. Schad, N. (1977). Non-traumatic assessment of left ventricular wall motion and regional stroke volume after myocardial infarction. *J. Nucl. Med.*, **18,** 333
14. Buddemeyer, E. V. and Mitchell, T. G. (1974). Instrumentation. In Strauss, H. W., Pitt, B. and James, A. E. (eds.).*Cardiovascular Nuclear Medicine*, pp. 9–35 (St Louis: Mosby)
15. Zaret, B. L., Strauss, H. W., Hurley, P. J., Natarajan, T. K. and Pitt, B. (1971). A non-invasive scintiphotographic method for detecting regional ventricular dysfunction in man. *N. Engl. J. Med.*, **284,** 1165
16. Burow, R. D., Strauss, H. W., Singleton, R., Pond, M., Rehn, T., Bailey, I. K., Griffith, L. C., Nickoloff, E. and Pitt, B. (1977). Analysis of left ventricular function from multiple gated acquisition cardiac blood pool imaging. Comparison to contrast angiography. *Circulation*, **56,** 1024
17. Cohn, P. F., Gorlin, R., Adams, D. F., Chahine, R. A., Vokonas, P. S. and Herman, M. V. (1974). Comparison of biplane and single plane left ventriculograms in patients with coronary artery disease. *Am. J. Cardiol.*, **33,** 1
18. Marshall, R. C., Berger, H. J., Costin, J. C., Freedman, G. S., Wolberg, J., Cohen, L. S., Gottschalk, A. and Zaret, B. L. (1977). Assessment of cardiac performance with quantitative radionuclide angiocardiography. Sequential left ventricular ejections fraction, normalized left ventricular ejection rate and regional wall motion. *Circulation*, **56,** 820
19. Bodenheimer, M. M., Banka, V. S., Fooshee, C. M., Hermann, G. A. and Helfant, R. H. (1978). Quantitative radionuclide cineangiography in the right anterior oblique view: comparison with contrast ventriculography. *Am. J. Cardiol.*, **41,** 718
20. Dymond, D. S., Jarritt, P. H., Britton, K. E. and Spurrell, R. A. J. (1979). Detection of post-infarction left ventricular aneurysms by first-pass radionuclide ventriculography using a multicrystal gamma camera. *Br.Heart J.*, **41,** 68
21. Gough, J. N., Davis, R. and Stacey, A. J. (1968). Radiation doses delivered to the skin, bone marrow and gonads of patients during cardiac catheterization and angiocardiography. *Br. J. Radiol.*, **41,** 508
22. Folse, R. and Braunwald, E. (1962). Determination of fraction of left ventricular volume effected per beat, and of ventricular end-diastolic and residual volumes. *Circulation*, **25,** 674
23. Strauss, H. W., Zaret, B. L., Hurley, P. J., Natarajan, T. K. and Pitt, B. (1971).

A scintiphotographic method for measuring left ventricular ejection fraction in man without cardiac catheterization. *Am. J. Cardiol.*, **28**, 575
24. Parker, J. A., Secker-Walker, R. H., Hill, R., Siegel, B. A. and Potchen, E. J. (1972). A new technique for the calculation of left ventricular ejection fraction. *J. Nucl. Med.*, **13**, 649
25. Secker-Walker, R. H., Resnick, L., Kunz, H., Parker, J. A., Hill, R. L. and Potchen, E. J. (1973). Measurement of left ventricular ejection fraction. *J. Nucl. Med.*, **14**, 798
26. Schelbert, H. R., Verba, J. W., Johnson, A. D., Brock, G. W., Alazraki, N. P., Rose, F. J. and Ashburn, W. L. (1975). Nontraumatic determination of left ventricular ejection fraction by radionuclide angiocardiography. *Circulation*, **51**, 902
27. Jengo, J. A., Mena, I., Blaufuss, A. and Criley, J. M. (1978). Evaluation of left ventricular function (ejection fraction and segmental wall motion) by single pass radioisotope angiography. *Circulation*, **57**, 326
28. Green, M. V., Brady, W. R., Douglas, M. A., Borer, J. S., Ostrow, H. G., Line, B. R., Bacharach, S. L. and Johnston, G. S. (1978). Ejection fraction by count rate from gated images. *J. Nucl. Med.*, **19**, 880
29. Weaver, W. D., Hamilton, G. W., Williams, D. L., Trobaugh, G. B. and Ritchie, J. L. (1976). Reproducibility of the ejection fraction measured by first transit radionuclide studies. *J. Nucl. Med.*, **17**, 556
30. Marshall, R. C., Berger, H. J., Reduto, L. A., Gottschalk, A. and Zaret, R. L. (1978). Variability in sequential measures of left ventricular performance assessed with radionuclide angiography. *Am. J. Cardiol.*, **41**, 531
31. Cohn, P. F., Gorlin, R., Cohn, L. F. and Collins, J. J. Jr. (1974). Left ventricular ejection fraction as a prognostic guide in surgical treatment of coronary and valvular heart disease. *Am. J. Cardiol.*, **34**, 136
32. Rackley, C. (1976). Quantitative evaluation of left ventricular function by radiographic techniques. *Circulation*, **54**, 862
33. Pierson, R. N. Jr., Alam, S., Kemp, H. G. and Friedman, M. I. (1977). Radiocardiography in clinical cardiology, *Sem. Nucl. Med.*, **7**, 85
34. Maddox, D. E., Holman, B. L., Wynne, J., Idoine, J., Parker, J. A., Uren, R., Neill, J. M. and Cohn, P. F. (1978). Ejection fraction image: a noninvasive index of regional left ventricular wall motion. *Am. J. Cardiol.* **41**, 1230
35. Bodenheimer, M. M., Banka, V. S., Fooshee, C. M., Hermann, G. A. and Helfant, R. H. (1979). Comparison of wall motion and regional ejection fraction at rest and during isometric exercise: concise communication. *J. Nucl. Med.*, **20**, 724
36. Dymond, D., Camm, J., Stone, D., Rees, S., Rees, G. and Spurrell, R. (1980). Dual isotope stress testing in congenital atresia of the left coronary ostium: applications before and after surgical treatment. *Br. Heart J.* **43**: 270
37. Jones, R. H., Sabiston, D. C. Jr., Bates, B. B., Morris, J. J., Anderson, P. A. W. and Goodrich, J. K. (1972). Quantitative radionuclide angiocardiography for determination of chamber to chamber cardiac transit times. *Am. J. Cardiol.*, **30**, 855
38. Steele, P. P., VanDyke, D., Trow, R. S., Anger, H. O. and Davies, H. (1974). Simple and safe bedside method for serial measurement of left ventricular ejection fraction, cardiac output and pulmonary blood volume. *Br. Heart J.*, **36**, 122
39. Maltz, D. and Treves, S. (1973). Quantitative radionuclide angiocardiography: determination of Qp : Qs in children. *Circulation*, **47**, 1049
40. Zierler, K. L. (1965). Equations for measuring blood flow by external monitoring of radioisotopes. *Circ. Res.*, **16**, 309
41. Mullins, C. B., Mason, D. T., Ashburn, W. L. and Ross, J. Jr. (1969). Determination of ventricular volume by radioisotope angiography. *Am. J. Cardiol.*, **24**. 72

42. Sullivan, R. W., Bergeron, D. A., Vetter, W. R., Hyatt, K. H., Haughton, V. and Vogel, J. M. (1971). Peripheral venous scintillation angiocardiography in determination of left ventricular volume in man. *Am. J. Cardiol.*, **28,** 563
43. Kostuk, W. J., Ehsani, A. A., Karliner, J. S., Ashburn, W. L., Peterson, K. L., Ross, J. and Sobel, B. E. (1973). Left ventricular performance after myocardial infarction assessed by radioisotopic angiocardiography. *Circulation* **47,** 242
44. Dymond, D. S., Stone, D. L., Elliott, A. T., Britton, K. E., Banim, S. O. and Spurrell, R. A. J. (1979). Comparison of single plane and biplane radionuclide ventriculography performed in oblique projections in patients with acute myocardial infarction. *Br. Heart J.*, **42,** 671
45. Gault, J. H., Ross, J. Jr. and Braunwald, E. (1968). Contractile state of the left ventricle in man. *Circ. Res.*, **22,** 451
46. Steele, P., LeFree, M. and Kirch, D. (1976). Measurement of left ventricular mean circumferential fibre shortening velocity and systolic ejection rate by computerised radionuclide angiocardiography. *Am. J. Cardiol.*, **37,** 388
47. Steele, P., Kirch, D., Matthews, M. and Davies, H. (1974). Measurement of left heart ejection fraction and end diastolic volume by a computerised scintigraphic technique using a wedged pulmonary arterial catheter. *Am. J. Cardiol.*, **34,** 179
48. Henning, H., Schelbert, H., Crawford, M. H., Karliner, J. S., Ashburn, W. and O'Rourke, R. A. (1975). Left ventricular performance assessed by radionuclide angiocardiography and echocardiography in patients with previous myocardial infarction. *Circulation*, **52,** 1069
49. Schelbert, H. R., Henning, H., Ashburn, W. L., Verba, J. W., Karliner, J. S. and O'Rourke, R. A. (1976). Serial measurements of left ventricular ejection fraction by radionuclide angiography early and late after myocardial infarction. *Am. J. Cardiol.*, **38,** 407
50. Rigo, P., Murray, M., Strauss, H. W., Taylor, D., Kelly, D., Weisfeldt, M. and Pitt, B. (1974). Left ventricular function in acute myocardial infarction evaluated by gated scintigraphy. *Circulation*, **50,** 678
51. Feild, B. J., Russell, R. O. Jr., Dowling, J. T. and Rackley, C. E. (1972). Regional left ventricular performance in the year following myocardial infarction. *Circulation*, **46,** 679
52. Sobel, B. E., Bresnahan, G. F., Shell, W. E. and Yoder, R. D. (1972). Estimation of infarct size in man and its relation to prognosis. *Circulation*, **46,** 640
53. Mathey, D., Bleifeld, W., Hanrath, P. and Effert, S. (1974). Attempt to quantitate relation between cardiac function and infarct size in acute myocardial infarction. *Br. Heart J.*, **36,** 271
54. Bruschke, A. V. G., Proudfit, W. L. and Sones, F. M. (1973). Progress study of 590 consecutive non-surgical cases of coronary disease followed 5–9 years. II. Ventriculographic and other correlations. *Circulation*, **47,** 1154
55. Rigo, P., Murray, M., Strauss, H. W. and Pitt, B. (1974). Scintiphotographic evaluation of patients with suspected left ventricular aneurysm. *Circulation*, **50,** 985
56. Friedman, M. L. and Cantor, R. E. (1979). Reliability of gated heart scintigrams for detection of left ventricular aneurysm: concise communication. *J. Nucl. Med.*, **20,** 720
57. Key, J. A., Aldridge, H. E. and MacGregor, D. C. (1968). The selection of patients for resection of left ventricular aneurysm. *J. Thorac. Cardiovasc. Surg.*, **56,** 477
58. Watson, L. E., Dickhaus, D. W. and Martin, R. H. (1975). Left ventricular aneurysm: pre-operative haemodynamics, chamber volume and results of aneurysmectomy. *Circulation*, **52,** 868
59. Dymond, D. S., Stephens, J. D., Stone, D. L., Jarritt, P. H., Elliott, A. T., Britton, K. E. and Spurrell, R. A. J. (1980). Assessment of the function of contractile seg-

ments in patients with left ventricular aneurysms by quntitative first pass radionuclide ventriculography. Haemodynamic correlations at rest and exercise. *Br. Heart J.*, **43,** 125

60. Graber, J. D., Oakley, C. M., Pickering, B. N., Goodwin, J. F., Raphael, M. J. and Steiner, R. E. (1972). Ventricular aneurysm: an appraisal of diagnosis and surgical treatment. *Br. Heart J.*, **34,** 830
61. Sesto, M., Schwarz, F., Thiedemann, K. U., Flameng, W. and Schlepper, M. (1979). Failure of aneurysmectomy to improve left ventricular function. *Br. Heart J.*, **41,** 79
62. Dymond, D. S., Stephens, J. D., Stone, D. L., Elliott, A. T., Britton, K. E., Banim, S. O., Rees, G. M. and Spurrell, R. A. J. (1980). Combined radionuclide and haemodynamic evaluation of the results of left ventricular aneurysmectomy. in preparation)
63. Lee, D. C. S., Johnson, R. A., Boucher, C. A., Wexler, L. F. and McEnany, J. T. (1977). Angiographic predictors of survival following left ventricular aneurysmectomy. *Circulation*, **55, 56** (Suppl. II), II-12
64. Rogers, W. J., Oberman, A. and Kouchoukos, N. T. (1978). Left ventricular aneurysmectomy in patients with single *vs.* multivessel coronary artery disease. *Circulation*, **58** (Suppl. I), I-50
65. Mason, D. T. (1973). Regulation of cardiac performance in clinical heart disease. Interactions between contractile state, mechanical abnormalities and ventricular compensatory mechanisms. *Am. J. Cardiol.*, **32,** 437
66. Botvinick, E. H., Shames, D., Hutchinson, J. C., Roe, B. B. and Fitzpatrick, M. (1976). Non-invasive diagnosis of a false ventricular aneyrysm with radioisotope gated cardiac blood pool imaging. Differentiation from true aneurysm. *Am. J. Cardiol.*, **37,** 1089
67. Dymond, D. S., Elliott, A. T. and Banim, S. O. (1979). Detection of a false left ventricular aneurysm by first-pass radionuclide ventriculography. *J. Nucl. Med.*, **20,** 851
68. Sweet, S. E., Sterling, R., McCormick, J. R., Klein, M. D., Berger, R. L. and Ryan, T. J. (1979). Left ventricular false aneurysm after coronary bypass surgery. Radionuclide diagnosis and surgical resection. *Am. J. Cardiol.*, **43,** 154
69. Davidson, K. H., Paris, A. F., Harrington, J. J., Barsamian, E. M. and Fishbein, M. C. (1977). Pseudoaneurysm of the left ventricle: an unusual echocardiographic presentation. Review of the literature. *Ann. Intern. Med.*, **86,** 430
70. Berman, D. S., Salel, A. F., Denardo, G. L., Bogren, H. G. and Mason, D. T. (1975). Clinical assessment of left ventricular regional contraction patterns and ejection fraction by high-resolution gated scintigraphy. *J. Nucl. Med.*, **16,** 865
71. Hellman, C., Blau, F., Johnson, W. D. and Schmidt, D. (1978). Evaluation of myocardial viability by first pass nitroglycerin radionuclide angiography. *Proc. VIIIth World Congress of Cardiology, Tokyo, Japan*, p. 545
72. Salel, A. F., Berman, D. S., DeNardo, G. L. and Mason, D. T. (1976). Radionuclide assessment of nitroglycerin influence on abnormal left ventricular segmental contraction in patients with coronary heart disease. *Circulation*, **53,** 975
73. Helfant, R. H., Pine, R., Meisier, S. G., Feldman, M. S., Trout, R. G. and Banka, V. S. (1974). Nitroglycerin to unmask reversible asynergy: correlation with post coronary bypass ventriculography. *Circulation*, **50,** 108
74. Borer, J. S., Bacharach, S. L., Green, M. V., Kent, K. M., Johnston, G. S. and Epstein, S. E. (1978). Effect of nitroglycerin on exercise-induced abnormalities of left ventricular regional function and ejection fraction in coronary artery disease. Assessment by radionuclide cineangiography in symptomatic and asymptomatic patients. *Circulation*, **57,** 314

75. Marshall, R. C., Berger, H. J., Reduto, L. A., Cohen, L. S., Gottschalk, A. and Zaret, B. L. (1978). Assessment of cardiac performance with quantitative radionuclide angiocardiography. Effects of oral propranolol on global and regional left ventricular function in coronary artery disease. *Circulation*, **58**, 808
76. Battler, A., Ross, J. Jr., Slutsky, R., Pfisterer, M., Ashburn, W. and Froelicher, V. (1979). Improvement of exercise-induced left ventricular dysfunction with oral propranolol in patients with coronary heart disease. *Am. J. Cardiol.*, **44**, 318
77. Alexander, J., Dainiak, N., Berger, H. J., Goldman, L., Johnstone, D., Reduto, L., Duffy, T., Schwartz, P., Gottschalk, A. and Zaret, B. L. (1979). Serial assessment of Doxorubicin cardiotoxicity with quantitative radionuclide angiocardiography. *N. Engl. J. Med.*, **300**, 278
78. Borer, J. S., Bacharach, S. L., Green, M. V., Kent, K. M., Epstein, S. E. and Johnston, G. S. (1977). Real-time radionuclide cineangiography in the non-invasive evaluation of global and regional left ventricular function at rest and during exercise in patients with coronary artery disease. *N. Engl. J. Med.*, **296**, 839
79. Stone, D. L., Dymond, D. S., Elliott, A. T., Britton, K. E., Banim, S. O. and Spurrell, R. A. J. (1980). The use of first pass radionuclide ventriculography in the assessment of wall motion abnormalities induced by incremental atrial pacing in patients with coronary artery disease. *Br. Heart J.* 43: 369
80. Jengo, J. A., Oren, V., Conant, R., Brizendine, M., Nelson, T., Uszler, J. M. and Mena, I. (1979). Effects of maximal exercise stress on left ventricular function in patients with coronary artery disease using first pass radionuclide angiocardiography. A rapid non-invasive technique for determining ejection fraction and segmental wall motion. *Circulation*, **59**, 60
81. Stone, D. L., Dymond, D. S., Elliott, A. T., Britton, K. E., Banim, S. O. and Spurrell, R. A. J. (1980). Exercise first pass radionuclide ventriculography detection of coronary artery disease. *Br. Heart J.* 44: 208
82. Bodenheimer, M. M., Banka, V. S., Fooshee, C. M., Gillespie, J. A. and Helfant, R. H. (1978). Detection of coronary heart disease using radionuclide determined regional ejection fraction at rest and during handgrip exercise: correlation with coronary arteriography. *Circulation*, **58**, 640
83. Wainwright, R. J., Brennand-Roper, D., Cueni, T. A., Sowton, E., Hilson, A. J. W. and Maisey, M. N. (1979). Cold pressor test in detection of coronary heart disease and cardiomyopathy using Technetium-99m gated blood-pool imaging. *Lancet* **2**, 320
84. Schmidt, D. H., Hellman, C., Anholm, J., Kamath, M. L. and Johnson, W. D. (1979). Bypass graft surgery in severe left ventricular dysfunction. *Circulation*, **59, 60** (Suppl. II), II-237
85. Stone, D. L., Dymond, D. S., Elliott, A. T., Britton, K. E., Rees, G. M., Banim, S. O. and Spurrell, R. A. J. (1980). Exercise first pass radionuclide ventriculography in the assessment of coronary artery bypass surgery. *British Heart Journal* 43: 108
86. Morch, J. E., Klein, S. W. and Richardson, P. (1972). Mitral regurgitation measured by continuous infusion of ^{133}Xenon. *Am. J. Cardiol.*, **29**, 812
87. Kirch, D. L., Metz, C. E. and Steele, P. P. (1974). Quantitation of valvular insufficiency by computerised radionuclide angiocardiography. *Am. J. Cardiol.*, **34**, 711
88. Rigo, P., Alderson, P. O., Robertson, R. M., Becker, L. C. and Wagner, H. N. Jr. (1979). Measurement of aortic and mitral regurgitation by gated cardiac blood pool scans. *Circulation*, **60**, 306
89. Borer, J. S., Bacharach, S. L., Green, M. V., Kent, K. M., Henry, W. L., Rosing, D. R., Seides, S. F., Johnston, G. S. and Epstein, S. E. (1978). Exercise-induced left

ventricular dysfunction in symptomatic and asymptomatic patients with aortic regurgitation: assessment with radionuclide cineangrography. *Am. J. Cardiol.*, **42,** 351

90. Freedman, G. S. (1974). Radionuclide angiocardiography in the adult. In Strauss, H. W., Pitt, B. and James, A. E.) (eds.). *Cardiovascular Nuclear Mecicine*, pp. 101–120. (St Louis: Mosby)
91. Alazraki, N. P., Ashburn, W. L., Hagan, A. and Friedman, W. F. (1972). Detection of left-to-right cardiac shunts with the scintillation camera pulmonary dilution curve. *J. Nucl. Med.*, **13,** 142
92. Strauss, H. W. (1972). Detection and quantification of intracardiac shunts. In Strauss, H. W., Pitt, B. and James, A. E. (eds.). *Cardiovascular Nuclear Medicine*, pp. 128–37 (St Louis: Mosby)
93. Greenfield, L. D. and Bennett, L. R. (1973). Detection of intracardiac shunts with radionuclide imaging *Sem. Nucl. Med.*, **3,** 139
94. Maltz, D. L. and Treves, S. (1973). Quantitative radionuclide angiocardiography. Determination of Qp : Qs in children. *Circulation*, **47,** 1049
95. Ashkenazi, J., Ahnberg, D. S., Korngold, E., LaFarge, C. G., Maltz, D. L. and Treves, S. (1976). Quantitative radionuclide angiocardiography: detection and quantitation of left to right shunts. *Am. J. Cardiol.*, **37,** 382
96. Wesselhueft, H. L., Hurley, P. J., Wagner, H. N., Jr. and Rowe, R. D. (1972). Nuclear angiography in the diagnosis of congenital heart disease in infants. *Circulation*, **45,** 77
97. Treves, S. and Collins-Nakai, R. L. (1976). Radioactive tracers in congenital heart disease. *Am. J. Cardiol.*, **38,** 711
98. Ferlinz, J. (1977). Measurements of right ventricular volumes in man from single plane cineangiograms. A comparison to the biplane approach. *Am. Heart J.* **94,** 87
99. Starr, I., Jeffers, W. A. and Meade, R. H., Jr. (1943). The absence of conspicuous increments of venous pressure after severe damage to the right ventricle of the dog, with a discussion of the relation between clinical congestive failure and heart disease. *Am. Heart J.*, **26,** 291
100. Cohn, J. N., Guiha, N. H., Broder, M. I. and Limas, C. J. (1974). Right ventricular infarction. Clinical and haemodynamic features. *Am. J. Cardiol.*, **33,** 209
101. Isner, J. M. and Roberts, W. C. (1978). Right ventricular infarction complicating left ventricular infarction secondary to coronary heart disease. Frequency, location, associated findings and significance from analysis of 236 necropsy patients with acute or healed myocardial infarction. *Am. J. Cardiol.*, **42,** 885
102. Berger, H. J., Matthay, R. A., Loke, J., Marshall, R. C., Gottschalk, A. and Zaret, B. L. (1978). Assessment of cardiac performance with quantitative radionuclide angiocardiography. Right ventricular ejection fraction with reference to findings in chronic obstructive pulmonary disease. *Am. J. Cardiol.*, **41,** 897
103. Tobinick, E., Schelbert, H. R., Henning, H., Lewinter, M., Taylor, A., Ashburn, W. L. and Karliner, J. S. (1978). Right ventricular ejection fraction in patients with acute anterior and inferior myocardial infarction assessed by radionuclide angiography. *Circulation*, **57,** 1078
104. Maddahi, J., Berman, D. S., Matsuoka, D. T., Waxman, A. D., Stankus, K. E., Forrester, J. S. and Swan, H. J. C. (1979). A new technique for assessing right ventricular ejection fraction using rapid multiple gated equilibrium cardiac blood pool scintigraphy: description, validation and findings in chronic coronary artery disease. *Circulation*, 60, 581
105. Sharpe, D. N., Botvinick, E. H., Shames, D. M., Schiller, N. B., Massie, B. M., Chatterjec, K. and Parmley, W. W. (1978). The noninvasive diagnosis of right ventricular infarction. *Circulation*, **57,** 483

106. Steele, P., Kirch, D., Ellis, J., Vogel, R. and Battock, D. (1977). Prompt return to normal of depressed right ventricular ejection fraction in acute inferior infarction. *Br. Heart J.*, **39,** 1319
107. Johnson, L. L., McCarthy, D. M., Sciacca, R. R. and Cannon, P. J. (1979). Right ventricular ejection fraction during exercise in patients with coronary artery disease. *Circulation*, **60,** 1284
108. Ellis, R. J., Born, M., Feit, T. and Ebert, P. A. (1978). Potassium cardioplegia. Early assessment by radionuclide ventriculography. *Circulation*, **58** (Suppl. I), I-57
109. Pohost, G. M., Pastore, J. O., McKusick, K. A., Chiotellis, P. N., Kapbuakis, G., Meyers, G. S., Dinsmore, R. E. and Block, P. C. (1977). Detection of left atrial myxoma by gated radionuclide cardiac imaging. *Circulation*, **55,** 88
110. Treves, S., Kulprathipanja, S. and Hnatowich, D. J. (1976). Angiocardiography with Iridium-191m: an ultra-short-lived radionuclide ($T_{\frac{1}{2}}$ 4.9 sec). *Circulation*, **54,** 275

SECTION II

Aspects of Cardiopulmonary Bypass and Anaesthesia

16
Historical review and introduction

D. G. MELROSE

In this introduction I apologize for being unashamedly nationalistic, for while open heart surgery is very properly a worldwide affair and is particularly the result of North American skill, determination and investment, we in Britain can claim a useful share in its pioneering, particularly in regard to cardiopulmonary bypass and anaesthesia. If we take our starting-point from the first clinical use of a heart–lung machine by Clarence Dennis and others in 1951[1], you will note that Britain is represented by the sixth recorded case in the world and the fourth survivor (Table 1).

The equipment used was developed at the Royal Postgraduate Medical School between 1949 and 1952, and a production version was made available for sale in 1954 by New Electronic Products Ltd – the first machine to be so offered (Figure 1). Subsequent models were delivered to many countries and undoubtedly contributed to the spread of cardiac surgery throughout the world.

Coincident with our experimental work leading to the design of a machine for clinical use, others at the Royal College of Surgeons Research Farm at Downe were also to make an important contribution to heart surgery. Andreasen and Watson[2] were determining the least cardiac output that would prove sufficient to maintain safely the circulation of a dog for half an hour. They decided that 10% of the normal cardiac output was the lowest figure possible – a quantity that became known as the Azygos flow because it was achieved by leaving only the azygos vein to fill the right atrium; the superior and inferior vena cavae being clamped. This work, though apparently unimportant of itself, was to have considerable influence subsequently.

An interesting detail in the technique used by us at that time for perfusing dogs was to substitute 6% dextran in saline for blood in the machine prime. Donor blood was used in the first five experiments and on each occasion initial delivery from the machine produced a fall in arterial blood pressure which persisted throughout the perfusion. In the subsequent 25 experiments when dextran in saline was used, the introduction, maintenance, and termination of the perfusion was accomplished without untoward events,

Table 1 Developments 1951–3

Author		*Age of patient (years)*	*Condition*	*Operation details*	*Result*
1951	Dennis, C., *et al.* (1951). *Ann. Surg.*, **134,** 709	6	ostium primum	40 min total bypass	died
1951	Dogliotti, Mario (1952). *Bull. Johns Hopkins Hosp.*, **90,** 131	49	mediastinal tumour	20 min partial bypass	survived
1952	Dodrill, F. D., *et al.* (1953). *J. Thorac. Surg.*, **26,** 584	16	pulmonary stenosis	25 min total right heart bypass	survived
1953	Helmsworth, J. A. (1953). *J. Thorac. Surg.*, **26,** 617	4	VSD	33 min total bypass	died
1953	Gibbon, J. H. Jr. (1954). *Minnesota Med.*, **37,** 171	18	ASD	26 min total bypass	survived
1953	Aird, I., *et al.* (1954). *Br. Med. J.*, **1,** 1284	32	aortic stenosis and mitral incompetence	97 min partial bypass	survived

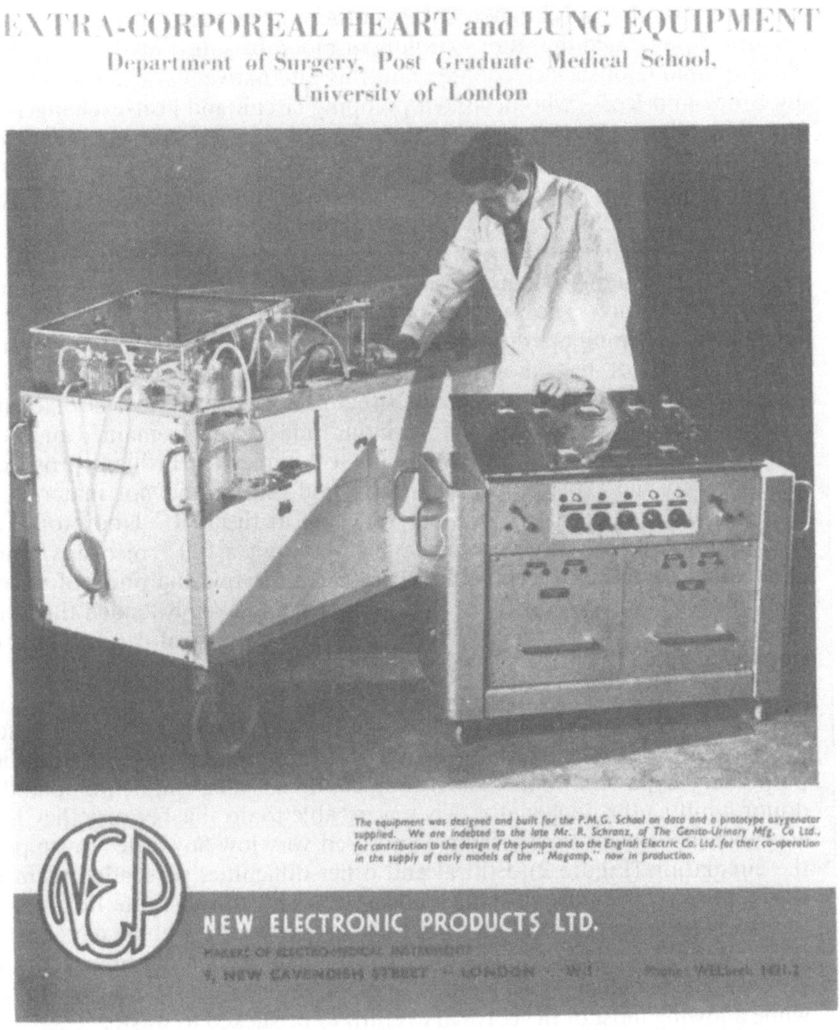

EXTRA-CORPOREAL HEART and LUNG EQUIPMENT
Department of Surgery, Post Graduate Medical School,
University of London
The equipment was designed and built for the P.M.G. School on data and a prototype oxygenator supplied. We are indebted to the late Mr. R. Schranz, of The Genito-Urinary Mfg. Co Ltd., for contribution to the design of the pumps and to the English Electric Co. Ltd. for their co-operation in the supply of early models of the "Magamp," now in production.
NEW ELECTRONIC PRODUCTS LTD.

Figure 1 The first production heart/lung machine

with blood pressure, pulse, and respiratory rates remaining virtually constant. Regrettably when the first patients were operated on, normal clinical practice prevailed and this demonstrably safer technique was rejected. Indeed it was many years before more adventurous priming fluids superseded fresh blood drawn into heparin.

It is important at this point to consider the influence of Bigelow's[3] suggestion and experimental proof in 1950 that the period during which an animal could withstand circulatory arrest could be greatly prolonged by hypothermia. This had led to intense research activity culminating in successful clinical intracardiac operations by both Lewis and Taufic[4], and Swan and Zeavin[5] in 1953. In this country several workers made important contributions to the development of hypothermia in these formative years. Delorme[6] suggested that direct cooling of blood be substituted for the standard technique of surface cooling, and this alternative was extensively used by Brock and Ross[7] who devised a pumping circuit and heat-exchanger for this. This allowed better control of the temperature especially in fat patients, and led to the development by Drew *et al.*[8] of what came to be called profound hypothermia. They used two pumps without an oxygenator to carry the right and left circulations while reducing body temperature to below 15 °C. At this point the circulations were discontinued and surgery proceeded in cadaveric conditions, with no intracardiac suction, a still heart, and of course excellent exposure. The method produced good results at the time, but demanded very long operation times and was as complex as using a heart–lung machine. It had, however, the merit of circumventing the major disadvantage of simple hypothermia – that of a very short intracardiac time limit. In spite of much determined work this time limit has remained an essential and limiting feature of the standard technique: the brilliant prospects suggested by the experiments of Andjus and Smith[9] did not materialise, and have not materialised, in man. Working at the MRC laboratories in Mill Hill they nearly succeeded in 1955 in obtaining a 100 % recovery in rats after surface cooling to temperatures close to the freezing point of water, with circulatory arrest for more than an hour, and even extended this time in hamsters. Hypothermia nevertheless is as much part of cardiac surgery today as is the heart–lung machine, and in many roles it plays a vital part in ensuring its safety.

The spring of 1954 saw the real beginning of open heart surgery, when Lillehei and Varco at the University of Minnesota began using cardiopulmonary bypass in infants and young children with a simple pump and a donor adult as the oxygenator. They were able to do this because they had accepted the Azygos flow principle and used very low flow rates to support the circulation (Figure 2). Ethical and other difficulties persuaded them to abandon cross-circulation by the end of 1954 and to substitute first a continuous 'arterialized' blood infusion and then to use the bubble oxygenator of De Wall. They continued to use the low-flow technique, however, and were also accustomed to using quite large quantities of 'arterialized' blood while allowing most of the coronary return to be sucked to waste.

Meanwhile in 1955 at the Mayo Clinic in Rochester, Kirklin *et al.*[10] began to do open heart surgery with a modified version of Gibbon's machine which used vertical screens and roller-pumps. They preferred to attempt to support the circulation in as normal a way as possible and to retrieve the coronary blood.

The helpful rivalry between the two Minnesota schools became known as the high-flow–low-flow controversy. Many took sides but inevitably this conflict was eventually resolved by a merging of views as technique improved and equipment became safer. Disc oxygenators came to predominate, as did full-flow perfusions at 2.4 l/m^2 of body surface through roller-pumps, though several pulsatile pumps were available and some centres used them. The pulsatile versus non-pulsatile controversy waned quickly in favour of convenient roller-pumps, but it is to be hoped that the more rigorous ex-

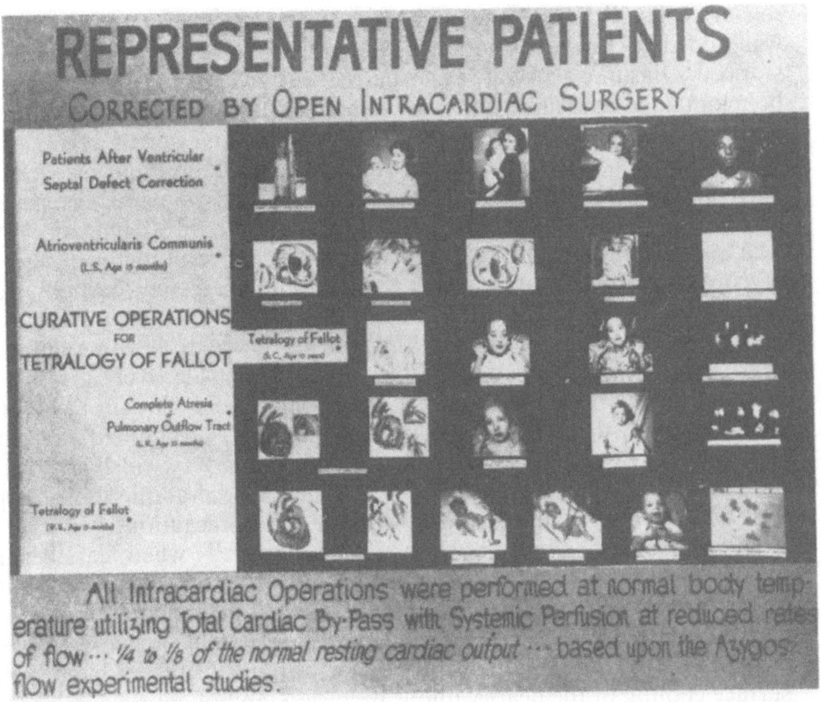

Figure 2 The first successful series by Lillehei and Varco

perimental methods available now will be again turned to examine this problem.

Cardiac surgery spread rapidly in clinical range and also geographically. We entered a period of relatively high mortality for these reasons, and also because more complex surgery called for longer perfusion times and a higher proportion of patients in chronic heart failure came to be accepted.

The problem of the protection of the myocardium had been obvious from the outset. Whole-body perfusion of itself did not ensure a dry heart or even adequate surgical vision, and the danger of trapping air in the cardiac cavities after cardiotomy was clearly recognized. A quote from that time reads: 'The ideal solution will be reached only when the surgeon is able to work on hearts from which all blood flow is excluded and which are quite inactive.' Senning had suggested in 1952[11] that it might be safer to induce ventricular fibrillation, even accepting the risk entailed of failure to restore normal beating rather than to allow the ventricles to beat. Another solution proposed by Swan was to fill the chest with Ringer's solution before closing the cardiac incision.

To solve these problems we had begun in London to work on what became known as elective cardiac arrest. By 1955 we were able to publish[12] the results of a large number of experiments in dogs and on the isolated hearts of several species which indicated that the heart beat could be stopped and re-started at will. When potassium citrate in a concentration of over 1 mg/ml was added to Locke's solution used to perfuse the heart, cardiac action stopped. Diastolic arrest always occurred within 20 s of injection and could be maintained as long as the heart contained this solution. Coronary flow was usually stopped for 15 min. Spontaneous beating started again, usually within 90 s following reperfusion with Locke's solution and recovery was normally complete within 3 min. This series of events was perfectly repeatable and the time of arrest could be prolonged to more than 30 min. By contrast hearts in which the beat was stopped by asphyxia, resulting from cessation of coronary flow, recovered very slowly – and then only partially – even after very short periods of arrest.

Perhaps I have laboured the last point but it was to have an important bearing on subsequent events. Effler *et al.*[13] first electively arrested the human heart with potassium citrate in a 17-month-old child on 17 February 1956, and by early 1957 had used it in 97 patients. Kirklin had also enthusiastically taken up the technique and it had spread very widely throughout the USA. Cooley, however, found that it added several minutes of bypass time and began to clamp the aorta without other precautions.

His simpler arrest in asphyxia prevailed, especially when fears began to be expressed that the high concentration of potassium salts might of itself be responsible for myocardial damage. The experimental findings on asphyxia were ignored. Several schools emerged: simple asphyxia, individual coronary perfusion at normal temperature or at varying degrees of hypothermia, surface cooling of the heart without perfusion, and of course combinations of these. It was only when the so-called stone heart was recognized to be exhibiting a form of rigor mortis that simple asphyxia was abandoned, and it is only now that a consensus is being re-established giving elective cardiac arrest and hypothermia pride of place in the management of the myocardium.

Several other developments deserve particular note. One is the gradual replacement of equipment made of materials designed for continued re-use, by disposable items guaranteed pyrogen-free, sterile, and increasingly blood-compatible. Bubble oxygenators perhaps represent this trend best, and the continuing improvement in design and construction is a very welcome feature of the present time. Their use has also been made a great deal safer by the adoption of non-blood primes with resulting haemodilution, and by greater attention to the ratio of gas flow to blood flow through them. Equally important has been the development of practical membrane oxygenators, and if we are to extend the period in which we may safely oxygenate blood extracorporeally it will be using such membrane devices. In fact both types were proposed and tried at the very outset of cardiac surgery; now they deservedly dominate the field.

Continuing improvements in the quality of the surfaces exposed to blood, a better understanding of sterilizing techniques, and an increasing awareness of the consequences of microemboli are also beginning to contribute to safety. Better blood filtration, improvements in anticoagulant regimes, a deeper understanding of the role of platelets and new studies of the effect of different perfusion regimes on organ function must also add up to safer cardiac surgery.

These matters form the substance of our session, 'Aspects of Cardiopulmonary Bypass and Anaesthesia'. Individually each is important, but it is when ideas combine in synergy that real momentum is established. May we strive for that today.

References

1. Dennis, C., Spreng, D. S. Jr., Nelson, G. E., Karlson, K. E., Nelson, R. M., Eddy, F. D. and Sanderson, D. (1951). Development of pump-oxygenator to replace heart and lungs, an apparatus applicable to human patients, and application to one case. *Ann. Surg.*, **134**, 709
2. Andreasen, A. T. and Watson, F. (1953). Experimental cardiovascular surgery; discussion of results so far obtained and report on experiments. *Br. J. Surg.*, **41**, 195
3. Bigelow, W. G., Lindsay, W. K. and Greenwood, W. F. (1950). Hypothermia; its possible role in cardiac surgery; investigation of factors governing survival in dogs at low body temperatures. *Ann. Surg.* **132**, 849
4. Lewis, F. J. and Taufic, M. (1953). Closure of atrial septal defects with aid of hypothermia; experimental accomplishments and report of one successful case. *Surgery*, **33**, 52
5. Swan, H. and Zeavin, I. (1954). Cessation of circulation in general hypothermia; technics of intracardiac surgery under direct vision. *Ann. Surg.*, **139**, 385
6. Delorme, E. J. (1952). Experimental cooling of blood-stream; preliminary communication. *Lancet*, **2**, 914
7. Ross, D. N. (1954). Venous cooling; new method of cooling blood-stream. *Lancet*, **1**, 1108
8. Drew, C. F., Keen, G. and Benazon, D. B. (1959). Profound hypothermia. *Lancet*, **1**, 745
9. Andjus, R. K. and Smith, A. U. (1955). Reanimation of adult rats from body temperatures between 0 and +2 °C. *J. Physiol.*, **128**, 446
10. Kirklin, J. W., Dushane, J. W., Patrick, R. T., Donald, D. E., Hetzel, P. S., Harshbarger, H. G. and Wood, E. C. (1955). Intracardiac surgery with aid of mechanical pump-oxygenator system (Gibbon type): report of 8 cases. *Proc. Staff Meet. Mayo Clin.*, **30**, 201
11. Senning, A. (1952). Ventricular fibrillation during extracorporeal circulation; used as a method to prevent air embolism and to facilitate intracardiac operations. *Acta Chir. Scand.*, **105**, 390
12. Melrose, D. G., Dreyer, B., Bentall, H. H. and Baker, J. B. E. (1955). Elective cardiac arrest. *Lancet*, **2**, 21
13. Effler, D. B., Knight, H. F. Jr., Groves, L. K. and Kolff, W. E. (1957). Elective cardiac arrest for open-heart surgery. *Surg. Gynaecol. Obstet.*, **105**, 407

17
Anaesthesia for coronary artery surgery

D. W. BETHUNE, J. M. COLLIS, I. HARDY AND R. D. LATIMER

The increase in the number of patients presenting with angina for coronary artery vein bypass grafting has led to an increasing awareness of those factors involved in the maintenance of myocardial viability during the intra-operative period. The successful management of this type of patient depends on co-operation between cardiologists, anaesthetists and surgeons to ensure optimum results and it would appear that the actual anaesthetic technique used has little bearing on the results achieved. From the point of view of the cardiothoracic anaesthetist the management of these patients has led to a change of emphasis in the period between induction of anaesthesia and initiation of bypass. Previously the main hazards to the patient were related to the direct effects of surgical intervention, such as haemorrhage, whereas in the patient with a compromized coronary circulation, more emphasis needs to be placed on the control of the circulation to ensure an optimum ratio between myocardial work and myocardial oxygen consumption. The normal concept of the relationship between the systolic pressure time interval which is proportional to the myocardial work and the diastolic pressure time interval[1] which is proportional to the sub-endocardial coronary blood flow (Figure 1) needs to be modified in the patient who has critical stenosis of the coronary arteries resulting in angina. In these patients it is obvious that even with an apparently normal relationship between these two pressure time intervals, the myocardial oxygen needs may not be fully met and any factors which may either increase the oxygen consumption or reduce the period of time for coronary blood flow in diastole must be promptly recognized and treated.

PRE-OPERATIVE PREPARATION OF THE PATIENT

The development by Black[2], working at ICI, of the original β_1-antagonists resulted in a major advance in the medical management of the patient with angina and there are now a very wide range of β-blockers available in the United Kingdom (Table 1). Most of these β-blockers are non-selective as in

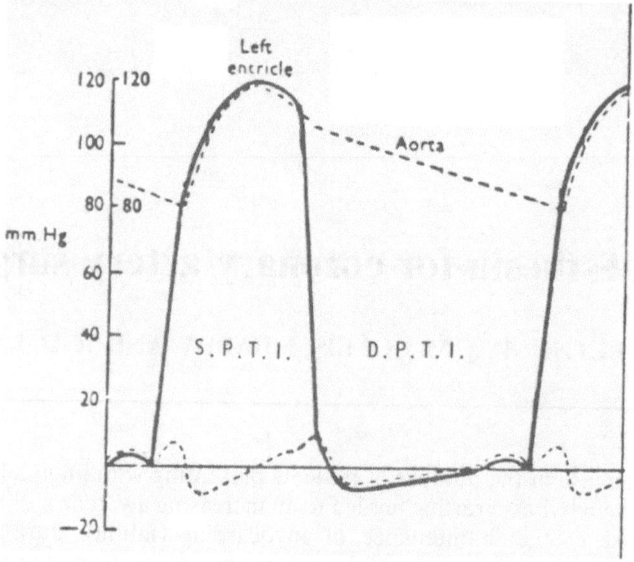

Figure 1 SPTI – Systolic Pressure Time Interval. DPTI is proportional to myocardial work and DPTI is proportional to subenducardial blood flow

addition the β_1-receptors in the myocardium, they also have widespread β_2-blocking actions. The selection of a β-blocker for a patient appears to be related to the prescribing physicians preference, and though some patients will tolerate a particular β-blocker better than an alternative one, no single β-blocker seems to be ideal in all cases.

Early reports in the literature suggested that the continuation of β-blockade up to the time of coronary artery bypass grafting and associated cardio-pulmonary bypass would result in a significant incidence of patients with depressed myocardial function following the surgical period. This led to recommendations that the β-antagonists should be withdrawn prior to surgical intervention[3 5]. With increasing experience[4,6 10] it has become obvious that the β-adrenergic blockade can, with benefit, be continued up to the time of surgery and our practice is to give the last dose of the β-antagonist on the morning of surgery to ensure full β-blockade during the period in the operating theatre. There are now numerous reports testifying to the danger to patients resulting in the abrupt withdrawal of β-adrenergic blockade[5,11,12]. Following abrupt withdrawal of β-adrenergic blockade in patients who are being treated for angina, their anginal symptoms will be accentuated, this may be due to an increased sensitivity of the myocardium to adrenergic stimuli or may result from a progression of the coronary artery disease during the time of treatment. Our initial experience with patients presenting for coronary artery surgery, where we had adopted a policy of discounting β-blockade 48 h before surgery, confirmed these reports of an increased severity of the anginal symptoms and led to our present policy of continuing β-blockade up to the time of bypass. It is possible to advance a very cogent argument for continuing β-blockades through the whole of the perioperative period and then slowly discontinuing in the postoperative period as there is a definite incidence of tachydysrhythmias in patients who have had coronary artery surgery in whom β-blockers are discontinued at the time of surgery.[10] These tachydysrhythmias are not as hazardous as a preoperative tachydysrhythmias but is none the less an unnecessary complication of the postoperative period. In the preoperative assessment of the patient one of the pertinent points that the anaesthetist has to consider is the contractility of the left ventricular muscle mass as shown on the left ventriculogram. This is usually expressed as the ejection fraction and our experience is that patients with an ejection fraction greater than 40% will not present any undue problems either intra-operatively or after revascularization of the myocardium, and even patients with ejection fractions below 30% will normally have an uneventful postoperative recovery. The results of preoperative exercise testing are invaluable as a guide for the safe intraoperative management of the patient as from the results of the test the rate pressure product (RPP)[13] (systolic pressure × pulse rate) which produced symptoms can be determined. With knowledge of this critical RPP product the anaesthetist can manipulate the afterload in the patient to ensure that the value does not reach this level during the pre-bypass period. With full β-blockade, tachy-

Table 1 β-Adrenergic antagonists

		ISA	*Membrane Stabilising*	*Alpha Block*	
Beta 1	Practolol	×			Eraldin
	Metoprolol				Lopressor Betaloc
	Atenolol				Tenormin
Beta 1 and Beta 2	Propanolol		×		Inderal
	Oxprenolol	×	×	×	(Slow) Trasicor
	Acebutolol	×	×		Sectral
	Labetolol	×	×	×	Trandate
	Timolol				Blocadren
	Pindolol				Visken
	Sotalol				Sotacor Beta-cardone

ISA: Intrinsic Sympathetic Activity.

cardia should not occur but it is inevitable that an increased RPP from tachycardia is potentially more damaging than the same increase resulting from a higher systolic pressure.

ANAESTHETIC MANAGEMENT

It appears that in most cardiothoracic units anaesthetists have adopted the techniques that they previously used successfully with other forms of heart disease in dealing with this new group of patients who have critical coronary artery insufficiency. Many drugs and techniques are used satisfactorily[9,14–18], and this probably means that the mode of administration and the administrator have a greater importance than the actual pharmacological cocktail used. However, some general principles would appear to be relevant in the anaesthetic management of these patients.

The desirability of continuing β-blockade up to the time of surgery has already been mentioned. Anxiety and apprehension are obviously undesirable in these patients and night sedation for the patients during their hospitalization is often desirable. Additional oral sedation on the morning of surgery may also be useful particularly if the patient is scheduled for operation in the afternoon. Premedication should be generous, again many combinations of drugs are used, our preference being for the use of Omnopon (0.25–0.3 mg/kg) and Scopolomine (0.05–0.06 mg/kg) with the addition of Phenergan (0.3–0.35 mg/kg). This is given intramuscularly an hour and a half before the patient comes to the anaesthetic room.

MONITORING

In many centres direct intravascular monitoring is started before the induction of anaesthesia. It is not our routine practice to insert the arterial cannula before the patient has been induced, and we are not convinced there would be any definite benefit resulting from the routine use of invasive monitoring at this time. More controversial is the recommendation from some units that a float pulmonary artery catheter should be inserted routinely in all patients presenting for coronary artery surgery[19]. We believe the advocates of this more invasive monitoring must produce definite evidence of considerable benefit from the practice as even though the morbidity from pulmonary artery catheterization is quite low, the cost of using such catheters routinely would form a significant addition to the revenue costs of any cardiothoracic unit.

INDUCTION AND MAINTENANCE OF ANAESTHESIA

Virtually all methods of induction and maintenance of anaesthesia have been recommended as being suitable for patients undergoing coronary artery bypass grafting[14–18]. Our technique is to use an inhalation induction using nitrous oxide and oxygen with the addition of trichloroethylene. As far as we are aware this is unique and would be taken by some workers to prove that any method can work satisfactorily in the right hands. Other workers have described techniques based on the use of large doses of analgesics plus diazepam or thiopentone. The doses of intravenous inductions agents such as thiopentone which have been recommended in β-blocked patients presenting for coronary artery surgery are quite small, averaging 1.1 mg/kg[9] in one study and this seems to confirm the idea that the desired object is a minimal hypnotic level of the anaesthetic agent with adequate analgesia provided by other agents. There are a similar variety of methods recommended for the maintenance of anaesthesia but there is general agreement on the need for the provision of good analgesiac in these patients. Our practice is to use nitrous oxide and oxygen plus trichloroethylene with the addition of Omnopon intravenously in a dose of 0.25–0.5 mg/kg given in the period before sternotomy.

HAEMODYNAMIC MANAGEMENT OF PATIENTS

The period between induction and the initiation of cardiopulmonary bypass is a critical period for these patients. If their preoperative preparation has been satisfactory there should be no problem with the pulse rate, the continuing β-blockade ensuring low pulse rates. Some workers have advocated the use of the pulse pressure product as an indirect index of the balance between myocardial work and oxygen consumption. However experimental work has demonstrated that for a given pulse pressure product hypertension with a slow rate is not as injurious as the same pulse product produced with a lower blood pressure and a higher pulse rate[20]. The definition of hypertension in this context is somewhat arbitary, in some centres systolic pressures greater than 120 mmHg are routinely controlled with hypotensive agents, whereas in other centres pressures of up to 150 mmHg systolic would be accepted before hypotensive therapy is started. It is at this time that the results of preoperative exercise testing are particularly valuable in enabling the anaesthetist to determine the critical rate pressure product for the particular patient he is managing. Hypertension is normally easily controllable with an infusion of nitroprusside and reports from other centres would suggest that the use of nitroglycerine may be equally useful. Occasionally in a patient with refractory hypertension α blockade is of help. The addition of Halothane to the anaesthetic mixture could also be considered as experimental work has demonstrated the beneficial effects of Halothane on both the myocardial work and oxygen demands[18]. Some caution must be used in applying the results from animal experimental work to the clinical situation. Reports from animal experimental work suggested that the combination of β-blockade and trichloroethylene was potentially hazardous.[21] Our clinical experience using this combination has not confirmed these animal experimental studies and we feel that the results from studies in other species must, as always, be interpreted with some caution.

MYOCARDIAL REVASCULARISATION AND CARDIOPULMONARY BYPASS

The management of cardiopulmonary bypass in these patients is essentially similar to that in other forms of heart disease. While we have no hard evidence to support the practice we prefer to have slightly higher mean arterial pressures during perfusion with these patients on the suspicion that patients with coronary atheroma may also have significant cerebral atheroma and for this reason we prefer to see a mean arterial pressure on bypass greater than 70 mmHg. In the conduct of the cardiopulmonary bypass accurate control of the pressures on the left side of the heart is essential. For this reason a pressure monitoring line is inserted in the left atrium and an easily controlled and monitored left atrial venting system is used. The left atrial vent is used to prevent distension of the left side of the heart but accurate control is needed as if a negative pressure is created in the left atrium air may be entrained into the heart which would represent an additional unnecessary hazard to the patient as the actual surgical intervention is a totally extra-cardiac procedure. The distal anastomoses to the coronary vessels are normally undertaken with the aorta cross-clamped. The technique used for myocardial preservation during this period of aortic cross clamping will obviously depend on the surgeon's particular preference. The method used in our unit is to use a single dose of cardioplegia immediately after clamping the aorta giving a maximum of 500 ml of the solution.

Table 2 Cardioplegic solution as used at Papworth Hospital. The solution is made up by adding a stock solution to non-lactated Ringer's 10 ml/kg to maximum of 500 ml

	mmol/l
Mg^{++}	16
Na^{+}	149
K^{+}	20
Ca^{++}	2
Cl^{-}	172
HCO^{-}	1.5
Procaine	1.2

This induces a metabolic arrest of the heart and as the cardioplegic solution is administered at 4 °C rapid cooling of the myocardium results (Figure 2). Myocardial cooling is then continued using a re-circulating system for the topical cooling fluid introduced into the pericardial cavity[22]. Experimentally the combination of cardioplegia and topical cooling has been shown to give adequate myocardial preservation for periods of up to 16 h. Our clinical practice confirm that periods of aortic cross clamping of 3 h can be tolerated without apparent myocardial injury. The use of the aortic cross clamping

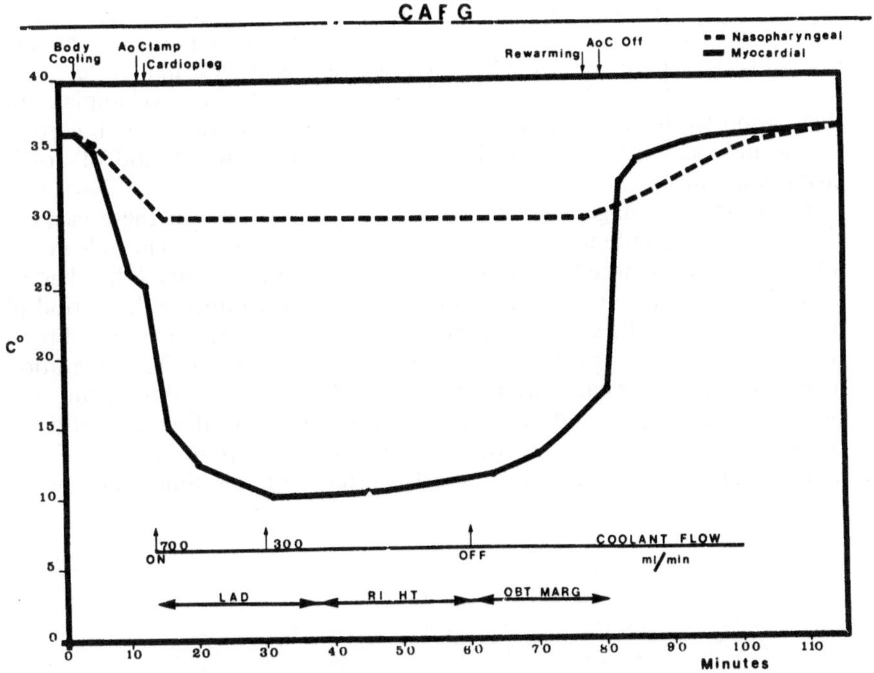

Figure 2 Cooling curve using a combination of cold cardioplegia and profound topical myocardial cooling. Cooling flow initially at 700 ml/min which is reduced when myocardial temperature reaches 10–12 °C. Pericardial cooling has to be discontinued when the obtuse marginal graft is being performed and a rise of 5 °C myocardial temperature occurs during the anastemosis of this graft

without either the protection afforded by cardioplegia or by cooling is similar to the historical techniques used for correction of simple congenital defects, where surface cooling was combined with in-flow occlusion. Both techniques are severely limited by time restriction before irreversible damage occurs. In the case of surface cooling and in-flow occlusion the damage was immediately apparent in organs which are more sensitive to anoxic damage than the heart. In the case of aortic cross clamping without myocardial preservation the damage which is undoubtedly produced in the myocardium by any periods of normathermic ischaemia of greater than 20 min is unlikely to be sufficient to affect the immediate mortality of the procedure but may influence subsequent myocardial function and rehabilitation. Myocardial preservation with a combination of cardioplegia and myocardial cooling does not add to the time of operation or time on bypass and it is now well established that it has a beneficial effect in preserving myocardial function. This is particularly important in patients who are presenting with inadequate coronary circulation, as in these patients areas of the myocardium may already be anoxic before the aorta is cross clamped. For this reason we believe that adequate myocardial preservation with cardioplegia and pericardial cooling is mandatory during the period of aortic cross clamping.

The general management of cardiopulmonary bypass in these cases is similar to that in patients with other forms of cardiac disease. The only major difference we have noted is in that patients with a non-selective β-blockade a paradoxical rise in serum potassium may be observed during the period of bypass[23]. The results shown in Figure 3 were from a patient who had been receiving 240 mg of propranolol daily before operation. The operation involved triple coronary artery bypass grafting. Serum potassium rose steadily during bypass and on the first occasion when the discontinuation of bypass was attempted myocardial contractility was poor. Dextrose and insulin and calcium chloride were administered at this time and a weak

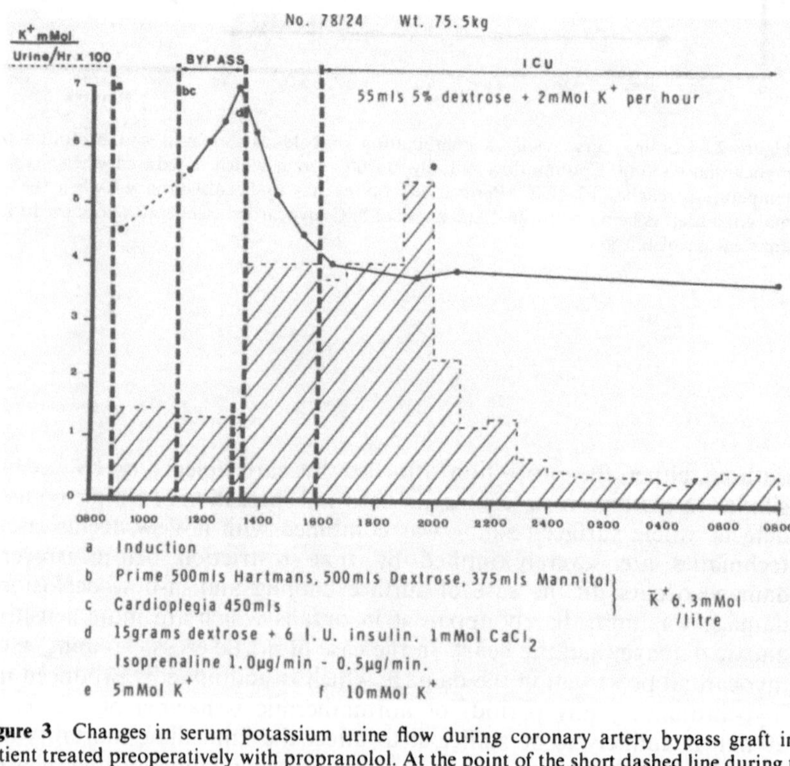

Figure 3 Changes in serum potassium urine flow during coronary artery bypass graft in a patient treated preoperatively with propranolol. At the point of the short dashed line during the bypass period an attempt was made to discontinue bypass which was unsuccessful due to poor myocardial contractility. The administration of dextrose and insulin induced a prompt recovery in myocardial contractility. The shaded area represents hourly urinary flow

isoprenaline infusion was commenced. Despite continuing high serum potassium levels bypass was then successfully and easily discontinued and the myocardium contracted well. The serum potassium fell rapidly during the postoperative period and the patient's further postoperative course was uneventful. Following this observation we undertook a prospective study of two groups of patients undergoing coronary artery bypass grafting[24]. One group was treated preoperatively with propranolol and the other group treated preoperatively with Metoprolol. There was a progressive rise in serum potassium in the patients who had been treated with Propranolol. Before bypass their mean serum potassium was 4.09 mmol/l and after 85 min it had risen to 5.22 mmol/l. In the metoprolol patients the prebypass level was 4.04 mmol/l and at 85 min it was 4.16 mmol/l. The difference between these two groups of patients is significant at the 1% level. Two patients in the propranolol group had peak serum potassium levels greater than 6.3 mmol/l. Urinary potassium loss was similar in both groups of patients and no difference was discernible between bypass time, severity of preoperative disease or duration of ischaemia and the only difference between them appeared to be in the choice of preoperative β-antagonist. It has been shown that after non-selective β-blockade total body potassium increases and there may be some alteration in the renal handling of potassium. However this did not appear to be so in our group of patients and the most cogent explanation for the paradoxical rise in potassium that we observed in the patients treated with propranolol would appear to be modification of the adrenergic[25,26] response which occurs during non-pulstile cardiopulmonary bypass. The non-selective β-blocker by its β_2-blocking action prevented the β_2-mediated uptake of potassium by both skeletal and cardiac muscle[27] in response to the adrenergic stimulus whereas the hepatic release of potassium in response to that stimulus would be unaffected by such β-blockade[28,29]. Experimental work in both animals[28] and human volunteers[30] has demonstrated disturbance of potassium handling in subjects who have a β_2-blockade and are under stress and reports from other centres where propranolol is used preoperatively have confirmed that this effect is commonly seen[31]. In the prospective study of the two groups of patients a significant difference in the levels of blood glucose 85 min after the start of bypass was also seen. The patients in the propranolol group had a significantly lower level of blood glucose when compared to those in the Metoprolol group. This can be taken to indicate that the effects of β_2-blockade which have been observed in insulin dependant diabetics[32,33] must also be occurring during the period of cardiopulmonary bypass. Current policy in most units and in ours is to discontinue β-blockers at the time of surgery and recommence them postoperatively only if there is a definite clinical indication. Tachdysrhythmias occur in a significant percentage of these patients in the postoperative period and while this does not cause angina if the myocardial revascularization is adequate it is nonetheless a troublesome complication which is probably iatrogenic and related to the abrupt discontinuation of β-blockers at the time of surgery. It would appear to bc more logical to continue β-blockade through the surgical and postoperative period[34] and then discontinue the β-blockers gradually 4–5 days after operation.

DISCUSSION

The anaesthetic management of the patient for coronary artery bypass grafting is interesting as it presents a combination of pharmocological and physiological derangements in the perioperative period. The range of drugs and techniques recommended for anaesthesia are extremely wide and suggest that expertise in dealing with the underlying problems is more important than the actual drugs and techniques used. One fascinating aspect of the management of these patients is the changes that have occurred in a comparatively brief period of time. The reports of intractable cardiac failure following coronary artery bypass grafting in patients preoperatively treated with propranolol by Viljoen *et al.* in 1972[3] obviously represented a real and life-threatening syndrome. Their experience was not unique and it is interesting to speculate on why there has been an apparently major change in the post-cardiopulmonary bypass state of these patients. It is difficult to believe that it is related to anaesthetic or surgical expertise as in the early reports good results were reported following the withdrawal of β-blockers some time prior to surgery which would seem to exonerate the anaesthetic and surgical management. The early withdrawal of β-blockers did however lead to undesirable problems in the preoperative period. Our view is that the explanation of this radical change in postbypass course must be related to the greatly improved myocardial preservation during the period when the distal coronary anastomoses are performed. Viljoen comments in his paper that coronary perfusion was not used during the cardiopulmonary bypass, presumably meaning that aortic cross clamping was used and this would inevitably lead to some myocardial hypoxic acidosis. This hypoxic acidosis occurring in a patient who already had a coronary circulation which was sufficiently compromised to cause angina, would certainly lead to definitive myocardial injury. Similar results would occur with the practice of ventricular fibrillation during the period of performing the distal anastomoses as numerous studies have demonstrated that regional myocardial blood flow is disturbed in the fibrillating heart. It would appear that the only radical change which has occurred in the practice of coronary artery bypass grafting is the use of cardioplegia and/or topical cooling to produce a virtual total metabolic inhibition of the myocardial metabolism during the period of aortic cross clamping and in our view this is sufficient to account for the clinical difference which is now seen in the postperfusion state of these patients. The safe management of patients having surgery for ischaemic heart disease is obviously a problem for a multidisciplinary team and this is emphasized by the results of a survey carried out by the Society of Thoracic and Cardiovascular Surgeons into mortality following open heart surgery where there was a very significant negative correlation between the number of cases operated on with ischaemic heart disease and the mortality in the individual units in the United Kingdom.

The safe management of these patients is dependant more on an understanding of the haemodynamic effects of the disease and the pharmocological effects of the treatment rather than on any particular anaesthetic agent or technique. It also depends on the co-operation of the surgical team as even with perfect anaesthetic and haemodynamic management of the patient, a surgeon who insists on elevating the heart prior to bypass to palpate and inspect the circumflex system will undoubtedly cause profound hypotension which can only have a deleterious effect on the myocardial perfusion. The improvement in the results of surgery in these patients is undoubtedly related to the better use of β-adrenergic blockade, more understanding and control of the SPTI : DPTI ratio and better myocardial preservation with cooling and cardioplegia. The problem therefore of safe management in these patients must remain a co-operative venture between anaesthetists, surgeons and cardiologists.

ACKNOWLEDGEMENTS

We would like to acknowledge the help of the Sims Woodhead Laboratory and financial assistance from Astra Pharmaceutical and Ciba Geigy, UK.

References

1. Hoffman, J. I. E. and Buckberg, G. D. (1975). Pathophysiology of subenducardial ischaemia. *Br. Med. J.*, **1**, 76
2. Black, J. W., Crowther, A. F., Shanks, R. G., Smith, L. H. and Dornhurst, A. C. (1964). A new adrenergic beta receptor antagonist. *Lancet*, **1**, 1080
3. Viljoen, J. F. (1972). Estafanous, F. G., Kellner, G. A. (1972). Propranolol and cardiac surgery. *J. Thorac. Cardiovasc. Surg.*, **64**, 827
4. Romagnoli, A. and Keats, A. S. (1975). Plasma and atrial propranolol after pre-operative withdrawal. *Circulation*, **52**, 1123
5. Shand, D. G. (1975). Propranolol withdrawal. *N. Engl. J. Med.*, **293**, 449
6. Boudoulas, H., Lewis, R. P., Snyder, G. L., Karayannacos, P. E. and Vasko, J. S. (1979). Beneficial effect of continuation of propranolol through coronary artery bypass surgery. *Clin. Cardiol.*, **2**, 87
7. Kopriva, C. J., Guinazu, A. and Barash, P. G. (1978). Massive propranolol therapy and uncomplicated cardiac surgery. *J. Am. Med. Assoc.*, **239**, 1157
8. Kaplan, J. A., Dunbar, R. W., Bland, J. W., Sumpter, R. and Jones, E. L. (1975). Propranolol and cardiac surgery. *Anaesth. Analg.*, **54**, 571
9. Manners, J. M. and Walters, F. J. M. (1979). Beta adrenoceptor blockade and anaesthesia. *Anaesthesia*, **34**, 3
10. Oka, Y., Frishman, W., Becker, R. M., Kadish, A., Strein, J., Matsumoto, M., Opkin, L. and Frater, R. (1980). Clinical pharmacology of the new beta adrenergic blocking drugs. Part 10 Beta adrenoceptor blockade and coronary artery surgery. *Am. Heart J.*, **99**, 255
11. Alderman, E. L., Coltart, D. J., Wettach, G. E. and Harrison, D. C. (1974). Coronary artery syndromes after sudden propranolol withdrawal. *Ann. Intern. Med.*, **81**, 625
12. Miller, R. R., Olson, H. G., Amsterdam, E. A. and Mason, D. T. (1975). Propranolol withdrawal rebound phenomenon. *New Engl. J. Med.*, **293**, 416
13. Barash, P. G. (1980). The rate pressure product in clinical anaesthesia: boon or bane? (Editorial). *Anaesth. Analg.*, **59**, 229
14. Tyden, H. and Westerholm, C. J. (1979). Cardiovascular effects of neurolept anaesthesia in patients with coronary artery disease. (1979). *Acta Anaesth. Scand.*, **23**, 471

15. Kistner, J. R., Miller, E. D., Lake, C. L. and Ross, W. T. (1979). Indices of myocardial oxygenation during coronary artery revascularization in man with morphine versus halothane anaesthesia. *Anaesthesiology*, **50,** 324
16. Reves, J. G., Samuelson, P. N., Lell, W. A., Allarde, R. R., Younes, H. M. and Oget, S. (1977). Anaesthesia for coronary artery surgery: an evolution in anaesthetic management. *Alabama J. Med. Sci.*, **14,** 394
17. Lell, W. A., Walker, D. R., Blackstone, E. H., Kouchoukos, N. T., Allarde, R. and Roe, C. R. (1977). Evaluation of myocardial damage in patients undergoing coronary artery bypass procedures with halothane–N_2O anaesthesia and adjuvants. *Anaesth. Analg.*, **56,** 556
18. Delaney, T. J., Kistner, J. R., Lake, C. L. and Miller, E. D. (1980). Myocardial function during halothane and enflurane anaesthesia in patients with coronary artery disease. *Anaesth. Analg.*, **59,** 240
19. Swan, H. J. C. and Granz, W. (1980). Flotation catheters. *Br. J. Clin. Equipm.*, **5,** 48
20. Wilkinson, P. L., Tyberg, J. V., Moyers, J. R. and White, A. E. (1980). Correlates of myocardial oxygen consumption when after load changes during halothane anaesthesia in dogs. *Anaesth. Analg.*, **59,** 233
21. Roberts, J. G., Foex, P., Clarke, T. N. S., Bennett, M. J. and Saner, C. A. (1976). Haemodynamic interactions of high dose propranolol and anaesthesia in the dog III. The effects of haemorrhage during halothane and trichlorethylene anaesthesia. *Br. J. Anaesth.*, **48,** 411
22. Wheelden, D. R., Bethune, D. W., Gill, R. D. and English, T. A. H. (1976). A simple cooling circuit for topical cardiac hypothermia. *Thorax*, **31,** 565
23. Bethune, D. W. and McKay, R. (1978). Paradoxical changes in serum potassium during cardiopulmonary bypass in association with non-cardio-selective beta-blockade. *Lancet*, **2,** 380
24. Petch, M. C., McKay, R. and Bethune, D. W. (1981). The effect of β_2 adrenergic blockade on serum potassium and glucose levels during open heart surgery. *Eur. Heart J.* (In press)
25. Anton, A. H., Gravenstein, J. S. and Wheat, M. W. (1964). Extracorporeal circulation and endogenous epinephrine and norepinephrine in plasma atrium and urine in man. *Anaesthesiology*, **25,** 262
26. Butler, M. J., Brittan, B. J., Wood, W. G., Mainwaring Burton, R. and Irving, M. H. (1977). Plasma catecholamine concentrations during operation. *Br. J. Surg.*, **64,** 786
27. Clausen, T. and Flatman, J. A. (1977). The effect of catecholamines on Na–K transport and membrane potential in rat soleus muscle. *J. Physiol.*, **270,** 383
28. Lockwood, R. H. and Lum, B. K. B. (1974). Effects of adrenergic agonists and antagonists on potassium metabolism. *J. Pharm. Exp. Ther.*, **189,** 119
29. Guthrie, S. D. and Murphy, Q. R. (1976). Epinephrine induced hepatic potassium movements before and after adrenergic blockade. *Can. J. Physiol. Pharmacol.*, **54,** 347
30. Carlsoon, E., Fellenius, E., Lundberg, P. and Svensson, L. (1978). β-Adrenoceptor blockers plasma potassium and exercise. *Lancet*, **2,** 424
31. Todd, E. P., McAllister, R. G., Campbell, H. C. *et al.* (1977). Effects of propranolol on hypokalemia induced by cardiopulmonary bypass. (Abstract) *Circulation*, **55,** Suppl. 3, 60
32. Davidson, N. McD, Corrall, R. J. M., Shaw, T. R. D. and French, E. B. (1977). Observations in man of hypoglycaemia during selective and non-selective beta blockade. *Scott. Med. J.*, **22,** 69
33. Lager, I., Blohme, G. and Smith, U. (1979). Effect of cardioselective and non

selective β-blockade on the hypoglycaemia response in insulin dependent diabetics. *Lancet*, **1**, 458

34. Boudoulas, H., Snyder, G. L., Lewis, R. P., Kates, R. E., Karayannacos, P. E. and Vasko, J. S. (1978). Safety and rationale for continuation of propranolol therapy during coronary bypass operation. *Ann. Thorac. Surg.*, **26**, 222

18
Hypothermic circulatory arrest in infants and children

G. JACKSON REES

Perhaps the most significant factor in the dramatic change in the age at which the correction of congenital cardiac defects is undertaken is the development of profound hypothermic techniques. The advantages of these techniques in the younger age groups are that it enables cardiopulmonary bypass to be conducted with very simple cannulation of the atrium and the aorta even in the presence of intracardiac shunts, and it enables the surgery to be undertaken on a still heart in a totally dry field with a high degree of myocardial protection against ischaemic damage.

I propose to deal with this topic by first and very simply running through the techniques which are used at the Royal Liverpool Children's Hospital and then to take certain components of this technique, describing in more detail its rationale. In general, we choose to use this approach to open heart surgery in children who are (a) under the age of one year or (b) under the weight of 10 kg.

The procedure is as follows:

(1) Induction of anaesthesia is by means of thiopentone 4 ml/kg and d-tubocurarine chloride 0.8 ml/kg. The infant is intubated and it is important that the endotracheal tube used should be a relatively slack fit. The reason for this is that during the period of circulatory arrest mucosal surfaces are very vulnerable to pressure damage.

(2) Monitoring lines are set up and the most convenient and readily cannulated sites are the femoral vein and artery. Even in the smallest infant it is usually possible to achieve this percutaneously using a Seldinger technique.

(3) The intravenous fluids are administered through the central venous line into the inferior vena cava. The fluid which we use is 12.5% of dextrose in half strength Hartman's solution. Such an infusion at the rate of 4 ml/kg per hour will provide approximately half the normal calorie requirement of an infant. It is important that attention should be paid to maintaining appropriate calorie input because, during the

course of prolonged operations infants and especially those infants who are malnourished pre-operatively, are prone to become hypoglycaemic. Another aspect of the infusion technique is that it is desirable to connect the infusion to the cannula through a capillary sized tube. This means that drugs may be injected from a remote point and gain rapid access to the circulation without the necessity of flushing volumes of fluid into the infant. The use of a long capilliary tube for the connection of the infusion demands that some sort of syringe pump should be used to overcome the resistance in the line and maintain a constant infusion rate.

(4) The child is castrized and is now ready for sternotomy.

(5) During the pre bypass period the child is given morphia 0.25 ml/kg glucose and insulin over a 30 minute period and receives 1 ml of 50% dextrose and 0.25 units of insulin per kg of body weight. The reason for using this latter will be discussed later on. Also during the pre infusion period alpha blockade is achieved by the administration of phenoxybenzamine 1 ml/kg.

(6) Following cannulation of the atrium and the aorta, cardiopulmonary bypass is established in the normal way and on bypass the infant is cooled. The rate of cooling is at about 1 °C per minute. The temperature is measured at two sites: (a) in the nasopharynx and (b) in the oesophagus and if the temperature differential between these two sites exceeds 6°C centigrade, the rate of cooling is reduced. When the nasopharyngeal temperature reaches that which is estimated is appropriate for the duration of the surgery which is anticipated, perfusion is maintained for another 4–5 minutes to reduce the temperature differentials in the body and to ensure that a stable temperature will be maintained in the nasopharynx during the procedure.

(7) At temperatures below 3°C, 10% carbon dioxide is added to the oxygenator gases. This will be discussed later.

(8) When the stable temperature is used the child is exsanguinated into the oxygenator and having snared the cavae and clamped both aorta and pulmonary artery the surgeon may proceed with the intracardiac correction. During the period of circulatory arrest, the blood in the oxygenator circulates slowly through a bypass in order to prevent dense sedimentation and on the re-establishment of perfusion the filling of the circulation with concentrated cells.

(9) On the completion of surgery, cardiopulmonary bypass is re-established by pumping blood into the arterial system until the venous pressure rises to about 15 cmH_2O and then opening the venous drainage. Rewarming is carried out at about the same rate as cooling.

(10) At 30°C blood is withdrawn for acid–base measurement and the sample having been taken, an amount of sodium bicarbonate is infused which would correct a base deficit of 6 mEq. Experience has shown that this quantity of bicarbonate is always necessary and is usually all that is necessary to restore the base to normal levels.

(11) At 30°C an attempt is made to re-establish the cardiac output having

corrected the base and usually calcium is necessary at this stage. At about 32 °C the perfusion is discontinued. During the post-perfusion period, fresh frozen plasma is infused to maintain the central venous pressure with the object of maintaining a haematocrit value of approximately 0.3.

The above is an outline of the technique which we adopt and there follows an account of the rationale behind certain of the procedures.

ARREST TIMES AT VARYING TEMPERATURES

Normally it is accepted that it is permissible to arrest circulation for 50 minutes at 23 °C, for 60 minutes at 20 °C and for 70 minutes at 17 °C. There have been several studies of intellectual performance after durations of circulatory arrest of this order at the various temperatures and all such studies appear to show that if these limits are set, there is little danger of neurological damage. However, there is a need to make every effort to decrease any possible danger of cerebral damage.

It is well known that in neonatal life, all species have a very high tolerance of anoxia. One of the differences between neonates and adults which might at least in part account for this, is the fact that the glycogen content of brain of neonates is very much greater than that of the adult of any species. Furthermore, it is known that carbohydrate depletion tends to reduce the tolerance of hypoxia. Experiments carried out by Clark and Rees have shown that adult rats that had been infused with glucose and insulin, continued to exhibit respiratory activity in the face of circulatory arrest for about twice as long as untreated animals. This suggests that this sort of treatment does ensure that neurological activity persists for a longer period after the establishment of high intracellular glycogen levels. Further work by Clark demonstrated that the infusion of glucose and insulin does in fact greatly elevate the glycogen content of the rat brain and furthermore, maintains ATP levels within the brain at higher values during periods of total ischaemia. These findings are the basis for the inclusion in our procedure of the infusion of glucose and insulin during the pre-perfusion period. Clark's work showed that during the early part of an ischaemic period, the utilization of the carbohydrate reserves was rather extravagant, and current work has suggested that the inclusion of barbiturates in the pretreatment of rats reduces the rate at which the carbohydrate reserves of the brain decline during the anoxic period. We have not used high dose barbiturate for brain protection in this situation but the reports on the remarkable protective effects of barbiturates suggests that probably in future, we will be using massive doses of barbiturates prior to our periods of circulatory arrest at low temperature.

ALPHA-BLOCKADE

The clinical picture which we describe as low output following cardiac surgery is well known. It has been suggested that this may be the result of high levels of circulating angiotensin II which occur following cardiopulmonary bypass using non-pulsatile pumps. For some years, we have induced alpha-blockade with phenoxybenzamine prior to perfusion in all our open heart cases, and this has virtually eliminated the occurrence of low output situations. There is no way in which alpha-blockade might antagonize vasocontrictive effects of angiotensin II. Therefore, if we accept that angiotensin is the factor giving rise to this situation, we must say that pretreatment with phenoxybenzamine reduces the post-perfusion levels of angiotensin II. This is the subject of study at the present moment. There is, however, little doubt that following profound hypothermia and circulatory arrest, the clinical condition of those infants treated with phenoxybenzamine is much better than that of those who are not. This is perhaps illustrated in a series of 50 Mustard procedures carried out under the age of 12 months at the Royal Liverpool Children's Hospital, where catacholamine myocardial support post-operatively was considered necessary in only three cases. It is our view that the inclusion of alpha-blockade in the regime contributes to the satisfactory cardiac performance of these cases during the post-operative period.

CARBON DIOXIDE

Equilibration of the blood with high tensions of carbon dioxide has been a part of hypothermic techniques for many years. It has not always been appreciated why this is necessary, although various reasons have been put forward. It was shown by the Australian workers that temperature gradients within the brain of rapidly cooled animals were reduced if the CO_2 tensions were maintained at high levels. It is also well known that high CO_2 levels can oppose the left shift of the oxygen dissociation curve which takes place at low temperatures. It is also known that CO_2 is a potent vasodilator, and might therefore be expected to contribute towards the uniformity of cooling of the body during rapid temperature changes.

The pharmacodynamics of carbon dioxide have recently been studied by us, using mass spectrometry to determine oxygen uptake and CO_2 output, under conditions of total body perfusion, during normothermic and hypothermic perfusion. In brief, our findings were that at normal temperatures, a new equilibrium for CO_2 following the introduction of an increased concentration of carbon dioxide to the oxygenator gases, was established in approximately 25 minutes. However, during a period of rapid cooling, the enhanced solubility of carbon dioxide prevents equilibration of the body with the carbon dioxide fed to the oxygenator, therefore, following rapid cooling over a period of 30 minutes, the body is still taking up carbon dioxide at a rapid rate in an attempt to establish equilibrium. The significance of this is that we can say that the mean tension of CO_2 in the body following a period of cooling, is very much less than the tension of CO_2 in the arterial blood which is fed to the body from the oxygenator. The corrolery of this is that if high tensions of CO_2 are not fed to the oxygenator, the mean PCO_2 in the body would be substantially lower than its normal value. I think that this is the explanation of the necessity to feed to the oxygenator high concentrations of carbon dioxide to avoid all the ill consequences, particularly in relation to cerebral circulation, of low PCO_2.

POST-OPERATIVE MANAGEMENT

The postoperative management of infants who have undergone cardiac surgery under profound hypothermia may perhaps be divided into five headings.

(1) The maintenance of gas exchange.
(2) The maintenance of blood volume and blood viscosity at appropriate levels.
(3) The maintenance of peripheral perfusion.
(4) The maintenance of urinary flow.
(5) The maintenance of energy reserves.

Maintenance of blood gases

Post-operatively, all our cases are ventilated and in view of the altered pulmonary haemodynamics which are inevitable following the correction of congenital heart defects, we consider that the tidal volumes and minute volumes which should be used, should be rather greater than those which are normal for infants of this size. In determining the tidal volume therefore, we increase the ventilator pressures until clinically there is good airation of all areas of the lungs. This inevitably results in low levels of PCO_2 unless compensatory steps are taken. In situations where a left-to-right shunt has been eliminated there is virtue in a low PCO_2, as it contributes towards the prevention of increases in pulmonary vascular resistance, but in most cases, the PCO_2 is kept at a value around 30 mmHg. In order to achieve this in the face of greater than normal minute volumes, we add CO_2 to the ventilating gas. This of course, is particularly valuable in infants who are being re-warmed in the recovery area, because it ensures that you have a stable PCO_2 in spite of big changes in VCO_2 which occur with increases in temperature.

It was shown many years ago, by McQuiston, in animal experiments, that following exposure to hypothermia there was a tendency for the haematocrit to rise and for a shrinkage of plasma volume to occur by virtue of loss of volume from the circulation to the extracellular space. This pattern of behaviour is well marked in infants who have undergone cardiac surgery under hypothermic techniques, and the haematocrit will rise unless active steps are taken to prevent this. Prevention of rises in the haematocrit can only be achieved by the infusion of plasma and as part of the routine and over and above any colloid which may be given to replace blood loss, we infuse during the first 24 post-operative hours fresh frozen plasma at the rate of about 1.5 ml/kg of weight per hour. We are anxious to maintain the haematocrit at about 0.3 and the choice of blood or plasma to replace blood losses is determined by the haematocrit measurements.

Peripheral blood flow and renal profusion

During the postoperative period, alpha-blockade is maintained by supplementary doses of phenoxybenzamine 6 and 12 hours postoperatively. This helps to maintain warm extremities and enhances the sensitivity of the kidney to diuretics.

Urinary flow

Diuretics are usually necessary in the postoperative period and one of the procedures which we have introduced to our postoperative management, which has improved our control over urinary output, is the almost routine use of frusemide infusions. This of course eliminates the cardiovascular effects which may follow bolus injections of diuretics and enables the urinary output to be very finely controlled. The order of dosage is about 0.2 ml/kg frusemide per hour. If this is given through a fine control infusion pump, it is possible to prescribe the urinary output in the same way as one prescribes the input of fluids. Using this approach, we aim to keep the fluid balance at zero. The use of infusion pumps has enabled nurses to adjust the urinary output in the same way as they adjust the input.

Nutrition

During the postoperative period, it is essential that the blood sugar should be monitored in infants at hourly intervals, by means of paper strips. Hypoglycaemia is treated with bolus injections of 50% dextrose, and high blood sugar levels in the face of the 12.5% glucose infusion which is continued into the postoperative period, are treated with insulin. If catacholamines are used, there is a tendency for high blood sugars to develop and insulin and dextrose in higher concentrations infusions may be necessary to maintain intracellular energy requirements to meet the increased demands made on the myocardium by catacholamines. It is interesting that if one gives glucose and insulin infusions in the early postoperative period, when the stress anti-insulin effects are at their peak, that the infant is insulin resistant. As the child improves, he becomes increasingly insulin sensitive. If therefore insulin infusions are used, it is essential that the insulin should be infused from a different syringe pump from the dextrose, so that each can be controlled independently and in response to careful monitoring of the blood sugar levels.

In summary, perhaps, one might say that the successful application of profound hypothermic techniques is dependent upon the meticulous attention to a wide variety of unrelated details. What I have tried to indicate in this paper is some of these details, which I consider to be important to the ultimately successful outcome of surgical intervention using this method.

19
Cerebral perfusion during cardiac surgery using cardiac bypass

J. C. SIMPSON

The serious causes of morbidity and mortality after cardiac surgery are still:

(1) low cardiac output
(2) surgical haemorrhage
(3) dysrhythmias
(4) brain damage.

The first three are, in the modern clinical environment, treatable; there is, however, little practical help to be offered to the patient with brain damage, and thus it must be prevented as far as possible.

The brain requires: (1) oxygen as a continuous supply – it has no facility for storing this molecule; (2) hexose sugar also as a continuous supply, as similarly no local storage mechanisms are available. Deprived of these two moieties brain damage will ensue. The supply of hexose sugars and oxygen is via the cerebral blood flow in the intracranial vasculature arising from the Circle of Willis in the human brain.

The maintenance of this blood supply and its controlling mechanisms has been the subject of a lot of research work since Kety and Schmidt first measured cerebral blood flow (CBF) in 1945. Blood flow homeostasis is maintained by autoregulation at arteriolar level within the calvalarium, thus for a changing range of mean arterial pressure (MAP) in the cerebral circulation the myogenic tone of the arterioles is able to alter to prevent a gross change in CBF. The limits of autoregulatory response in normal man[1] are between MAP 60 mmHg and 120 mmHg. Below and above this level the circulation becomes 'pressure-passive'. The mechanisms sustaining autoregulation are however modified by many factors (Table 1). All the above-mentioned factors change rapidly when a patient's circulation is 'taken over' by a heart-lung bypass machine during cardiac surgery, thus potentially CBF should be altered due to extensive modification of autoregulation, and the patient's brain may thus be at risk from

Table 1 Factors influencing cerebral blood flow

Change in:	P_aCO_2
	P_aO_2
	Temperature
	Pattern of flow
	Blood viscosity
	Cerebral metabolism
	Drugs

hypoxaemic damage due to changes in local blood flow. The distribution of the cerebral blood flow is not uniform and there are extensive variations of regional blood flow[2] aligned against metabolic activity. The areas of brain tissue depending on a higher blood-flow pattern are more vulnerable to infarction if autoregulatory responses are lost. Potentially the brain of the patient undergoing cardiac surgery with bypass procedure is at risk. These risks must be evaluated and a conclusion sought, whereby such 'physiological insults' can be minimized and the procedure made safer.

The techniques available for measuring CBF are many, indicating perhaps that no single method is accurate, reliable, and reproducible. They vary from interruption of the brain's blood supply, insertion of a rotameter and measuring the flow in this traumatic way, use of an electromagnetic flow probe outside the artery, counting glass spheres of varying size passing through the cerebral circulation, autoradiographic techniques, measurement of cerebral arteriovenous oxygen tension gradients, use of implanted hydrogen electrode system, to analysis of washout curve of intra-arterially injected or inhaled, radioactive isotope of xenon or krypton. These latter two techniques are clinically applicable in the human, but are invasive and tissue-destructive. The future success for measurement of CBF in man lies in refining the use of analysis of the cerebral washout curve obtained by the 'one-breath' inhalation technique[3]. This is potentially applicable to patients undergoing cardiopulmonary bypass procedures.

REVIEW OF PUBLISHED WORK

The measurement of CBF during heart–lung bypass was first undertaken by Halley and his colleagues in the USA[4]. Their technique was to measure CBF using the traumatic rotameter method and quantitate the global flow before and during extracorporeal circulation using a 'Sigmarotor' pump. Thus the anaesthetized dogs were exposed to non-pulsatile flow with haemodilution and a constant P_aCO_2. There results indicated that there was no change in CBF until the MAP (= perfusion pressure) fell to below 55 mmHg. At this level CBF fell and did not rise again with an increase in MAP. However an infusion of noradrenaline, begun at this low pressure, increased the CBF dramatically. These results in the dog suggest loss of autoregulation at MAP

50 mmHg and development of a pressure-passive state and with continuing low flows; but with augmented pressure, an improvement in CBF.

We repeated this experiment using the less traumatic xenon 133 washout analysis (Simpson, J. and Cronje, N. (1973), unpublished data). Before submitting the dogs to extracorporeal circulation we tested the range of autoregulation, instituted bypass and measured the CBF at 'full flow' and decrements of this flow state mimicking a clinical situation. The results indicated the circulation became pressure-passive at the lower limit of autoregulation and similarly did not return to the control value after 15 min of $\frac{1}{4}$ flow. However increasing the P_aCO_2 did increase the CBF significantly, as did an infusion of noradrenaline at this low flow rate; in the latter circumstance there was an expected rise of MAP. These results indicate that, despite loss of autoregulation, the CBF may be improved by increasing P_aCO_2 above normal values or use of noradrenaline. This work was done using non-pulsatile flow, but Simeone[5] had previously shown that if pulsatile flow was used in the same experimental protocol CBF was improved with a similarly low MAP and flow rate, suggesting perhaps that autoregulation may be retained at low MAP if the flow offered to the cerebral circulation is pulsatile in form. These results are further amplified by the work of Sanderson *et al.*[6], again working with the standard dog preparation. This group of workers studied the histology of the canine brain after periods of extracorporeal circulation – one group with genuine pulsatile flow, the second group without pulsatile flow – and found greater histological damage in the second group of dogs.

The assessment of CBF in man during extracorporeal circulatory states was first undertaken by Woolman and his colleagues[7] in Philadelphia. They used cerebral arteriovenous oxygen difference as a measure of CBF in six patients submitted to non-pulsatile flow, steady hypothermia to 30 °C. They came to the conclusion, assuming the cerebral metabolic rate (O_2 consumption) was steady, that P_aCO_2 was the most important factor influencing CBF at steady 'pump' flow rates.

A further study in man was undertaken by Margaret Branthwaite[8] whose methodology included the use of jugular bulb thermovelocity probes. Her measurements were performed in the period of transition to extracorporeal circulation and during the first 15 min of bypass at normothermia, non-pulsatile flow and with haemodilution, but with a steady P_aCO_2. The conclusions extrapolated from this study, especially in those patients whose MAP fell during the onset of bypass, was that the perfusion pressure was an important determinant of CBF and directly related to it.

Perhaps tentative conclusions drawn from the results of these two studies are: (1) during hypotension (i.e. below the lower limit of autoregulation in man) the circulation of the brain becomes pressure-passive; (2) that at these levels of MAP (= perfusion pressure), CBF can be influenced by changes in P_aCO_2.

The neuropathological[9] and neurological[10] sequelae of extracorporeal techniques have been extensively documented, but it may not always be easy to separate the effects of infarction due to microemboli from infarction due to inadequate regional cerebral blood flow. EEG studies and clinical neurological examination have a very limited application in differentiating the aetiological factor. The EEG is, however, valuable as a monitoring tool to detect aberration in cerebral perfusion and metabolism during bypass. Maynard and Prior have developed a single-channel EEG, the integrated cerebral function monitor[11] and its routine use during cardiac surgery is to be recommended. Stockard and his associates[12] correlated perfusion pressure, EEG changes and postoperative abnormal neurology in patients undergoing bypass surgery with constant flow rates, P_aCO_2 and hypothermia (30 °C). They showed that perfusion pressures below 50 mmHg caused neurological abnormalities in 60 % of the group, but the incidence decreased with increasing perfusion pressure and was apparently 'safe' at a perfusion pressure of 70 mmHg. They concluded that neurological sequelae were related, not only to the duration and depth of hypotension, but to the age of the patient and degree of atherosclerosis in the cerebral blood vessels.

A retrospective analysis of consecutive cases at the National Heart Hospital gives a crude incidence of 16.6 % of patients suffering from neurological deficit (Table 2). The group of patients with CNS disorder were subdivided into:

Group I: psychoses only;
Group II: neurological deficit;
Group III: brain death.

It is clinically impossible to be certain what part microembolization played in the production of neurological disease. Thus the groups of patients were further examined retrospectively for any periods of hypotension, during bypass, of 50 mmHg pressure for 20 min or longer. Cases with pre-bypass hypotension of this order were excluded from analysis. Patients below the age of 18 years were excluded from the total analyses. The percentage of patients who suffered from this hypotensive period is shown in Table 3.

The results would support the previously quoted work indicating a need for perfusion pressure, with a constant adequate pump flow, to be kept within

Table 2 Incidence of neurological disorder

		No.	*Percentage*
Total cases		480	100
Total neurological disorder		73	16.6
Group I	Psychoses	41	
Group II	Neurological deficit	29	
Group III	Brain death	3	

Table 3 Incidence of 'hypotensive' damage

Group	*Total No.*	*No. 'hypotensive' cases*	*Percentage*
Group I	41	26	63
Group II	29	19	64
Group III	3	3	100

the range of autoregulation of human cerebral circulation to prevent neurological disaster during bypass. When the changes in human CBF during the period of extracorporeal circulation have been studied adequately, it will be possible to add further guidelines to this simple statement.

References

1. Ingvar, D. and Lassen, N. (1967). The human cerebral circulation. *Acta Physiol. Scand.*, **62,** 164
2. Olesen, J. *et al.* (1971). Measurement of regional cerebral blood flow. *Stroke*, **2,** 519
3. Obrist, W., Thompson, H., *et al.* (1975). Cerebral blood flow, atraumatic methodology. *Stroke*, **6,** 245
4. Halley, M., Reemtsa, K. and Creech, O. (1958). Cerebral blood flow, metabolism and brain volume in extra-corporeal circulation. *J. Thorac. Surg.*, **36,** 506
5. Simeone, F. (1970). Pulsatile flow in extra-corporeal circulatory techniques. *J. Am. Med. Assoc.*, **212,** 968
6. Sanderson, J., Wright, G. and Sims, F. (1972). Brain damage in dogs immediately following pulsatile and non-pulsatile blood flow. *Thorax*, **27,** 275
7. Woolman, H. *et al.* (1966). Cerebral blood flow in man during extra-corporeal circulation. *J. Thorac. Cardiovasc. Surg.*, **52,** 558
8. Branthwaite, M. (1974). Cerebral blood flow and metabolism during open heart surgery. *Thorax*, **29,** 633
9. Brierley, J. B. (1967). Brain damage complicating open heart surgery, a neuropathological study. *Proc. R. Soc. Med.*, **60,** 858
10. Javid, H. *et al.* (1967). Neurological abnormalities following heart surgery. *J. Thorac. Cardiovasc. Surg.*, **58,**
11. Maynard, D. and Prior, P. (1971). Monitoring cerebral function. *Br. Med. J.*, **2,** 736
12. Stockard, J., Bickford, R. and Schauble, J. (1973). Pressure dependent cerebral ischaemia during cardiopulmonary bypass. *Neurology*, **23,** 521

20
Towards safer cardiopulmonary bypass

Ch. R. H. WILDEVUUR

Safer cardiac surgery will depend to a large extent on future improvements in cardiopulmonary bypass. Right from the start of open heart surgery in the early 1950s, severe damage to the blood has been recognized as one of the consequences of extracorporeal circulation. Even today, after almost 30 years of extensive research, we still have a poor understanding of this blood damage: its principal causes, its effects on the patient and more importantly, its prevention.

The large scale of routine coronary surgery performed in recent years with low mortality rates might give the impression that cardiac surgery is safe. However, all patients need intensive care treatment after the operation and, especially after longer periods of bypass, poor peripheral circulation, haemorrhagic diatheses and organ dysfunctions still frequently occur. We should realize that all the disturbances mentioned are not caused by the operation itself, but by the consequences of the extracorporeal circulation of blood.

The complications are attributed to haemolysis, platelet damage, leukocyte destruction and protein denaturation. It should be realized that the importance that has been attributed to each of these blood components is merely dependent on the ability to perform quantitative measurements. In the early days haemolysis was the only quantitative measure of blood damage available and the degree of haemolysis was, and sometimes still is, considered as *the* indication of haemocompatibility. But this measure is certainly a crude one and is not indicative of the secondary effects caused by blood damage. Methods to determine platelet damage, in terms of counts and function, have become more reliable and are used as more appropriate parameters to define haemocompatibility. Though certainly associated with the bleeding problem, the method of platelet function still needs further sophistication and standardization before it can become a quantitative indicator of platelet damage. More recently biochemical methods have been developed to measure specific platelet release products which might refine the quantitative assessment of platelet damage. However, except for the bleeding problems, these measures are not likely to be related to the complication of organ dysfunction. This might be more closely associated with the damage to leukocytes and/or plasma proteins, as indicated by the work of Jacob and co-workers[1]. Activation of complement factor C5a by artificial surfaces induces leukocyte aggregation which in the lung can cause the so-called perfusion, or shock lung, syndrome.

Leukocyte aggregates plug the capillaries, release of free oxygen radicals damages the vascular endothelium, and lung oedema will develop. The endothelial damage will also activate platelets and so microthrombi are another consequence; all of these factors lead to disturbed microcirculation and respiratory insufficiency. This general pattern of reaction might also be responsible for the dysfunction of other organs and, as often observed after perfusion, for a disturbed peripheral circulation. The latter, however, might also be activated by the release of vasoactive substances from damaged blood elements. We have demonstrated experimentally that minimizing blood damage by membrane oxygenator perfusion is associated with improved oxygen supply to the tissues[2]. Now that an *in vitro* quantitative method of measuring leukocyte aggregation and an *in vivo* measure of oxygen supply to the tissue have become available, the main interest, presently concentrated on platelets, might divert to leukocytes.

The interaction of the various blood elements with the artificial surfaces is, however, not the only factor of blood damage; others, like mechanical trauma and shear stress, do play an important additional role. The effects of the various components of the extracorporeal circuit used for open heart surgery have been analysed in standardized animal experiments[3]. In particular, the contributions of priming solutions[4], tubing[5], pumps, oxygenators and cardiotomy suction[6], in causing haematological damage, have been evaluated.

All these factors have an effect on blood damage, but not to the same extent and with preference to different blood elments. For example, by using better haemocompatible tubing materials, like silica-free silicone rubber (sfsr) instead of polyvinylchloride (pvc), small differences were obtained in erythrocyte damage (Figure 1), but no measurable discrimination in platelet protection (Figure 2). Improvements obtained with new blood pumps, like the rotor pump of Rhône-Poulenc, appear to be equally related to erythrocytes (Figure 3) as to platelets (Figure 4). In regard to the extent of damage, the oxygenator and the cardiotomy suction play the most important roles in the destruction of blood elements.

We have demonstrated experimentally that the damage to blood caused by bubble oxygenators can be minimized by using a membrane oxygenator (Figure 5), but that this only makes sense if the effect of cardiotomy suction is additionally controlled (Figure 6). This can be achieved by means of a recently developed, electronically controlled suction system which prevents aspiration of air in the suction line[6,7].

When controlled suction is used in conjunction with a membrane oxygenator, one can ask if the one membrane material is superior to another. We have examined in animal experiments the differences between two commercially available membrane oxygenators: the Travenol TMO with microporous membranes, and the Sci-Med spiral coil with silicone rubber membranes. For the sake of strict comparison the additional slave pump, needed

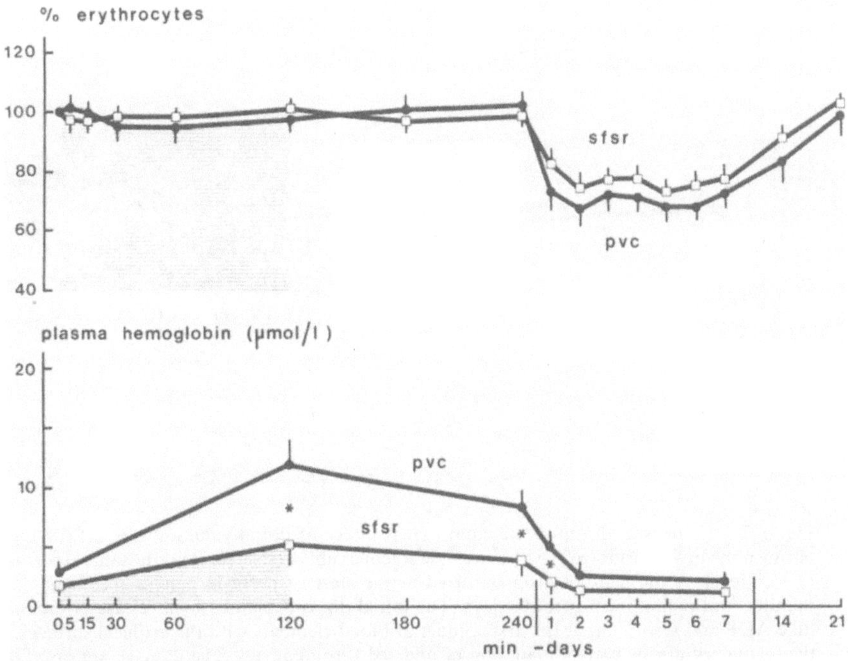

Figure 1 Changes in erythrocyte counts (percentage of initial values, mean ± SEM) and plasma haemoglobin (μmol/l, mean ± SEM) during and after veno-venous perfusion (3 l/min, during 2 h, shaded area) in dogs, comparing polyvinylchloride (pvc, $n = 6$) with silica-free silicone rubber (sfsr, $n = 6$) tubings (length 6 m). A non-occlusive roller-pump was used. No changes or differences are seen in the erythrocyte counts during perfusion, but a severe drop appeared in the first postoperative days, demonstrating early elimination of affected erythrocytes. The consistently higher level in the sfsr group (not significantly) is substantiated by the significantly ($p < 0.05$) lower levels of plasma haemoglobin as compared to the pvc group, indicating less erythrocyte damage in the sfsr tubing group

for the TMO, was also used for the otherwise one-pump system of the Sci-Med lung[3].

No differences were observed in erythrocyte damage but there were differences in platelet damage (Figure 7). Postoperatively no secondary dip in platelet counts was measured in the TMO on Day 1, whereas a secondary dip appeared in the Sci-Med group. This is explained by the early elimination of platelets affected during perfusion with the Sci-Med lung. This points to the superiority of the microporous membranes. The hypothesis that a microporous membrane acts as a microbubbler and that it does not prevent the blood–gas interface, is not supported by these results. It is more likely therefore that a thin albumin layer rapidly covers the micropores, thus preventing a blood–gas interface which is thought to be harmful for the blood elements, especially for the platelets. It is important to mention that these relatively small but significant differences between the two membrane oxygenators do not show up in differences in bleeding times[3].

The strict standardization of cardiopulmonary bypass (CPB) conditions obtainable in experiments, cannot be achieved in the clinical situation.

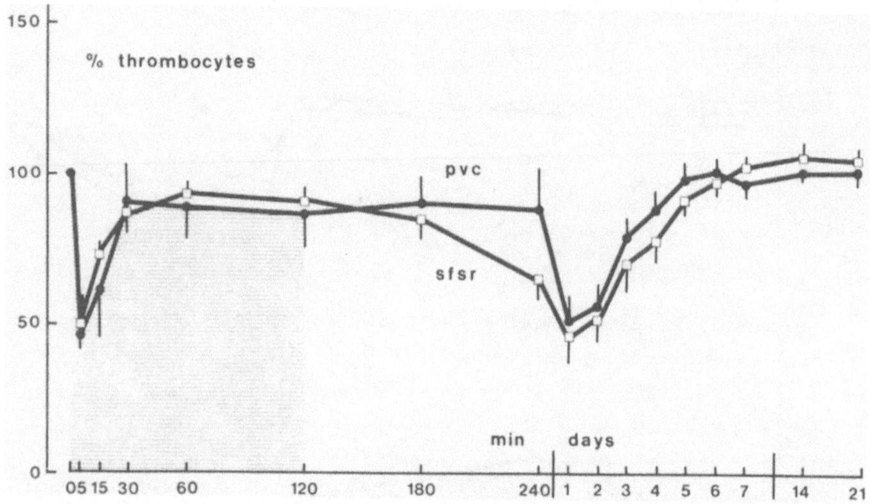

Figure 2 Changes in thrombocyte counts (percentage of initial values, mean ± SEM), comparing polyvinylchloride (pvc) with silica-free silicone rubber (sfsr) tubings (the same experiments of Figure 1). A momentary drop occurred at the start of perfusion and a secondary fall in numbers in the first postoperative days. The initial dip is explained by a release of bioamines (like ADP and serotonin) at the first contact of blood elements with the artificial surfaces, and the secondary dip by early elimination of affected thrombocytes. The damage appeared to be the same for the two tubing materials

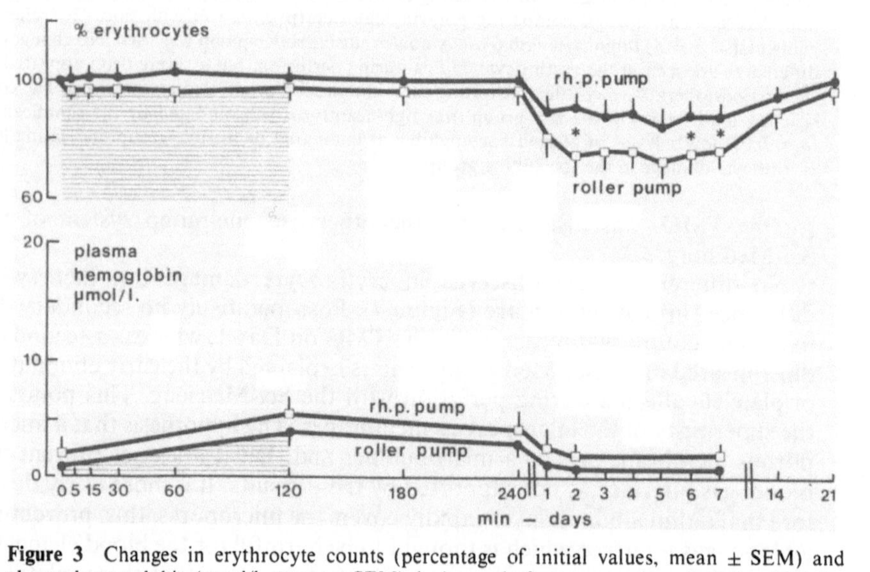

Figure 3 Changes in erythrocyte counts (percentage of initial values, mean ± SEM) and plasma haemoglobin (μmol/l, mean ± SEM) during and after veno-venous perfusion (3 l/min, during 2 h, shaded area) in dogs, comparing the Rhône-Poulenc rotor pump (rh.p., $n = 6$) with the Dreissen roller pump (non-occlusive, $n = 6$). Silica-free silicone rubber tubing was used. A significantly ($p < 0.05$) more pronounced postoperative anaemia occurred in the roller-pump group. This sublethal damage of the erythrocytes was not reflected in higher plasma haemoglobin levels during perfusion

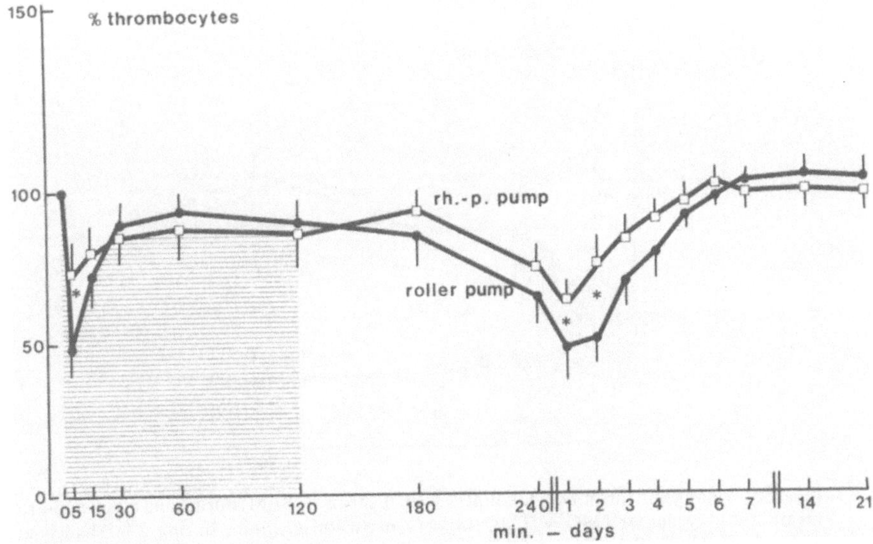

Figure 4 Changes in thrombocyte counts (percentage of initial values, mean ± SEM) comparing the Rhône-Poulenc rotor pump (rh.p.) with the Dreissen roller pump (the same experiments of Figure 3). The momentary drop, as well as the secondary dip in the first postoperative days, are significantly ($p < 0.05$) more expressed in the roller-pump group, indicating somewhat more damage caused by the conventional roller-pump than by the newly developed rotor pump of Rhône-Poulenc

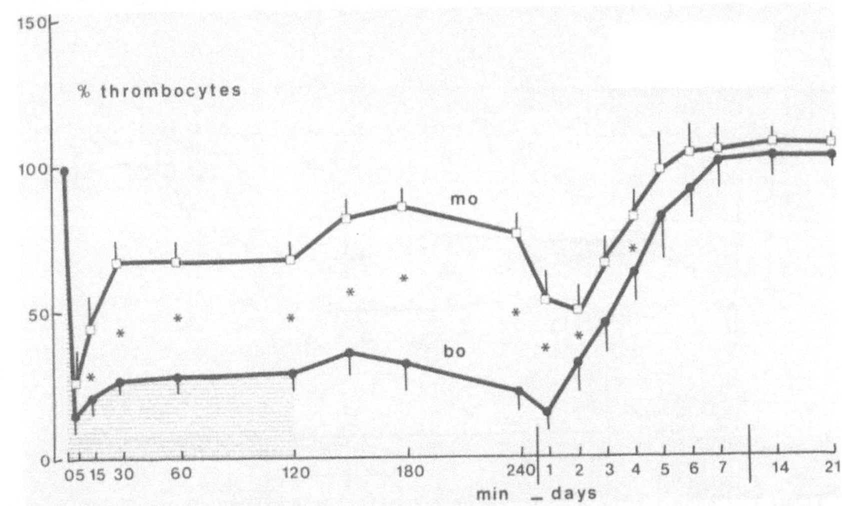

Figure 5 Changes in thrombocyte counts (percentage of initial values, mean ± SEM) during and after veno-arterial perfusion (3 l/min, during 2 h, shaded area) in dogs, comparing the Travenol TMO membrane oxygenator (MO) with the Bentley Temptrol bubble oxygenator (BO). Non-occlusive roller pumps and pvc tubing were used. The initial dip at the start of the perfusion is transient in the MO group and persistent in the BO group. Large and significant differences ($p < 0.05$) exist during and after perfusion. Platelets are clearly better preserved in MO than in BO perfusion

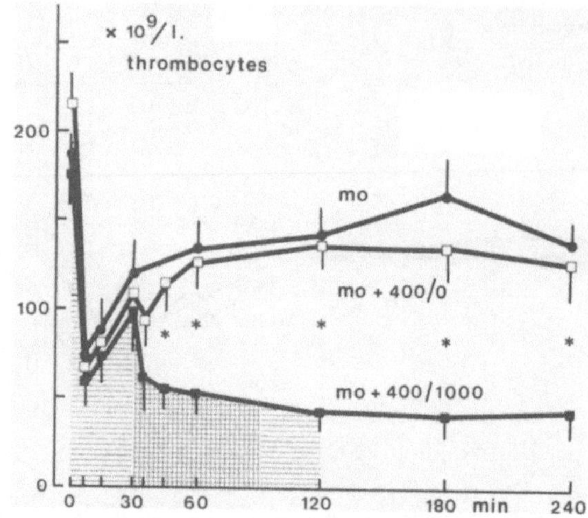

Figure 6 Changes in thrombocyte counts ($\times 10^9$/l, mean $\pm$ SEM) during and after veno-arterial membrane oxygenator (MO = TMO, n = 6) perfusion (3 l/min, during 2 h, shaded area), adding controlled (400/0, n = 6) or uncontrolled (400/1000, n = 4) cardiotomy suction (1 h, double-shaded area) in dogs. A non-occlusive roller pump and pvc tubing were used. Controlled suction (see text) does not affect the thrombocyte numbers additionally during MO perfusion, in contrast to uncontrolled suction ($p < 0.05$). In the MO + 400/1000 (uncontrolled) suction group the same low level as in the BO group without suction (compare Figure 5) is reached. The significant improvements of MO perfusion are abolished by uncontrolled suction

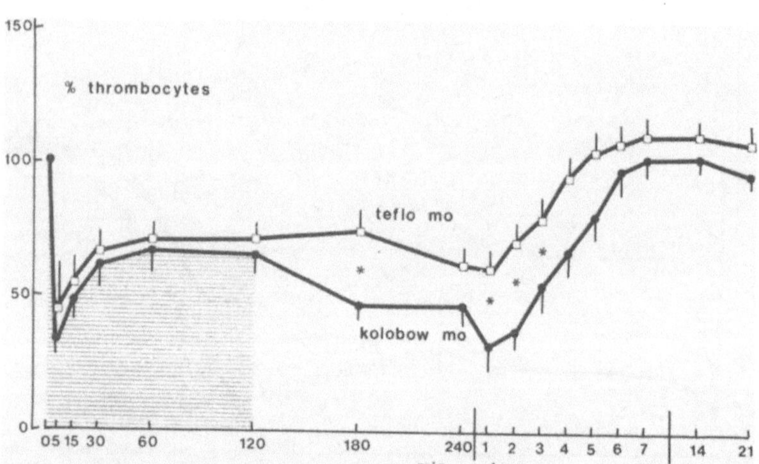

Figure 7 Changes in thrombocyte counts (percentage of initial values, mean $\pm$ SEM) during and after veno-arterial perfusion (3 l/min, during 2 h, shaded area), comparing the microporous membranes of the Travenol TMO (Teflo MO, n = 6) with the silicone rubber membranes of the Sci-Med (Kolobow MO, n = 6). Two non-occlusive roller-pumps with silica-free silicone rubber tubing were used in both groups. Significant differences ($p < 0.05$) appeared only after perfusion. The lower level in the Kolobow MO group postoperatively indicates that more sublethal damage of thrombocytes occurred in the Sci-Med lung with silicone rubber membrane than in the Travenol TMO with microporous membrane

However, categorizing the patients according to the main factors influencing blood damage renders it possible to make comparison between groups with a difference in only one major variable. These factors have been analysed in our patients undergoing CPB, using computer data acquisition[8]. From this the following guidelines can be given. One should only compare patients undergoing the same type of operation.

For example, operations done on the aortic side (aortic valve replacement (AVR) and coronary artery bypass graft (CABG)) require double the amount of whole blood transfusions as operations done on the venous side (mitral valve replacement (MVR)). This difference can be explained by more surgical bleeding in an area of high blood pressure.

There was also a three times higher blood loss when a large aortotomy (AVR) was made, as compared to a small aortotomy (CABG). More blood products were used in the AVR group, suggesting that impaired clotting was more frequently observed in the AVR than in the CABG patients. The CABG patients had the smallest standard deviation in all parameters associated with haemostasis, which implies that all the factors influencing haemostasis are pretty well the same in this well-standardized surgical technique. These patients are therefore the most attractive category for comparative studies.

In CABG patients the effect of perfusion time on blood loss and blood requirements in the operating room can be illustrated by a computer plot of these data in the individual patients (Figure 8). Perfusion times longer than 160 min showed more patients with blood losses over 2.5 l and blood requirements over 4.5 l; the mean values doubled after this period[9].

The effect of other factors, like suction, can be well demonstrated by the course of platelet function (ADP-induced platelet aggregation) (Figure 9).

In CABG operations platelet function was well maintained during membrane oxygenator perfusion (TMO) at a level of 60 % of the pre-bypass values for the first 2 h. However, a sharp decrease occurred after aortic cross-clamping was released and cardiotomy suction was intensified. We have measured the flow through the cardiotomy reservoir, which increased from an average of 206 ml/min to 526 ml/min during that time. It should be realized that in these patients the total amount of blood passing through the cardiotomy reservoir during CPB, including left ventricular decompression, averaged 34 l, with a range from 2 to 65 l. It is important to note that after CPB a second drop of platelet function occurred, reaching a level of less than 10 % of the initial values. This considerable drop, which is only partly reversible, is caused by the excess of protamine chloride, administered to neutralize the heparin effect[9,10]. The drop can be minimized if a dose of protamine, equivalent to the circulating heparin, is administered by means of titration with fractionated doses of protamine, using the activated clotting time[10].

It is obvious that the damaging effects of suction and protamine chloride counteract to a great extent the improvements that are likely to be obtained with a membrane oxygenator otherwise.

With these facts in mind little difference can be expected from comparative clinical studies of bubble versus membrane oxygenators, when strict categorization of patients, as proposed, has not been included.

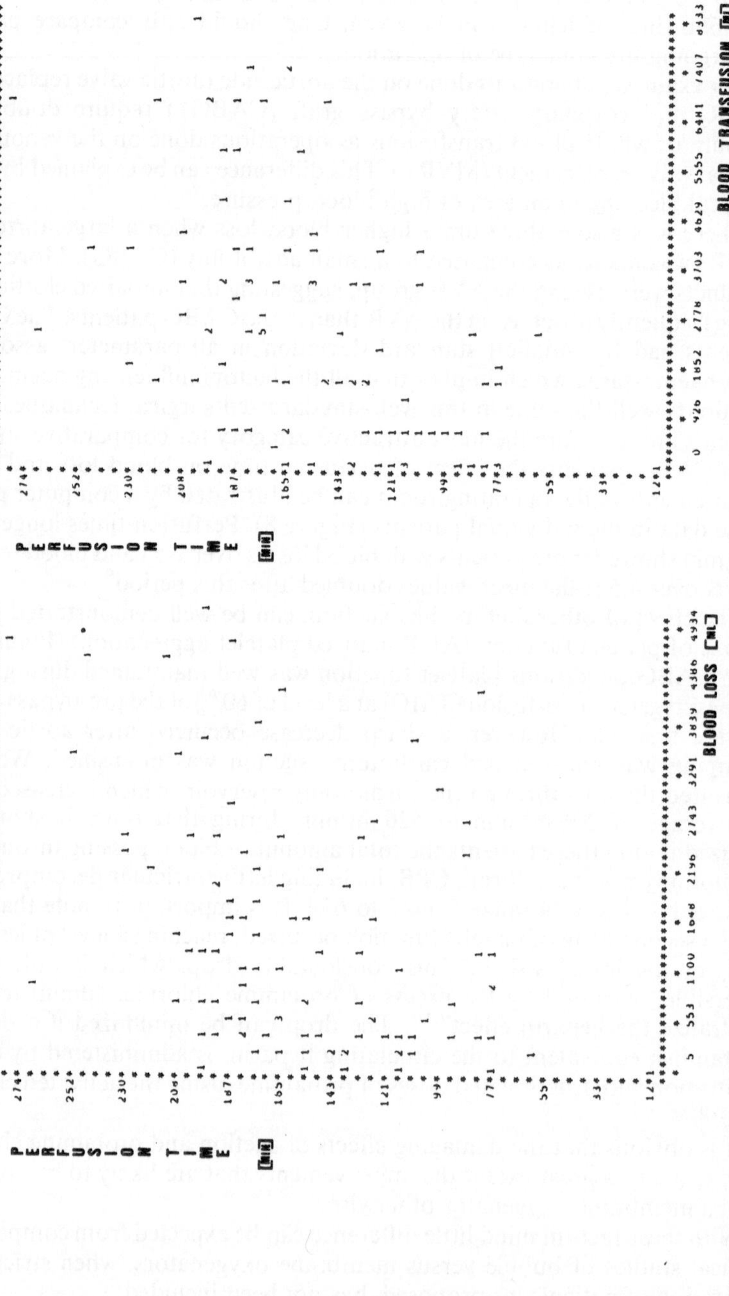

Figure 8 Perfusion time (min) related to blood loss (ml) and whole blood transfusion (ml) in the operating room of patients who received coronary artery bypass grafts. Total bypass was performed with membrane oxygenators (TMO). Perfusion times over 160 min resulted in more patients with blood losses over 2.5 l and blood requirements over 4.5 l.

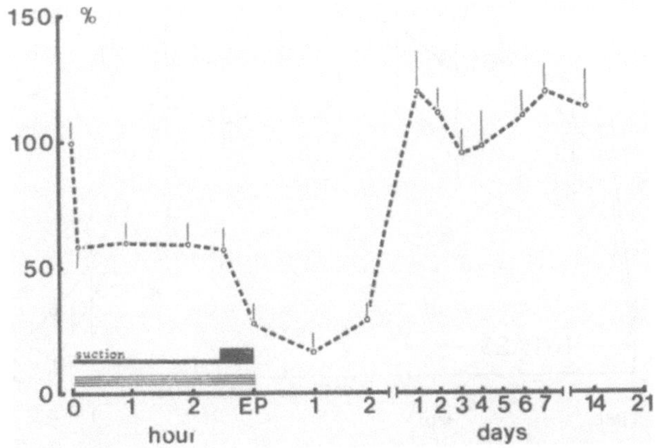

Figure 9 Changes in platelet function (maximal optical density loss (OD_{max}) of ADP-induced platelet aggregation) as a percentage of the initial value (mean ± SEM) in patients undergoing coronary artery bypass grafting ($n = 10$). Membrane oxygenators (TMO) were used. Platelet function was maintained at about 60 % during perfusion as long as aortic cross-clamping existed. A sharp fall in function was associated with intensified suction after release of aortic cross-clamping. A second fall occurred after protamine chloride administration at the end of perfusion (EP). Normal function was only restored after the day of operation. As a consequence low platelet function was experienced in the early postoperative period, despite the fact that initially the platelets were protected by the membrane oxygenator perfusion

I would like to present our recently completed prospective study[9] of 74 adult patients requiring CPB for CABG, comparing bubble oxygenators (BO) with membrane oxygenators (MO). The patients were perfused with the Polystan Venotherm 5000 bubble oxygenator ($n = 25$) or with the Travenol Total Bypass Membrane Oxygenator (TMO 5M 1430) with a polypropylene membrane ($n = 49$). Additionally extensive haematological data were obtained from 10 patients of both groups.

Erythrocyte damage, as expressed by plasma haemoglobin levels, appeared to be significantly higher (at 90 min) in the BO as compared to the MO group (Figure 10).

White blood-cell counts showed a similar pattern of changes and no significant differences occurred between both groups.

The platelet counts (Figure 11) showed a tendency of recovery in the MO group after an initial dip at the onset of bypass, but a gradual further decrease occurred in the BO group. Platelet counts were diminished in both groups after CPB and were only restored by a new population of platelets entering the circulation in the postoperative days. Although platelet counts were consistently higher in the MO group, no significant differences were noted compared with the BO group at any particular point.

The platelet function did show significant differences between the groups (Figure 12). Again an initial dip occurred at the onset of bypass in both groups but whereas the function remained low in the BO group, platelet function improved to normal levels in the MO group.

As pointed out earlier, after the release of aortic cross-clamping and consequently the start of intensified cardiotomy suction, platelet function

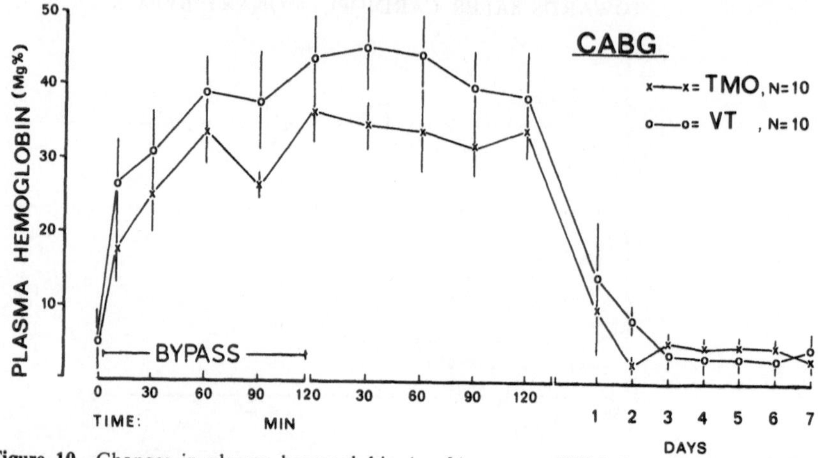

Figure 10 Changes in plasma haemoglobin (mg %, mean ± SEM) in patients undergoing coronary artery bypass grafting. Groups of patients treated with a membrane oxygenator (MO, $n = 10$) or a bubble oxygenator (VT, $n = 10$) are compared. The levels were consistently higher in the VT group, but only significantly ($p < 0.05$) different from the TMO group at 90 min of bypass

sharply decreased towards the end of perfusion. A second drop occurred immediately after perfusion and platelet function was equalized to the same low level of the BO group. This drop in function, due to protamine administration, is partly reversible in the MO group, but complete recovery of function is only initiated after Day 2, when a new population of platelets has begun to enter the circulation. The other clotting parameters, like fibrinogen and AT III, were affected in both groups but showed no significant differences.

In addition to the above haematological parameters, obtained from 10 patients only in each group, data of blood loss and blood requirements (mean ± SEM) in the whole group of 74 patients (BO, $n = 25$; MO, $n = 49$) were collected. Blood losses were significantly higher ($p < 0.01$) in the BO group (2.0 ± 0.1 l) as compared to the MO group (1.3 ± 0.1 l). Blood requirements (in units) consisted of whole blood transfusions (BO = 5.4 ± 0.8; MO = 3.8 ± 0.4), packed cells (BO = 1.3 ± 0.3; MO = 1.0 ± 0.2), platelet concentrate (BO = 3.6 ± 1.4; MO = 0.4 ± 0.3), cryoprecipitate (BO = 3.6 ± 1.6; MO = 0.4 ± 0.3) and fresh frozen plasma (BO = 3.2 ± 1.5; MO = 0.5 ± 0.2). All the whole blood and blood products requirements were significantly higher ($p < 0.05$) in the BO group, except for the packed cells.

These results, obtained in a well categorized group of patients, in which the varying clinical circumstances are more or less the same, showed that membrane oxygenators are indeed superior to bubble oxygenators, even for routine short-term CPB. This is not only demonstrated by the more sensitive parameters like platelet function, but also by the practical and clinical relevant measure of blood loss and blood requirements. The need of about 11 additional units of blood and blood products per patient, treated with a bubble oxygenator, is certainly of economic interest. This is despite the fact

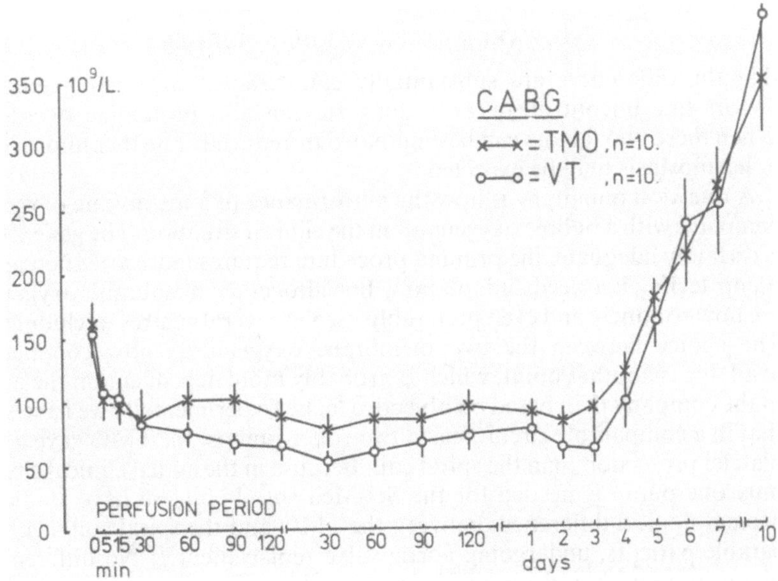

Figure 11 Changes in platelet counts ($\times 10^9$/l, mean $\pm$ SEM), comparing membrane oxygenators (TMO) with bubble oxygenators (VT) in the same group of patients described in Figure 10. After an initial equal decrease at the onset of bypass, numbers remained consistently higher in the TMO group than in the VT group. However, the differences were not significant

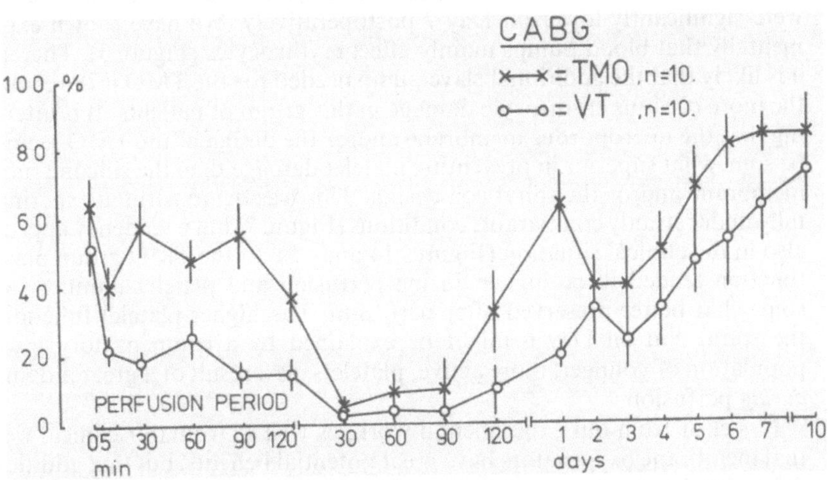

Figure 12 Changes in platelet function (maximal optical density loss of ADP-induced platelet aggregation, mean $\pm$ SEM), comparing membrane oxygenators (TMO) with bubble oxygenators (VT) in the same group of patients described in Figures 10 and 11. In the TMO group platelet function was significantly higher ($p < 0.05$) than in the VT group during perfusion. The stepwise fall in numbers after 90 min of perfusion and 30 min after the end of perfusion are caused by intensified cardiotomy suction (release of aortic cross-clamping) and protamine chloride administration respectively. Platelet function is rapidly restored in the TMO group, whereas in the BO group recovery of function depends on a new population of platelets which is achieved after 1 week

that the differences are substantially counteracted by existing damaging factors like uncontrolled cardiotomy suction and protamine overdosage. When these two factors can be eliminated or reduced, a further improvement in haemostasis may be expected.

A question remaining is how the performance of a membrane oxygenator compares with a bubble oxygenator in the clinical situation. The gas exchange is certainly adequate, the priming procedure requires more attention and the pump technician needs adaptation, but altogether membrane oxygenators are now routinely and even preferably used in several centres, including ours. The choice between the two membrane oxygenators now commercially available is another point, which is probably more dependent on the activity of the company than based on objective facts. Experimentally we have shown that in a comparable circuit, using two roller-pumps, the TMO gave a better platelet protection than the spiral coil. Because in the actual clinical situation only one pump is needed for the Sci-Med spiral coil, we have studied the haematological differences between the TMO and the spiral coil in 17 comparable patients, undergoing aortic valve replacement[11]. No differences in blood loss and blood requirements existed, and are perhaps not to be expected, between membrane oxygenators. However, haematological parameters do show significant differences.

Plasma haemoglobin (Figure 13) was significantly higher in the TMO group during perfusion and erythrocyte count, haemoglobin and haematocrit were significantly lower on Day 7 postoperatively. We have shown experimentally that blood pumps mainly affect erythrocytes (Figure 3). Therefore it is likely that the additional slave pump needed for the TMO is the cause of the more obvious erythrocyte damage in this group of patients. It is interesting that the microporous membrane and/or the design of the TMO seems to be somewhat superior in preventing platelet damage than the silicone rubber membrane and/or the spiral coil design. This was demonstrated experimentally under strictly comparable conditions (Figure 7) but a tendency appeared also in the clinical situation (Figures 14 and 15). In the TMO group platelet function tended to be higher during perfusion and platelet numbers were somewhat better preserved after perfusion. The higher platelet function in the spiral coil on Day 6 might be explained by a compensatory greater population of younger, more active, platelets, as a result of a greater damage *during* perfusion.

It is clear from our experimental work, as well as from our clinical work, that membrane oxygenators have great potential benefits, but that additional damaging factors compromise the ultimate results. On the other hand, the provision of the best components for extracorporeal oxygenation will not prevent the ongoing aggregation–desaggregation process of the platelets in contact with non-physiological surfaces.

The work of Vane and co-workers[12] has shown that even endothelial surfaces can only prevent this process by the local production of prostacyclin (PGI_2). Their work has stimulated another approach to prevent platelet damage by temporary inhibition of platelet aggregation[13]. The prostaglandins (PGE_1 and PGI_2) appeared to be the most promising ones[14]. PGE_1 is

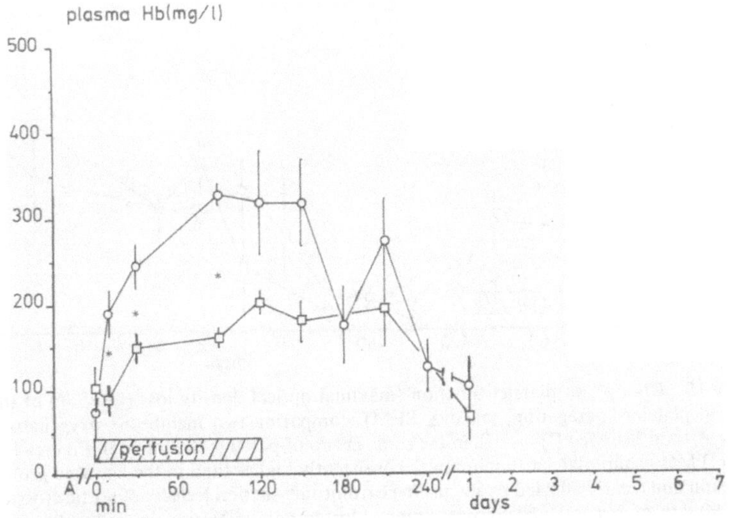

Figure 13 Changes in plasma haemoglobin (mg/l, mean ± SEM) in patients undergoing aortic valve replacement. Groups of patients treated with membrane oxygenators with microporous membranes O——O (Travenol TMO, $n = 10$) or silicone rubber membranes □——□ (Sci-Med spiral coil, $n = 7$) are compared. The values in the TMO group were significantly ($p < 0.01$) higher than in Sci-Med group during perfusion. This is most likely related to the additional roller pump needed for the TMO system (A = admittance)

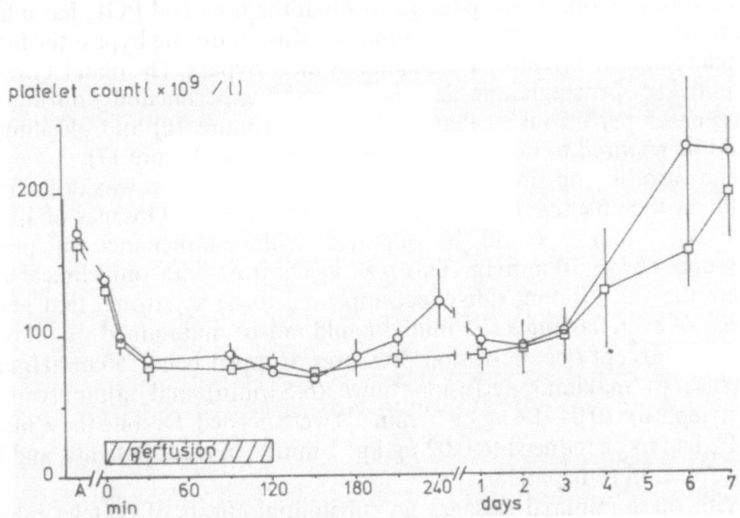

Figure 14 Changes in platelet counts (× 10^9/l, mean ± SEM), comparing two membrane oxygenators, TMO O——O and Sci-Med □——□, in the same group of patients described in Figure 13. Mainly due to the haemodilution, an equal drop in platelet numbers was observed in both groups. Numbers remained equally low until Day 4, before restoration occurred. No significant difference in platelet damage was observed between the two different membrane lungs (A = admittance)

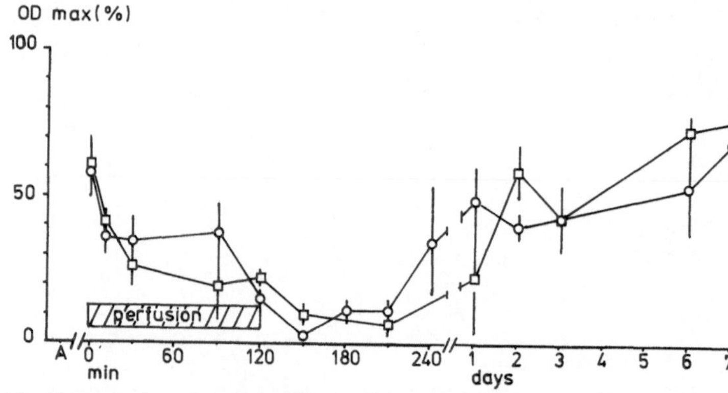

Figure 15 Changes in platelet function (maximal optical density loss (OD_{max})) of the ADP-induced platelet aggregation, mean ± SEM), comparing two membrane oxygenators, TMO ○——○ and Sci-Med □——□, in the same group of patients described in Figures 13 and 14. In the TMO group platelet function was consistently higher than in the Sci-Med group during perfusion and clearly affected by intensified cardiotomy suction (release of aortic cross-clamping after 90 min of bypass) and by protamine chloride administration immediately after bypass (A = admittance). Platelet function was also restored earlier in the TMO than in the Sci-Med group. However, all these differences were not significant. The higher platelet function in the Sci-Med group on Day 6 postoperatively was significant ($p < 0.05$) and indicates a compensatory greater population of younger, more active, platelets, as a result of greater damage *during* perfusion.

metabolized in one single passage through the lung and PGI_2 has a half-life of about 2–3 min. So, after a continuous infusion during bypass the inhibited platelet function is restored immediately after bypass. The platelet protective potentials of prostaglandin have been proven experimentally during bubble oxygenator perfusions[14]. Platelet function (Figure 16) and bleeding times could be restored to normal levels after perfusion (Figure 17).

The vasodilating side-effect of prostaglandin in dogs was not a limiting factor in the effective inhibition of platelet function. Dosages of 1–2 μg of PGE_1 kg^{-1} min^{-1} could be supplied with maintenance of perfusion pressures above 70 mmHg. This was in contrast with our clinical results, where the vasodilating side-effect appeared to be so strong, that generally a dose of even 0.05 μg kg^{-1} min^{-1} could not be maintained. In all patients ($n = 13$), except one, perfusion pressures dropped below 50 mmHg and an increase to maximal perfusion flows (6.5 l/min) and administration of phenylephrine (0.04–1.4 μg kg^{-1} min^{-1}) were needed. Despite these measures PGE_1 had to be reduced to 0.02 μg kg^{-1} min^{-1} in three patients, and had to be stopped in four patients.

With these minimal dosages no substantial effects of platelet inhibition during perfusion could be obtained, and no protective effects on platelets could be determined after perfusion. The influence of the negative effect of protamine on platelet function in this situation cannot be ruled out.

It is of interest that in a more detailed haemodynamic study[15] of PGE_1, given in a stable haemodynamic period before and during bypass, the hypotensive effects, although less expressed, were very variable, especially in the

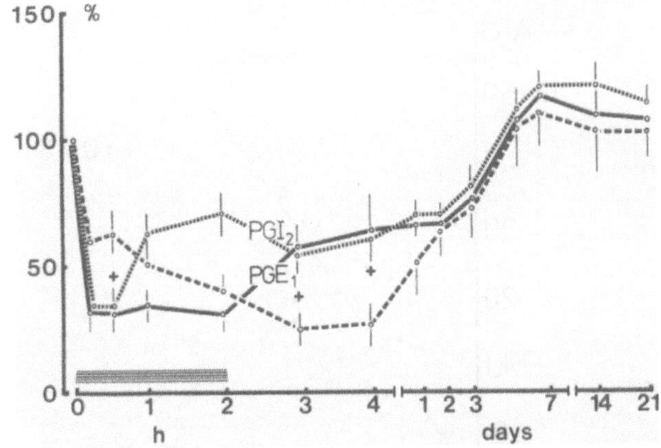

Figure 16 Changes in platelet function (percentage of the initial values, mean ± SEM, of the maximal optical density loss of the ADP-induced platelet aggregation) in dogs undergoing total bypass with a bubble oxygenator (BO, Temptrol Q 110, Bentley) during 2 h. The dogs were treated during perfusion with a continuous infusion of prostaglandin (PGE_1, 1–2 $\mu g\ kg^{-1}\ min^{-1}$) or prostacyclin (PGI_2, 0.5–1 $\mu g\ kg^{-1}\ min^{-1}$). The effects of platelet inhibition during perfusion are compared with a non-treated control group (dotted line). Postoperatively platelet functions in both treated groups (PGE_1 and PGI_2) were immediately restored to about normal levels, in contrast to the control group. Significant differences ($p < 0.05$) are marked (+)

period during bypass. It appeared that the drop in arterial pressure (ΔP_{art}) was dependent on the pre-existing systemic vascular resistance (SVR) (Figure 18). If the patient had a low SVR, the hypotensive effects were minimal.

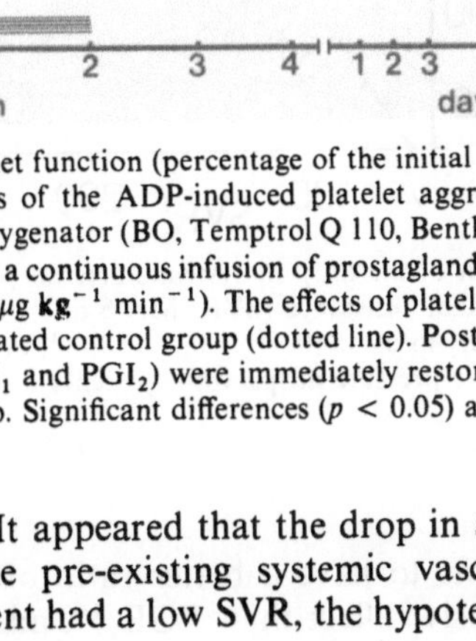

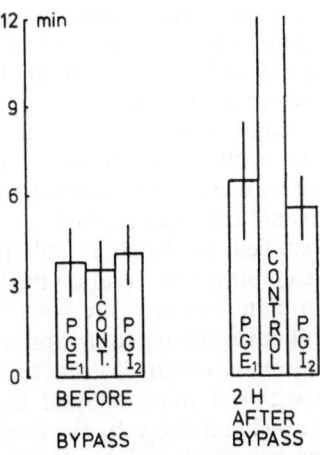

Figure 17 Changes in bleeding times (mean ± SEM), corresponding with the changes in platelet function in dogs treated with PGE_1 and PGI_2, as compared to the controls after bubble oxygenator perfusion. Preservation of platelet function by the PGE_1 and PGI_2 treatment (presented in Figure 16) was related to about normal bleeding times after perfusion, in contrast to the controls

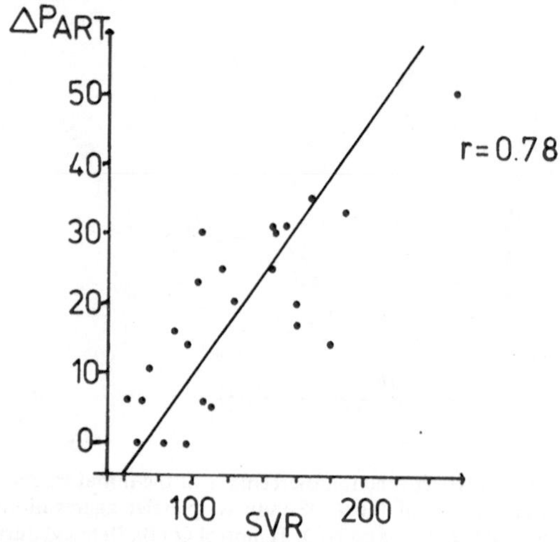

Figure 18 The correlation of the drop in systemic arterial pressures (ΔP_{art}, mmHg) and the pre-existing systemic vascular resistance (SVR, MN.S.m^{-5}) in patients on cardiopulmonary bypass, treated with a PGE_1 infusion (0.05 $\mu g\ kg^{-1}\ min^{-1}$, during 10 min). Patients with high pre-existing SVR had severe pressure drops, while patients with low SVR has a minimal or no drop in arterial pressures

Because PGI_2 seems to have a better ratio of platelet inhibitory effect compared to hypotensive effect than PGE_1[14], adequate platelet protection during CPB might be expected. Whether this will lead to better preserved haemostasis postoperatively, independent of the type of oxygenator (bubble or membrane) employed, cannot as yet be anticipated. Nevertheless, even when PGI_2 gives a maximal platelet protection, its effect on leukocytes is not clear.

I have already briefly pointed to the potential of artificial surfaces to activate complement C5a which causes leukocyte aggregation and might be the causative factor of disturbances in the microcirculation, leading to organ dysfunction[1]. This occurs with cellophane membranes of haemodialysers[16], and also with silicon rubber membranes, but not, however, in bubble oxygenators (H. S. Jacob, personal communication).

The mechanism described by Jacob is still hypothetical, but gives a plausible reason for the empirical observation made in extracorporeal circulation. It is important to note that there are several interactions between the cascade leading to leukocyte aggregation and platelet aggregation. For example, infusion of plasma in which C5a is activated by Zymosan, leads to severe leukocytopenia within 1 min, followed by thrombocytopenia after 5 min (Figure 19). Endothelial damage by the free oxygen radicals, released from the leukocyte aggregates, will activate platelet adherence and aggregation. Serotonin release from these aggregates in turn potentiates endothelial damage (Jacob, H. S., personal communication). However, prostaglandin synthesis from the leukocytes might on the other hand inhibit platelet adherence and aggregation[17]. No map of interaction between the two systems can be drawn yet, and the next steps have still to be guided by empirical observations. One of them is that methylprednisolone is advocated as a treatment for shock lung and as a prevention of the perfusion lung syndrome after open heart surgery. Recently Jacob *et al.* demonstrated *in vitro* and *in vivo* that leukocyte aggregation was inhibited by methylprednisolone[1]. This might point the way to prevention of organ dysfunction, caused by leukocyte aggregates during CPB, by giving high doses of methylprednisolone before or during bypass. The effect can now be measured quantitatively by the availability of the *in vitro* leukocyte aggregation test.

Another aspect of the uncontrolled complement granulocyte interaction in the described circumstances might be that chemotaxis and phagocytosis will be impaired, affecting the defence mechanism to infection. High incidence of infection has been reported after CPB[18]. We have shown experimentally that phagocytosis can be impaired by autotransfusion[19], by bubble oxygenator perfusion[20] as well as by membrane oxygenator perfusion, and might

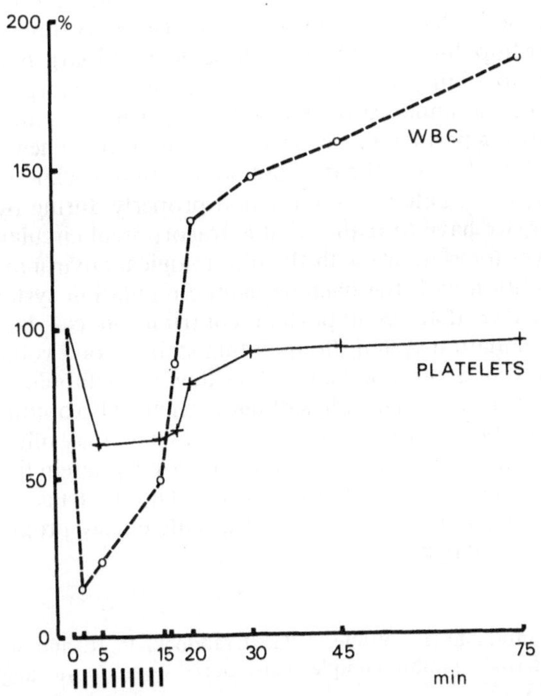

Figure 19 Changes in white blood cell (WBC) and platelet count induced by Zymosan-activated plasma infusion (200 ml in 15 min) in mongrel dogs (30–35 kg, mean of $n = 5$). Within 1 min after the start of perfusion WBC number dropped to 15 % of the initial value. Numbers restored to 50 % during the infusion period and raised to about 200 % after infusion. Platelet numbers dropped more gradually and less severely than the WBC. Numbers restored to normal after the infusion was stopped. The complement factor C5a in the plasma, activated by Zymosan, caused primarily a severe but transient leucocytopenia, followed by a moderate but also transient thrombocytopenia

cause sepsis[21]. Next to the possibility of impaired immune defence, patients on bypass have a great risk of airborne contamination[22]. This was also demonstrated recently in a prospective study, evaluating a cross-flow unit in our operating room[23]. It was found that in the normal conditions of an operating theatre after CPB, 79% of the oxygenators were contaminated, while only 17% were if the cross-flow unit was used. In an experimental set-up we could prove that cardiotomy suction was the open link to the air, causing contamination[24]. It is important to note that employing the previously described controlled suction system to reduce platelet damage, airborne contamination of the wound area and the circulating blood was also minimized. Furthermore, a reduction of sepsis was obtained in this animal model, probably as a result of reduced contamination and less-affected granulocyte function. The importance of reduced immune defence mechanism after CPB has still to be elucidated. Preliminary reports do suggest that immunoglobulins are reduced after bypass, and that phagocytosis can be impaired[20].

This, however, is only a part of the defence mechanism and the important role of the reticuloendothelial system that might become blocked by the extensive blood cell damage during bypass certainly deserves attention[25].

Safer cardiopulmonary bypass will be achieved largely by improvements in blood compatibility of each component in the extracorporeal circuit and/or inhibition of the unnecessary physiological reaction patterns of the blood elements during perfusion. I believe we are entering a new and exciting area in which, after 30 years of cardiopulmonary bypass experience, we have the perspectives to be able to handle blood properly during bypass.

However, we have to realize that extracorporeal circulation of blood not only involves interference with the physiological environment of blood, but also competition with the haemodynamic regulation system of the body. I strongly believe that an important contribution can be made by extracorporeal regulation systems to maintain stable blood volume[26], to regulate pressures and pressure pulses, to adapt flow to metabolic requirements and to control blood gases in the physiological range. Also optimal supplementary assistance of cardiac performance[27] after bypass may offer further benefits.

As we all have experienced, progress is slow; wherein lies the danger that we are satisfied with the situation of today. The challenge of the perspectives given in meetings like this one will eventually ensure progress towards safer cardiopulmonary bypass.

References

1. Hammersmith, D. E., White, J. G., Craddock, P. R. and Jacob, H. S. (1979). Corticosteroids inhibit complement-induced granulocyte aggregation. *J. Clin. Invest.*, **63**, 798
2. Pranger, R. L., Mook, P. H., Elstrodt, J. M., Kessler, M., Lübbers, D. W. and Wildevuur, Ch. R. H. (1980). Improved tissue perfusion (pO_2 histograms) in extracorporeal circulation (ECC) using membrane (MO) instead of bubble (BO) oxygenators. *J. Thorac. Cardiovasc. Surg.* **79**, 513
3. de Jong, J. C. F. and Wildevuur, Ch. R. H. (1980). Cardiopulmonary bypass: analysis of various components of the circuit in canine experiments. *Proc. 3rd Annual Symposium Red Cross Blood Bank Groningen-Drenthe: 'Open heart Surgery and Blood Transfusions'*. (In press)

4. Woltjes, J., de Jong, J. C. F., ten Duis, H. J. and Wildevuur, Ch. R. H. (1979). The priming of extracorporeal circuits: the effect on canine blood elements. *Transfusion*, **19,** 552
5. de Jong, J. C. F., Smit Sibinga, C. Th. and Wildevuur, Ch. R. H. (1979). Platelet behaviour in extracorporeal circulation. *Transfusion*, **19,** 72
6. ten Duis, H. J., de Jong, J. C. F., van Asseldonk, A. G. M., Smit Sibinga, C. Th. and Wildevuur, Ch. R. H. (1978). Improved hemocompatibility in open heart surgery. *Trans. Am. Soc. Artif. Intern. Organs*, **24,** 656
7. de Jong, J. C. F., ten Duis, H. J., Smit Sibinga, C. Th. and Wildevuur, Ch. R. H. (1980). Hematologic aspects of cardiotomy suction in cardiac operations. *J. Thorac. Cardiovasc. Surg.* **79,** 227
8. van den Dungen, J. J. A. M., Homan van der Heide, J. N., Karliczek, G. F. and Wildevuur, Ch. R. H. (1978). Clinical evaluation of blood damage related to cardiopulmonary bypass. *Proc. Eur. Soc. Artif. Organs*, **5,** 238
9. van den Dungen, J. J. A. M., Karliczek, G. F., Homan van der Heide, J. N. and Wildevuur, Ch. R. H. (1979). Clinical comparison of hemostasis in membrane (MO) and bubble oxygenator (BO) perfusion. *Br. J. Surg.*, **66,** 895
10. Velders, A. J., van den Dungen, J. J. A. M., Westerhof, N. J. W. and Wildevuur, Ch. R. H. (1979). Platelet damage by protamine administration: protection by reducing protamine or by prostacyclin (PGI_2) treatment. *Proc. Eur. Soc. Artif. Organs*, **6,** 194
11. van den Dungen, J. J. A. M., Boers, M., Homan van der Heide, J. N., Karliczek, G. F. and Wildevuur, Ch. R. H. (1980). Comparison of two membrane oxygenators and a bubble oxygenator in patients undergoing aortic valve replacement. (In preparation)
12. Moncada, S., Gryglewski, R., Bunting, S. and Vane, J. R. (1976). An enzyme isolated from arteries transforms prostaglandin endoperoxides to an unstable substance that inhibits platelet aggregation. *Nature* (*London*), **263,** 663
13. Weston, M. J., Woods, H. F., Ash, Gillian, Bunting, S., Moncada, S. and Vane, J. R. (1979). Prostacyclin as an alternative to heparin for hemodialysis in dogs. In Vane, J. R. and Bergstrom, S. (eds.). *Prostacyclin*, pp. 349–59. (New York: Raven Press)
14. van den Dungen, J. J. A. M., de Jong, J. C. F. and Wildevuur, Ch. R. H. (1979). Platelet preservation during cardiopulmonary bypass (CPB) with prostaglandins (PG). *Eur. Surg. Res.*, 2 (Suppl.), 51
15. Karlizcek, G. F., van den Dungen, J. J. A. M., Brenken, U., Eijsman, L., Kootstra, G. J., Homan van der Heide, J. N. and Wildevuur, Ch. R. H. (1980). Hemodynamic side-effects of prostaglandin in patients before and during cardiopulmonary bypass. (In preparation)
16. Craddock, P. R., Fehr, J., Brigham, K. L., Kronenberg, R. S. and Jacob, H. S. (1977). Complement and leukocyte-mediated pulmonary dysfunction in hemodialysis. *N. Engl. J. Med.*, **296,** 769
17. Flower, R. J. and Cardinal, D. C. (1979). Use of a novel platelet aggregometer to study the generation by, and actions of prostacyclin in whole blood. In Vane, J. R. and Bergstrom, S. (eds.). *Prostacyclin*, pp. 211–16. (New York: Raven Press)
18. Goodman, J. S., Schaffner, W., Collins, H. A., Battersby, E. J. and Koenig, M. G. (1968). Infections after cardiovascular surgery. *N. Engl. J. Med.*, **278,** 117
19. Woltjes, J., ten Duis, H. J., de Jong, J. C. F. and Wildevuur, Ch. R. H. (1976). Phagocytic capacity of neutrophilic leucocytes: standardization and application of a simple technique. *Proc. Eur. Soc. Artif. Organs*, **3,** 89
20. Deggeller, K., van den Dungen, J. J. A. M., Dankert, J., Marrink, J., Halie, M. R., Karliczek, G. F. and Wildevuur, Ch. R. H. (1979). Susceptibility to infections related to extracorporeal circulation: sources of infection, granulocyte function and immu-

noglobulins. *Proc. Workshop 'Basic Aspects of blood trauma in extracorporeal circulation'*, Aachen. pp. 365–379, (The Hague: Martin Nÿhoff Publishers)

21. de Jong, J. C. F., Woltjes, J., Paping, R. H. L. and Wildevuur, Ch. R. H. (1977). Impaired leucocyte function and postoperative infection in extracorporeal circulation (ECC). *Proc. Eur. Soc. Artif. Organs,* **4**, 523
22. Blakemore, W. S., McGarrity, G. J., Thurer, R. J., Wallace, H. W., MacVaugh, III, H. and Coriell, L. L. (1971). Infection by air-borne bacteria with cardiopulmonary bypass. *Surgery*, **70**, 830
23. Dankert, J. and Eijgelaar, A. (1978). The use of a mobile cross-flow unit in open-heart surgery: A bacteriological evaluation. *Antonie van Leeuwenhoek,* **44**, 247
24. Zijlstra, J. B., Logher, E., Dankert, J., van Asseldonk, A. G. M. and Wildevuur, Ch. R. H. (1978). Contamination and infection induced by autotransfusion: an experimental study in dogs. *Proc. Eur. Soc. Artif. Organs*, **5**, 222
25. Halie, M. R., Deggeller, K. and Wildevuur, Ch. R. H. (1980). Leucocytes and extracorporeal circulation. *Proc. 3rd Annual Symposium Red Cross Blood Bank Groningen-Drenthe: 'Open-heart Surgery and Blood Transfusions'*. (In press)
26. Mook, P. H., Oosting, P., Elstrodt, J. M. and Wildevuur, Ch. R. H. (1978). Automation of cardiopulmonary bypass for open heart surgery. *Proc. Eur. Soc. Artif. Organs*, **5**, 234
27. Wildevuur, Ch. R. H., Moulopoulos, S. D., Kolff, J., Crosby, M. J. and Nose, Y. (1968). Supplementary mechanically assisted circulation. An experimental study. *Ann. Thorac. Surg.*, **6**, 137

21
Haematological effects of cardiotomy suction

G. WRIGHT

Cardiotomy suction is generally recognized to be a traumatic part of the cardiopulmonary bypass procedure. Yet the severity of the blood cell damage generated by suction is not widely appreciated, and very little effort has been made to improve this part of the system.

As a result of a series of clinical experiences and experimental investigations, it was concluded that the cellular aggregation and trauma that can occur during blood collection, blood storage, circuit priming, admixture of the patient's blood with the circuit prime and extracorporeal circulation could be reduced to negligible values by the use of simple technical precautions[1-3]. However, the problem of cardiotomy suction was found to be more refractory. This system has now been investigated in order to evaluate the effects of contact of the blood with the pericardium, the differences between roller pump and vacuum suction, and the effects of air aspiration. As a result it has been possible to develop a theory to explain the mechanisms of cell trauma during cardiotomy suction and to offer some suggestions of ways to reduce this trauma.

The first step in the investigations was to obtain blood samples from patients undergoing open heart operations. A conventional non-pulsatile cardiopulmonary bypass procedure was used with bubble oxygenation. Low positive pressure (vacuum) suction was employed using a Travenol rigid cardiotomy reservoir. As shown in Table 1, the differences between blood samples obtained from the patient's radial artery and from the cardiotomy reservoir outlet at the termination of cardiopulmonary bypass were pronounced. The values in the table have been adjusted for haemodilution by corrccting to the patient's preoperative packed cell volume.

Following this, two sets of experiments were set up to examine the various factors involved. A set of *in vivo* experiments were performed on dogs to examine the effects of blood contact with the pericardium, the effects of cardiotomy suction *per se* and the differences between roller pump and vacuum suction. The circuits used for these experiments are shown in Figure

Table 1 Haematological values at the termination of cardiopulmonary bypass on human patients (means and standard errors of six measurements)

	Radial artery	*Cardiotomy reservoir*
Platelet count ($\times 10^9$/l)	103.7 ± 12.2	59.5 ± 4.7
Plasma haemoglobin concentration (mg/dl)	40.5 ± 7.6	383.7 ± 79.5
Plasma K^+ concentration (mmol/l)	6.2 ± 0.3	12.7 ± 2.2

1. These circuits permitted roller pump or vacuum suction to be applied either to the left atrium or to the pericardial well, into which blood was allowed to leak via a left atrial catheter.

Thirty animals were subjected to 1 h of cardiotomy suction and blood reinfusion. A further six animals were subjected to only 5 min of suction and reinfusion in order to mix the blood and circuit prime (Hartmann's solution). This latter group served as controls. Measurements were made of the suction line, cardiotomy reservoir, reinfusion line, arterial and venous pressures, heart rate, oesophageal and blood temperatures, and blood and air flow rates. The roller pump and vacuum suction source were adjusted so that all of the blood in the left atrium or pericardial well was aspirated along with an equal quantity of air.

Blood samples were taken from the left atrium and femoral artery for measurements of platelet and leucocyte aggregation by Swank's screen filtration pressure (SFP) technique[4]; platelet and leucocyte counts, packed cell volume, red cell osmotic fragility, whole blood and plasma haemoglobin concentrations[5]. The traumatic index was calculated according to Koller and Hawrylenko (1967)[6] and all haematological values were corrected for haemodilution to give values corresponding to a packed cell volume of 0.40.

Figure 2 shows the corrected changes in plasma haemoglobin concentration in the control group and in the experimental group composed of all dogs subjected to cardiotomy suction. The increase in the plasma haemoglobin concentration in the experimental group may be considered as fairly severe when the low flow rate ($\bar{x}$ = 450 ml/min) is considered. During the 1 h period of suction the plasma haemoglobin concentration increased by 17.4 ± SE 3.2 mg/dl compared with 5.2 ± SE 2.1 mg/dl in the control group. This difference was statistically significant at the 5% probability level by a Mann–Whitney U test. The change in platelet count was also statistically significant, decreasing by 23.3 ± SE 1.8 × 10^9/l in the suction group and increasing by 61.7 ± SE 49.4 × 10^9/l in the control group (Figure 3). The haematological differences between left atrial and pericardial aspiration, and between roller pump and vacuum suction, were not statistically significant.

During five preliminary experiments, it was found that it is important to wash the pericardial and epicardial surfaces with saline before allowing any blood to enter the suction circuit. Failure to do so resulted in immediate severe platelet and leucocyte aggregation.

(a)

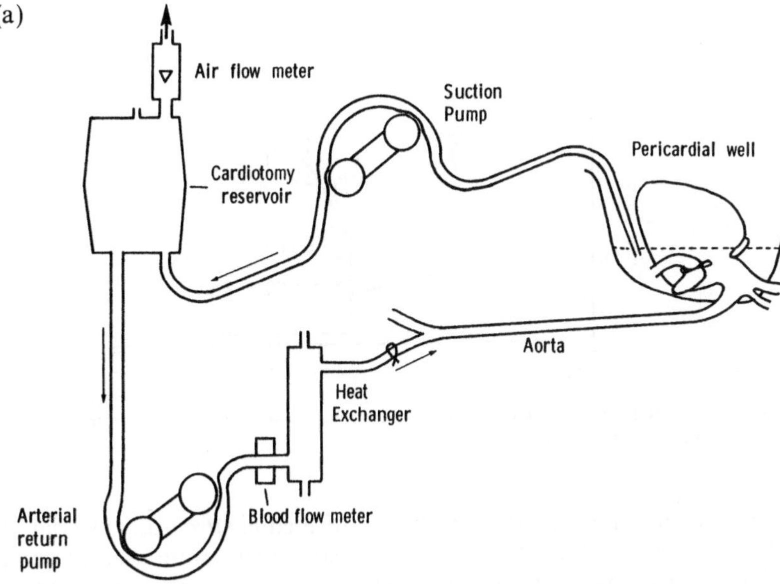

(b)

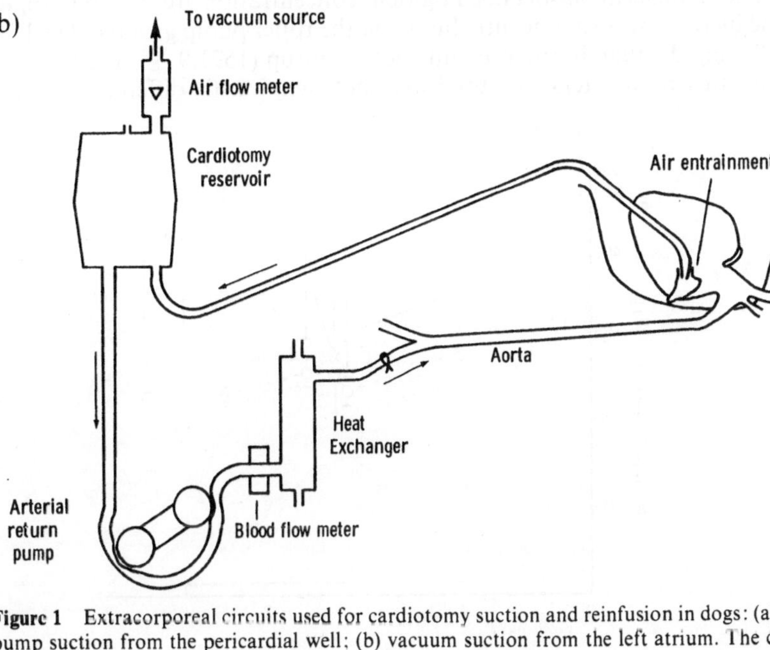

Figure 1 Extracorporeal circuits used for cardiotomy suction and reinfusion in dogs: (a) roller pump suction from the pericardial well; (b) vacuum suction from the left atrium. The circuits were also used for vacuum suction from the pericardial well and for roller pump suction from the left atrium

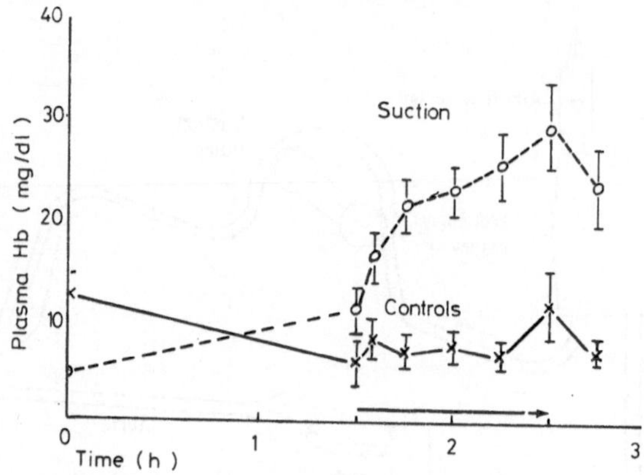

Figure 2 Plasma haemoglobin concentration during *in vivo* cardiotomy suction. The period of suction is indicated by the arrow

The second set of experiments was performed *in vitro* using arterial blood collected from 13 dogs. Seven of these experiments were used to compare roller pump and vacuum suction, and the other six were used to examine the effects of air aspiration. The circuits were identical to those shown in Figure 1 except that the position of the animal was occupied by a polyvinyl chloride reservoir.

The changes in plasma haemoglobin concentration are shown in Figure 4. The increase was significantly higher in the roller pump group (2238.1 ± SE 420.3 mg/dl) than in the vacuum suction group (1591.9 ± SE 293.5 mg/dl). The other parameters measured were not significantly different.

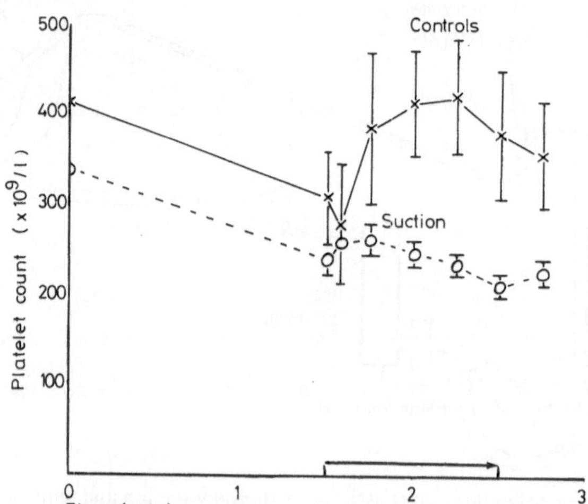

Figure 3 Platelet counts during *in vivo* cardiotomy suction. The period of suction is indicated by the arrow

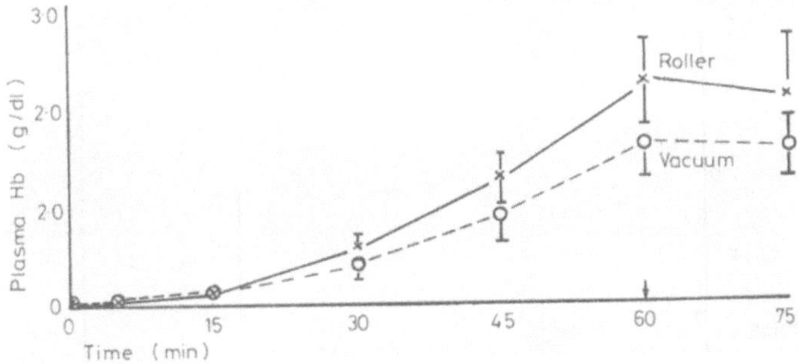

Figure 4 Plasma haemoglobin concentration during *in vitro* suction of blood and air using a roller pump and vacuum source. Suction was terminated after 60 min

The greatest differences were found in the experiments used to examine the effects of air aspiration. The two circuits were primed with blood from the same animal and circulated at the same blood flow rate, but in one circuit the vacuum source was adjusted to aspirate an equal quantity of air as before, while in the second circuit no air was aspirated. The differences in plasma haemoglobin concentration, screen filtration pressure and platelet counts shown in Figures 5–7 and Table 2 were all significant by Wilcoxon's rank sum test for paired data.

Table 2 Haematological changes during suction and recirculation of dog blood (means and standard errors of six experiments)

	Radial artery	*Cardiotomy reservoir*
Plasma haemoglobin concentration (mg/dl)	2168 ± 323	215 ± 121
SFP (mmHg)	39 ± 11	−2 ± 1
PCV	−0.12 ± 0.02	−0.01 ± 0.0
Platelet count ($\times 10^9$/l)	−264.7 ± 16.6	−100.5 ± 2.3

The question of the reason for the marked effects of air aspiration now arises. It is quite inadequate to answer this question by claiming that the cell damage is caused by the blood–air interface. A somewhat better hypothesis can be developed in the following manner:

It has been demonstrated that blood cells can withstand low positive pressures down to 150 mmHg absolute pressure[7]. On the other hand they are easily damaged by high shear stress[8–14] and wall impact[13]. These conditions are prevalent in turbulent flows[15]. There are several reasons for believing that the flow is turbulent in the suction system[17]:

(1) Direct observation and photography show that when a blood and air mixture is aspirated, the blood flows from the patient towards the cardiotomy reservoir in short boluses (Figure 8). The velocity profile in the tube appears to be parabolic. However this is not true of the

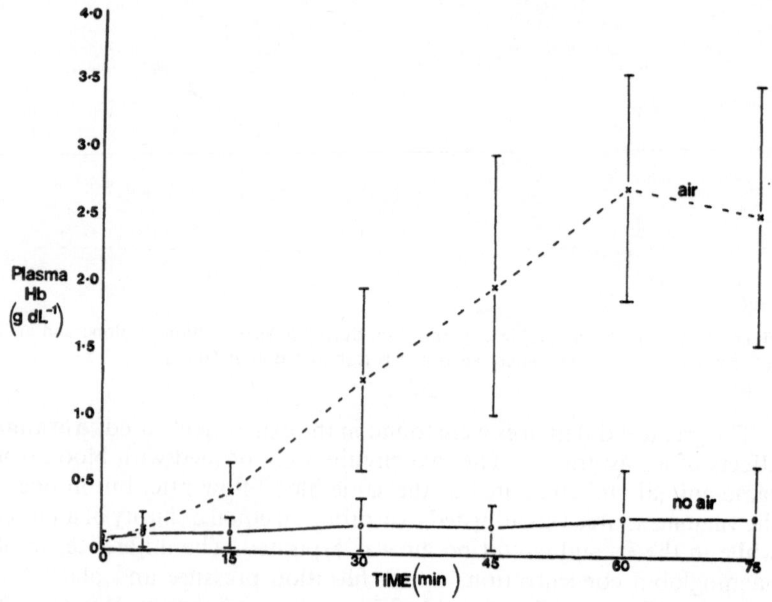

Figure 5 Plasma haemoglobin concentration during *in vitro* suction of blood and air and of blood alone. Suction was terminated after 60 min

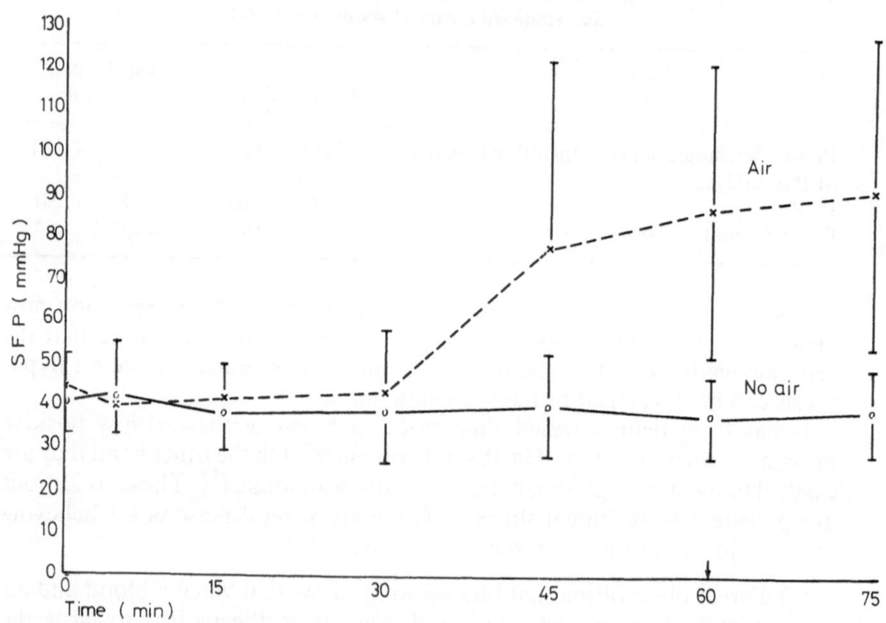

Figure 6 Screen filtration pressure during *in vitro* suction of blood and air and of blood alone. Suction was terminated after 60 min

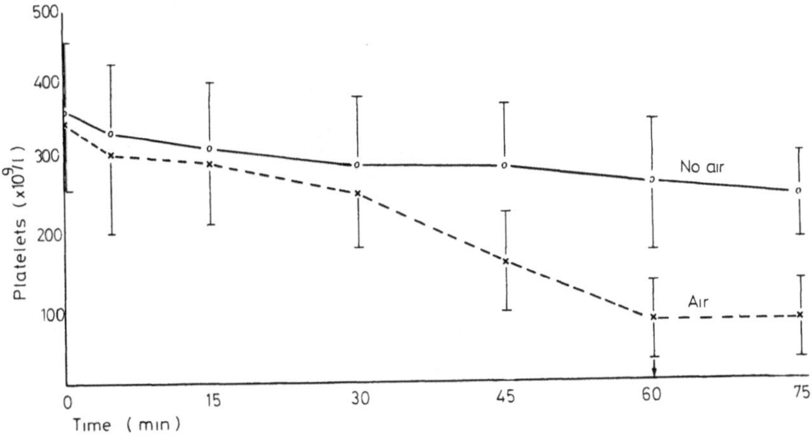

Figure 7 Platelet counts during *in vitro* suction of blood and air and of blood alone. Suction was terminated after 60 min

inlet region. The fully developed flow pattern is established approximately 10 cm from the inlet. Within this 10 cm region the flow appears to be turbulent.

(2) The measured inlet length of 10 cm lies between 26.7 cm and 1.8 cm, which are the calculated inlet lengths for the full development of laminar flow in the system when the reservoir is stationary and when it is turbulent. Thus the measured value is appropriate for a system in which the inlet region is not fully formed laminar flow and in which the reservoir (left atrium or pericardial well) is neither stationary nor turbulent but something between.
(3) The relationship between pressure drop from the inlet to a point in the suction tube 15 cm from the inlet and flow rate was parabolic. Laminar flow would give a linear relationship according to the Poiseuille formula.
(4) The flow is noisy – a characteristic of turbulence.

Shear stress for laminar flow (τ_1) can be calculated from measured data using the formula:

$$\tau_1 = \mu\frac{dv}{dr},$$ in which μ is absolute viscosity, v is fluid velocity, and r is tube radius.

Using this relationship, laminar shear stresses for whole blood in cannulae (or any other tubes) of 1–9 mm internal diameter are shown in Figure 9. Each line is terminated at the value corresponding to the critical Reynold's number of 2300, above which laminar flow cannot be maintained[16].

Turbulent flows are very much more difficult to analyse, but a formula for turbulent shear stress (τ_t) has been proposed by Schlichting (1960)[15] as

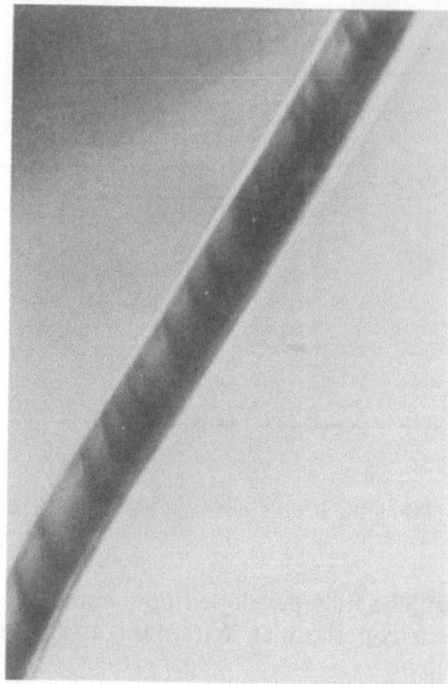

Figure 8 Photograph of blood and air flowing in the cardiotomy suction line between the patient and cardiotomy reservoir

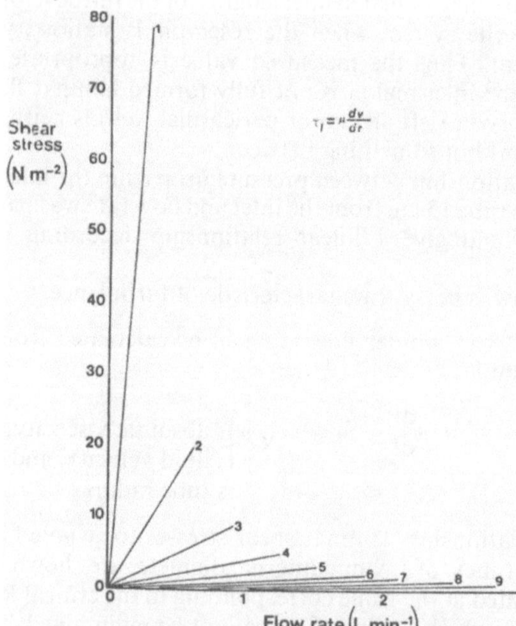

Figure 9 Laminar shear stresses calculated for whole blood flowing through cannulae 1–9 mm internal diameter. Each line terminates at the point corresponding to a Reynolds number of 2300

follows:

$$\tau_t = e\varepsilon\frac{dv}{dr} = 0.03\frac{2\Delta P}{e},$$

where e is fluid density,
ε is eddy current kinematic viscosity, and
ΔP is pressure drop.

Thus the turbulent shear stress for bulk flow can be calculated from the pressure drop data. The results calculated from a set of measurements on the suction system are shown in Figure 10. Notice that the turbulent shear stresses are about 100 times those of the corresponding laminar shear stresses. A survey of the recent literature on the effects of shear stress on blood cells reveals that this model can be used to correctly predict that red cells and platelets would be damaged under normal conditions of cardiotomy suction.

Of course the model suffers from the limitations that we do not know the precise value of blood viscosity, or of the density, of a variable blood and air mixture. Also it does not include wall impact effects, local turbulence (microvortices) or long exposure times (>1 s). However, these effects would only increase the differences between laminar and turbulent shear stresses, and the unknown values are not critical to the conclusion that the traumatic

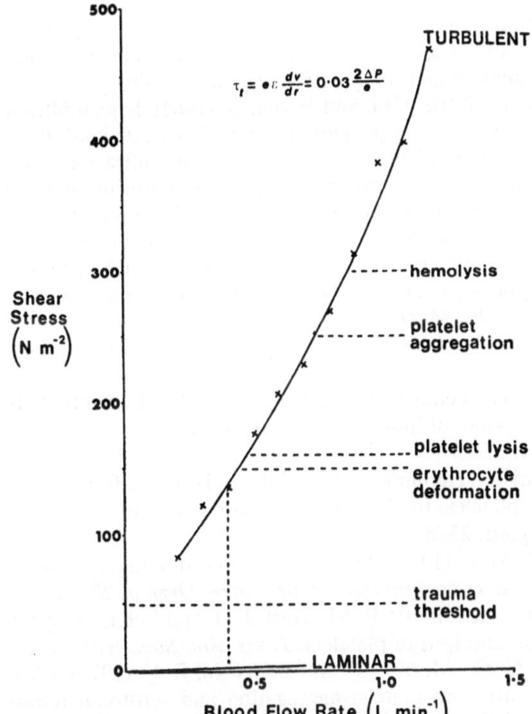

Figure 10 Laminar and turbulent shear stresses for blood and air flowing through cannulae of 4 mm internal diameter

effect of aspirating a blood and air mixture is very much greater than that of aspirating blood alone. We are in the process of developing a regulated suction system which minimizes the air aspiration and similar systems have been described by others[18,19]. However, until these systems become available we may derive some benefit by reducing the blood flow rate, by increasing the diameter of the suction cannula, and by reducing the amount of applied suction. The use of vacuum rather than roller pump suction, and an initial washing of the pericardial and epicardial surfaces, are also likely to be beneficial.

Acknowledgments

Technical advice given by Dr K. H. Parker of the Imperial College of Science and Technology, and the assistance of Mrs Margaret Riley, are gratefully acknowledged. Most of the work was performed under a grant from the British Heart Foundation. Permission to reproduce Figures 1–7 and 9, from *Thorax*, **34**, was kindly given by the British Medical Association.

References

1. Wright, G. (1976). L'aggrégation cellulaire au cours d'une circulation extra-corporelle. *Les Cahiers du Cercle d'Etude de la Circulation Extracorporelle*, **6**, 27
2. Wright, G. (1977). The avoidance of blood cell aggregation during extracorporeal circulation for open-heart surgery. *Proc. Eur. Soc. Artif. Intern. Organs*, **3**, 102
3. Wright, G. and Sanderson, J. M. (1976). Cellular aggregation and destruction during blood circulation and oxygenation. *Thorax*, **31**, 405
4. Swank, R. L., Roth, J. G. and Jansen, J. (1964). Screen filtration pressure method and adhesiveness and aggregation of blood cells. *J. Appl. Physiol.*, **19**, 340
5. Crosby, W. H. and Furth, F. W. (1956). A modification of the benzidine method for measurement of haemoglobin in plasma and urine. *Blood*, **11**, 380
6. Koller, T. and Hawrylenko, A. (1967). Contribution to the *in vitro* testing of pumps for extracorporeal circulation. *J. Thorac. Cardiovasc. Surg.*, **54**, 22
7. Wielgorski, J. W., Cross, D. E. and Nevadike, E. V. O. (1975). The effects of subatmospheric pressure on the haemolysis of blood. *J. Biomech.*, **8**, 321
8. Bernstein, E. F., Marzec, V. and Johnston, G. G. (1977). Structural correlates of platelet functional damage by physical forces. *Trans. Am. Soc. Artif. Intern. Organs*, **23**, 617
9. Brown, C. H., Lemuth, R. F., Hellums, J. D., Leverett, J. B. and Alfrey, C. P. (1975). Response of human platelets to shear stress. *Trans. Am. Soc. Artif. Intern. Organs*, **21**, 35
10. Colantuoni, G., Hellums, J. D., Moake, J. L. and Alfrey, C. P. (1977). The response of human platelets to shear stress at short exposure time. *Trans. Am. Soc. Artif. Intern. Organs*, **23**, 626
11. Goldsmith, H. L. (1974). The effects of flow and fluid mechanical stress on red cells and platelets. *Trans. Am. Soc. Artif. Intern. Organs*, **20**, 21
12. Hung, T. C., Hochmuth, R. M., Joist, J. H. and Sutera, S. P. (1976). Shear-induced aggregation and lysis of platelets. *Trans. Am. Soc. Artif. Intern. Organs*, **22**, 285
13. Johnston, G. G., Marzec, V. and Bernstein, E. F. (1975). Effects of surface injury and shear stress on platelet aggregation and serotonin release. *Trans. Am. Soc. Artif. Intern. Organs*, **21**, 413
14. Nevaril, C. G., Lynch, E. C., Alfrey, C. P. and Hellums, J. D. (1968). Erythrocyte damage and destruction induced by shearing stress. *J. Lab. Clin. Med.*, **71**, 784

15. Schlichting, H. (1960). *Boundary Layer Theory*, 4th Edn. (New York: McGraw-Hill)
16. McDonald, D. A. (1974). *Blood Flow in Arteries*, 2nd Edn. (London: Edward Arnold)
17. Wright, G. and Sanderson, J. M. (1979). Cellular aggregation and trauma in cardiotomy suction systems. *Thorax*, **34**, 621
18. Barthelemy, R., Vives, M., Couzy, H., Morucci, J. P., Puel, P. and Enjalbert, A. (1978). Dispositif de controle automatique des aspirations chirurgicales en chirurgie cardiaque. *Med. Biol. Eng. Comp.*, **16**, 165
19. ten Duis, H. J., de Jong, J. C. F., van Asseldonk, A. G. M., Smit Sibinga, C. T. and Wildevuur, C. R. H. (1978). Improved hemocompatibility in open heart surgery. *Trans. Am. Soc. Artif. Intern. Organs*, **24**, 656

22
Gaseous microemboli during open heart surgery

D. T. PEARSON, R. F. CARTER, M. B. HAMMO, and P. S. WATERHOUSE

INTRODUCTION

Several investigators have described the deleterious effects resulting from the functional replacement of the heart and lungs by a pump oxygenator during open heart surgery[1-6]. The brain appears to be most susceptible to damage in this context. Many reports indicate the high incidence and wide variety of disturbances in cerebral function, ranging from mild delirium and psychosis to overt focal or diffuse neurological deficits[5,7,8] which can nullify the benefits of open heart surgery. Although during recent years there has been a reduction in the incidence of major cerebral damage there remain signs that cardiopulmonary bypass causes subclinical cerebral injury leading to intellectual impairment which can only be detected by careful psychometric testing[2,4].

Table 1 summarizes the more important aetiological factors which have been described as causing neurological dysfunction following open heart surgery.

As well as disturbances produced by systemic arterial hypotension[8-10] reduction in cerebral blood flow[11] and non-pulsatile flow[12,13] the incidence of neurological dysfunction is increased if the patient is over 50 years old and if the duration of bypass exceeds 120 min[8,10]. Alterations in cerebral physiology caused by a variety of microemboli are well documented[14-17]. Emboli of denatured protein[18], silicone anti-foam[19], calcium[20], fat[21,22], and aggregated blood elements[23] have been implicated as causative factors in the widespread organ dysfunction which may follow open heart surgery. Gaseous microemboli originating from the heart, the pulmonary veins, or the pump oxygenator system can also cause alterations in myocardial and cerebral physiology during cardiac surgery[24-28]

Table 1 Cerebral dysfunction during open heart surgery. Aetiological factors

A. Embolic
- GASEOUS MICROEMBOLI from:
  - (i) heart and pulmonary veins
  - (ii) pump oxygenator
- Foreign material from:
  - (i) oxygenator (cotton fibres, silicone, plastic chips)
  - (ii) pump (spallation of pump tubing)
  - (iii) operative equipment (talc, thread, dust, cloth particles)
- Red cell, platelet and leukocyte aggregates
- Fibrin
- Calcium and arteriosclerotic debris
- Denatured protein
- Fat globules

B. Haemodynamic
- Age of patient
- Duration of bypass
- Systemic arterial pressure on bypass
- Pulsatile versus non-pulsatile flow

GASEOUS MICROEMBOLI DETECTION USING ULTRASOUND

Gaseous microemboli originating from the pump oxygenator system during cardiopulmonary bypass have been described by Selman and his colleagues using a transparent chamber in the arterial line[29]. Following a preliminary report by Austen and Howry in 1965[30], describing the use of ultrasound to detect bubbles and particulate matter, many other workers have used this technique[25,31-35].

Detection of gaseous microemboli in blood vessels and extracorporeal circuits by ultrasound has many limitations and problems[36,37]. The use of Doppler-based instruments incorporating filters which attempt to specifically discriminate the bubble-derived signals from those of the blood flow signals[25,36] may give rise to errors in measuring the size and population density of the gaseous microemboli. These errors cannot be completely eliminated by the use of pulsed ultrasound. Transducer coupling and angulation of the transducer in relationship to the blood flow may also introduce errors. In spite of these limitations it is agreed that whilst the techniques currently available do not completely quantify and determine the size of the gaseous microemboli, they provide a representative sample of those passing the transducer[31,32]. However, as a result of the many different devices used it is difficult to compare studies from different surgical centres.

We report our experience in the detection of gaseous microemboli during open heart surgery using cardiopulmonary bypass, and an *in vivo* and *in vitro* analysis of the performance characteristics of various commercially available extracorporeal components.

A transcutaneous Doppler ultrasonic blood flow detector producing a 2 MHz beam of ultrasound has been used to detect gaseous microemboli in the systemic arterial circulation during open heart surgery[25]. The transducer of this device was fixed over the left carotid artery by adhesive strapping, using olive oil for acoustic coupling. The left carotid artery was chosen to avoid interference from ventilator and intravenous therapy tubing. The optimal position of the transducer was indicated by maximal pulsatile blood flow signals. In order to minimize the lower-frequency signals caused by blood flow, the signals from the detector were passed through an active high-pass filter with a cut off frequency of 1.6 kHz. This permitted the higher frequency signals of gaseous microemboli to be amplified and graphically displayed. Simultaneous recordings of systemic arterial pressure, electrocardiograph and cerebral electrical activity[38] were made.

Original work in this department[25] involved the use of the ultrasonic transducer placed over the carotid artery. During detailed observation on many patients undergoing open heart surgery for a wide variety of congenital and acquired heart disease, gaseous microemboli were detected in the systemic arterial circulation. They originated from the pump oxygenator system and from recognized surgical procedures on the heart.

SOURCES OF 'SURGICAL' GASEOUS MICROEMBOLI

Cannulation of the heart

Cannulation of the ascending aorta before the start of cardiopulmonary bypass may admit gaseous microemboli into the systemic arterial circulation. This is a consistent finding in every case monitored, and appears to be independent of the level of the arterial pressure and whether the cannula is primed with saline.

Insertion of caval or right atrial cannulae through the right atrial wall in the presence of an atrial septal defect results in systemic arterial gaseous microemboli even when there is a left-to-right shunt at atrial level.

The placement of a left atrial, or apical left ventricular vent may introduce gaseous microemboli into the systemic arterial circulation. During closed mitral valvotomy both digital exploration of the valve and the introduction of the dilator through the left ventriculotomy may produce similar results.

Following removal of the aortic clamp

If the left heart is opened air may collect between the aortic clamp and aortic valve, and even when the root of the aorta is vented through the aortic suture line or by aspiration using a wide-bore needle, gaseous microemboli will be released into the systemic arterial circulation when the clamp is removed.

Entrainment of air at venous cannulation sites

Air may be entrained into the venous line leading to the oxygenator as a consequence of inadequate snaring of the site of insertion of the right atrial cannulae, and during venting of cardioplegic solution through an incision in the right atrium. This air will pass into the oxygenator, and it has been demonstrated that a large proportion will pass through both bubble and membrane oxygenators to enter the arterial line. Increased numbers of gaseous microemboli can be detected in the carotid artery when there are visible bubbles in the venous line. Whilst it is uncertain how much of this air is removed by the defoamer of a bubble oxygenator, it must be recognized as a major source of systemic gaseous microemboli during cardiopulmonary bypass.

Following restoration of effective heart action

Following cardiotomy for a septal defect, or during exposure of left-sided cardiac valves, cardiac ejection is prevented until the heart is filled with blood, air pockets are displaced, and bubbles trapped in muscular trabeculae are finally removed. Many techniques have been described to avoid the hazards of systemic air embolism, and they include the insertion of a drain in the apex of the left ventricle attached to suction[39]. This may be combined with induced ventricular fibrillation[40,41], flooding of the operative field with carbon dioxide[42,43], and aspiration of pulmonary veins and cardiac chambers with a needle[44]. Vents have been placed in the right superior pulmonary vein, and air removed from the aorta using a wide-bore needle, either free-draining or attached to suction. In spite of all attempts to remove entrapped air all patients so far monitored demonstrate a variable amount of systemic gaseous microemboli when effective heart action is restored at the end of cardiopulmonary bypass. Electrocardiographic demonstration of myocardial ischaemia provides indirect evidence of coronary artery embolism.

The total number of gaseous microemboli entering the systemic circulation during cannulation of the heart and removal of the aortic clamp is relatively small. Residual air trapped in the heart at the end of the operation contributes the greatest number of gaseous microemboli from surgical sources, and may exceed in total the number originating from the pump oxygenator system.

Figure 1 demonstrates many of the features described, and it is the record of electrocardiograph, systemic arterial blood pressure, quantity of gaseous microemboli detected in the left carotid artery, and cerebral electrical activity in a 65-year-old male during open heart surgery for aortic valve replacement. The record is typical of many of the cases so far monitored. The valve replacement was carried out under moderate hypothermia at 28 °C with the addition of cold cardioplegic solution. A bubble oxygenator (Bentley Laboratories BOS 10) was used with pulsatile flow at 4.5 l/min from a Stockert roller-pump. Admission of bubbles into the systemic arterial circulation is demonstrated to occur:

(1) During aortic cannulation.
(2) At onset of cardiopulmonary bypass.
(3) During insertion of the left ventricular vent.
(4) During release of the aortic clamp.

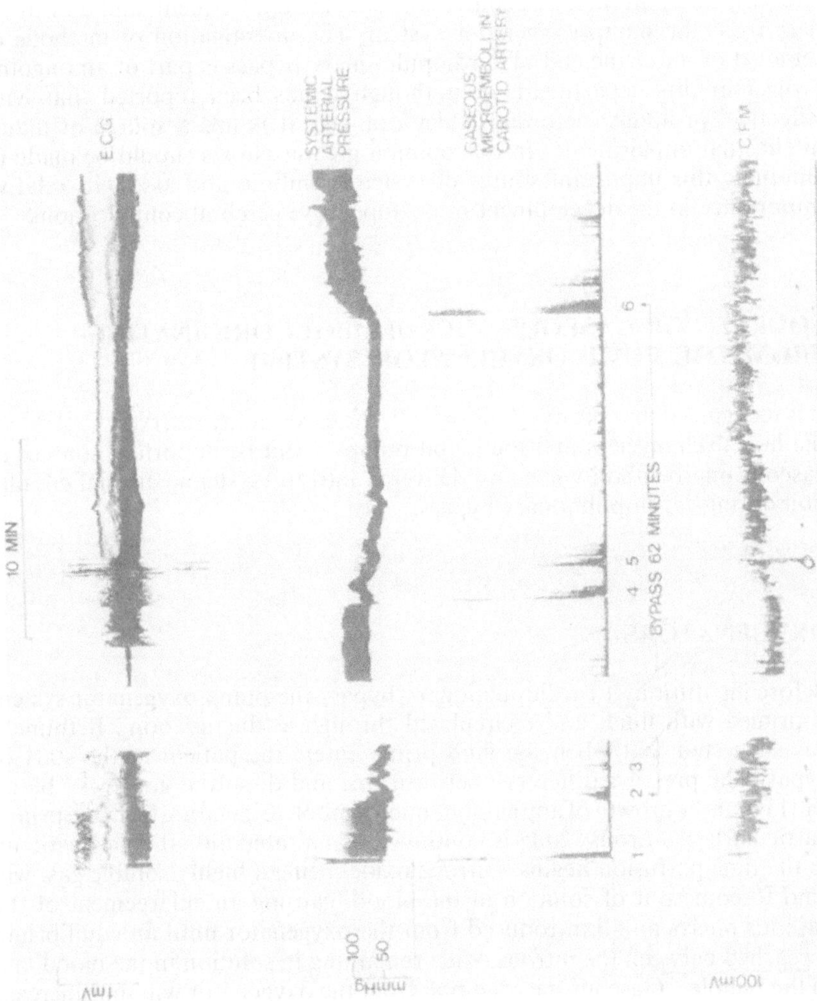

Figure 1 Intraoperative recording of gaseous microemboli in carotid artery during open heart surgery for aortic valve replacement (see text)

(5) Following the restoration of normal cardiac electrical activity by defibrillation.
(6) At restoration of effective cardiac ejection of blood.

Signals attributable to gaseous microemboli occuring between these definitive surgical events are, by comparison, small and infrequent, and they originate from the pump oxygenator system. The investigation of methods of removal of air at the end of cardiopulmonary bypass is part of an ongoing project in this department, even though it has been reported that with 'effective' prolonged left ventricular drainage it is not a source of major intellectual impairment[2]. In our opinion greater efforts should be made to eliminate this important source of systemic emboli, and assess its relative importance in the development of postoperative cerebral complications.

SOURCES OF GASEOUS MICROEMBOLI ORIGINATING FROM THE PUMP OXYGENATOR SYSTEM

It is recognized that the oxygenator[25,31], the cardiotomy reservoir[25,31,33,35], the heat exchanger[46], and the blood pumps[45] can be important sources of gaseous microemboli which are delivered into the systemic arterial circulation during cardiopulmonary bypass.

OXYGENATORS

Before institution of cardiopulmonary bypass the pump oxygenator system is primed with fluid, and recirculated through a 'ductus loop'. Bethune[47] has suggested that when the fluid prime enters the patient at the start of bypass, the pressure difference between free and dissolved gas in the blood will favour the growth of any gaseous microemboli originating from the prime, particularly if nitrous oxide is continued as an inhalational anaesthetic up to the time perfusion begins. Nitrous oxide, being a highly soluble gas, will tend to come out of solution in the blood, causing an enlargement of the gaseous microemboli introduced from the oxygenator until an equilibrium is reached between the nitrous oxide remaining in solution in the blood and in the bubbles. Gaseous microemboli from the oxygenator will thus increase in size. To prevent this complication it is recommended by Bethune that the bypass circuit should be flushed with carbon dioxide, a highly soluble gas, prior to priming with warmed fluids. Recirculation of the priming fluid should take place without introduction of gas into the oxygenator, and nitrous oxide should be discontinued 10 min prior to institution of perfusion, thus allowing most of the nitrous oxide to be eliminated via the lungs. The number of gaseous microemboli originating from the oxygenator is usually high at the beginning of perfusion, decreasing rapidly with time[46], but the numbers and size might be reduced by applying the techniques described above.

Disc oxygenators

The production of gaseous microemboli by disc oxygenators was described by Gallagher and Pearson in 1973[25]. Increasing the rate of disc rotation and maintaining a low or excessively high level of blood in the oxygenator are factors which increase the number of gaseous microemboli in the perfusion fluid. Close spacing of the discs in the oxygenator increased the production of gaseous microemboli.

Membrane oxygenators

The membrane oxygenator, having no direct blood/gas interface or defoamer, is claimed to produce less gaseous microemboli than do bubble oxygenators[34,48,49]. If gaseous microemboli are introduced into a membrane oxygenator from cardiotomy suction (see below), entrainment of air around the venous cannulae, or infusion of cold fluids – or are produced by excessive temperature gradients between the water inflow and patient blood during rewarming – then they will pass through the oxygenator into the arterial line.

Bubble oxygenators

The improvement in the design of bubble oxygenators resulting in a reduction in oxygen/blood flow ratios has also been reported to have decreased the number of gaseous microemboli remaining in the perfused blood following oxygenation and defoaming[50]. The numbers of gaseous microemboli originating from several different types of oxygenator have produced widely varying results[29,50–52] presumably due to differences in monitoring techniques. The factors which have been reported to increase the number of gaseous microemboli originating from bubble oxygenators[25,31] include:

(1) Increase in oxygen to blood flow ratios.
(2) Introduction of cardiotomy suction blood.
(3) Transfusion of cold donor blood into the oxygenator.
(4) Vibration of the oxygenator.
(5) Low level of blood in the oxygenator.
(6) Addition of fluid or medications to the oxygenator.

An *in vivo* analysis of six commercially available bubble oxygenators has recently been carried out in this department in an attempt to correlate their gas transfer characteristics with gaseous microemboli production. The oxygenators (see Appendix) were used during clinical perfusion for prosthetic valve replacement.

METHOD

A TM8 microbubble activity monitor was fixed over the arterial line leading from the oxygenator. This device generates a continuous narrow beam of ultrasound which is propagated by the transducer into the blood passing through the tubing. When gaseous microemboli pass this beam, the receiving transducer picks up modifications in the signal which are then processed by an electronic unit to provide a digital display in the size range selected on the sensitivity control. The output from the bubble activity monitor was then fed into an electronic processor which divided the signals into bubble counts in the 10, 15 and 20+ μm range. Each range was scanned for 1 s periods, and the output was displayed on a Devices M2R-35 chart recorder. Samples of venous and arterial blood were analysed for PCO_2 and PO_2 using a Corning 175 blood gas analyser, and the results were corrected for patient temperature.

All patients were maintained at a pulsatile blood flow rate of 4 l/min from the oxygenator using a Stockert pump, and data were collected when the patient temperature had been reduced from 37 °C and stabilized at 28 °C. During this period there was no addition of fluid from the cardiotomy reservoir, and counts of gaseous microemboli originating from the priming fluid or heat-exchanger would not interfere with the results. During the period of analysis, the blood gases of the venous inflow blood to the oxygenator were monitored and found to be constant. Gas flow rates to the oxygenator were carefully monitored using back-pressure-compensated anaesthetic rotameters to provide accurate gas/blood flow ratios.

RESULTS

Gaseous microemboli during recirculation of the priming fluid

All oxygenators were primed with 1000 ml of 5% dextrose and 1000 ml Ringer lactate. This priming solution was circulated through the oxygenator at 3.4 l/min via a 'ductus loop', the temperature of the priming solution being maintained at 37 °C. The level of priming fluid in each oxygenator was maintained at the 1000 ml indicated level on the arterial reservoir of the oxygenator and the oxygen inflow to the oxygenating column adjusted to 1.0 l/min. We have included the results from an early model of the Bentley Laboratories BOS 10 which has since been modified by the insertion of a polyurethane defoamer plug in the mixing chamber.

The values for bubble counts for each oxygenator are shown in Figure 2 and indicate a wide variation in the numbers of gaseous microemboli in the priming solution in different oxygenators.

Level in oxygenator

With a constant gas/blood flow ratio, each oxygenator was assessed regarding its ability to defoam oxygenated blood when the level in the oxygenator was altered. All oxygenators showed a decrease in the number of gaseous microemboli as the level in the arterial reservoir was increased. The most dramatic changes occurred in the Shiley S100 oxygenator. Little change in the numbers of gaseous microemboli with respect to level in the arterial reservoir occurred with the Bentley Q200A oxygenator (Figure 3).

Gas/blood flow ratio

With the patient temperature maintained constant at 28 °C, and no admission of cardiotomy suction blood to the oxygenator, correlation of the numbers of gaseous microemboli in the arterial line were made with sampling of arterial blood for PCO_2 and PO_2. The blood flow rate from the oxygenator was maintained constant during the analysis at 4.0 l/min and the gas flow to the oxygenator increased progressively in 1.0 l increments from 1.0 to 4.0 l/min. The level of blood in the oxygenator was kept at the 1000 ml mark during the analysis.

The results (Figure 4) show that in each oxygenator tested, an increase in gas/blood ratio resulted in a rise in arterial PO_2 with an associated fall in PCO_2 when venous inflow PO_2 and PCO_2 were constant. Simultaneously, there was a rise in the numbers of gaseous microemboli detected in the arterial

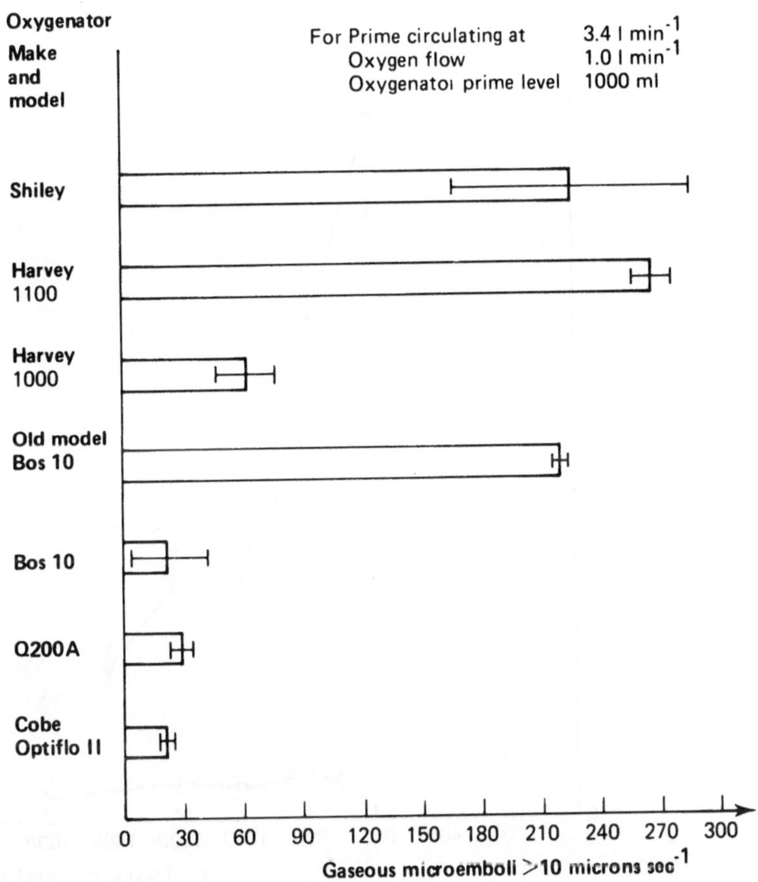

Figure 2 Numbers of gaseous microemboli detected in the arterial line of various oxygenators during recirculation of priming solution

line as the flow rate of gas to the oxygenator increased. There were marked differences between different oxygenators: (i) in their ability to produce physiological blood gas levels, and (ii) in their defoaming capabilities at a given gas/blood flow ratio.

Membrane oxygenators

We have been unable to detect gaseous microemboli originating from the Travenol membrane oxygenator.

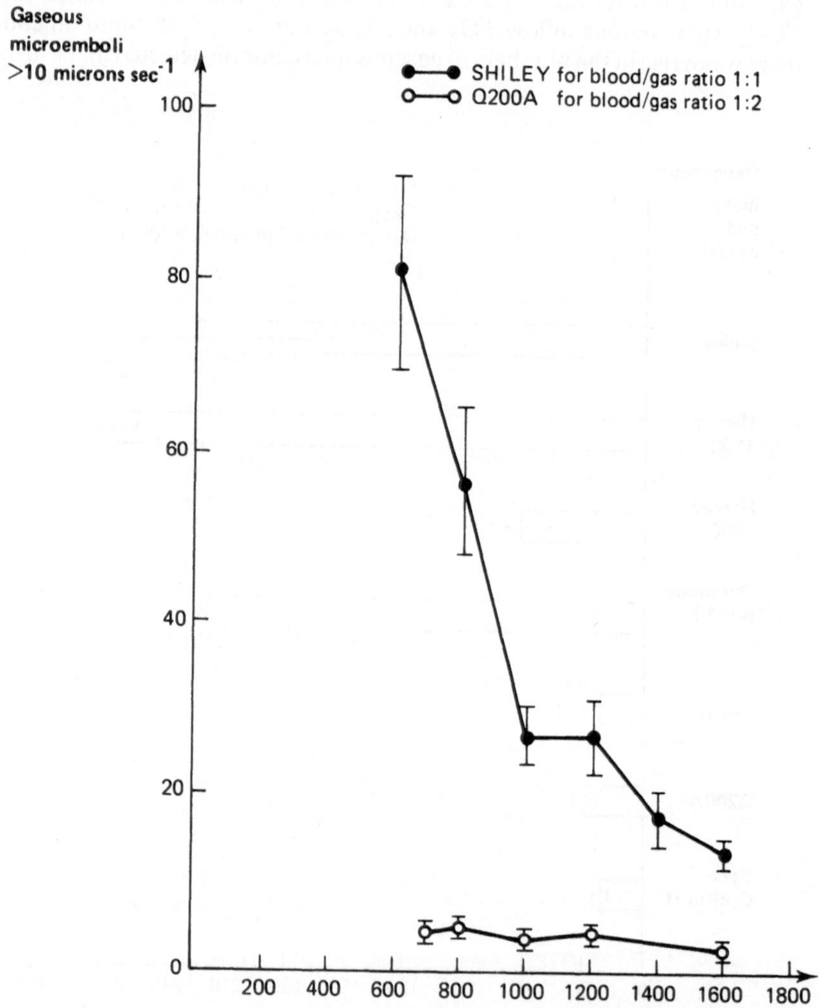

Figure 3 Numbers of gaseous microemboli (mean ± SD) detected in arterial line of two oxygenators with respect to level of blood in arterial reservoir

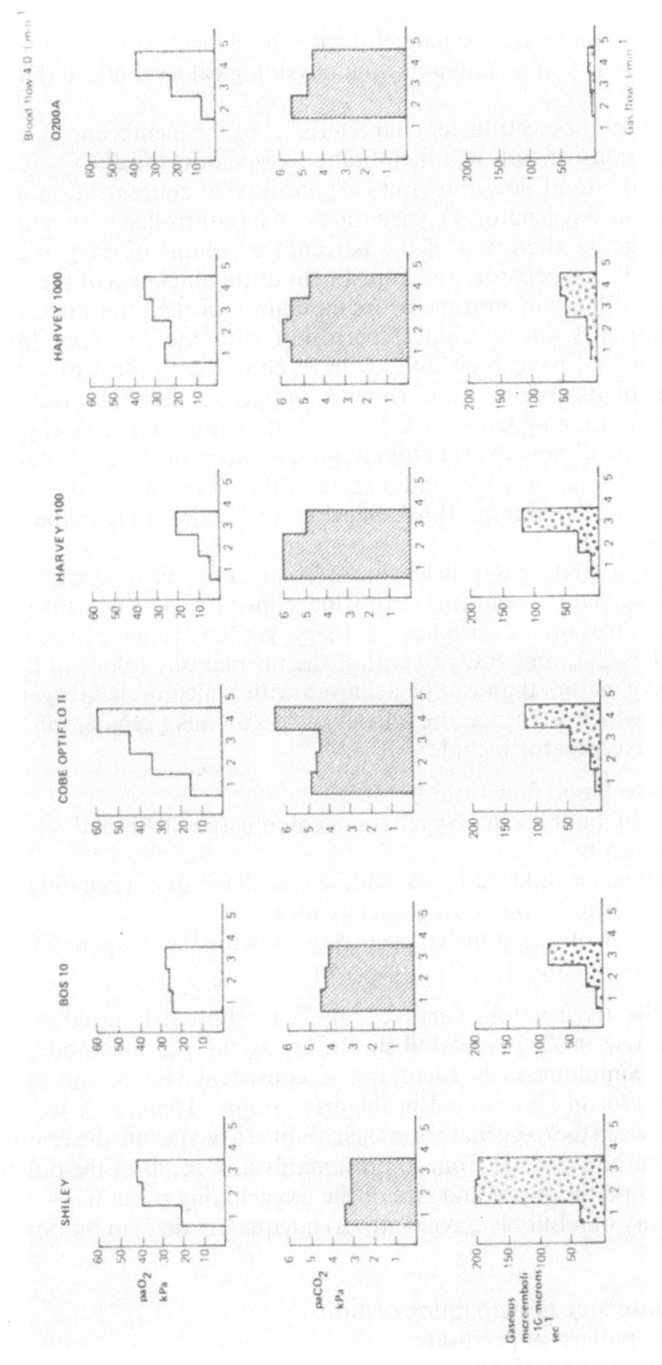

Figure 4 Relationship between numbers of gaseous microemboli detected in arterial line of various oxygenators and arterial blood gases with changing blood/gas flow ratios

COMMENT

The major role of a gas exchanger device for clinical perfusion during open heart surgery is to maintain a normal physiological level of arterial PO_2 and PCO_2.

Apart from the gas transfer characteristics of the membrane material, and method of construction in a membrane oxygenator, the P_aCO_2 is inversely related to the total flow rate and carbon dioxide concentration of the gas passing to the oxygenator. Oxygenation can be controlled within the physiological range by alteration of the percentage volume of oxygen in the gas passing to the oxygenator, and adjustment of the thickness of the blood film in contact with the membrane by manipulation of the shim pressure. Using these techniques during clinical perfusion with the Travenol Membrane Oxygenators we have been able to have complete control of P_aCO_2 and P_aO_2 in patients ranging from neonates to overweight adults and at patient temperatures ranging from 18 °C to 37 °C. If venous and arterial pumps are used in the membrane oxygenator circuit it is theoretically possible to induce a degree of venous or arterial admixture of the blood by altering the relative flow rate of the two pumps, thus achieving further flexibility in the control of P_aCO_2 and P_aO_2.

The analysis of the gas transfer characteristics of six commercially available bubble oxygenators confirms our wide clinical experience during extracorporeal perfusion for open heart surgery. We have found a lesser degree of control of P_aCO_2 and P_aO_2 to within the normal physiological range with bubble oxygenators than can be achieved with a membrane oxygenator.

Factors which influence the efficiency of gaseous exchange in a bubble dispersion oxygenator include:

(1) Gas to blood flow ratio.
(2) Size of bubbles in oxygenation column (gas to blood surface area interface).
(3) Turbulence induced by gas inflow and shape of oxygenating column.
(4) Time spent by blood in contact with gas.
(5) Amount of gas transfer occurring outwith the oxygenating column (in defoamer and arterial reservoir).

Each of the oxygenators surveyed at 28 °C showed a progressive trend towards a rise in P_aO_2 and fall in P_aCO_2 as the gas to blood flow ratio increased. Simultaneously there was a consistent rise in the number of gaseous microemboli detected in the arterial line. There were marked differences between the oxygenators in their ability to oxygenate the venous blood and clear carbon dioxide from it, presumably as a result of the different gas dispersers, and the shape and size of the oxygenating column.

The ability of a bubble oxygenator to adequately defoam blood is related to:

(1) Surface area of defoaming section.
(2) Flow pattern of perfusate.
(3) Configuration of defoamer.

(4) Level in arterial reservoir.
(5) Dynamic hold-up (resident time) in defoamer.
(6) Number and size of bubbles entering defoaming section.

It was discovered that the Harvey H1000 and Bentley Q200A oxygenators could produce acceptable P_aCO_2 and P_aO_2 with the generation of less gaseous microemboli in the arterial line at higher gas/blood flow ratios than the other oxygenators tested.

The trend towards a reduction in the gas/blood flow ratios of current 'more efficient' bubble oxygenators does not always result in a reduction in the numbers of gaseous microemboli in the effluent from the oxygenator. It is based on a misconception that the less gas that enters the oxygenator the less that must come out. We have noted during clinical perfusion, particularly during rewarming and at normothermic conditions, a need to increase the gas/blood flow ratio in order to achieve a normal P_aCO_2 in this group of oxygenators. This is often at the expense of an excessively high P_aO_2 outwith the physiological range and a dramatic rise in the number of gaseous microemboli in the perfusate.

The large numbers of gaseous microemboli found in the priming fluid when gas was passed into the oxygenators tested lend support to the recommendations of Bethune[47] as to means of reducing the number of gaseous microemboli entering the systemic arterial circulation at the start of cardiopulmonary bypass. Although there was a marked variation between the oxygenators tested each showed a consistent inverse relationship between level of blood in the arterial reservoir and number of gaseous microemboli in the perfusate. Each have different amounts and configuration of defoamer, thus a wide difference is to be expected.

Care should be exercised during clinical perfusion to maintain an adequate level of blood in the arterial reservoir of the oxygenator, though the manufacturer's recommended minimum levels may be too low to prevent an excessive number of gaseous microemboli in the perfusate.

HEAT-EXCHANGER

It has been demonstrated *in vitro*, and inferred during clinical perfusion, that a temperature gradient between water inflow to the heat-exchanger and blood of greater than 10 °C on rewarming causes a significant increase in the number of gaseous microemboli in the perfusate[21]. It is, therefore, important to maintain as low a gradient as possible commensurate with the rate of rise of patient temperature. Most currently available bubble oxygenators have heat-exchangers in the oxygenating column so that any gaseous microemboli generated during rewarming are presented to the defoamer of the oxygenator. We have not been able to confirm the theoretical benefits of this heat-exchanger position. However when membrane oxygenators, which have no defoaming capabilities, are used for clinical perfusion, caution should be exercised in minimizing temperature gradients during rewarming if an excessive gaseous microemboli load is not to be presented to the patient.

ROLLER-PUMPS

Bass and Longmore[45] have reported that negative pressures which develop behind each pump roller are potentially capable of causing microbubble formation by cavitation. During *in vitro* experiments with different arterial PO_2, variation in roller occlusion settings and pulsatile/non-pulsatile flow using a Stockert roller-pump we have been unable to confirm their findings.

CARDIOTOMY RESERVOIRS

During cardiopulmonary bypass, venous blood is drained into a pump oxygenator, arterialized and returned to the systemic arterial circulation. Since both vena cavae can be cannulated separately through the right atrium, if the veins are occluded around the cannulae, it is possible to withdraw the systemic venous blood by gravity into the oxygenator even when the right heart is opened. In operations on the left side of the heart a single cannula placed in the right atrium will suffice. In this latter situation, and when the vena cavae are cannulated, but not occluded around the cannulae, the venous blood returning directly to the right heart cavities, including that from the Thebesian veins, anterior coronary veins, and coronary sinus will be included in the venous drainage to the oxygenator.

If no cardiotomy is performed any blood entering the right atrium, and not draining via the venous cannulae, will fill the right ventricle and be ejected into the pulmonary vascular bed to return to the left heart and be ejected into the aorta. If the heart is arrested and no ejection is possible acute cardiac dilatation will ensue. Flooding of the pulmonary circulation and pulmonary oedema will occur. Total cardiopulmonary bypass and a dry operative field require the removal of coronary sinus blood by suction through the right atrial or ventricular cardiotomy, or by vents placed in the left atrium or left ventricle. Bronchial venous blood returning to the left atrium presents similar problems since, if the heart is arrested and no cardiac septal defect permits blood to drain into the right heart, pulmonary and cardiac damage will occur if no venting of this blood takes place.

Under normal circumstances, coronary and bronchial blood flow amount to 10% of cardiac output. The collateral circulation through the lungs may be increased in cardiac disease, and some 20–50% of the output from the pump oxygenator may pass through the pulmonary systemic anastomoses in cyanotic congenital heart disease. This is a similar situation to the one which pertains when a patent ductus arteriosus and surgically produced systemic/pulmonary shunt is present. The heart and lungs will be flooded with blood at systemic arterial pressure during cardiopulmonary bypass.

A patent ductus arteriosus or artificially produced anastomosis must be ligated or clamped during perfusion, and a left-sided superior vena cava clamped or drained via a separate cannula. Any distension of the left ventricle due to aortic incompetence can be prevented by cross-clamping the aorta or venting the left ventricle.

Intracardiac blood from collateral anastomosis often cannot be reduced during clinical perfusion and exceeds the normal 10% of cardiac output coronary sinus and bronchial return to the heart.

It is essential that any cardiotomy drainage system can cope with large volumes of blood aspirated from the cardiac chambers. It must be possible to compensate for blood loss via cardiotomy suction by a comparable increase in the output from the pump oxygenator. Myocardial contractility must be sufficient to ensure that the heart does not distend when cardiotomy suction and left ventricular venting have not been established or have been removed.

When gravity venous drainage to the oxygenator is inadequate, or when there is a need to aspirate blood from the open heart, the blood will be mixed with air before being discharged into a cardiotomy reservoir.

A cardiotomy suction system will require[52]:

(1) Large storage capacity.
(2) Minimal degree of suction to avoid blood trauma.
(3) Minimal admixture with air.
(4) Reliable defoaming capacity.
(5) Incorporation of filter material[33,35].

Several authors have identified cardiotomy suction as a potent source of both particulate[46,49] and gaseous microemboli[25,31,33,35]. Various cardiotomy reservoirs have been designed incorporating defoaming chambers and filters to remove these emboli. Bubbles created by suction are quantitatively different from those generated in a bubble oxygenator consisting mainly of nitrogen, which is a relatively insoluble gas. The admission of a volume of blood collected over a short period from a cardiotomy reservoir into a bubble oxygenator results in an increase in gaseous microemboli detected in the arterial line[25]. The persistence of these microemboli, after passage through both the defoamer in the cardiotomy reservoir and oxygenator, indicates their relative stability.

The increase in numbers of gaseous microemboli in the arterial line of the oxygenator after admission of a volume of cardiotomy suction is shown in Figure 5.

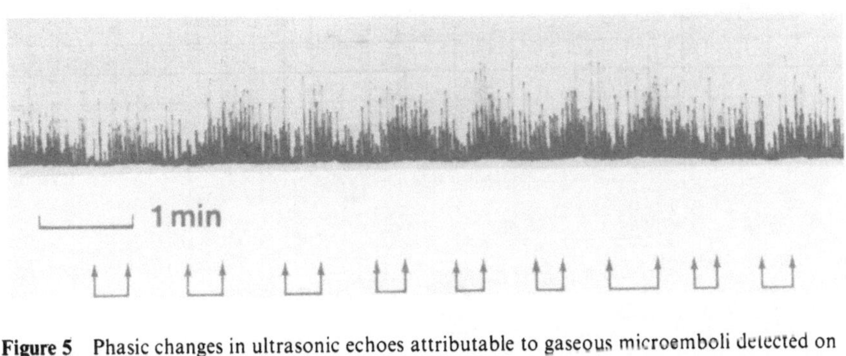

Figure 5 Phasic changes in ultrasonic echoes attributable to gaseous microemboli detected on the arterial line from the oxygenator following intermittent admission of cardiotomy suction blood from the cardiotomy reservoir

Recent work in this Unit[35] has enabled a comparison to be made of the efficiency of various commercially available cardiotomy reservoirs, and micropore blood filters (see Appendix) to remove gaseous microemboli from coronary suction blood. It has also enabled us to define perfusion techniques which influence the performance of the reservoirs and minimize the gaseous microemboli load to the patient.

METHOD

An *in vitro* cardiopulmonary bypass circuit was constructed as shown in Figure 6. The main circuit consisted of a polycarbonate disc oxygenator with arterial and venous connections joined by a loop of $\frac{3}{8}$ inch diameter tubing. The circuit was primed with heparinized acid-citrate-dextrose blood which was circulated at a flow rate of 2.5 l/min by a double-arm non-pulsatile roller-pump (pump A). The temperature of the blood was maintained at

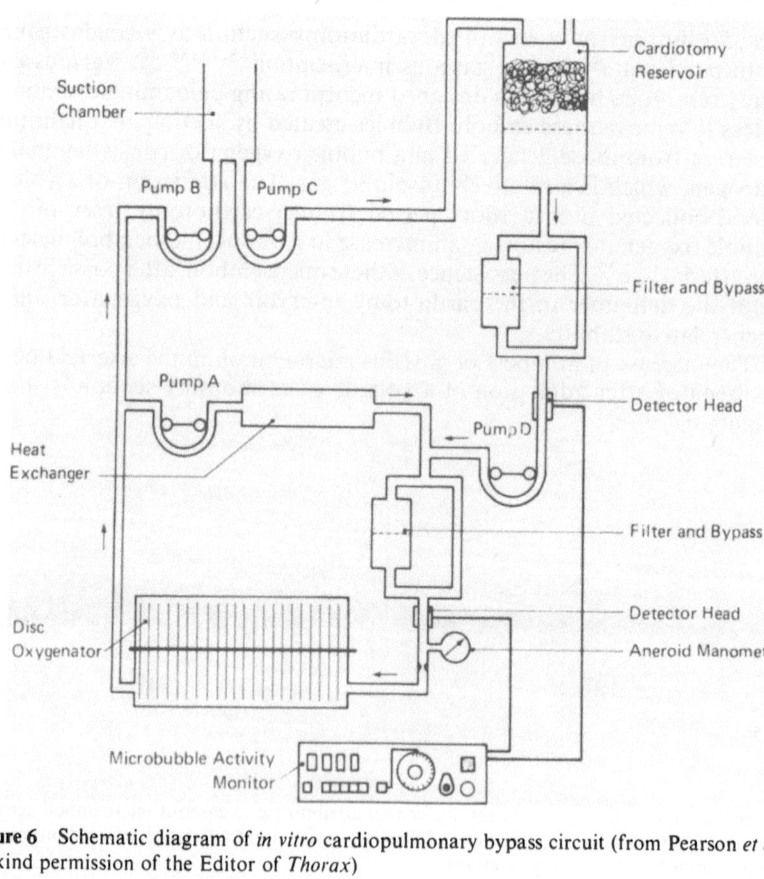

Figure 6 Schematic diagram of *in vitro* cardiopulmonary bypass circuit (from Pearson *et al.*[35] by kind permission of the Editor of *Thorax*)

37 °C by a heat-exchanger. The detector head of a TM8 Microbubble Activity Monitor was applied to the external surface of the circuit tubing.

The blood in the circuit was circulated without rotation of the discs in the oxygenator until free of gaseous microemboli. Blood was then pumped at 0.5 l/min from the main circuit to the base of an open-ended jar by pump B. At the same time a mixture of blood and air was aspirated from the jar by pump C, whose flow rate could be adjusted to vary the proportion of blood and air. This mixture, simulating cardiotomy suction, was discharged into the cardiotomy reservoir under investigation.

When a suitable volume of blood had collected in the cardiotomy reservoir it was returned to the main circuit either directly or via a micropore blood filter at 0.5 l/min by pump D. The microbubble monitor was applied distal to the cardiotomy reservoir, micropore filter and bypass loop to assess the number of gaseous microemboli remaining in the blood.

Initial experiments demonstrated that with a given cardiotomy reservoir, the numbers of gaseous microemboli varied by less than 5% in successive experiments. In view of this consistency it was possible to compare the efficiency of microbubble removal of different types of cardiotomy reservoir and to measure the further improvement produced by micropore filtration either below the reservoir or in the main circuit. Each experiment was repeated three times and the main circuit allowed to become bubble-free between each experiment.

RESULTS

Using a Polystan HL282DF cardiotomy reservoir sequential experiments were carried out following collection of blood in the reservoir. This blood was pumped without micropore filtration past the detector head immediately following collection, or after it had remained in the reservoir for varying periods of time. The decline in numbers of gaseous microemboli greater than 10 μm in diameter remaining in the blood, in relationship to increasing storage time, is shown in Figure 7.

The relative speeds of Pumps B and C determine the blood/gas volume ratio of the simulated cardiotomy suction blood. The effluent from a Polystan HL 282DF cardiotomy reservoir showed an increasing number of gaseous microemboli as the proportion of air in the blood injected into the reservoir increased (Figure 8).

Using a blood/gas volume ratio of 1/2.7 in the simulated cardiotomy suction blood an equal volume was successively injected into 12 commercially available cardiotomy reservoirs. The effluent was immediately pumped past the detector head without micropore filtration or following passage through an Ultipor filter. The results (Figure 9) show a wide variation in the ability of the reservoirs to remove gaseous microemboli but in all cases an improvement in performance was achieved by using a micropore filter below the reservoir. This experiment has recently been updated to reassess previously investigated reservoirs, and to compare their efficiency with design modifications carried out by the manufacturer (Figures 10 and 11). Cardiotomy

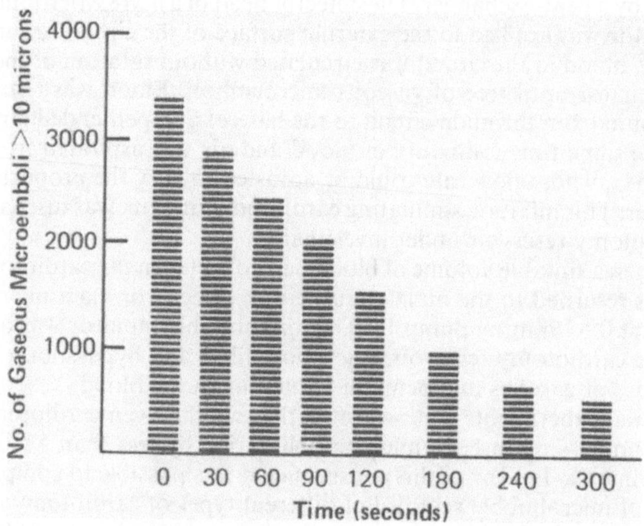

Figure 7 Numbers of gaseous microemboli $>10\ \mu m$ remaining in effluent from Polystan HL 282DF cardiotomy reservoir in relation to duration of storage time (from Pearson *et al.*[35] by kind permission of the Editor of *Thorax*)

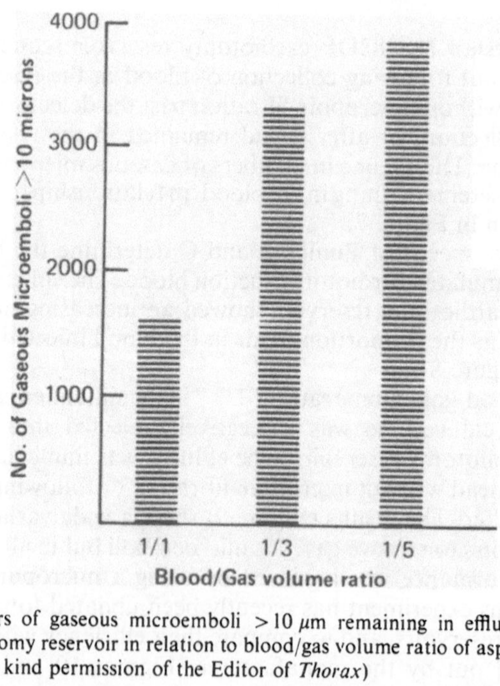

Figure 8 Numbers of gaseous microemboli $>10\ \mu m$ remaining in effluent from Polystan HL 282DF cardiotomy reservoir in relation to blood/gas volume ratio of aspirated blood (from Pearson *et al.*[35] by kind permission of the Editor of *Thorax*)

reservoirs are also included which were not assessed for efficiency in the original work. The results again indicate a wide variety in performance (Figure 12).

When a micropore filter and bypass are inserted in the main circuit, the effluent from the cardiotomy reservoir can be discharged directly into this circuit with the detector applied to the tubing distal to the filter (Figure 6). In this way the ability of the microfilter to retain gaseous microemboli when sited in the simulated arterial line can be compared with its efficiency when sited below the cardiotomy reservoir. In that the priming volume of the main circuit exceeded 3 l and the flow rate of pump A was 2.5 l/min no gaseous microemboli were counted twice if the duration of counting did not exceed 1 min. An anaeroid manometer was placed in the main circuit and the line pressure adjusted to 13.3 kPa (100 mmHg) distal to the filter by means of a screw clamp. The results (Figure 13) show that the numbers of gaseous microemboli from a Polystan HL 282DF cardiotomy reservoir were reduced by micropore filtration situated in the 'arterial line' but a greater reduction was achieved by inserting the filter below the cardiotomy reservoir. A greater overall reduction in numbers of gaseous microemboli was obtained when the

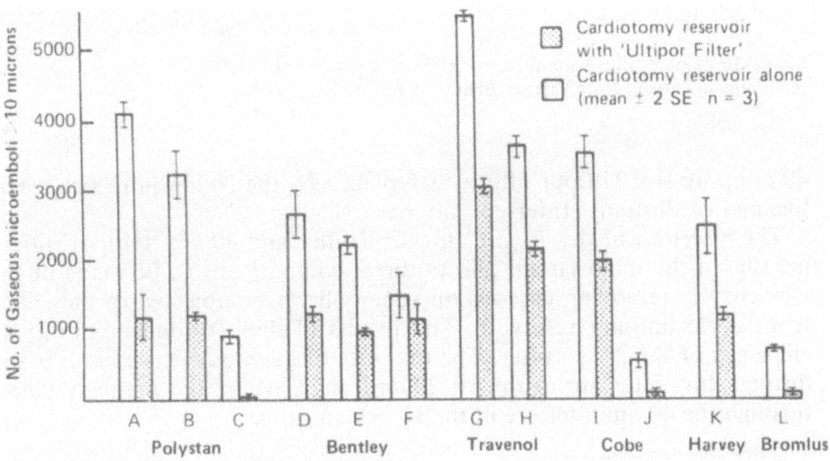

Figure 9 Comparative numbers of gaseous microemboli $>10\ \mu m$ remaining in effluent from various cardiotomy reservoirs with and without filtration by a 40 μm Ultipor filter (from Pearson *et al.*[35] by kind permission of the Editor of *Thorax*).

A. Polystan HL 282DF cardiotomy reservoir
B. Polystan HL 280DF cardiotomy reservoir
C. Polystan 40 cardiotomy reservoir
D. Bentley Q220 disposable expanded volume cardiotomy reservoir
E. Bentley Q120 disposable cardiotomy reservoir
F. Bentley Q220F disposable expanded volume cardiotomy reservoir with filter
G. Travenol 2-litre cardiotomy blood reservoir 5MO391
H. Travenol rigid cardiotomy reservoir 5MO305
I. Cobe cardiotomy reservoir 42/301
J. Cobe cardiotomy reservoir with Swank filter 42/300
K. Harvey disposable cardiotomy reservoir model H500
L. Bromlus cardiotomy suction filter and defoamer

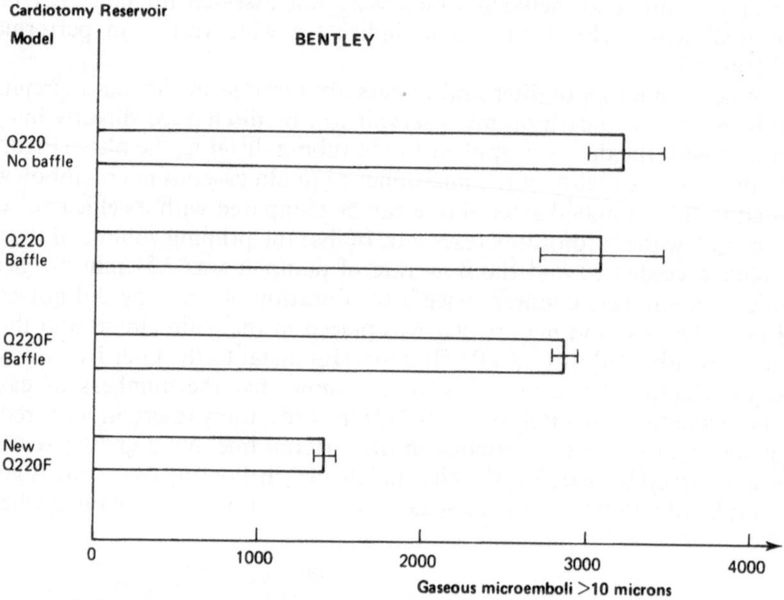

Figure 10 Comparative numbers of gaseous microemboli >10 μm (mean ± 2 SE, n = 3) remaining in effluent from various Bentley cardiotomy reservoirs

40 μm pore size Ultipor filter was replaced by the 20 μm pore size arterial line and cardiotomy 'Intersept' filters.

The insertion of the 20 μm 'Intersept' filter and 40 μm 'Ultipor' filter in parallel in the main circuit allows direct comparisons to be made of their efficiency in removing gaseous microemboli when subjected to the effluent from a cardiotomy reservoir. The results (Table 2) confirm the greater efficiency of the 20 μm filter. The majority of gaseous microemboli passing through this filter are in the 10–20 μm range, whilst the majority passing through the 40 μm filter are in the 10–30 μm range.

Table 2 Size profile of gaseous microemboli detected beyond 'arterial line' filter

	40 μm *'Ultipor' filter*		20 μm *'Intersept' filter*	
Bubble size	*Number*	*Percentage of total*	*Number*	*Percentage of total*
>10	13609	100	6064	100
11–20	8025	59	5372	88
21–30	5064	37	658	11
31–40	470	3	34	1
>41	50	1		

COMMENT

Alterations in perfusion technique will influence the performance of a cardiotomy reservoir. If the blood is stored for as long as possible within the confines of an adequate oxygenator level, not only will the maintenance of a high level reduce splashing of the defoamed blood, but gaseous microemboli will have time to settle out. The greater proportion of air to blood in the aspirate from the heart and pericardium, the more difficult it is for the cardiotomy reservoir to remove completely gaseous microemboli. The speed of the suction pumps should be continuously monitored to allow as low an admixture of air with the blood as is commensurate with the surgical technique. Filtration of blood after passage through a cardiotomy reservoir has been shown to further reduce the numbers of gaseous microemboli. The size and number of gaseous microemboli remaining are related to the pore size of the filter used. A simulated 'arterial line' filter is not as effective at removing gaseous microemboli as is the same filter situated below the cardiotomy reservoir.

This study shows the wide variation in the ability of commercially available cardiotomy reservoirs to defoam aspirated blood and produce an effluent relatively free from gaseous microemboli. Many of the previously described features which influence the ability of a bubble oxygenator to defoam blood

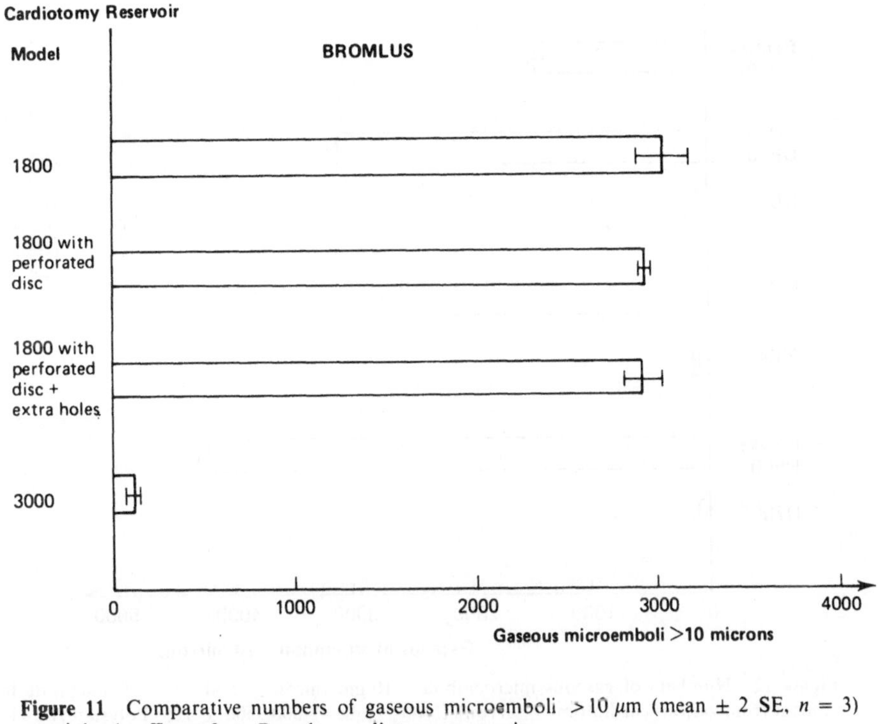

Figure 11 Comparative numbers of gaseous microemboli $>10\ \mu m$ (mean $\pm$ 2 SE, $n = 3$) remaining in effluent from Bromlus cardiotomy reservoirs

are equally applicable to cardiotomy reservoirs. The design of a cardiotomy reservoir can affect its performance:

(a) Some of the reservoirs tested induced turbulence and frothing prior to admission of blood to the defoamer. The addition of a baffle to the Bentley Q200A blood-entry ports did not significantly influence its

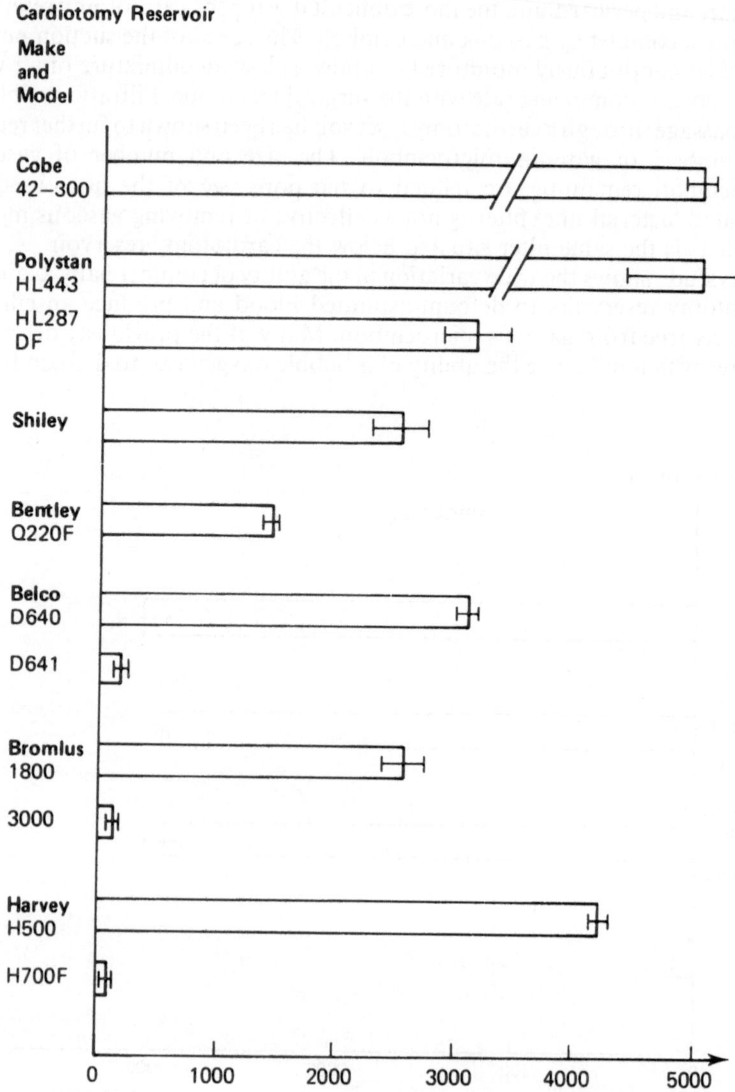

Figure 12 Numbers of gaseous microemboli $>10\ \mu m$ (mean $\pm$ 2 SE, $n = 3$) remaining in effluent from various cardiotomy reservoirs (Note: Cobe 42/300 9500 ± 125; Polystan HL 443 10 000 ± 625)

performance, but this has been improved by a redesign of the blood entry ports (Figure 10).

(b) A proportion of aspirated blood can bypass the defoaming substance in some reservoirs. The Travenol 5MO391 suffers from this design fault. The Bromlus 1800 series cardiotomy reservoir performed better during initial experiments than in the update series. It is understood that the shape and amount of the defoaming substance has been reduced in the later model allowing some aspirated blood to bypass the defoamer. The efficiency of the reservoir could not be improved by attempting to alter the pattern of blood flow through the defoamer by insertion of various holed baffles (Figure 11). The addition of micropore filtration to this reservoir in the Bromlus model 3000 has improved its performance.

(c) Some reservoirs, having defoamed the blood, allow it to fall into the storage part of the reservoir with splashing. The Bentley series of cardiotomy reservoirs, including the model with integral micropore filtration, did not perform as well as expected for this reason. Other reservoirs are similarly inefficient.

(d) Of the reservoirs tested those which incorporated integral micropore filtration performed best. The three Polystan reservoirs are essentially similar in overall design but show progressive improvement in efficiency as the pore size of the filter is reduced from 180 through 120 to 40 μm (Figure 9). The Bentley Q200F reservoir, incorporating a 27 μm filter, did not perform as well as other cardiotomy reservoirs with filters since excessive turbulence was induced at the blood inlet ports and splashing occurred in the storage part of the reservoir.

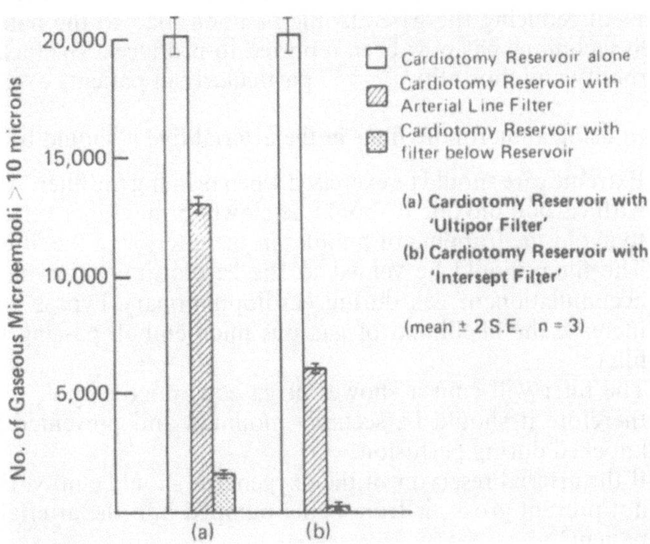

Figure 13 Comparison of efficiency of micropore filters sited below cardiotomy reservoir and in a simulated arterial line (from Pearson *et al.*[35] by kind permission of the Editor of *Thorax*)

No reference has been made to the ability of cardiotomy reservoirs to deal with non-gaseous microemboli and surgical debris. Other workers have evaluated various devices used in the cardiotomy reservoir system in this respect[31,33]. We have not tested the long-term use of the cardiotomy reservoirs and filters.

An analysis of the design features of the cardiotomy reservoirs, assessed by correlation of their *in vitro* performance, overall configuration, type of defoamer and pore size of the incorporated filter material, suggests that optimal efficiency can be achieved by direct injection of aspirated blood into the defoamer and filtration with 20 μm nylon mesh. Defoamed and filtered blood should not be allowed to fall into the storage part of the reservoir.

MASSIVE AIR EMBOLISM

The dangers of massive arterial air embolism from extracorporeal equipment are well recognized and frequently result in a fatal outcome for the patient. Devices to prevent accidental emptying of the oxygenator arterial reservoir include:

(1) An audible and visual level alarm attached to the oxygenator, which may include a device which shuts off the arterial pump.
(2) An intra-arterial line ball valve[53].

MICROPORE BLOOD FILTERS

Several authors have recommended the use of arterial line microfiltration as a means of reducing the gaseous microemboli load to the patient[31,54–56], and this technique has now been reported to produce a significant decrease in morbidity and mortality[1,9,23,31] particularly in patients over 65 years of age.

When using a micropore filter in the arterial line it should be noted that:

(1) Extreme care should be exercised when priming the filter. After flushing with carbon dioxide it should be slowly primed in a vertical position to avoid the trapping of bubbles in the interior of the filter medium.
(2) The filter should be vented to the cardiotomy reservoir to prevent accumulation of gas during cardiopulmonary bypass which would increase the likelihood of gaseous microemboli passing through the filter.
(3) The filter will emit a shower of gaseous microemboli when tapped, therefore it should be securely mounted and prevented from being knocked during perfusion.
(4) If the arterial reservoir of the oxygenator should empty, the filter will not prevent gross air from being pumped into the arterial line to the patient[54].
(5) Filters with a 20 μm pore size and depth filters are more effective in removing gaseous microemboli than filters with larger pore size.

Not all investigators are convinced of the need for arterial line filtration[1,57]. Heimbecker *et al.*[57] have demonstrated that an arterial line micropore filter is a grave source of platelet and fibrin destruction due to excessive turbulence and high-frequency vibration of the filter mesh induced by the high blood flow through the filter. This phenomenon did not occur when the filter was placed below the cardiotomy reservoir. In the patients investigated there was an improvement in platelet counts and reduction in postoperative bleeding when an arterial line filter was not used. Postoperative neurological changes did not occur in the absence of an arterial line filter.

Much of the published work on arterial line filtration does not include details of monitoring of heparin therapy. Many of the established protocols for heparin and protamine therapy during extracorporeal circulation are inadequate[58]. The numbers of microemboli detected distal to the arterial line may increase as the activated clotting time decreases[34], and the addition of heparin to the extracorporeal circuit may release gaseous microemboli throughout the extracorporeal circuit[56].

In this Unit we prefer to rely on the integral filtration material within a bubble oxygenator and not add additional arterial line micropore filtration. Using ultrasound as a monitor we have found it difficult to debubble the arterial line filter, and we feel that it gives a false sense of security during perfusion. It is more important to choose the extracorporeal components with care, being aware of their functional characteristics, and to conduct the perfusion in a manner which minimizes the introduction of gaseous microemboli into the arterial line.

CONCLUSION

All patients having open heart surgery using cardiopulmonary bypass receive a variable amount of gaseous microemboli from extracorporeal components and surgical sources. The tolerance of patients to large numbers of these emboli is indicated by the absence of gross psychiatric or neurological damage in the majority of patients subjected to this procedure. It is possible, by careful choice of extracorporeal components and meticulous conduction of perfusion, that elimination of gaseous microemboli will result in a low level of clinical cerebral complications and may reduce subclinical cerebral damage.

A great deal of attention is paid to the analysis of oxygenator and cardiotomy reservoir design and function with respect to microemboli (both gaseous and particulate), and less emphasis has been directed towards surgical sources of gaseous microemboli because it is extremely difficult to standardize and control currently available techniques for removal of surgical air.

There is no doubt that careful attention to the management of equipment during perfusion can be negated by injection of gaseous microemboli into the systemic arterial circulation when the aortic cross-clamp is released, and from the left heart when cardiopulmonary bypass is terminated. Gaseous microemboli from surgical sources are not prevented by arterial line filtration, and can have serious clinical implications. The relative importance of gaseous microemboli originating from the heart needs further assessment and the development of controlled, proven techniques to reduce the amount of 'surgical air', if the safety of cardiac surgery is to be improved.

Acknowledgments

One of us (Dr D. T. Pearson) is in receipt of a research grant from the Department of Health and Social Security.

We are grateful to Mr M. P. Holden, FRCS, for his constructive criticism of the manuscript and for permission to publish the case report. We acknowledge the help of the Department of Photography, Newcastle University, in the preparation of diagrams. Mr A. Sibbald, Department of Anaesthetics, Newcastle University and Mr P. Weatherston, Department of Medical Physics, Freeman Hospital, provided valuable assistance and advice on electronic equipment. Mrs P. Holliday typed the manuscript.

APPENDIX

Avon Medicals Ltd, 1649 Pershore Road, Birmingham B30 3DR
- Bromlus cardiotomy filter and defoamer 1800
- Bromlus cardiotomy filter and defoamer 3000

Bentley Laboratories Ltd, 267 Cranbook Road, Ilford, Essex IG1 4TG
- Q220 disposable expanded volume cardiotomy reservoir
- Q220F disposable expanded volume cardiotomy reservoir
- Q120 disposable cardiotomy reservoir
- BOS 10 bubble oxygenator
- Q200A bubble oxygenator

Albert Browne Ltd, Chancery House, Abbey Gate, Leicester LE4 0AA
- Polystan HL 282DF cardiotomy reservoir
- Polystan HL 280DF cardiotomy reservoir
- Polystan 40 cardiotomy reservoir
- Polystan HL 443 cardiotomy reservoir
- Polystan HL 287DF cardiotomy reservoir

Cobe Laboratories Ltd, 11 Chancel Close, Eastern Avenue, Gloucester GL4 7SN
- Cobe cardiotomy reservoir 42/301
- Cobe cardiotomy reservoir with Swank filter 42/300
- Cobe Optiflo II bubble oxygenator
- Stockert roller-pump

Corning Medical, Corning Ltd, Halstead, Essex CO9 2DX
- Corning 175 automatic pH/blood gas system

Definox Ltd, 12 Brambleton Avenue, Farnham, Surrey
- Belco cardiotomy reservoir D 640
- Belco cardiotomy reservoir D 641

Devices Instruments Ltd, Welwyn Garden City, Hertfordshire
Devices M2R-35 chart recorder

GU Manufacturing Co. Ltd, Plympton St, London NW8 8AB
Harvey cardiotomy reservoir with filter H700F
Harvey disposable cardiotomy reservoir H500
Harvey bubble oxygenator H1000
Harvey bubble oxygenator H1100

Johnson and Johnson Ltd, 260 Bath Road, Slough, Berks SL1 4EA
Intersept arterial extracorporeal blood filter
Intersept cardiotomy extracorporeal blood filter

Pall Biomedical Ltd, Walton Road, Portsmouth PO6 1TD
Pall Ultipor blood filter

Shiley Ltd, Shiley House, 42 Thames St, Windsor, Berks SL4 1PR
Shiley cardiotomy reservoir
Shiley bubble oxygenator S100

Technique Laboratories Ltd, 1 High St, Hartley Wintney, Hants RG27 8PE
TM8 microbubble activity monitor

Travenol Laboratories Ltd, Caxton Way, Thetford, Norfolk IP24 3SE
2 l cardiotomy blood reservoir 5MO391
Rigid cardiotomy reservoir 5MO305
TMO membrane oxygenator

References

1. Aberg, T. (1974). Effect of open heart surgery on intellectual function. *Scand. J. Thorac. Cardiovasc. Surg.*, Suppl. 15
2. Aberg, T. and Kihlgren, M. (1977). Cerebral protection during open heart surgery. *Thorax*, **32,** 525
3. Aguilar, M. J., Gerbode, F. and Hill, J. D. (1971). Neuropathological complications of cardiac surgery. *J. Thorac. Cardiovasc. Surg.*, **61,** 676
4. Branthwaite, M. A. (1975). Prevention of neurological damage during open heart surgery. *Thorax*, **30,** 258
5. Branthwaite, M. A. (1972). Neurological damage related to open heart surgery. *Thorax*, **27,** 748
6. Brennan, R. W., Patterson, R. H. and Kessler, J. (1971). Cerebral blood flow and metabolism during cardiopulmonary bypass. *Neurology*, **21,** 665
7. Lee, W. H., Jr., Brady, M. P., Rowe, J. M. and Miller, W. C. Jr. (1971). Effects of extracorporeal circulation upon behaviour, personality and brain function. 2. Haemodynamic metabolic and psychometic correlations. *Ann. Surg.*, **173,** 1013
8. Tufo, M., Ostfeld, A. M. and Shekelle, R. (1970). Central nervous system dysfunction following open heart surgery. *J. Am. Med. Assoc.*, **212,** 1333
9. Branthwaite, M. A. (1973). Detection of neurological damage during open heart surgery. *Thorax*, **28,** 464
10. Javid, H., Tufo, H. M., Najafi, H., Dye, W. S., Hunter, J. A. and Julian, O. C. (1969). Neurological abnormalities following open heart surgery. *J. Thorac. Cardiovasc. Surg.*, **58,** 502

11. Branthwaite, M. A. (1974). Cerebral blood flow and metabolism during open heart surgery. *Thorax*, **29**, 633
12. Sanderson, J. M. Wright, G. and Sims, F. W. (1972). Brain damage in dogs immediately following pulsatile and non-pulsatile blood flows in extracorporeal circulation. *Thorax*, **27**, 275
13. Wright, G. and Sanderson, J. M. (1972). Brain damage and mortality in dogs following pulsatile and non-pulsatile blood flows in extracorporeal circulation. *Thorax*, **27**, 738
14. Allardyce, D. B., Yoshida, S. H. and Ashmore, P. G. (1966). The importance of microembolism in the pathogenesis of organ dysfunction caused by prolonged use of the pump oxygenator. *J. Thorac. Cardiovasc. Surg.*, **52**, 706
15. Editorial. (1975). Brain damage after open heart surgery. *Lancet*, **2**, 399
16. Patterson, R. H. and Kessler, J. (1969). Microemboli during cardiopulmonary bypass detected by ultrasound. *Surg., Gynaecol. Obstet.*, **129**, 505
17. Solis, R. T., Noon, G. P., Beall, A. C. and DeBakey, M. E. (1974). Particulate microembolism during cardiac operation. *Ann. Thorac. Surg.*, **17**, 332
18. Lee, W. H., Krumhaar, D., Fonkalsrud, E. W., Schjeide, O. A. and Maloney, J. V. (1961). Denaturation of plasma proteins as a cause of morbidity and death after intracardiac operations. *Surgery*, **50**, 29
19. Cassie, A. B., Riddell, A. G. and Yates, P. O. (1960). Hazard of antifoam emboli from a bubble oxygenator. *Thorax*, **15**, 22
20. Baglio, C. M. and Hunter, W. C. (1959). Calcific arterial embolisation accompanying commisurotomy. *J. Thorac. Surg.*, **37**, 490
21. Caguin, F. and Carter, M. G. (1963). Fat embolisation with cardiotomy with the use of cardiopulmonary bypass. *J. Thorac. Cardiovasc. Surg.*, **46**, 665
22. Evans, E. A. and Wellington, J. S. (1964). Emboli associated with cardiopulmonary bypass. *J. Thorac. Cardiovasc. Surg.*, **48**, 323
23. Osborn, J. J., Swank, R. L., Hill, J. D., Aguilar, M. J. and Gerbode, F. (1970). Clinical use of a Dacron wool filter during perfusion for open heart surgery. *J. Thorac. Cardiovasc. Surg.*, **60**, 575
24. Fishman, N. H., Carlsson, E. and Roe, B. B. (1969). The importance of the pulmonary veins in systemic air embolism following open heart surgery. *Surgery*, **66**, 655
25. Gallagher, E. G. and Pearson, D. T. (1973). Ultrasonic identification of sources of gaseous microemboli during open heart surgery. *Thorax*, **28**, 295
26. Groves, L. K. and Effler, D. B. (1964). A needle-vent safeguard against systemic air embolism in open heart surgery. *J. Thorac. Cardiovasc. Surg.*, **47**, 349
27. Lawrence, G. H., McKay, H. A. and Sherensky, R. T. (1971). Effective measures in the prevention of intraoperative aeroembolus. *J. Thorac. Cardiovasc. Surg.*, **62**, 731
28. Starr, A. (1960). The mechanism and prevention of air embolism during correction of congenital cleft mitral valve. *J. Thorac. Cardiovasc. Surg.*, **39**, 808
29. Selman, M. W., McAlpine, W. A. and Ratan, R. D. (1967). The effectiveness of various heart lung machines in the elimination of microbubbles from the circulation. *J. Thorac. Cardiovasc. Surg.*, **53**, 613
30. Austen, W. G. and Howry, D. H. (1965). Ultrasound as a method to detect bubbles of particulate matter in the arterial line during cardiopulmonary bypass. *J. Surg. Res.*, **5**, 283
31. Loop, F. D., Szabo, J., Rowlinson, R. D. and Urbanek, K. (1976). Events related to microembolism during extracorporeal perfusion in man. Effectiveness of in line filtration recorded by ultrasound. *Ann. Thorac. Surg.*, **21**, 412
32. Patterson, R. H. and Kessler, J. (1969). Microemboli during cardiopulmonary bypass detected by ultrasound. *Surg. Gynaecol. Obstet.*, **129**, 505

33. Solis, R. T., Scott, M. A., Kennedy, P. S. and Wilson, R. K. (1976). Filtration of cardiotomy reservoir blood. *J. Extracorp. Technol.*, **8,** 69
34. Abts, L. R., Beyer, R. T., Galletti, P. M., Richardson, P. D., Karon, D., Massimino, R. and Karlson, K. E. (1978). Computerised discrimination of microemboli in extracorporeal circuits. *Am. J. Surg.*, **135,** 535
35. Pearson, D. T., Watson, B. G. and Waterhouse, P. S. (1978). An ultrasonic analysis of the comparative efficiency of various cardiotomy reservoirs and micropore blood filters. *Thorax*, **33,** 352
36. Moulinier, H. and Masurel, G. (1978). Detection of bubbles in blood vessels and the evaluation of their flow. *Med. Biol. Eng. Comput.*, **16,** 585
37. Furness, A., Wright, G. and Sanderson, J. M. (1979). Detection of bubbles in blood vessels and extracorporeal circuits. Letter to the Editor. *Med. Biol. Eng. Comput.*, **17,** 534
38. Maynard, D., Prior, P. F. and Scott, D. F. (1969). Device for continuous monitoring of cerebral activity in resuscitated patients. *Br. Med. J.*, **4,** 545
39. Miller, B. J., Gibbon, J. H., Greco, V. F., Cohn, C. H. and Allbritten, F. F. (1963). The use of a vent for the left ventricle as a means of avoiding air embolism to the systemic circulation during open cardiotomy with the maintenance of the cardio-respiratory function of animals by a pump oxygenator. *Surg. For.*, **4,** 29
40. Nicks, R. (1969). Air embolism in cardiac surgery: incidence and prophylaxis. *Austr. N.Z. J. Surg.*, **38,** 328
41. Senning, A. (1952). Ventricular fibrillation during extracorporeal circulation used as a method to prevent air embolisms and to facilitate intracardiac operations. *Acta Chir. Scand.*, Suppl. 171
42. Burbank, A., Ferguson, T. B. and Burford, T. H. (1965). Carbon dioxide flooding of the chest in open heart surgery. *J. Thorac. Cardiovasc. Surg.*, **50,** 691
43. Nichols, H. T., Morse, D. P. and Hirose, T. (1958). Coronary and other air embolisation occurring during open cardiac surgery. *Surgery*, **43,** 236
44. Taber, R. E., Maraan, B. M. and Tomatis, L. (1970). Prevention of air embolism during open heart surgery. A study of the role of trapped air in the left ventricle. *Surgery*, **68,** 685
45. Bass, R. M. and Longmore, D. B. (1969). Cerebral damage during open heart surgery. *Nature* (*London*), **222,** 30
46. Clark, R. E., Dietz, D. R. and Miller, J. G. (1976). Continuous detection of microemboli during cardiopulmonary bypass in animals and man. *Circulation*, **54,** 74
47. Bethune, D. W. (1976). Organ damage after open heart surgery. (Letter). *Lancet*, **2,** 1410
48. Karlson, K. E., Murphy, W. R., Kakvan, M., Anthony, P., Cooper, G. N., Richardson, P. D. and Galletti, P. M. (1974). Total cardiopulmonary bypass with a new microporous Teflon membrane oxygenator. *Surgery*, **76,** 935
49. Solis, R. T., Kennedy, P. S., Beall, A. C., Jr., Noon, G. P. and DeBakey, M. E. (1975). Cardiopulmonary bypass. Microembolisation and platelet aggregation. *Circulation*, **52,** 103
50. Simmons, E., MaGuire, C., Lichti, E., Helvey, W. and Almond, C. (1972). A comparison of the microparticles produced when two disposable-bag oxygenators and a disc oxygenator are used for cardiopulmonary bypass. *J. Thorac. Cardiovasc. Surg.*, **63,** 613
51. Kessler, J. and Patterson, R. H., Jr. (1970). The production of microemboli by various blood oxygenators. *Ann. Thorac. Surg.*, **9,** 221
52. Miller, D. R. and Allbritten, F. F. (1960). Coronary suction as a source of air embolism: an experimental study using the Kay–Cross oxygenator. *Ann. Surg.*, **151,** 75
53. Burgess, M. F. (1977). A new anti-air embolism device. *AMSECT Proc.*, **23**

54. Mandl, J. P. and Wise, E. A. (1978). Comparison of the Agger with the Intersept arterial line filter at removing gaseous microemboli. *J. Extracorp. Technol.*, **10,** 187
55. Miller, S. S. and Mandl, J. P. (1977). Comparison of the effectiveness of various extracorporeal filters at reducing gaseous emboli. *AMSECT Proc.*, **55**
56. Streczyn, M. V. (1977). Gas emboli arterial line filtration. Efficiency of Pall and J–J filters under stress conditions. *AMSECT Proc.*, **6**
57. Heimbecker, R., Robert, A. and McKenzie, F. N. (1976). The extracorporeal pump filter – saint or sinner? *Ann. Thorac. Surg.*, **21,** 55
58. Bull, B. S., Korpman, R. A., Huse, W. M. and Briggs, B. D. (1975). Heparin therapy during extracorporeal circulation. 1. Problems inherent in existing heparin protocols. *J. Thorac. Cardiovasc. Surg.*, **69,** 674

23
The value of prostacyclins in cardiopulmonary bypass

D. B. LONGMORE

Cardiopulmonary bypass has been a routine procedure for a quarter of a century. Until the advent of prostacyclin, there has been no opportunity for revolutionary changes in technique. To improve safety surgical results have gradually improved because of small incremental refinements of technique. Better prosthetic implants and a better understanding of homograft materials have also helped. From the late 1950s to the early 1970s, open heart surgery was still a specialist procedure too difficult and too expensive to be undertaken outside specialized centres. It was routine only on adults with well-advanced disease, and on children and infants with congenital deformities. The indications for surgery were strict. Only patients with disease so advanced that it was potentially lethal were referred for operation and then only when cardiac failure was imminent. The possibilities of bacterial endocarditis or advancing pulmonary hypertension were also indications for surgery.

The patient spectrum has changed over the past 5 years. One of the most common cardiac operations now is the coronary vein graft. In 1979 over 90 000 coronary vein graft operations were done in the USA where it is nearly as common as appendicectomy. Frequently, this procedure is carried out on the fit patient who only complains of chest pain. This operation, because of the patients which present, is mainly done on active males in the prime of their working life. Figure 1 shows the incidence of deaths from coronary artery disease compared with all other causes of death in England and Wales and the USA in a typical year.

Coronary artery blockage is usually part of a generalized occlusive vascular disease. Accordingly, it is naive to assume that any surgery which is undertaken can be anything but palliative. Figure 1 also shows the relative incidence of coronary artery disease and cerebrovascular disease in England and the USA. The figures for deaths from these two diseases added together in a typical year are similar in the two countries at over 52 %. The histogram shown in Figure 1 is further subdivided to separate the mortality of males

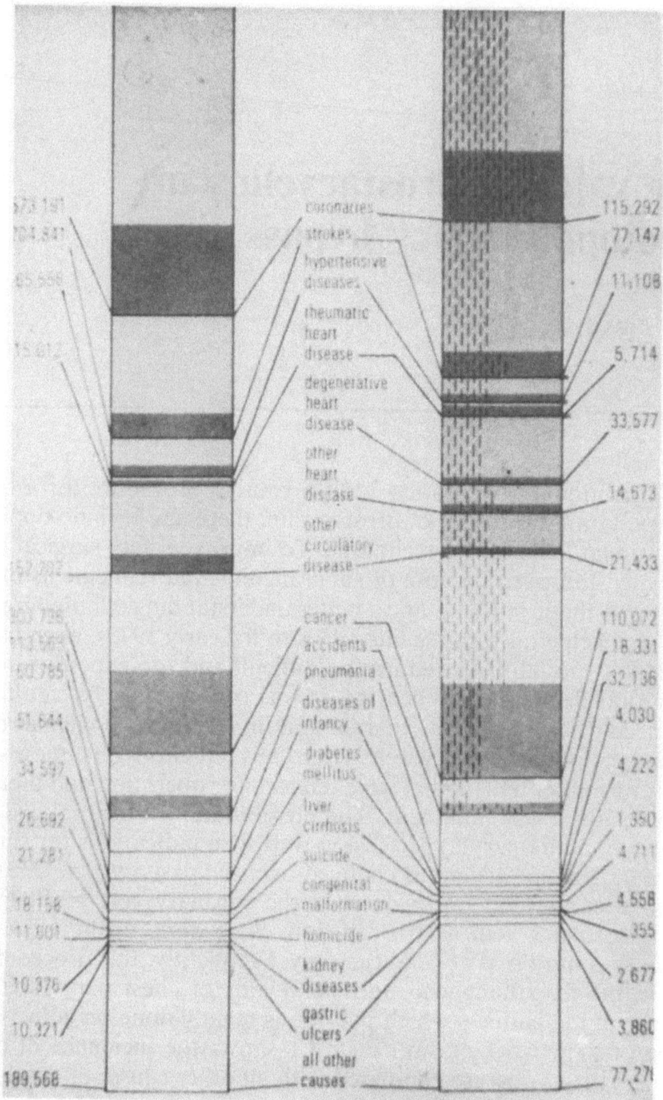

Figure 1 The histogram shows the causes of death in England and Wales and the United States in a typical year. The vertical hatching is for males and the dark shading relates to the working age group. It may be seen that coronaries are the biggest single cause of death in the males in the working age group and that cardiovascular disease accounts for 52% of all deaths

from females, and the working age group aged 16–64 years from deaths at all ages. This breakdown shows that the commonest cause of death in the working male is coronary artery disease. The figures also suggest that cerebrovascular disease is frequently associated with coronary disease in that group.

Figure 2 shows the inexorable increase in the incidence of coronary artery deaths in the United Kingdom since 1931 when reliable figures became available for the first time. Not only is coronary artery disease now numerically the most important cause of death, but because of the steady increase it promises to be an even more sinister threat to productive life in future. Statistics on follow-up results show that coronary artery surgery can now offer an increased life-expectancy. Elimination of pain on exertion and an increased exercise tolerance are expected. The hospital mortality in good centres is now below 5%. Nevertheless surgical triumphs of this kind are worthless if the patient's brain is so damaged during operation that he is unable to hold down his job, or unable to live in harmony with his family. He may even become irresponsible and a burden to the community. Many of these patients have become accustomed, preoperatively, to pain and physical limitations, and cope well with these. Postoperative cerebral damage and severe psychiatric disturbances are far more difficult for the patient and family to manage. Sometimes the low hospital mortality figures conceal many postoperative problems. A patient who leaves hospital may have undergone a second operation for bleeding, or have had to endure many painful hours of intensive care.

A multi-million-dollar industry has been built up around cardiopulmonary bypass. Physicians, surgeons, and manufacturers of equipment are conscious that something needs to be done to make heart surgery easier and safer, and to eliminate brain injury and psychiatric disturbance. The difficulty has always been that the causes of complications are manifold. The manufacturers of equipment tend to blame the surgeon for any complications which occur. The surgeon, on the other hand, has so many ancillary products and procedures to whom he can attribute his potentially disastrous difficulties that he may overlook his own shortcomings of technique. There has never before been a medical problem of such complexity and importance. There are two entities the manifestations of which are not easy to separate. On the one hand, a patient's decreased postoperative cerebral function may be due to organic brain damage; whilst on the other, apparently similar symptoms can arise entirely from psychological damage and stress. To compound the problem, the brain injury and disturbance may pre-exist either as a complication of the heart disease or as a result of carotid artery disease. Furthermore, it can occur in the preoperative, operative, and postoperative periods. The discovery of prostacyclin (PGI_2) by John Vane and his group in the Wellcome Research Laboratories in 1977 gives us a new hope for safer cardiac surgery and the reduction of the problem of brain injury. Its use eliminates many causes of cerebral embolization. Prostacyclin also promises to eliminate propagating thrombus associated with embolization. It is the first major conceptual advance in cardiopulmonary bypass since the technique was introduced.

Prostacyclin is a prostaglandin. It is one of the metabolites of arachidonic acid. It is now recognized as the natural substance which prevents intravascular clotting. Arachidonic acid, its precursor, metabolizes in two ways: (1) in the platelet, to form thromboxane A2, which is a vital component of the clotting cascade and a powerful vasoconstrictor; (2) in the vessel wall, to form prostacyclin which is secreted into the plasma adjacent to the endo-

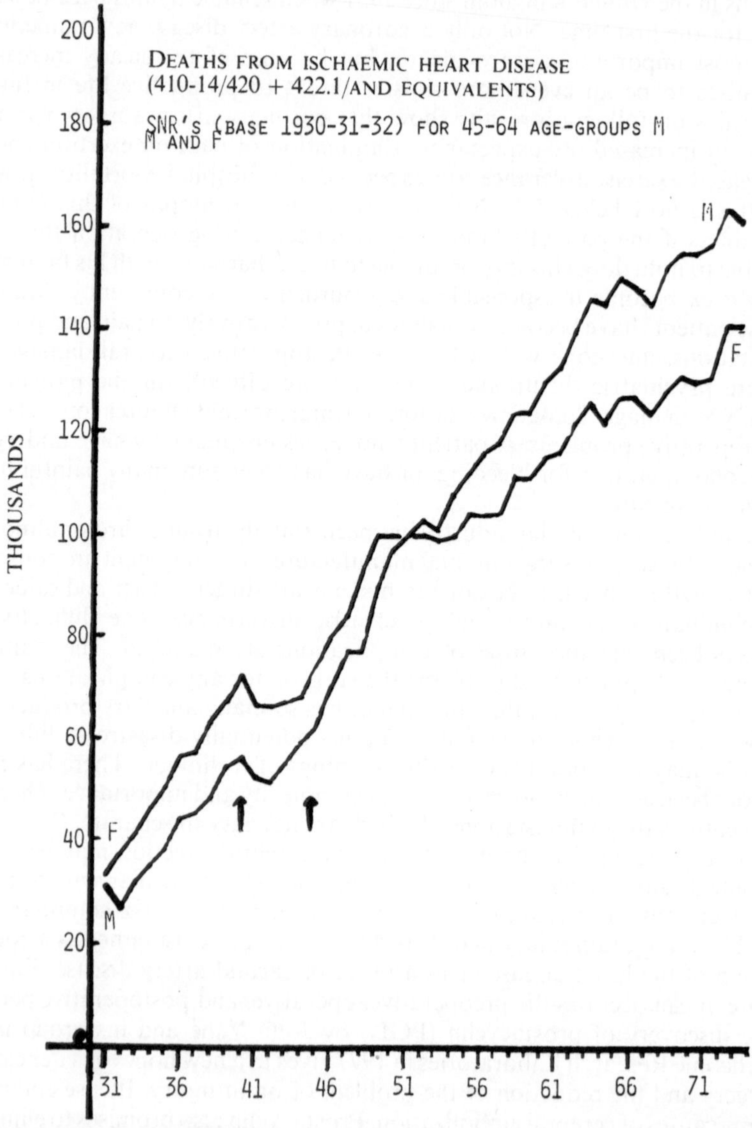

Figure 2 Shows the increase in the incidence of coronaries in males and females since 1931. The two arrows cover the period of World War II. It should be noted that in 1950, co-incidental with the introduction of drugs to control hypertension there was a decrease in the acceleration of the incidence of coronaries in females

thelium. Prostacyclin interacts with the surface of platelets to stabilize them. The effect is to prevent platelet aggregation and breakdown. It is also a vasodilator.

Platelet loss and aggregation in open heart surgery has always been linked with postoperative disorders, including bleeding and cerebral damage. Uncontrollable bleeding is even more pronounced when extracorporeal oxygenation is used for long-term respiratory support. Attempts to overcome the bleeding diathesis associated with bypass have included the use of less traumatic oxygenation methods, other improvements in the extracorporeal apparatus, inclusion of 20–40 μm filters in the arterial lines, removal of arterial filters from the circuit and the use of other less effective inhibitors of platelet aggregation including dipyrimadole (Persantin) and PGE_1 – all without success.

Although the use of heparin during cardiopulmonary bypass prevents gross clotting of blood, the clotting system, even in the presence of heparin, is stimulated when blood passes over a foreign surface such as the extracorporeal tubing. During a typical 90-min bypass, blood passes through approximately 20 miles of tubing. The blood also passes over vast areas of non-physiological, often bio-incompatible material. Platelet adhesion and activation start immediately after contact between blood and a foreign surface, and results in formation of platelet aggregates enmeshing white and red blood cells. Figure 3 shows a typical thrombus formation 2 minutes after exposure of a silicone rubber membrane to heparinized blood. There is release of anti-heparin activity and pro-coagulant activity from platelets and leukocytes after contact with foreign surfaces, causing fibrin deposition despite the presence of heparin.

Platelets adhere to, and aggregate on, any surface other than normal vascular endothelium even if heparinization is adequate. Now we know that endothelium is not inert and that it actively generates prostacyclin. Prostacyclin added to the blood in the extracorporeal apparatus should be beneficial, for several reasons: it should prevent the initiation of the clotting mechanism and prevent embolism from blood products; it should also prevent small emboli from foreign material from enlarging, and prevent clots from propagating. Platelet aggregates and microthrombi are always present in the blood leaving an extracorporeal circuit, and on return to the patient are known to be responsible for thrombotic occlusion of the microvasculature. Defibrination leads to severe postoperative bleeding problems. The use of inhibitors of platelet activity, particularly persantin and prostaglandin E_1, during extracorporeal circulation have been reported previously but with variable results. Prostacyclin generated by the vessel walls is the most potent anti-aggregating agent yet discovered. Like prostaglandin E_1, it acts by increasing platelet cyclic AMP. It is, however, approximately 30 times more potent than PGE_1; this is because it is the natural mechanism whereby the healthy blood vessel resists the deposition of platelet aggregates and consequent thrombus formation.

The value of the addition of prostacyclin to the extracorporeal circuit to inhibit platelet activity has been previously demonstrated in animal experiments, in renal dialysis and charcoal haemoperfusion.

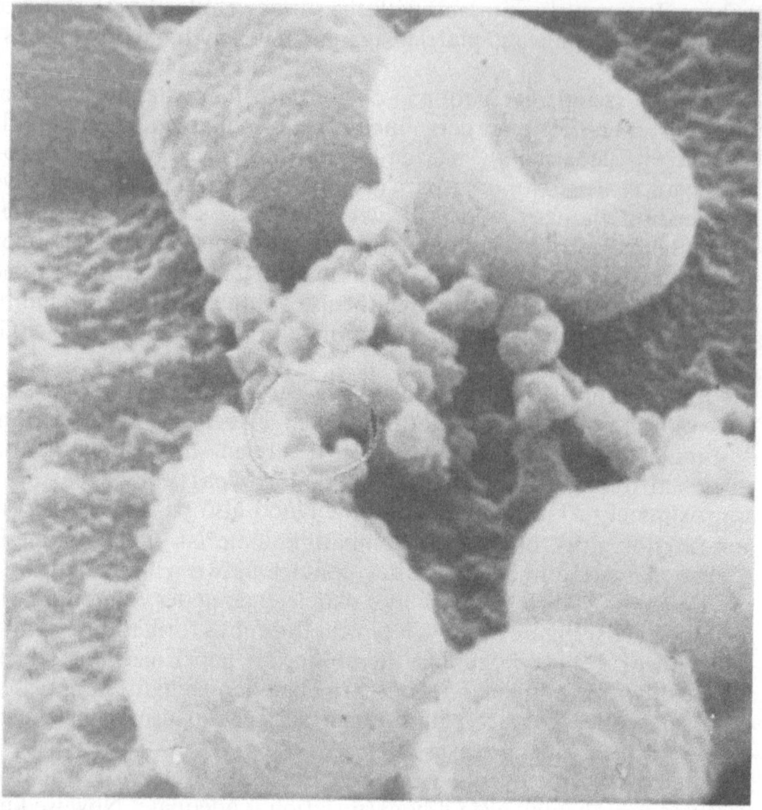

Figure 3 Shows clot on the surface of a silicone rubber membrane when heparinized blood has been exposed to it for less than 5 minutes

We have studied its use in extracorporeal circulation in dogs. Our experimental results were so encouraging that we have now started a human clinical trial. In our experimental work we studied the use of prostacyclin alone, heparin alone and a combination of both at various dose levels. We also tried unsuccessfully to repeat the work reported by Fletcher on cardiopulmonary bypass in primates using haemodilution alone – without the use of any anticoagulants.

For the experiments we used a simple cardiopulmonary bypass apparatus with a Bentley Temptrol Paediatric Oxygenator, a single-roller arterial pump with two filters in series in the arterial line. The animals were bypassed for 2 hours. Serial platelet counts, platelet aggregations and fibrinogen levels were done in 15-minute intervals. Samples of blood were also taken 5 minutes after bypass was started and 5 minutes before the end of bypass to study protein denaturation, using the fetal heart toxicity test. This technique is fully described in Chapter 28.

In addition to these studies, the haematocrit was measured, screen filtration pressure tests were done to demonstrate the presence of platelet aggregates, and the pressure differential across the two arterial filters was measured. Figure 4 shows the bypass apparatus with the pressure take-off points proximal to the first filter and distal to the first and the second filters. An increasing pressure gradient between these two points indicates that the

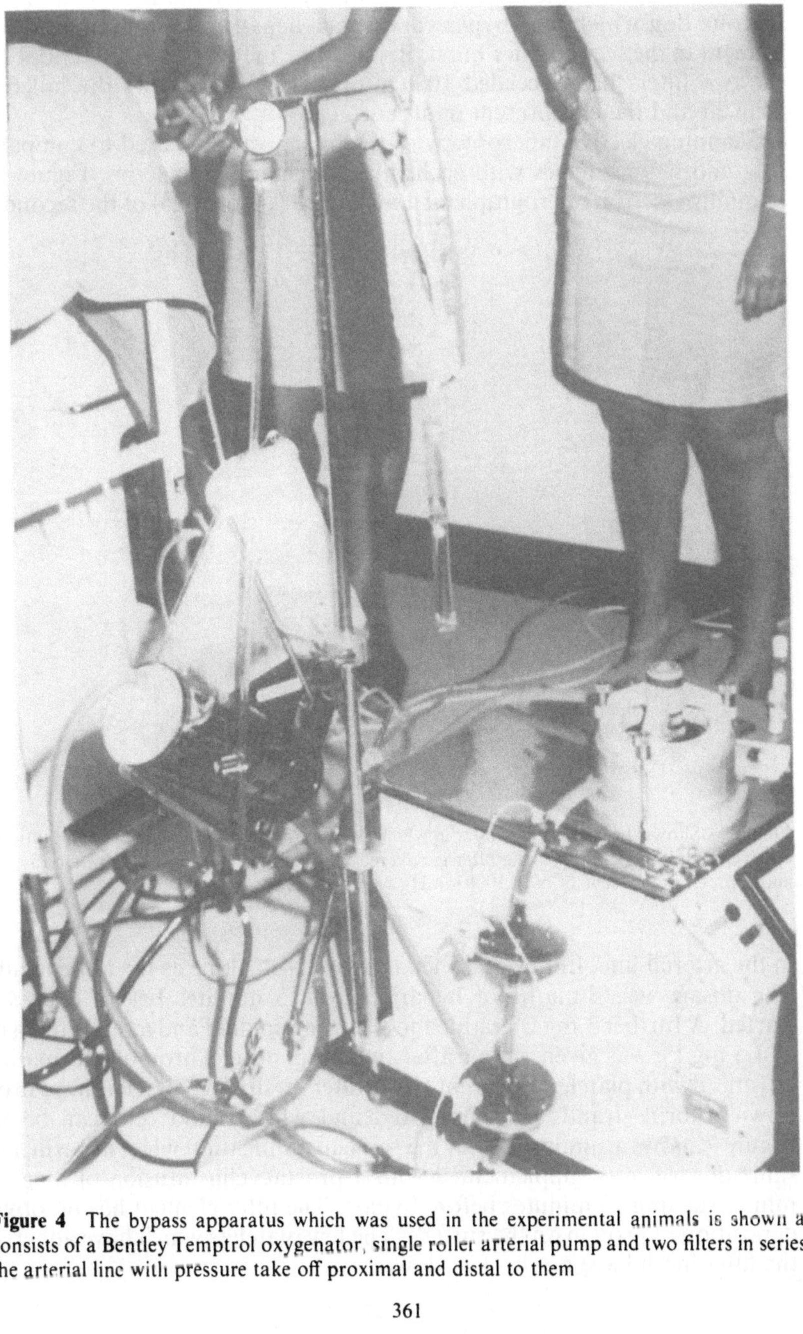

Figure 4 The bypass apparatus which was used in the experimental animals is shown and consists of a Bentley Temptrol oxygenator, single roller arterial pump and two filters in series in the arterial line with pressure take off proximal and distal to them

filters are becoming blocked either with clot or platelet aggregates. When the pressure gradient across one or both of the filters was seen to rise slowly and then fall suddenly, it was assumed that the filter had blocked and unloaded the deposits blocking its mesh into the arterial line. When this happened in the proximal filter, the pressure drop was transferred to the second filter. In the one dog which was bypassed without heparin or protamine, the filter element in the second filter burst. By this time the pressure differential across the two filters had exceeded 1000 mmHg. Figure 5 shows the failed filter element and the clot present on its surface.

Scanning electron microscopy of the filters was also used to compare the first and second filters with each other in each of the series. Figure 6 is a scanning electron micrograph (at a magnification of 3125) of the second filter

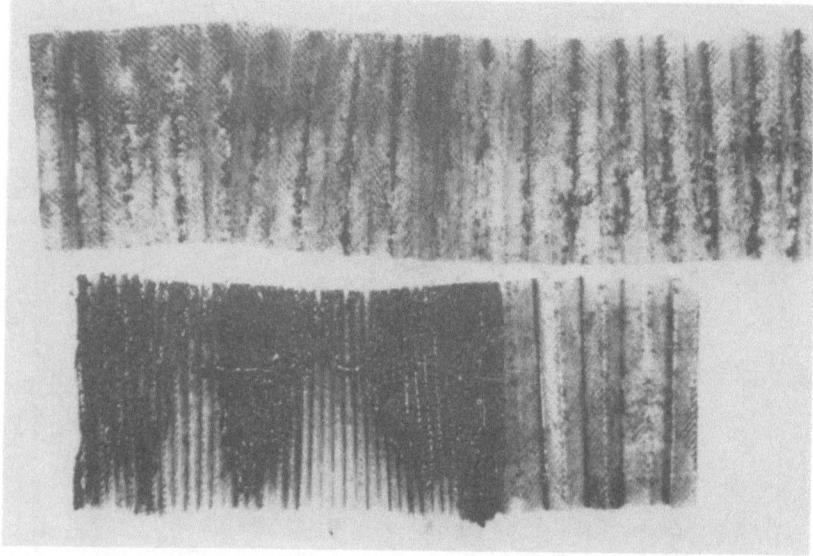

Figure 5 Shows the element of a filter in which an attempt was made to use haemodilution only in cardiopulmonary bypass. The filter is covered with massive clot and burst after 15 minutes and a pressure gradient of over 1000 mmHg was recorded

in the arterial line. In this case, heparin was used alone as the anticoagulant. The dosage was 3 mg/kg of heparin, given 5 minutes before bypass was started. A further 3 mg was added to the priming fluid and a reinforcing dose of 1.5 mg/kg was given 1 hour after the initial dose. Thrombus formation is advanced with platelets adherent to the filter mesh. The platelets have broken down. Fibrin strands enmeshing red and white blood cells can be seen. Figure 7 shows a similar filter at the same magnification when heparin, at the same dosage, was supplemented with a prostacyclin infusion of 8 ng kg^{-1} min^{-1} starting 15 minutes before bypass. The filter element has no obvious deposition of protein on the surface. The few platelets which have adhered to the filter mesh have not broken down.

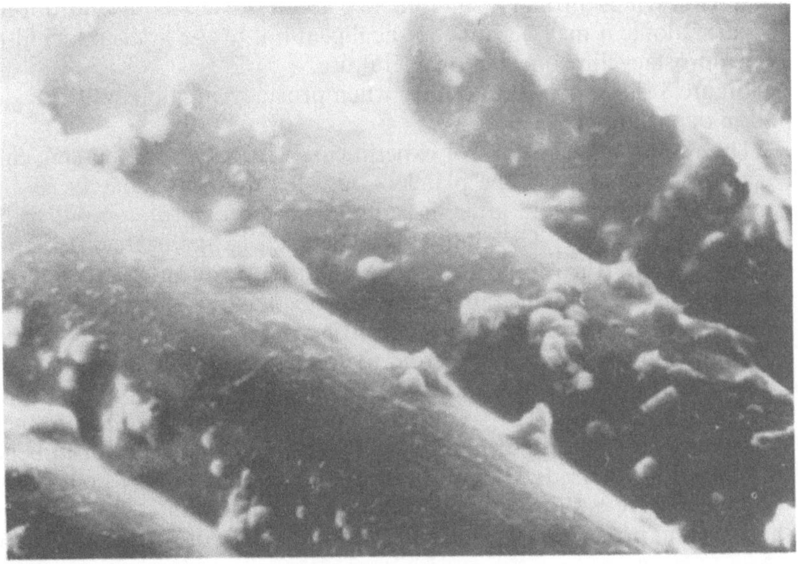

Figure 6 Scanning electron micrograph, magnification × 3125 of the surface of the second filter in the arterial line when heparin alone was used. Note the amount of platelet emboli and thrombus formation

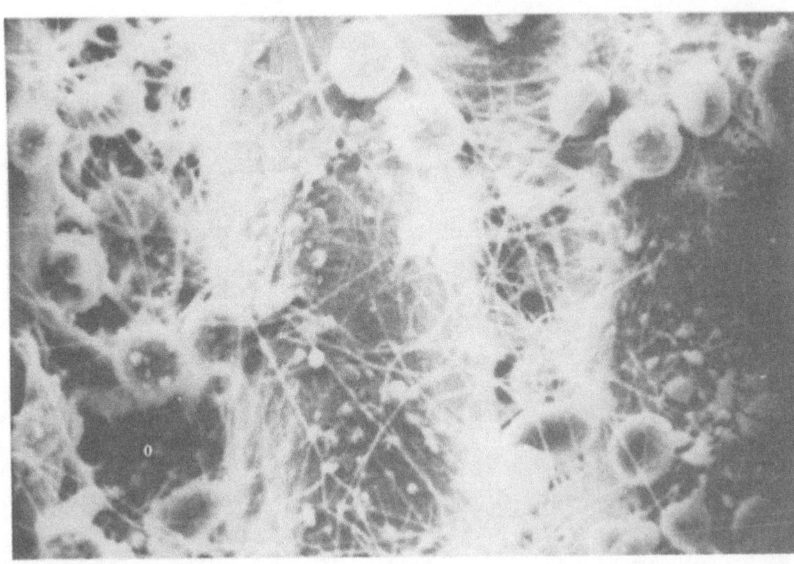

Figure 7 Scanning electron micrograph, magnification × 3125 of the second filter in the arterial line when PGI_2 was added to the heparin showing occasional deposition of platelets but no clot

Whereas it is probably malpractice to use arterial line filtration with heparin alone, it may be similarly negligent not to use arterial line filtration when prostacyclin comes into general use.

Figure 8 shows the second filter when prostacyclin alone was used. Some fibrin deposits were seen.

The results of this series of experiments were clear. In the conventional 'heparin alone' bypass, the platelet count fell to approximately 30% of its preoperative figure and after the administration of protamine there was a further drop to 25%. The ability of the platelets to aggregate was reduced to about 15% of their preoperative level, thus confirming the well-known clinical observation that after bypass with heparin and neutralization of heparin with protamine, the blood clotting mechanism is severely impaired. There was pressure build-up across the filters and scanning electron microscopy of both filters showed massive platelet deposition, thrombus formation and partial blockage. The second filter was as severely involved as the first, suggesting that the use of filters in the arterial line is of doubtful benefit if heparin alone is used. The filters appear to create as many emboli as they remove. Figure 9 shows the comparative platelet counts with heparin and heparin plus prostacyclin. Figure 10 shows the return of normal aggregation in

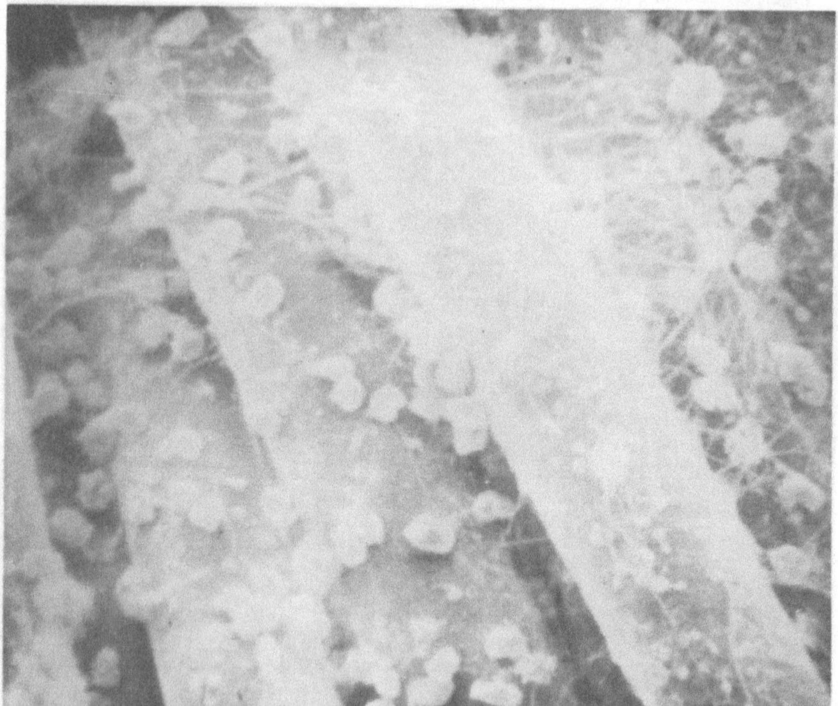

Figure 8 Shows the surface of the second filter when PGI_2 alone was used showing some platelet deposition and some fibrin strands

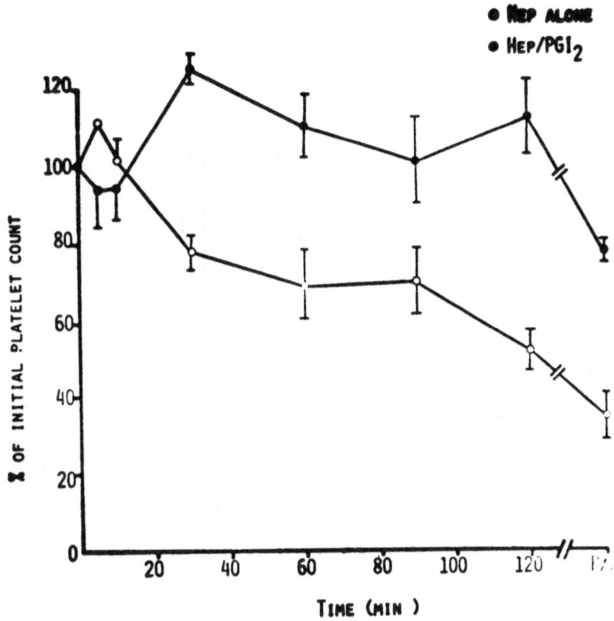

Figure 9 Shows the comparative platelet counts in heparin alone and heparin and PGI_2. It should be noted that protamine further reduces the platelet count. The // line indicates the administration of protamine.

the heparin and prostacyclin bypass. There was virtual elimination of platelet activity after administration of protamine in the conventional heparin bypass. Figure 11 shows the comparison of the beating rate and the survival time in the fetal heart test, with blood taken from animals with conventional heparinization. Figure 12 compares fibrinogen levels in the three groups. The fall in plasma fibrinogen in the prostacyclin-alone bypass is due to clot formation in the stagnant areas of the oxygenator which was used. The clot formation can be prevented by gentle agitation of the oxygenator.

Careful examination of the micrographs of the filters shows that, in addition to the absence of clot formation, there is no visible protein film on the fibres of the second filter when prostacyclin is used, suggesting that prostacyclin might be counterproductive when microporous membranes are used. Scanning electron microscopy of membrane oxygenators in the presence of prostacyclin shows a protein layer.

The positive results of the animal study have led us to start a clinical trial. We are at present undertaking a double-blind study. The 60 patients in the study undergo psychometric testing 2 days before operation and post-operatively at 3 and 6 days. We also do neurological examinations at the same intervals. The following tests are done preoperatively, postoperatively, and at 15-min intervals during the bypass:

haematocrit; haemoglobin; platelet count; corrected platelet count; fibrinogen levels; thrombin clotting time; PTTK; prothrombin time; euglobin clot lysis time; fibrinogen degradation products; white blood

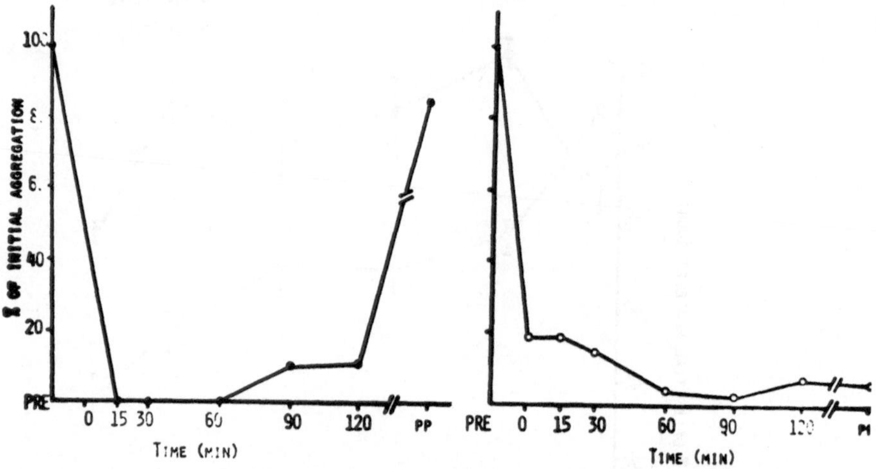

Figure 10 The left hand side of this graph shows the percentage of initial aggregation of ADP in the presence of PGI_2. There is almost complete inhibition of platelet function during bypass with recovery after cessation of administration of PGI_2. On the right the failure of platelet function to recover is shown.

count; platelet aggregation; percentage initial platelet aggregation; haemochron time; antithrombin III; screen filtration pressure; heparin levels; plasma haemoglobin levels; blood pressure recording before, during, and after prostacyclin infusion; perfusion pressure; perfusion flow rates; Coulter counted platelets; CK total; CKMB; thromboxane A_2; heart rate; blood loss 0–6 h, 6–12 h, 12–18 h; blood given; urine output; fluids given; rewarming time; protein denaturation and damage test (fetal heart culture method); particle counts in pump washings; particle counts in pump prime; particle counts in any drugs which are administered.

I will now review the place of prostacyclin in cardiopulmonary bypass, emphasizing its potential for preventing brain injury. To do this it is necessary to define the main causes of multi-organ and cerebral injury in the pre-operative period, and postoperatively. The significance of the presence of prostacyclin is described with relation to each of the common causes of organ damage.

Table 1 The main preoperative period causes of brain damage

1. *Cerebral emboli* from clot in the left side of the heart
2. *Paradoxical embolization* through defects in the cardiac septa
3. *Septic emboli* from infection in the heart
4. *Stroke and transient ischaemic attacks* due to carotid obstruction

Note: The causes of brain damage which are eliminated or potentially reduced by prostacyclin are italicized in this and in all subsequent tables.

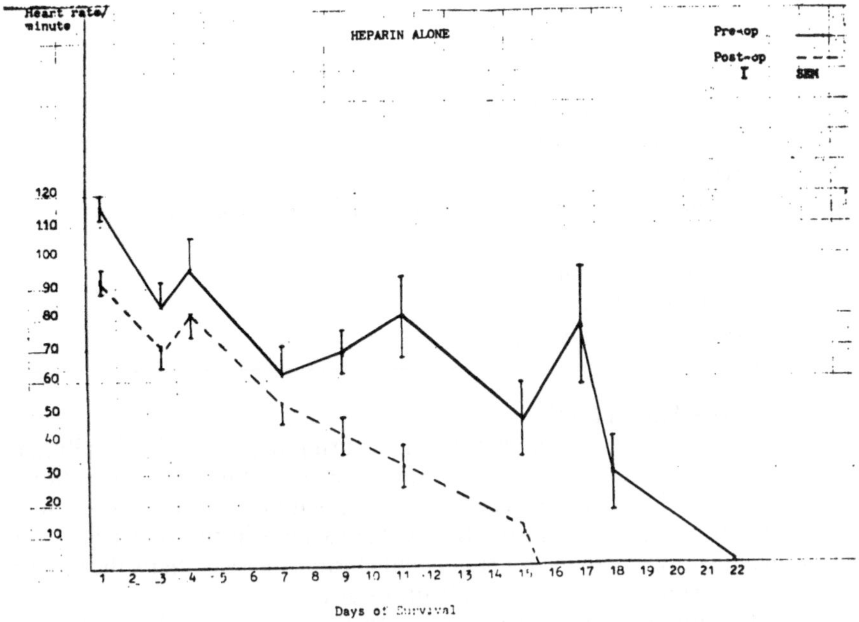

Figure 11 The foetal heart toxicity test shows the diminution of the beating rate and a reduction in survival time in animals which were bypassed with heparin alone. This was not seen when PGI_2 was used.

Although the use of prostacyclin does not avoid all possible sources of brain damage in these three phases of the patient's treatment, many of the commoner and most of the more serious causes are partially or completely eliminated with prostacyclin.

It is easy for the surgeon who is evaluating the patient for operation and for the referring physician to overlook the existence of a history of previous cerebral disturbances. There is always a tendency for the surgical team to concentrate only on the purely cardiac aspects of the diagnosis. The surgeon has to decide whether the muscle of the heart on which he is planning to operate will in fact still function as an effective pump after the insult of surgery and cardiopulmonary pass. This problem may exercise him so much that he may overlook warning features in the medical history. In any case, a history of psychiatric illness and transient stroke is frequently glossed over or suppressed by the patient who wants an operation. There is less justification for a surgeon failing to detect the presence of previous cerebral emboli, but it can be overlooked even in cases of mitral stenosis and left atrial myxoma where it classically occurs. It is usually overlooked in patients with previous myocardial infarcts. The reason for this is that neurological recovery is often fairly complete and the patient may appear to be normal. A careful neurological examination will reveal residual disabilities, but usually this is not done.

Organ damage during operation is very much more common than pre-operative causes of injury, the main ones being listed in Table 2.

Table 2

1.	*Air embolization*
2.	*Particle embolization*
3.	*Embolization from blood products*
4.	Toxins from the extracorporeal apparatus
5.	Haemolysis
6.	Toxins due to protein denaturation caused by mechanical damage
7.	Hypotension
8.	Biochemical disturbances
9.	Abnormal blood gases
10.	Inadequate anaesthesia

AIR EMBOLIZATION

The commonest cause of embolization during bypass is air, usually termed surgical air, which is left in, or let into, the heart during the operation. The inside of the heart is roughened and ridged with the presence of the musculi pectinati in the atria and the trabeculae carneae in the ventricles. Any air which is allowed into the heart is usually beaten into a froth by the movement of the heart and is extremely difficult to dislodge.

Air commonly enters the aorta when the aortic cannula is inserted and when cold cardioplegic solutions are introduced under pressure. Figure 13 shows how dangerously cardioplegic solutions are introduced. Figure 14 reminds us of the dangers of taking pressure measurements on the left side

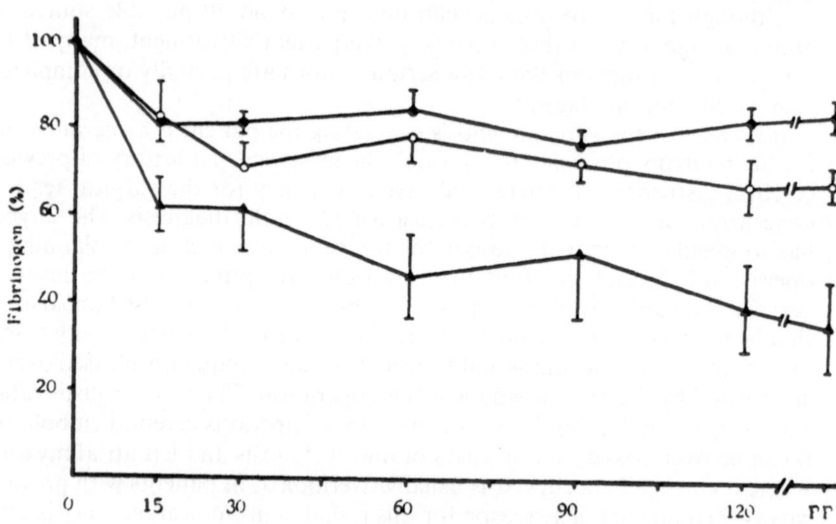

Figure 12 Plasma fibrinogen expressed as a percentage of the original level is shown. The top line is heparin and PGI_2, the middle line is heparin alone and the lower line is PGI_2 alone showing that some clotting was taking place in the extracorporeal bypass when PGI_2 alone was used.

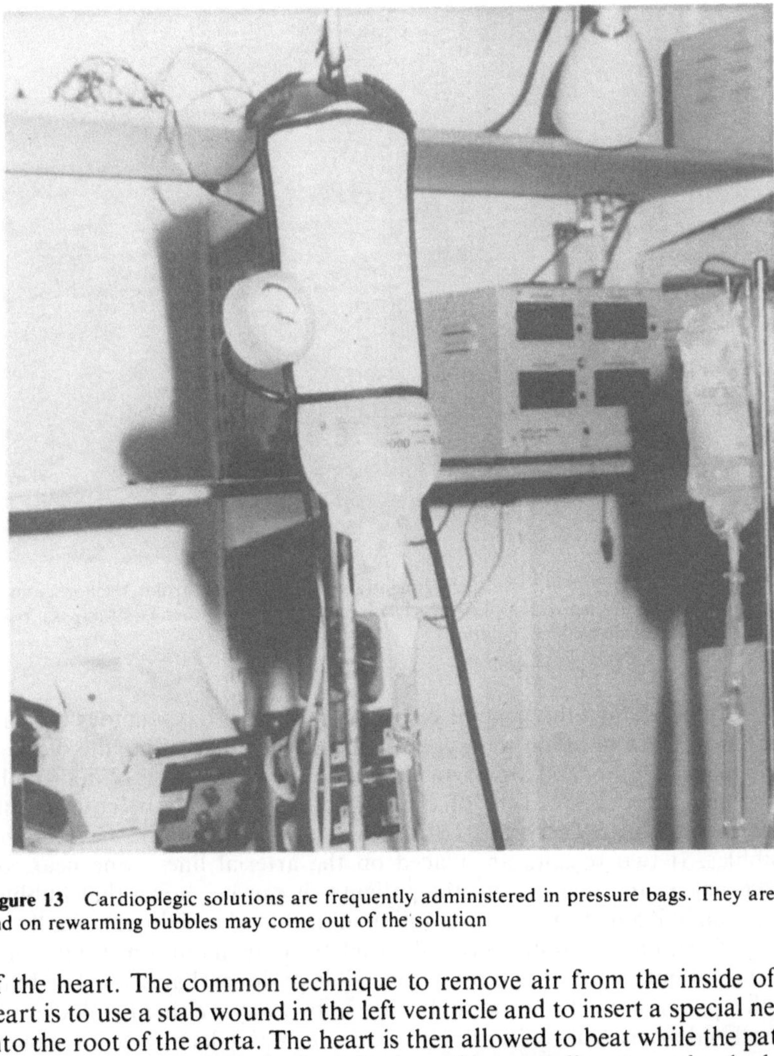

Figure 13 Cardioplegic solutions are frequently administered in pressure bags. They are cold and on rewarming bubbles may come out of the solution

of the heart. The common technique to remove air from the inside of the heart is to use a stab wound in the left ventricle and to insert a special needle into the root of the aorta. The heart is then allowed to beat while the patient is on bypass to expel froth. An injection of isoprenaline, to make the heart beat vigorously and to drive air through the coronary vessels, is often used. In spite of all these precautions bubbles frequently reach the brain and small air bubbles remain on the endocardial surface for many hours and act as a focus for platelet aggregates. The embolus may either consist of platelets surrounding a bubble or streams of pure platelet emboli separating from the bubble surface. The administration of prostacyclin will reduce this problem. Another common source of large bubbles, which can lodge in the brain and similarly act as a site for platelet emboli, is air which is entrained in the arterialized blood leaving the oxygenator when the levels are allowed to drop below the recommended level. Prostacyclin prevents platelet aggregates around these bubbles. All bubble oxygenators pass varying numbers of

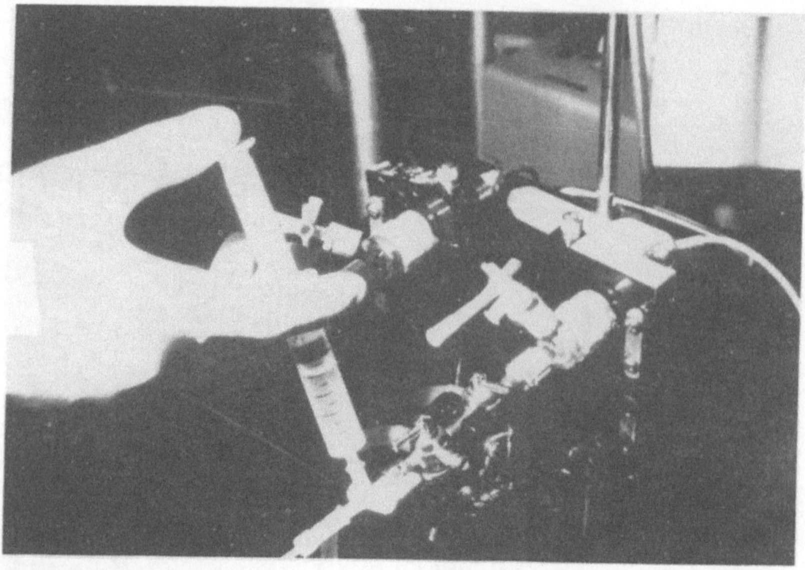

Figure 14 The pressure line which is frequently placed in the left atrium, the aorta and the left ventricle may be flushed with a pressure system or a syringe. In either case there is a risk of air entering the left side of the circulation

microbubbles into the general circulation. Bubble oxygenators depend on making a froth of blood to oxygenate it and then defoaming the blood over silicone anti-foam, and are particularly dangerous. Streams of microbubbles pass into the patient. Tens of thousands of these may be counted in the arterial line during a bypass. Ultrasound equipment can be used to size the bubbles. If two sensors are placed on the arterial line – one near to the oxygenator, and one near to the patient – it can be shown that bubbles of less than half a micron go into solution in the blood and do not usually reach the patient. Larger bubbles not only reach the patient but can also be counted in the patient's carotid and other accessible peripheral arteries. The bubbles which pass into the brain cause damage in two ways: either by blocking vital small end arteries or by forming foci on which platelet aggregates can form. Prostacyclin will eliminate these platelet aggregates.

Membrane oxygenators produce few air-bubbles if they are used properly. Cardiotomy reservoirs are used in most membrane oxygenator circuits. These are a major source of air emboli. Nevertheless most contemporary membrane osygenators use Celgard 2402 or 2502 polypropylene membranes which are made as two-ply microporous membranes, with pore sizes ranging between 200 and 400 Å. To work properly, these membranes depend on a coating of protein which covers the water meniscus bridges across the micropores in the membrane. Figure 15 shows this situation schematically, approximately to scale. The deposition of the protein layer probably depends to some extent on platelet adhesion to the surface and platelet breakdown. In oxygenators with microporous membranes, the administration of prosta-

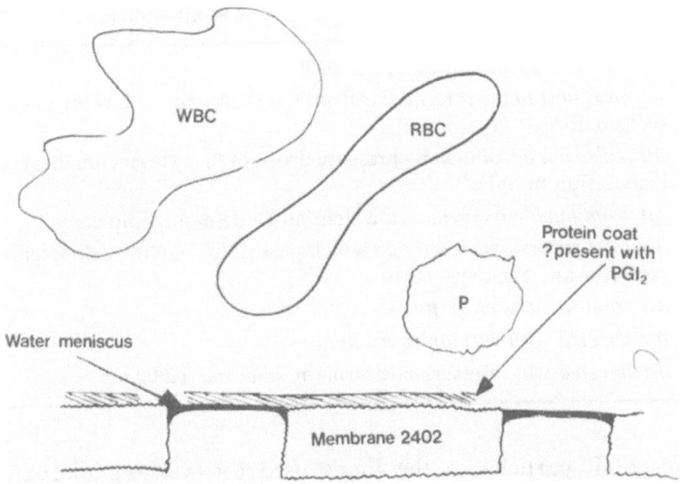

Figure 15 Shows microporous membrane related to the white blood cell, the red blood cell and platelet, approximately to scale. In order to oxygenate properly a protein layer is required to bridge the water meniscus across the pores. It was thought on theoretical grounds that PGI_2 would prevent this taking place. Experimental work has shown that the protein layer is still deposited

cyclin theoretically might not be advantageous. In practice our experimental studies indicate that the formation of the protein layer is independent of platelet activity. The beneficial effect of prostacyclin is to reduce platelet deposition, platelet loss and the thickness of the protein layer, which itself diminishes oxygenating capacity. The beneficial effect may be to allow better gas transference through the membrane because the protein barrier is thinner. The answer to this has yet to be found. We are actively examining membranes at the moment.

There are two other sources of microemboli from the extracorporeal apparatus. Figure 16 shows the changing solubility of dissolved gases in clear fluids at various temperatures. Warming the prime in the bypass apparatus is likely to produce massive gaseous embolization and platelet deposition on the surface of the bubbles. Prostacyclin is beneficial in this situation.

The most dangerous form of air from the extracorporeal apparatus results from the formation of 'cavitation' bubbles in zones of low pressure in the arterial pumps. If the pump is incorrectly adjusted, or if the tubing is dimensionally inaccurate, cavitation bubbles will form.

PARTICLE EMBOLIZATION

There are many sources of particles which pass into the patient during bypass. When bubble oxygenators are used up to 7 g of silicone anti-foam may pass into the patient. This usually enters the patient as a coating on red cells, white cells, and platelets. Prostacyclin should have no influence on the damage which is done to the brain by silicone anti-foam until the anti-foam emboli become foci for platelet thrombi.

Table 3 The main causes of air embolism

1.	*Air left in or let into heart by the surgeon*
2.	*Air entrained in the arterial line* from the pump due to low levels in the oxygenator
3.	*Air pulled out of solution* by pressure drops in the extracorporeal system ('cavitation bubbles')
4.	*Air from bubble oxygenators* which fail to defoam completely
5.	*Air from cardiotomy reservoirs* which passes through the defoamers of the reservoir and the oxygenator
6.	*Air from warmed clear fluids*
7.	*Air injected with cardioplegia solutions*
8.	*Air injected with pressure-measuring needles and cannulae*

We count particles in the fluids used for washing the extracorporeal apparatus in the prime and in any drugs which are added to the extracorporeal apparatus. These particles arise from the closures and rubber aspirating sites as well as from the manufacture of the drugs and precipitates. The number of particles found even after preliminary flushing of the heart lung apparatus is frighteningly large. Nevertheless, the number of particles in the prime is small compared with the vast number produced by spellation

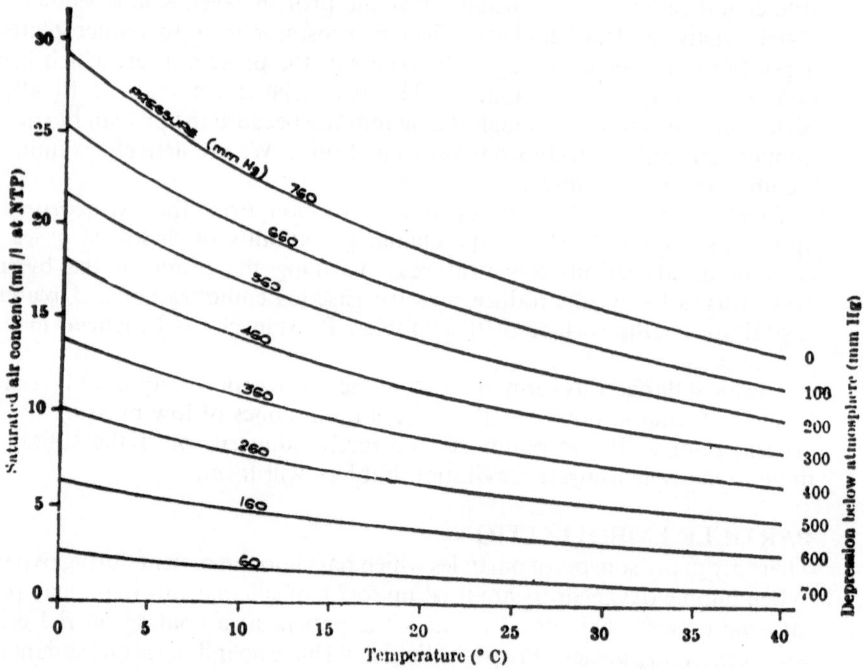

Figure 16 Relates solubility on the vertical axis to the temperature on the horizontal axis. Normal saline at room temperature can hold less dissolved gas than at blood temperature

from the inside of the arterial tubing due to wear and distortion in the plastic pump tube. Whatever the source of particle microemboli all are equally dangerous, and all can be the centre of thrombus formation. Prostacyclin significantly reduces the danger of particle emboli from the apparatus because it prevents enlargement of these due to deposition of platelets on them.

Table 4 The main causes of particle embolization

1.	*Silicone antifoam* from cardiotomy reservoirs and bubble oxygenators
2.	*Plastic debris* in the extracorporeal apparatus left in by manufacturers
3.	*Precipitates and particles* in the prime and added fluids
4.	*Plastic debris due to spellation from the arterial pump tube*

EMBOLIZATION FROM BLOOD PRODUCTS

The prevention of embolization from blood products during bypass is the most obvious area in which prostacyclin would be expected to be beneficial. Prostacyclin, with effect on platelet aggregates, removes a major source of embolization from the extracorporeal apparatus. This alone must significantly reduce the incidence of brain and multi-organ damage. Furthermore, prostacyclin prevents the formation of platelet aggregates on filters in the arterial line. This makes it possible and safe to place filters in this site to remove other potential emboli. In the past alters have been counterproductive, producing more emboli on their own account than they have eliminated.

During conventional bypass operation, even with adequate heparinization, intravascular clotting takes place in recesses of the vascular system and in

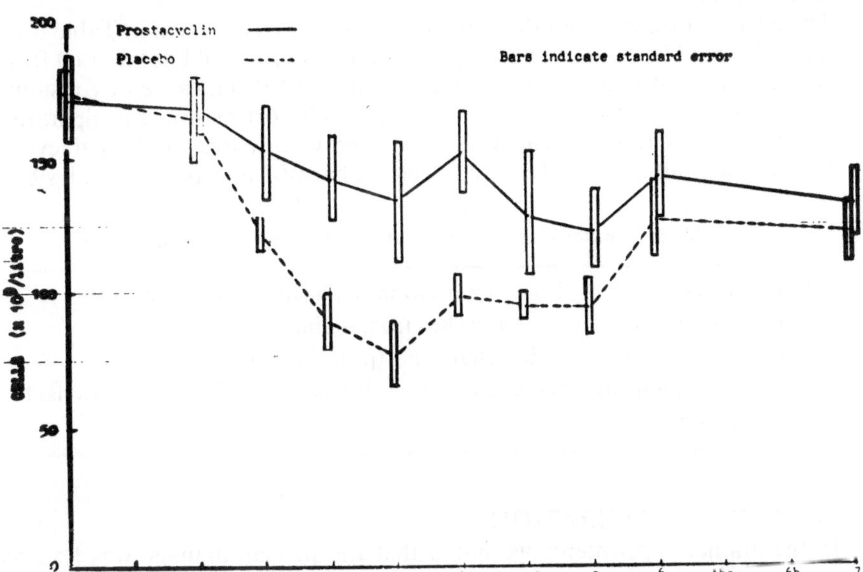

Figure 17 Shows maintenance of normal platelet count during bypass when PGI_2 is used

areas where any vortex or eddy formation is present. In this situation platelets aggregate and liberate an anti-heparin agent causing clot to form. This clot will propagate as more platelets adhere and eventually block important vessels. Prostacyclin completely eliminates this dangerous complication when heparin is used as an anticoagulant.

Another valuable contribution of prostacyclin is reduction in the dose of heparin required; the heparin-sparing effect of prostacyclin. Heparin itself is prepared from several biological sources (animal lung, gut, and liver). Heparin is not a single molecular species. At least some constituents of commercial heparin actually cause the formation of platelet aggregates and microemboli. Prostacyclin eliminates heparin-induced platelet aggregation. The other beneficial effect is that prostacyclin, by reducing the dose level require, eliminates the formation of heparin–protamine macromolecules.

Table 5 The sources of embolization from blood

1. *Platelet aggregates* in the patient
2. *Platelet aggregates from the extracorporeal apparatus* and formed on the arterial filter elements
3. *Whole blood clots from extracorporeal apparatus*
4. *Intravascular clotting*
5. *Heparin–protamine macromolecules*
6. *Heparin-induced platelet aggregates*

TOXINS LIBERATED FROM THE EXTRACORPOREAL APPARATUS

The effects of toxins from the extracorporeal apparatus listed in Table 6 are not influenced by the presence of prostacyclin. This should not detract from consideration of their dangers. Many deaths have been caused by residual ethylene oxide, and freons and plasticizers from the extracorporeal apparatus. When red blood cells are haemolysed the products are toxic, but prostacyclin has no contribution to make in reducing the harmful effects of haemolysis.

Table 6 Toxins from the extracorporeal apparatus during bypass

1. Residual ethylene oxide and freons from sterilization procedures
2. Plasticizers (phthalates, etc.) leached from tubing
3. Drugs administered via the arterial line (penicillin fits, etc.)
4. Changes in tonicity when non-isotonic substances are added to the arterial blood
5. Haemolysis

PROTEIN DENATURATION

In the animal experiments we noted that the protein damage was less, as measured by the very sensitive fetal heart toxicity test, when prostacyclin was used. The reason for this is probably that there were less platelet breakdown products which are thought to be harmful to plasma proteins. This point is not proven.

HYPOTENSION DURING BYPASS

The dose level of prostacyclin is critical, since it is a very potent naturally occurring substance. A high level of circulating prostacyclin can cause hypotension. A dose rate of 2–5 ng kg^{-1} min^{-1} has an anti-platelet effect without dropping the blood pressure. Higher concentrations sometimes cause hypotension. In the conscious subject headache and colic sometimes occur when a dose rate of 9 ng kg^{-1} min^{-1} of prostacyclin is exceeded. In the clinical trail we use a dose level of 8 ng kg^{-1} min^{-1} before bypass, and double this dose when bypass is commenced. We usually see an obvious effect on the platelets with these dose levels. Hypotension is not a problem and vasopressors are not required. Although, theoretically, prostacyclin might be expected to increase brain damage due to any hypotension, this has not been our experience.

Table 7 The causes of hypotension during bypass

1. Low pressures due to anaesthetic and other drugs
2. Low pressures due to inadequate flow
3. Relative hypotension (when patient was hypertensive before operation)
4. Low pressures due to cannulae blocking vessels and reducing cardiac output before going on bypass
5. Non-pulsatile flow causing organ underperfusion

Table 8 The biochemical disturbances which occur during bypass; these are not affected by prostacyclin

1. Due to dilution of blood-reducing enzyme and trace element levels
2. Relative biochemical abnormalities due to distortion by hypothermia of CO_2 levels and selective enzyme inhibition by hypothermia
3. Metabolic or respiratory acidosis

Table 9 The causes of abnormal blood gases which are also not affected by prostacyclin

1. Inadequate oxygenation
2. Over-oxygenation
3. Low CO_2 levels
4. High CO_2 levels

One other cause of brain dysfunction during operation is inadequate anaesthesia during bypass. Anaesthetic agents are diluted when the patient goes on bypass. A patient may be paralysed and awake during substantial periods of the operation, with consequential psychiatric trauma.

Table 10 The causes of brain damage after operation

1.	Hypotension
2.	*Air released from inside the heart*
3.	Excessive drug therapy (hypnotics, diuretics)
4.	Sleep-deprivation, pain and fear in intensive care
5.	*Embolization from clot* on a cardiac implant or disintegration of an implant

Postoperative hypotension due to bleeding sometimes leading to reoperation is a distressingly frequent occurrence when heparin is used. Many surgeons legislate for up to 2 h to be spent obtaining haemostasis before closing the chest after bypass is finished. This is because the few remaining platelets have lost the power to coagulate. When prostacyclin is present, the platelets are protected. Prostacyclin has no influence on the other postoperative causes of brain damage.

Because we have the potential for eliminating, with the use of prostacyclin, so many of the known causes of brain damage, it is now necessary for us to refine our techniques for logging causes of brain damage. By doing this, we should be able to detect, early, any single new cause which appears.

I have set up a dedicated computer to collate data, and I suggest the need for an international study. Preliminary results are now available from the first part of the double-blind trial of prostacyclin and placebo.

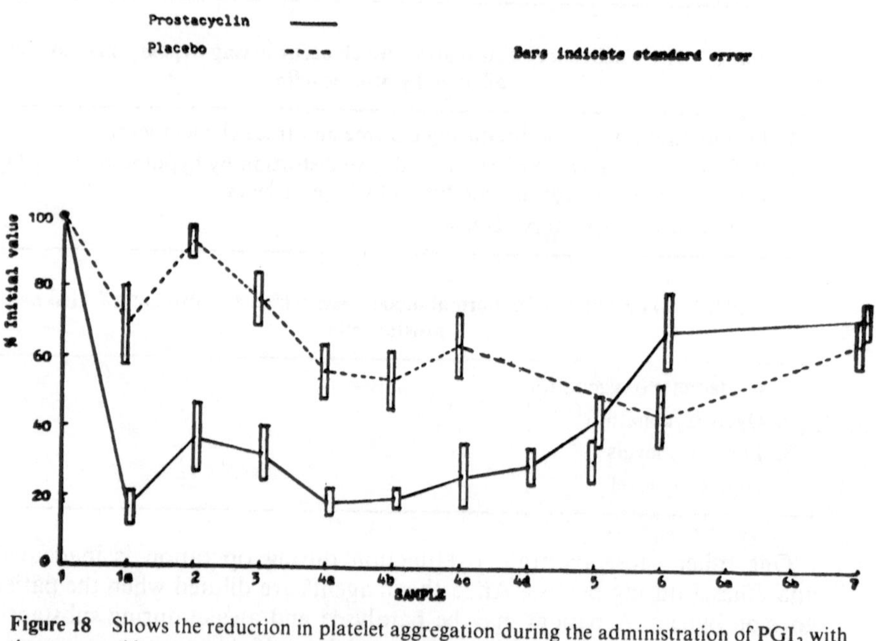

Figure 18 Shows the reduction in platelet aggregation during the administration of PGI_2 with the more rapid return to normal aggregation post bypass

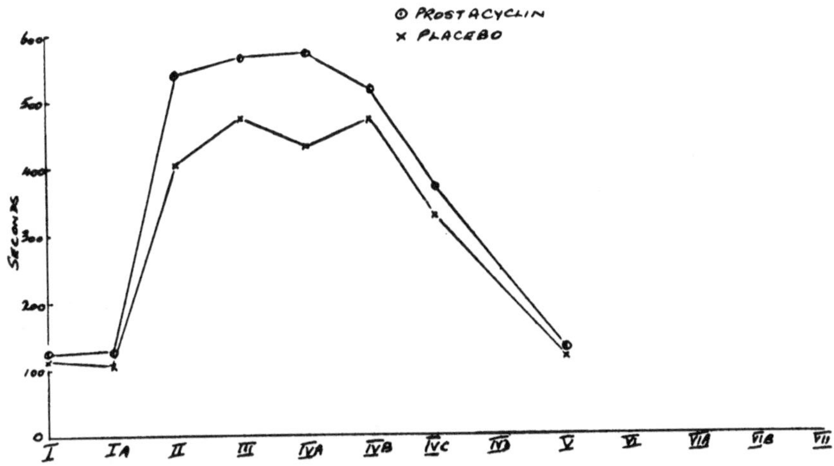

Figure 19 Shows higher haemachron times when PGI_2 is used than when heparin alone is used in similar cases, illustrating the heparin sparing effect of PGI_2.

The results of platelet counts, Figure 17; aggregation, Figure 18; and fibrinogen levels, Figure 19, are similar to those found in the dog experiments. The heparin-sparing effect of prostacyclin is well shown in the haemochron times, which are significantly higher when prostacyclin is used.

The postoperative blood loss is reduced when prostacyclin is used.

Urine output is greater in the prostacyclin group, suggesting that there is better organ perfusion when it is present. The results of psychometric testing and of other tests in the battery are not yet significant, except for the higher CK total levels also suggesting better organ perfusion.

CONCLUSION

We hope now to enter a new era of cardiac surgery. Dry operative fields, no postoperative bleeding, better extracorporeal apparatus which will not fill the patient with emboli, all promise to virtually eliminate organic brain damage, renal failure – which is already uncommon – and other organ damage. International cooperation in the collection of data about the remaining psychopathological complications will enable us to detect any flaws in design of extracorporeal apparatus and operations. Any lapses in manufacturing or sterilizing techniques will become immediately apparent; it is now up to us to continue to seek cooperation and to maintain a multidisciplinary approach. A pusillanimous approach to the huge problem of complications of cardiopulmonary bypass will not suffice in the last two decades of the twentieth century. A new generation of apparatus must be designed to take advantage of prostacyclin. Apparatus which does not require heparinization of the patient will make heart surgery with prostacyclin as complication-free as conventional general surgery.

24
Features of cardiac myocytes in culture: characterisation of the failing cell

JOCELYN W. DOW and ELAINE J. WALKER

Current problems in cardiac surgery have led us to study events at the level of the single cardiac cell. At present those patients with the best functional hearts are selected for surgery. The range of patients could usefully be extended either if we could protect a high risk system, where spontaneous myocardial work is unlikely to be resumed after surgery, or if we knew how to prepare the poorer prognosis patients biochemically for successful surgery. Secondly, increasing use of successful organ grafts requires the longest maintenance interval between excision and implant of the donor heart. Optimum conditions for organ graft survival have yet to be established.

The isolated myocardial cell has advantages for studying these problems.

(1) The environment of cultured myocytes can be manipulated readily in a defined manner so that oxygenation and other nutrients can be altered simultaneously for all cells.

(2) Similarly drugs can be administered to, and subtracted from the culture in a homogeneous manner.

(3) Environmental temperature can be controlled precisely and quickly.

(4) Uniform samples can be taken from the culture over the time course of an experiment for analysis of cells or culture medium.

ISOLATED CARDIAC MYOCYTES

Isolation of intact cells from the myocardium would not have seemed feasible before recognition of the cellular, rather than syncytical, nature of the myocardium. Membranous intercalated disc structures were first reported by van Breeman[1] and subsequently by Sjostrand *et al.*[2], and Price *et al.*[3]. These observations pointed to the role of intercalated discs as junctions between neighbouring cells. More recently Muir[4] has established that, from the earliest stages of differentiation of the myocardium, intercalated discs are present, acting as specialized regions of adhesion between cells. Adhesion between myocardial cells is maintained by calcium. Muir[5] demonstrated that in rat hearts perfused with calcium-free medium, intercellular separation occurs at the disc. Subsequent addition of calcium to this preparation precipitates many cells into severe and irreversible contractures associated with disorganization of myofibrils and extrusion of mitochondria from between the fibre bundles. This phenomenon, the calcium paradox[6], is assumed to result from influx of calcium through the damaged membranes, but there is as yet no molecular explanation.

Calcium depletion was first used as a method of preparing individual myocardial cells by Yokoyama *et al.*[7] and subsequently by Muir[8]. Muir noted that the intercalated disc junction remained attached entirely to one of the two contributing cells. Clearly there is a precarious balance of calcium ion concentration for maintaining cell adhesion on the one hand, and on the other for separating cells which are subsequently able to maintain structural integrity when calcium is added to the medium. It was not until 1972 that Gould and Powell[9] reported a method for isolating adequate yields of single cardiac myocytes which were tolerant to calcium. We confirm Dr Powell's findings[10] that individual cardiac myocytes can be isolated in an environment of carefully regulated calcium ion concentration to produce cells free of the calcium paradox. This has been a crucial milestone in producing normal, beating cardiac cells (Figure 1).

Biochemically these cells are stable at 37 °C for periods in excess of 5 hours. It is particularly noteworthy by comparison with other recent reports[11, 12] that our cells sustain concentrations of high energy phosphates (ATP and CP) consistent with those of intact myocardial tissue so long as they are maintained in an aerobic nutrient-replete environment (Walker, Burns and Dow, manuscript in preparation). Our single cardiac myocyte preparation thus mirrors the biochemical properties of the whole heart.

Structure of isolated cardiac myocytes

The intercalated disc is a complex membranous structure which crosses each myofibril at the level where a Z-line would be expected. Adjacent myofibrillar bundles within a single cell are crossed at different Z-line levels creating a step-like profile across the fibre. Myofibrils terminate by insertion of the actin (thin) filaments into the disc structure. These structural features are faithfully reproduced at the ends of isolated myocytes (Figure 1).

Individual myocytes are rod-shaped, most being 80–150 μm, in length, with 30–60 sarcomeres making up this length. Cells as long as 90 sarcomeres (225 μm) are not uncommon. Cell diameter varies between 8 and 20 μm. Our studies of size distribution, are in agreement with those of Powell *et al.*[13]. Some cells have irregular 'branched' shapes (Figure 2) similar to those first reported by Muir.[8] The dark and light striations defining the sarcomere are clearly visible in rod cells. Round cells lack organized structure and are assumed to arise during tissue digestion, being those cells which do not retain the intercalated disc structure.

HYPOXIA AND CELL STRUCTURE

Under hypoxic conditions the striated appearance of the rod-shaped cells deteriorates within a few minutes and the beat pattern changes. These cells assume a less elongated appearance, thickening in diameter. While the myofibrillar bundle structure running the length of the cells is still apparent, it is no longer possible to distinguish individual sarcomere banding. During shortening, contractile cell volume remains constant, there being simply an increase in the inter-filament spacing across the diameter of the cell to accommodate the shortening process. At rest length the sarcomere has a length of 2.4 μm, decreasing to 1.6 μm in a fully contracted cell. Thus a cell which at rest length is 150 μm long and 15 μm in diameter, will fully shorten to a length of 100 μm and a diameter of 18.4 μm. This appears as a relatively small change in diameter under the microscope compared with the length change.

Isolated hypoxic cells in this irreversibly contracted state rapidly thereafter lose cellular material. These changes appear first as small balloon-like protrusions from the cell (Figure 3A) which progressively enlarge as more cellular material is extruded (Figure 3B, C, D). Ultimately these cells round up and are surrounded by a substantial halo of intracellular material. Structural degeneration parallels our enzyme measurements which show a high rate of loss of cytoplasmic enzymes during development of the irrever-

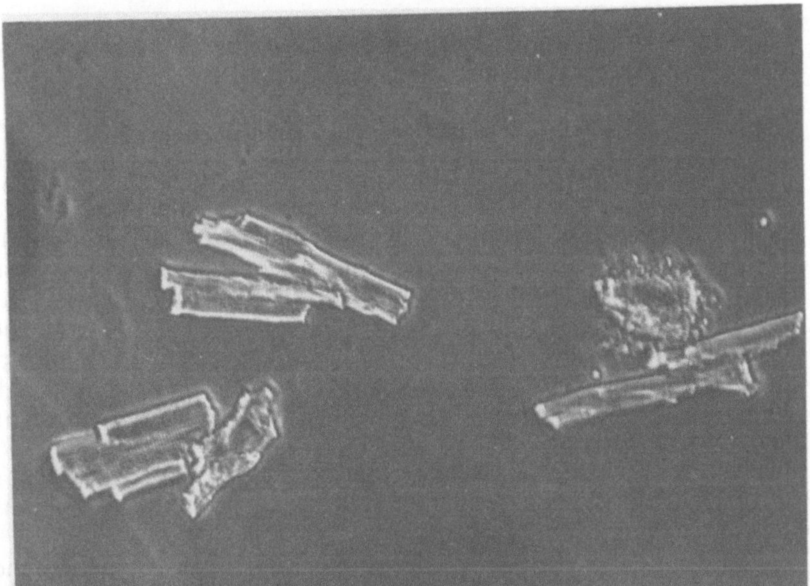

Figure 1 Single rod-shaped myocytes from adult rat heart. The alternate light and dark banding of the sarcomere structure is seen. Intercalated disc structure is reflected in the step-like ends of each cell. The field includes one round myocyte which clearly lacks organized myofibrillar structure

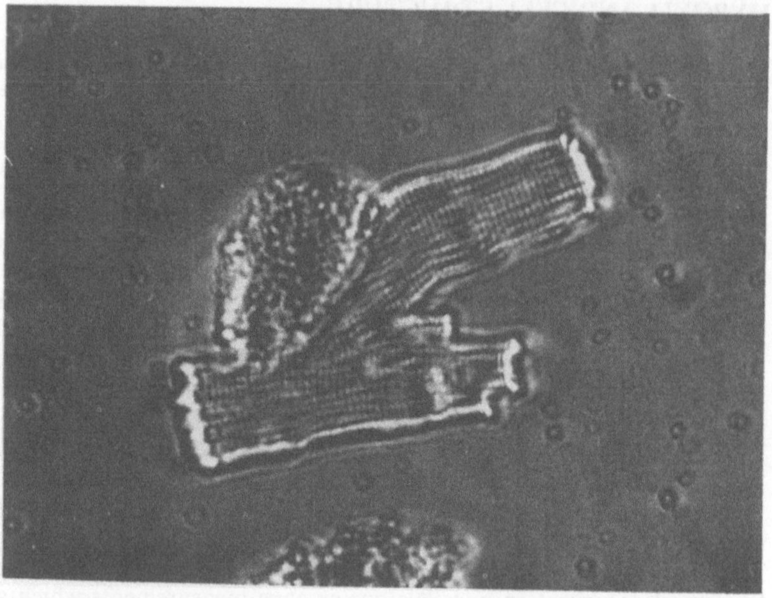

Figure 2 High power magnification of a single 'branched' rod cell, with a round cell lying alongside. The existence of these 'branched' cells was first reported by Muir[8]

sible loss of integrated cell structure, there being a somewhat slower loss of enzymes of partly mitochondrial origin such as CPK.

Hypoxia in cardiac myocytes during open heart surgery

Morales *et al.*[14] first reported the appearance of contracture bands in the myocardial tissue of patients dying with low cardiac output syndromes after cardiac surgery. It is clearly seen by re-examining Morales' pictures that a small number of fully contracted sarcomeres may occur within cells of otherwise normal appearance, and cells containing contracture bands may be surrounded by normal cells. Overall changes were similar to those in infarct patients except for the patchy, irregular distribution of necrosis, an appearance of numerous contraction bands, and marked interstitial haemorrhage in the larger necrotic areas. These abnormalities were more common at the apex and in areas of decreased vascularity. Deterioration progressed, in patients dying at longer intervals after surgery, to partial dissolution of contractile fibres, and subsequently to the laying down of collagen in these areas.

Morales observations give rise to questions about the condition of individual myocytes within the myocardium in patients surviving cardiac surgery. Clearly long-term survival postoperatively must be influenced by the overall state of the myocardium, the sum of its constituent cells.

Plasma enzyme concentrations have been monitored throughout the duration of hospitalization in cardiac surgery patients at the Western

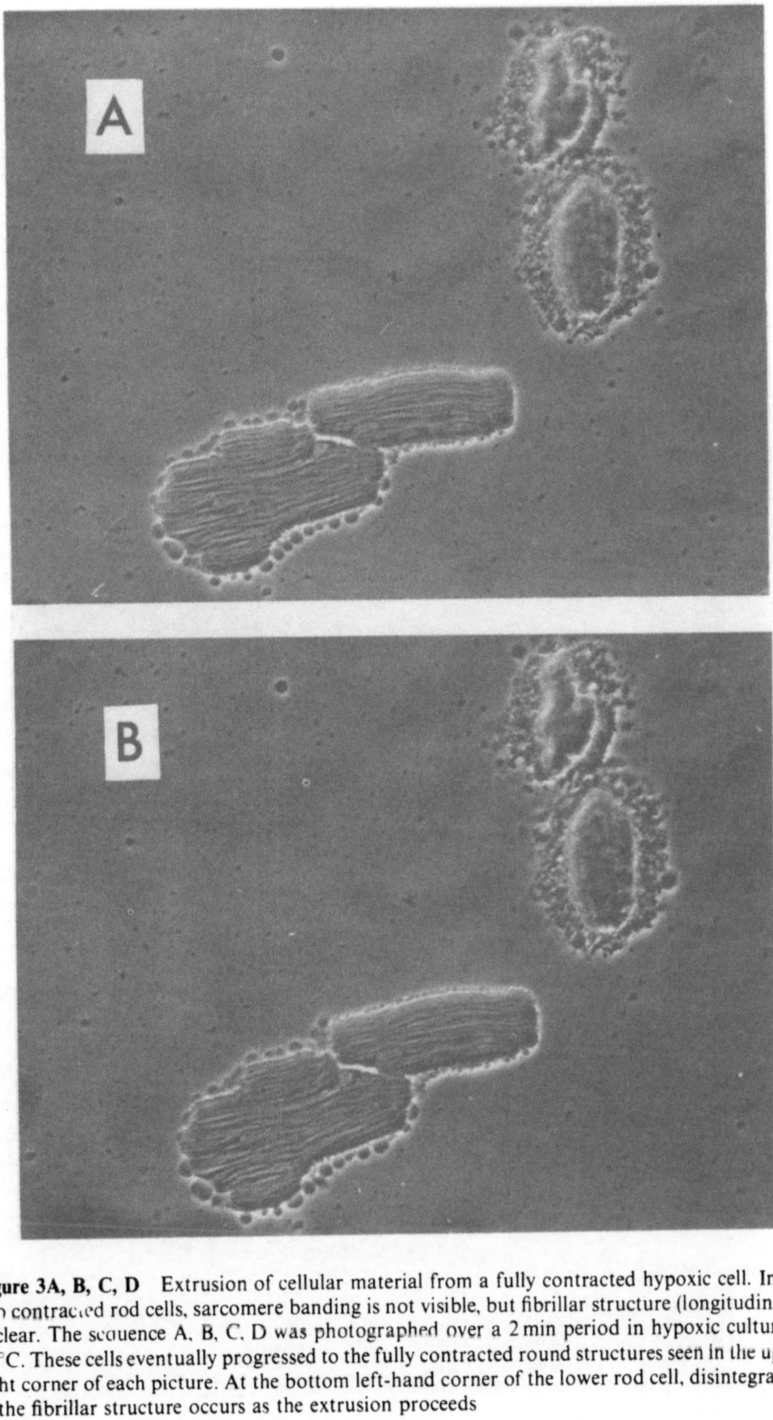

Figure 3A, B, C, D Extrusion of cellular material from a fully contracted hypoxic cell. In the two contracted rod cells, sarcomere banding is not visible, but fibrillar structure (longitudinally) is clear. The sequence A, B, C, D was photographed over a 2 min period in hypoxic culture at 37 °C. These cells eventually progressed to the fully contracted round structures seen in the upper right corner of each picture. At the bottom left-hand corner of the lower rod cell, disintegration of the fibrillar structure occurs as the extrusion proceeds

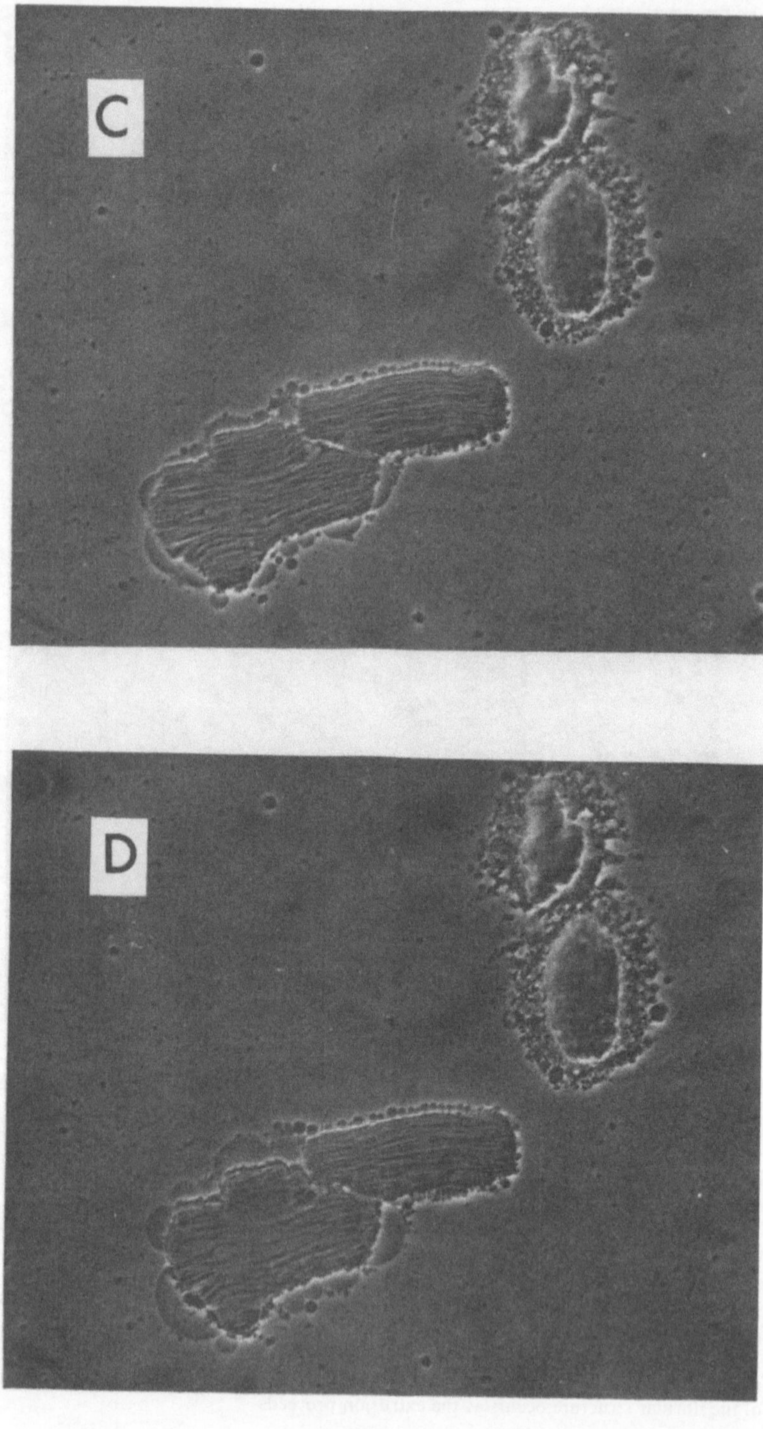
C
D

Infirmary, Glasgow. Our data suggest that enzyme losses from damaged myocardial cells may be substantial, occurring early in relation to surgery and being expressed on a time scale considerably longer than is normal for infarct patients. An example is given for one typical patient in Figure 4.

MOLECULAR EVENTS IN STRESSED CELLS

Cardiac cells in an hypoxic environment undergo a sequence of degenerative structural change, reversible only in the earliest stages. In heart preparations the sequential changes have been described in physiological terms by measurements of changes in the length–tension relationships[15, 16, 26] and in structural terms by electron microscopic observations of fixed and sectioned tissue[17]. Major advantages of using the isolated myocyte preparation for studying this

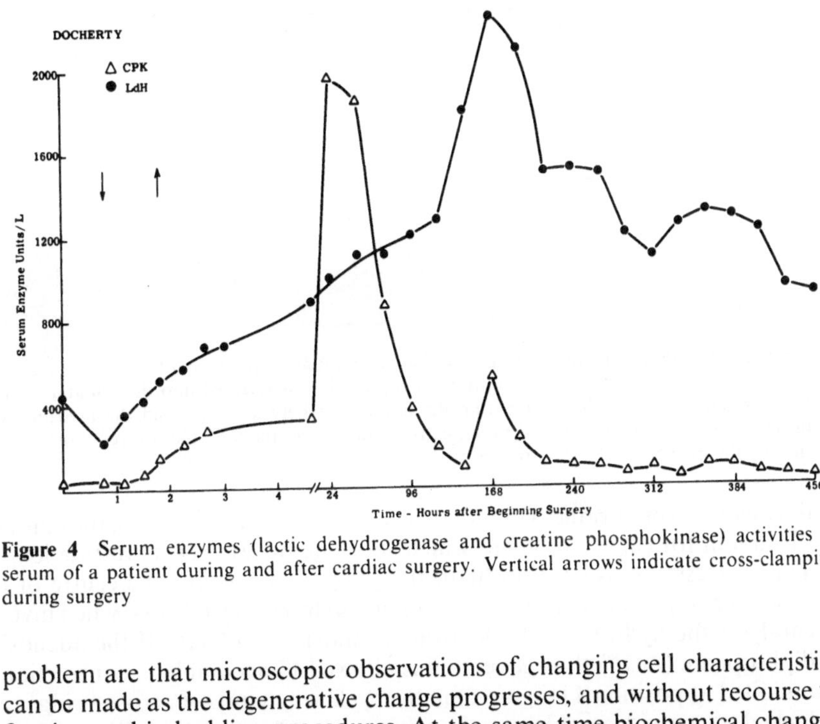

Figure 4 Serum enzymes (lactic dehydrogenase and creatine phosphokinase) activities in serum of a patient during and after cardiac surgery. Vertical arrows indicate cross-clamping during surgery

problem are that microscopic observations of changing cell characteristics can be made as the degenerative change progresses, and without recourse to fixation and imbedding procedures. At the same time biochemical changes can be monitored. Conditions in the cell culture medium can be altered readily by nutrient or drug additions, by oxygenation or pH changes, or changes in temperature.

Hypoxic structural degeneration is grossly expressed when cells can be seen to develop severe contractures. Our work to date indicates that the cells are irreversibly committed to this state. In molecular terms it seems that a progressive number of sarcomeres become fully contracted so that the cells seem unable to complete the normal 'beat' cycle by relaxing. An important question is therefore, what underlies this contractile failure?

The phenomenon can be explained, as follows, by classical contraction theory[18], and the known kinetic parameters of the actin–myosin interaction [19]. The processes of contraction and relaxation of muscle filaments are determined by the cytoplasmic concentration of calcium, and the availability of both ATP and ADP. Contraction is initiated by an increase in the cytoplasmic calcium ion concentration, derived from both extracellular sources and from the cellular storage sites of the sarcoplasmic reticulum. Binding of calcium to the thin filament receptor protein, troponin (Figure 5) triggers a sequence of molecular changes which permit sarcomere shortening. The progressive overlap of thick and thin filaments required for contraction, and described by the Sliding Filament Theory[20–22], is generated by a repeated cycling of

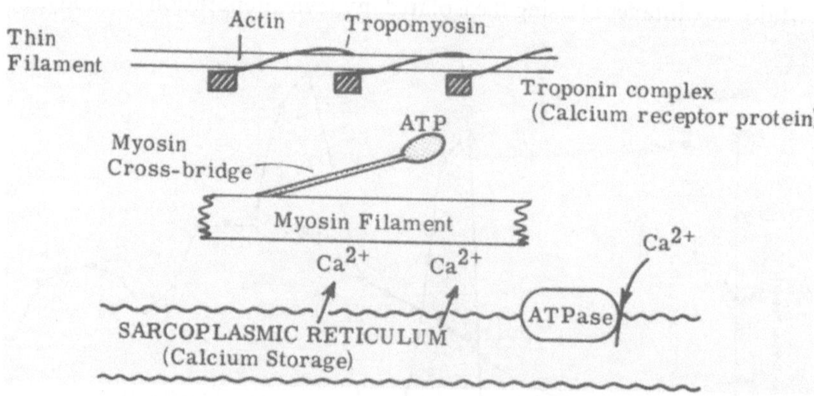

Figure 5 The thin filament has three proteins: actin, tropomyosin, and troponin (the calcium receptor complex). Contraction is initiated when calcium is released into the cell and binds to the troponin complex, thus permitting the interaction between actin and the myosin cross-bridges. The fibres relax when calcium is actively pumped to the sarcoplasmic reticulum storage sites by the membrane ATPase pump

the myosin cross-bridges (Figure 6), five or six cycles completing the contractile action for each sarcomere which shortens by 30% of its resting length. This process, by which thin filaments are pulled towards the centre of the sarcomere is powered at each cycle (Figure 6) by energy released when myosin catalyses the hydrolysis of adenosine triphosphate (ATP). If the adenosine diphosphate (ADP) thus generated is allowed to accumulate, contraction is inhibited at position 4 (Figure 6) in the cycle where myosin cross-bridges are locked as a rigid complex to the actin molecules in a thin filament as an actomyosin–ADP–Pi complex. The accumulating ADP inhibits ADP release from actomyosin[19] (the transition from state 4 to state 1 in Figure 6). Tension developed during each 'beat' is a measure of the force exerted by interactions between actin and myosin, and depends upon the number of active actin-myosin interactions.

In summary, the tension development phase of a beat consists of five or six repeated contractile cyclings (Figure 6) of actin and myosin which results in shortening of the sarcomeres. Tension is released by a passive sliding apart of the overlapped filaments until they return to the sarcomere rest length.

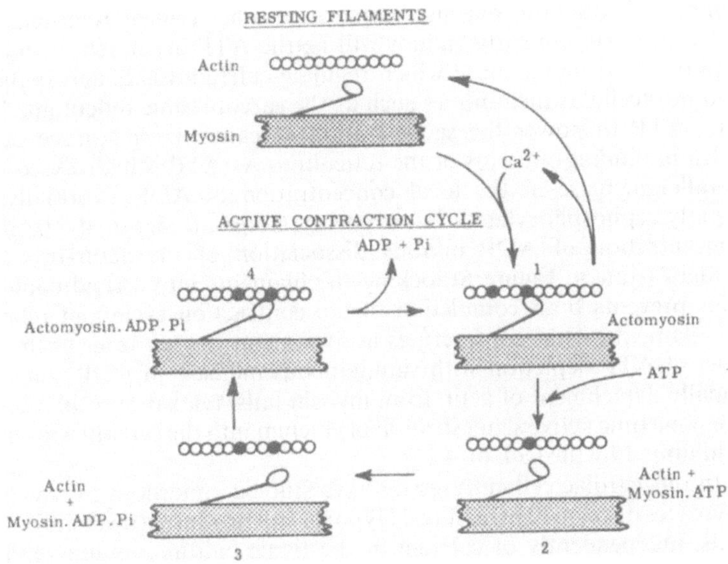

Figure 6 Cross-bridge cycle and the utilization of ATP. The cross-bridge cycle and accompanying hydrolysis of ATP is described in four states. Filaments are activated when calcium binds to the troponin complex allowing actin and myosin to interact (state 1). Binding of ATP to the myosin head is followed by a very rapid dissociation of actin from myosin (state 2). ATP is hydrolysed by myosin, ADP and Pi remaining bound to the catalytic site (state 3), which assumes a high energy state. The transition from state 3 to state 4 depends upon myosin–ADP–Pi interacting with actin. Energy is released as the cross-bridge pulls the thin filament towards the centre of the sarcomere, simultaneously releasing ADP and Pi while the cross-bridge returns to the low energy conformation

Relaxation is preceded by active sequestration of cell calcium, lowering the calcium concentration by two orders of magnitude.

In hypoxic myocardial tissue, the early reduction in peak tension occurs because fewer myosin heads make active links with actin. The subsequent progressive increase in resting tension is paralleled by a rise in peak tension, yet the tension amplitude is small. Indeed the tension amplitude is barely sufficient to account for a single active cross-bridge cycle per 'beat', compared with the normal five to six active cycles. A likely explanation for this is that co-ordination of cross-bridge cycling, within a single sarcomere, fails and random cross-bridge formation occurs. The asynchronous oscillation of individual cross-bridges is nevertheless sufficient to maintain a slowly increasing tension. Relaxation to the resting equilibrium position fails progressively as fewer complexes are dissociated at any one time.

Contraction and energy supply

The normal ATP content of myocardial cells is sufficient, if not constantly regenerated by metabolic processes, to allow 12–15 beats/cell. In hypoxic cells, where metabolic production of ATP is severely limited, contractile activity will rapidly deplete ATP reserves. Depletion of ATP not only inhibits contraction, but also jeopardizes other critical ATP-requiring cell processes. Among early victims will be the ATP-dependent membrane ion pumps, particularly those which regulate calcium fluxes across the plasma and intracellular membranes such as the sarcoplasmic reticulum. The latter uses ATP to power the sequestration of calcium for storage on specific calcium binding proteins of the reticulum. As ATP is hydrolysed there is a parallel increase in the local concentration of ADP. Normally ADP is rapidly rephosphorylated, but if energy stores are depleted, the increasing concentration of ADP inhibits dissociation of the actin–myosin cross-bridges (state 4, Figure 6) locking the filaments into a rigid configuration. This prevents both completion of the contraction cycle and relaxation of the filaments. Thus contractures in hypoxic myocytes occur as the end-product of ATP depletion with simultaneous increase in ADP concentration. Finally detachment of actin from myosin fails, relaxation is blocked, and at the same time active sequestration of calcium into the sarcoplasmic reticulum is inhibited by the lack of ATP.

In our cardiac cell cultures we have studied conditions in which isolated myocytes develop contractures. Hypoxia will produce irreversibly contracted cells, independently of calcium in the tissue culture medium. Evidence of this type argues against the hypothesis that changes in the length–tension relationship during the development of hypoxia can be explained primarily by failure of the sarcolemmal system to regulate the amount of calcium entering and leaving cells. It argues rather for an explanation predominantly based upon changes in the relationship between actin, myosin, ATP, ADP and calcium.

Myocyte protein balance

The irreversible phase of hypoxic stress is characterized by disintegration of myofibrillar structure and loss of cell and mitochondrial membrane integrity – generalized necrosis. A primary cause of this pattern of functional cell death is the action of proteolytic enzymes of the myocyte. These enzymes are responsible for the scavenging processes of the cell, and their action is normally balanced by the synthesis of new protein. During hypoxia, lysosomal acid hydrolases are released into the cytoplasm, whilst in contrast hypothermia alone does not have this deleterious effect[23]. Hypoxia induces a generalized disorganisation of cell structure including disruption of lysosomal enzyme storage structures. In such cases the resulting increase in the rate of protein catabolism is not balanced by an increase in the rate of synthesis of new protein. The end product of protease activity is clearly seen as dissolution of myofibrils and organelles in the history of the hypoxic or ischaemic heart.

Several biochemical processes impinge upon the problem of maintaining protein balance in the myocyte. Amino acids are largely supplied from extracellular sources, and enter the cell by active (energy-requiring and temperature-dependent) processes. The rate at which proteins are synthesized depends upon the availability of amino acids as well as upon a high degree of organisational integrity within the cell. In hypoxic cells, particularly those where energy reserves are falling, both amino acid transport and protein synthesis are jeopardized. Our experiments suggest that early in the development of hypoxia it may no longer be possible to sustain these processes in an effective manner. Thus if cellular material is to be preserved the most effective intervention may be to inhibit the proteolytic destruction of structural proteins and membranes.

We have begun a programme to define the sequence of events in stress-induced acceleration of catabolism. Understanding of the cardiac specific proteases has advanced considerably[24, 25] but less is known of the control of these enzymes within the myocyte, or of factors which precipitate failure of the normal regulatory processes. These problems must be understood in order that we may develop rational approaches to protection of the myocardium during hypoxia. Within the programme, rates of synthesis and of degradation for individual proteins of the myofibril, the calcium regulating membrane systems, and the energy producing enzymes of the cells, are being measured. It has become apparent that many of the structural proteins are normally long-lived. In these cases the synthesis of new molecules should not be critical on the time scale during which the decreased myocardial temperature during surgery will slow down protein synthesis. However catabolic destruction appears rapid during hypoxia, even at reduced tissue temperatures. In contrast, the synthesis of some metabolic proteins is quite rapid, and it may be that we will find one or more of these rapid turnover proteins have critical roles in for example, calcium regulation.

These considerations are important in cardiac surgery where the myocardium may be at risk for two reasons. Firstly pre-existing vascular disease leaves clusters of cells unable to cope with the overall surgical procedures because they will be working at the limits of their energy reserve and secondly such cells will doubtless also be at risk if conditions for cardioplegia are not optimum.

ACKNOWLEDGMENTS

This work was supported by grants from the British Heart Foundation and the Medical Research Council. We are also grateful to the Astra Chemical Co., for financial support, to Dr Nigel Harding and Mr Patrick Doherty for use of their photomicroscope, to Mr Murdo Turner and Dr Peter Wallace for clinical samples, and to Professors T. D. V. Lawrie and R. M. S. Smellie for their continued encouragement.

References

1. Van Breeman, V. L. (1953). Intercalated discs in heart muscle studied with the electron microscope. *Anat. Rec.*, **117**, 49
2. Sjostrand, F. S. and Andersson, E. (1954). Electron microscopy of the intercalated discs of cardiac muscle tissue. *Experientia*, **10**, 369
3. Price, K. C., Weiss, J. M., Hata, D. and Smith, J. R. (1955). Experimental needle biopsy of the myocardium of dogs with particular reference to histologic study by electron microscopy. *J. Exp. Med.*, **101**, 687

4. Muir, A. R. (1957). An electron microscope study of the embryology of the intercalated disc in the heart of the rabbit. *J. Biochem. Biophys. Cytol.*, **3,** 193
5. Muir, A. R. (1967a). The effects of divalent cations on the ultrastructure of the perfused rat heart *J. Anat.*, **101,** 239
6. Muir, A. R. (1967b). A calcium-induced contracture of cardiac muscle cells. *Proc. Anat. Soc.*, **102,** 148
7. Yokoyama, H. A., Jennings, B. B. and Wartman, W. B. (1961). Intercalated disks of dog myocardium. *Exp. Cell. Res.*, **23,** 29
8. Muir, A. R., (1965). Further observations on the cellular structure of cardiac muscle. *J. Anat.*, **99,** 27
9. Gould, R. P. and Powell, T. (1972). Intact isolated muscle cells from the adult rat heart. *J. Physiol.*, **225,** 16P
10. Powell, T. (1979). Isolation of cells from adult mammalian myocardium. *J. Mol. Cell. Cardiol.*, **11,** 511
11. Farmer, B. B., Harris, R. A., Jolly, W. W., Hathway, D. R., Katzberg, A., Watanabe, A. M., Whitlow, A. L. and Besche, H. R. (1977). Isolation and characterisation of adult rat heart cells. *Arch. Biochem. Biophys.* **179,** 545
12. Clark, M. G., Gannon, B. J., Bodkin, N., Patten, G. S. and Berry, M. N. (1978). An improved procedure for the high-yield preparation of intact beating heart cells from the adult rat. Biochemical and morphological study. *J. Mol. Cell. Cardiol.*, **10,** 1101
13. Powell, T., Steen, E. M., Twist, V. W. and Woolf, N. (1978). Surface characteristics of cells isolated from adult rat myocardium. *J. Mol. Cell. Cardiol.*, **10,** 287
14. Morales, A. R., Fine, G. and Taber, R. E. (1967). Cardiac surgery and myocardial necrosis. *Arch. Path.*, **83,** 71
15. Brooks, W. W.. Sturckow, B. and Bing, O. H. L. (1974). Myocardial hypoxia and reoxygenation, electrophysiologic and mechanical correlates. *Am. J. Physiol.* **226,** 523
16. Dhalla, N. S., Yates, J. C., Walz, D. A., McDonald, V. A. and Olson, R. E. (1972). Correlation between changes in the endogenous energy stores and myocardial function due to hypoxia in the isolated perfused rat heart. *Canad. J. Physiol. Pharmacol.*, **50,** 333
17. Hatt, P. Y. and Moravec, J. (1971). Acute hypoxia of the myocardium. Ultrastructural changes. *Cardiology*, **56,** 73
18. Hanson, J. and Huxley, H. E. (1953). Structural basis of the cross-striations in muscle. *Nature*, **172,** 530
19. Lymn, R. W. and Taylor, E. W. (1971). Mechanism of adenosine triphosphate hypoxia and hypothermia on the release of lysosomal enzymes in the fog heart.
20. Huxley, A. F. and Niedergerke, R. (1954). Structural changes in muscle during contraction. *Nature*, **173,** 971
21. Huxley, H. E. (1971). The structural basis of muscular contraction. *Proc. Roy. Soc. London. B.*, **178,** 131
22. Huxley, H. E. and Hanson, J. (1954). Changes in the cross-striations of muscle during contraction and stretch and their structural interpretation. *Nature*, **173,** 973
23. Leighty, E. G., Ressallat, M. M., Passananti, G. T. and Sirak, H. D. (1966). Effects of hypoxia and hypothermia on the release of pysosomal enzymes in the dog heart. *Surgical Forum*, **27,** 181
24. Decker, R. S., Poole, A. R., Griffin, E. E., Dingle, J. T. and Wildernthal, K. (1977). Altered distribution of lysosomal cathepsin D in ischaemic myocardium. *J. Clin. Invest.* **59,** 911
25. Murakami, U. and Uchida, K., (1978). Purification and characterisation of a myosin-cleaving protease from rat heart myofibrils. *Biochim. Biophys. Acta.* **525,** 219
26. Ekblom, B. and Bing, O. H. L. (1975). Tolerance of isolated cardiac muscle to hypoxia: Force-frequency interrelationships. *Proc. Soc. Exp. Biol. Med.*, **148,** 484

25
Factors influencing the origin and cycling of hydrogen ions in cardiac surgery

JOCELYN W. DOW, N. G. L. HARDING, G. N. C. KENNY, M. A. TURNER AND P. G. WALLACE

INTRODUCTION

Knowledge of the origin of hydrogen ions (protons) is central to their therapeutic regulation. It is the purpose of this paper to indicate which factors are involved in the origin and control of hydrogen ions in order to optimize the biochemistry of patients undergoing cardiac surgery.

Relatively small concentrations of protons such as those at pH 7.4 (40 nmol/l) and pH 6.8 (158 nmol/l), have considerable metabolic effects. These concentrations are appreciably less than those of therapeutically effective drugs and are similar to those of some hormones. A current problem in biochemistry is to identify the acidifying reactions in aerobic, hypoxic and hypothermic cells.

Cardiac surgery is associated with procedures which are known to have profound effects on proton flux, buffering, and loss, namely anaesthesia and artificial ventilation, tissue injury, hypothermia, and the administration of exogenous hydrogen ions. For instance, severe metabolic acidosis can be produced by inadequate tissue oxygenation or the provision of an acid load such as may occur with transfusion of blood. Whatever the origin of the protons, even a mild metabolic acidosis may adversely affect myocardial function and decrease the effectiveness of vasopressor agents[1]. During the course of surgery, perfusion and maintenance of a normal acid–base equilibrium is associated with normal plasma adrenalin and noradrenalin[2]. This is important, for a rise in noradrenalin concentration will accentuate metabolic acidosis by increasing resistance to perfusion and accentuating tissue hypoxia.

THE ORIGIN AND CYCLING OF PROTONS

Release of protons is complicated at biological pH values by the fact that production of protons from ionizable hydrogen atoms is not necessarily a stoicheiometric process. The reason is that some ionizing groups may have a pK close to the biological pH value and so only a partial mole (more correctly gram atom) fraction of ionizable hydrogen will appear as protons. The amount released also depends upon temperature. All cells have reactions which can be written as proton generators from particular substrates on a $> 1:1$, $1:1$, or $< 1:1$ basis. For the present purposes it is convenient to consider these reactions as (1) glycolysis based, (2) energy-rich phosphate-linked, (3) respiratory-chain derived and (4) CO_2 based. The acidifying reactions will be those in which a proton is released and not consumed stoicheiometrically elsewhere. Other reactions can be identified in which there is a massive proton flux with no release to the exterior, and so are termed proton recycling reactions.

Glycolysis-based proton release

It is conventionally held that lactate is the source of protons which cause metabolic acidosis under conditions of oxygen deprivation. This is questionable because creation of the carboxyl ($COO^- \; H^+$) group of lactate occurs at an earlier stage of glycolysis.

The 1-carboxyl group created at 1,3-diphosophoglycerate $\rightleftharpoons$ 3-phosphoglycerate dissociates to form a hydrogen ion and is carried through to pyruvate. This is reduced to lactate if oxygenation is inadequate, or further transmuted to acetyl-CoA for aerobic oxidation in the tricarboxylic acid (TCA) cycle. The fate of the attendant proton would probably normally be to enter the respiratory chain for oxidation to water but under anaerobic conditions it appears as a cytoplasmic hydrogen ion.

A second carboxyl group, with its attendant proton, is created at the next step, the first of the TCA cycle, catalysed by citrate synthetase.

$$\text{oxaloacetate} + \text{acetyl-CoA} + H_2O \rightleftharpoons \text{citrate}$$

The carboxyl group appears as CO_2 in the TCA cycle, whilst the intramitochondrial proton released should enter the respiratory chain under aerobic conditions. The foregoing reactions can account for the origin of cytoplasmic and mitochondrial protons. Under hypothermic conditions the balance of proton production and disposal appears to be maintained for the short periods encountered in surgery.

No detailed calculations have yet been performed on proton release and flux during integrated operation of the glycolytic pathways and TCA cycle, particularly under hypoxic and hypothermic conditions. From the point of view of proton release these routes are highly conserved, giving a minimum proton yield per mole of substrate oxidized. This is achieved by transferring H atoms to the electron transport chain for oxidation. This forms a second potential source of protons which could accumulate under anaerobic conditions.

Energy-rich phosphates and proton release

Each time a molecule of ATP is hydrolysed, two potential protons appear, one on each of the ADP and P products. At neutral pH the stoicheiometry is complicated by the fact that both ATP and ADP have a pK of 7.2 at 25°C. Taking this into account, about 0.7 mol H^+ appear for each mole of ATP hydrolysed. Indeed, the reaction forms the basis for the pH-stat method of estimating ATPase activity. In contrast to the protons released by some other acidifying reactions, protons from ATP hydrolysis are recycled stoicheiometrically, being reabsorbed during ATP synthesis to create massive occult fluxes (Table 1). Release rather than cycling of these protons would create the problem of disposing of the equivalent of a Winchester of fuming HCl per day. Similar arguments apply to phosphocreatine protons.

Table 1 Fuels and proton cycling in the aerobic human heart

Glucose (amount used per day)	11 g (60 mmol) equivalent to 2100 mmol ATP
Lactate (amount used per day)	10 g (110 mmol) equivalent to 3630 mmol ATP
Protons	
released	570 μmol/min
cycled	4000 μmol/min

Calculated from data of Bernsmeier and Rudolph[34]

The transition from aerobic to normothermic, hypoxic conditions creates a problem of proton disposal because the protons are not recycled in the absence of ATP synthesis. In view of the massive nature of these fluxes, it is clinically important to ensure that there is hypothermic reduction in the proton flux rate before the possible development of hypoxic conditions as may occur in under-perfused regions.

Protons derived from the respiratory chain

Under aerobic conditions the passage of H atoms along the respiratory chain is associated with no net gain or loss of protons. Mitochondria are adapted for water, oxygen and carbon dioxide transport. The total oxygen handling capacity of human mitochondria is of the order of 10 mmol/min. Mechanisms of carbon dioxide transport are less well defined. Mitochondria possess a carbonic anhydrase[3], raising the question of whether carbon dioxide is exported as bicarbonate[4] or as dissolved CO_2

Provision of energy rich molecules by mitochondria is pH sensitive. Carriers linked to oxidative phosphorylation have been found in all mitochondria studied. The pH dependence of the adenine nucleotide (ATP,ADP) carrier ($pK = 7.2$) has considerable relevance to adequate control of intracellular pH. The important question of whether protons are exported by hypoxic mitochondria *in vivo* is not sufficiently clarified to be certain that intra-mitochondrial proton release is responsible for ultrastructural damage observed under hypoxic conditions.

Considerable evidence points to H^+/carrier coupling as a normal mitochondrial function. Experimental inhibition of sections of the electron transport chain is associated with proton release. For example, rotenone added to mitochondria inhibits NADH from reducing ubiquinone, and marked Ca^{2+}-coupled proton release is observed[5]. Nitroprusside, used in cardiac surgery as a vasodilator, can yield CN^- to inhibit terminal mitochondrial cytochrome oxidase. A profound fatal bicarbonate unresponsive acidosis can result but whether the proton source is extra- or intra-mitochondrial or both, is not clear.

Clinically, cardioplegic techniques must be designed to ensure minimum production of protons by decreasing metabolic rate with hypothermia, and by ensuring adequate oxygenation of intracellular myoglobin before cardioplegia. This raises the question of whether cardioplegic solutions could beneficially be both oxygenated and cooled.

Protons and carbon dioxide

In addition to evidence from subcellular diffusion studies, processes such as the red-cell Cl^--shift support the view that CO_2 is the principal terminal metabolite of aerobic energy production leaving the cells. Hydration of CO_2 in the blood maintains a cell–blood CO_2 gradient of some 15 mmHg for removal of tissue CO_2.

In the erythrocyte, carbonic anhydrase catalyses the hydration of CO_2 to result in an increase in H^+ concentration by the reaction:

$$CO_2 + H_2O \rightleftharpoons H_2CO_3 \rightleftharpoons H^+ + HCO_3^-$$

The total amount of CO_2 produced is of the order of 10 mmol/min (about 220 ml/min). The protons released are buffered by haemoglobin whilst about 70% of the intra-erythrocyte HCO_3^- formed diffuses into the plasma. Thus erythrocytes are central to proton–carbon dioxide homeostasis. At the lungs the reverse process occurs. The carbon dioxide diffuses into the alveoli and is exhaled, causing the equilibrium to shift to the left. the protons recombining as water. The net production of H^+ by this route is of the order of 10 mmol/min at 37°C or 15000 mmol/day.

For this reason if adequate elimination of CO_2 is not maintained, protons produced by the hydration of tissue CO_2 rapidly contribute to a decrease of blood pH.

PUMP PRIMES AND PROTON REGULATION

Clear fluid primes remove the problem of introducing an acid load with the priming blood. Nevertheless there remains the issue of a transfusional acidosis. Also, clear fluid primes have not yet been optimized from the point of view of proton control and they introduce problems of haemodilution and fluid shifts.

The pH of acid citrate dextrose (ACD) blood can decrease to 6.5 after 21 days' storage[6] and the extracellular K^+ concentration increases to about 25 mmol/l as a result of hypothermic failure of membrane potassium transport[7]. Several hours after an ACD infusion an initial acidosis may be replaced by an alkalosis[8] as the citrate is metabolized (17 mmol/l ACD blood), leaving a Na^+ excess (36 mmol/l ACD blood). The alkalosis can reach its peak at around 24–48 h after administration. Aerobic metabolism of citrate can have advantages for regulating proton homeostasis. Malm *et al.*[9] observed negligible metabolic acidosis using ACD + Tris compared with heparinized control blood. However, this raises questions of calcium control, because ACD-preserved blood may reduce the Ca^{2+} below 0.5 mmol/l, a level incompatible with cardiac activity[10]. Also there is the question of how the hypothermic and posthypothermic kidney can handle the sodium load.

Proton release and haemoglobin oxygenation are related. Factors which alter the position of the oxyhaemoglobin dissociation curve include pH, PCO_2, and temperature[11]. In transfused blood there is a loss of capacity to release oxygen caused by loss of 2,3-diphosphoglycerate[12].

Use of clear fluid pump primes results in haemodilution on mixing with the patient's blood. This affects the oxygen carrying and buffer capacities of the diluted blood. For example, at a haemoglobin concentration of 15 g/100 ml, 196 ml oxygen/l blood can be carried at a PaO_2 of 100 mmHg, but at 8 g/100 ml only 110 ml oxygen is transported[13,14,15,16]. This is still adequate in the resting state. Whole body oxygen consumption does not fall until the haematocrit is less than 10 %. Before that occurs, excess lactate begins to appear at a haematocrit of 15–20 %[17] but it is not clear where this lactate arises. The degree of acidosis is a function of haemodilution, but paradoxically, Neville[18] has observed that less acidosis occurred with Ringer–lactate than with other fluids. As with citrate, the explanation may again lie with the co-administered sodium load. Nevertheless, haemodilution has beneficial effects upon liver[19], brain[20] and kidney perfusion[21]. A further complication has been observed in that a combination of haemodilution and severe hypocapnia ($PCO_2 < 11$ mmHg) markedly reduces cerebral oxygen uptake[20].

HYPOTHERMIA

In terms of the regulation of metabolism, there are two questions posed by using hypothermia in surgery. Firstly the nature of the biochemical effects related to the period of hypothermia and secondly, any long term or 'flywheel' effects following its use during surgery.

The homoiothermic animal responds to cold by erecting its hair, by peripheral vasoconstriction and later by a temperature-sensitive centre in the hypothalmus activating shivering and noradrenalin release. This increases the metabolic rate. If the cold continues, the anterior pituitary produces adrenotropic and thyrotropic hormones. In addition, cellular sensitivity to the hormone increases as temperature falls.

From the point of view of the metabolic effects of hypothermia, man does not have the adaptive mechanisms of the hibernator. Regional blood flow control mechanisms have been known to exist since the investigation of Mares[22]. In hibernating animals these appear to be based on a guardian vasomotor mechanism, apparently deriving its control from a central clock. In man, clinical observations suggest that such clock-based regional perfusion mechanisms do not exist. Further, the hibernator is adapted to slow its heart rate in relation to the environmental temperature. In contrast, man is threatened with ventricular fibrillation as cooling intensifies[23]. The metabolic effects of man being a non-hibernator are profound. Generalized vasoconstriction mechanisms in response to cold essentially mean that there is stasis of blood in under-perfused regions. Thus metabolite exchange, and hydrogen ion concentration, vary according to the degree of perfusion, and vasoconstriction. There may be temperature-dependent variations in regional blood flow and in the effects on metabolism. The picture is thus complicated and presently incomplete from the point of view of understanding the origin and disposal of hydrogen ions in hypothermia.

Renal function in hypothermia

Normally the kidney contributes much less than the lung to the acute disposal of H^+ ion. In cardiac surgery, renal function is important during the operative and postoperative periods not only for continuance of normal renal electrolyte and H^+ ion controls but also because titration of excess H^+ ion by bicarbonate may be required. This introduces the problem of disposal of excess Na during correction of plasma pH with bicarbonate.

The kidney is affected by hypothermia, studies indicating that there is depression of a variety of renal functions. However, the impression that renal function is reduced to insignificance by cooling to even 25°C is not correct. At this temperature the following mechanisms operate in the kidney.

(a) Renal plasma flow is markedly reduced and there is a comparable reduction in the glomerular filtration rate (GFR); the filtration fraction remains unchanged.

(b) Tubular secretory activity is reduced to a similar extent so the tubular perfusion ratio is unaltered.

(c) Renal oxygen extraction and renal blood flow are decreased in parallel, so their ratio and the renal arteriovenous oxygen difference is unchanged.

(d) Tubular Na reabsorption and renal oxygen uptake are proportionally reduced so that the Na/O_2 ratio is constant.

(e) Urine flow is maintained in hypothermia, despite a marked reduction in GFR, by the coincident suppression of Na and water reabsorption.

At 25°C, renal blood-flow falls to 25% of the 37°C value. Creatinine clearance behaves similarly. Under these conditions, plasma K^+ falls slightly, and the urinary potassium may rise. It is known[24], that for a given GFR nearly twice the amount of potassium can be excreted by the hypothermic kidney than the normothermic organ. Data for reduction of oxygen consumption is scant, but at 25°C consumption is one third the value at 37°C.

In terms of cardiac surgery, mechanisms for the handling of protons and bicarbonate by the hypothermic human kidney require further elucidation. The loss of potassium experienced in cardiac surgery may not be completely accounted for by the hypothermic renal enhancement of potassium loss.

Proton-potassium homeostasis in hypothermia

The interpretation of this relationship in cardiac surgery is complex. Normothermically, a decrease in extracellular pH would result in an increase in plasma K^+[25]. However, in hypothermia a decrease in temperature resulted in a decrease in arterial pH and a decrease in plasma K^+[26]. This paradoxical response remained after nephrectomy. It is possible that the driving force for this exchange is an increased intracellular H^+, which results in proton efflux and potassium influx in a non-stoicheiometric ratio. With renal function conserved or enhanced in hypothermia with respect to K^+ loss, it seems that other mechanisms result in a decrease in cellular and extracellular K^+, independently of an H^+–K^+ exchange.

The implications for man are that, in hypothermia, cellular proton efflux, i.e. fall in plasma pH, is only a crude measure of changes in plasma K^+ concentration. If the H^+ ion efflux is excessive, extrinsic control by titration with bicarbonate or other buffers may be required. This raises questions of cation and anion disposal by the hypo- and post-hypothermic kidney.

Disposal of bicarbonate in hypothermia

The hypothermic kidney can reabsorb nearly all the bicarbonate filtered at normal plasma HCO_3^- concentrations[27], despite the effects of cold on tubular transport. In the conditions of cardiac surgery it is not known whether there is elevation or depression of the threshold for bicarbonate reabsorption.

Bicarbonate loading in hypothermic dogs results in a marked excretion of alkali. In massive loading (infusion at 1.24 mmol/min), urine pH rises to 7.95 whilst arterial pH stabilizes at a maximum of 7.56 at 27 °C (corrected). In this experiment urine flow increased with a decrease in temperature. Thus the osmolar response of the kidney may be conserved in mild hypothermia. In addition there is a depressant effect of a bicarbonate load on potassium excretion by the hypothermic kidney[25,28].

Such factors as have been studied in hypothermic man indicate that changes in renal function parameters parallel those observed experimentally[29]. These changes may be a function of both metabolic temperature and perfusion, for in the human kidney at 28 °C, impedance to flow principally comprised an increase in the afferent arteriolar and venular resistances.

RELATIONSHIP BETWEEN INTRACELLULAR MYOCYTE PROTONS, POTASSIUM AND BICARBONATE

Proper control of potassium ion is essential, particularly in the post-surgical phase when patients may lose 100–200 mmol K^+ in 24 h. The mechanism of this kaluriesis is not clear, but K^+ movements are associated with changes in intracellular pH[30]. There is a significant linear relationship between proton and K^+ ion gradients across the muscle cell membrane[31]. Plasma potassium showed an inverse linear relationship to the proton gradient and to extracellular pH, and a negative exponential relationship to intracellular pH.

The shape of these profiles indicates that both skeletal muscle and cardiac myocytes are resistant to extracellular pH changes, but with an intracellular pH below about 7.1, myocytes lose their buffering capacity increasingly rapidly. This may represent failure of a proton pump. The two types of myocyte behave differently with respect to potassium. Skeletal myocytes act as a buffer for the plasma K^+, intracellular K^+ concentration falling with fall in the level of plasma K^+, whilst the cardiac intracellular K^+ concentration remains relatively conserved[32].

In applying these findings to man, the relative ability of cardiac myocytes to retain K^+ would have practical consequences. It may explain why in some patients cardioplegic K^+ is slow to wash from the heart. Secondly, the cardiac myocyte $K_i:K_e$ gradient increases as the plasma potassium level falls, changing the membrane potential and excitability. This explains why a postoperative plasma level of K^+ of 4–5 mmol/l seems optimum. The nature of the mechanism which relates potassium and proton fluxes is uncertain. Clancy and Brown[33] suggested that cardiac myocytes had a greater capacity to pump out protons than did skeletal muscle myocytes. By the Henderson equation proton export could be bicarbonate-dependent. In support of this, Irvine and Dow[32] found that cardiac intracellular bicarbonate increases by about 25 % as intracellular potassium is lost, whereas skeletal myocytes show little change in intracellular bicarbonate.

Thus from the point of view of cardiac proton efflux, bicarbonate may be an essential ion, particularly during cardioplegia.

SUMMARY AND CLINICAL CONCLUSIONS

(1) Priming solutions should be designed to support aerobic and anaerobic ATP production. Studies with precursors such as phosphoenolpyruvate may show advantages.

(2) Cardioplegic techniques should be designed to minimize H^+ ion production. An optimum technique may be prior cooling with an oxygenated solution containing glycolysis intermediates. Ionic cardioplegia then minimizes ATP utilization.

(3) Cardioplegic solutions may require bicarbonate in view of its known involvement in cardiac myocyte proton efflux.

(4) On-line monitoring of plasma lactate may provide early warning of the deleterious effects of excessive haemodilution and regional hypoperfusion.

(5) Precise control of H^+ and CO_2 tissue-plasma gradients is essential for optimizing proton disposal. Part of this control includes titration with exogenous bicarbonate.

(6) In the presurgical phase, plasma K^+ may not adequately represent the body buffer stores of potassium. In deep hypothermia this depletion may be masked by a passive leakage from cells as activity of the K^+ pumps decreases.

(7) In addition the hypothermic kidney retains ability to lose K^+ during and after surgery. Further, in hypothermia, paradoxical relationships between K^+ and H^+ occur.
For these reasons, careful regulation of K^+ is essential until the homeostatic mechanisms are restored.

References

1. Darby, T. D., Aldinger, E. E., Gasden, R. H. and Thrower, W. B. (1960). *Circ. Res.*, **8,** 1242
2. Malm, J. R., Manger, W. M., Sullivan, S. F., Pappas, E. M. and Nahas, G. G. (1966). *J. Am. Med. Ass.*, **197,** 121
3. Rossi, C. S. (1969). In *The Energy level and Metabolic Control of Mitochondria*, p. 74 (Adriatica Editrice)
4. Holton, F. A. (1969). *Biochem. J.*, **116,** 29P
5. Vercesi, A., Reynafarje, B. and Lehninger, A. L. (1978). *J. Biol. Chem.*, **253,** 6379
6. Wintrobe, M. M. (1967) *Clinical Hematology*. (Philadelphia: Lea and Febiger)
7. Leveen, H. M., Schatman, B. and Falk, G. (1959). *Surg. Gynecol. Obstet.*, **109,** 502
8. Litwin, M. S., Smith, L. L. and Moore, F. D. (1959) *Surgery St. Louis.*, **45,** 805
9. Malm, J. R., Sullivan, G. F., Patterson, R. W., Bowman, F. D. and Nahas, G. G. (1963). *Trans. Am. Soc. Artif. Intern. Org.*, **9,** 216
10. Salzman, E. and Britten, A. F. H. (1965). *Haemorrhage and Thrombosis.* (Boston: Little and Brown)
11. Shappell, S. D. and Lenfant, C. J. M. (1972). *Anesthesiology*, **37,** 127
12. Bunn, H. F. and Jandl, J. D. (1970). *N. Engl. J. Med.*, **282,** 1414
13. Kawashima, Y., Yamamoto, Z. and Manabe, H. (1974). *Surgery*, **76,** 391
14. Navari, R. M. and Gainer, J. L. (1973). In Gabelnick, H. L. and Litt, M. (Eds.) *Rheology of Biological Systems.* (Springfield, Illinois: C. Thomas)
15. Sanders, C. A., Kaulbach, M. G., Michalska, A. and Laver, M. B. (1966). *Circulation*, **23/24,** Suppl. III 205
16. Wright, C. J. (1974). *Surg. Forum*, **25,** 198
17. Cain, S. M. (1965). *Am. J. Physiol.*, **209,** 604
18. Neville, W. E. (1967). Extracorporeal Circulation. In Neville, W. E. (Ed.) *Current Problems in Surgery.* (Chicago: Yearbook Medical)
19. Kessler, M. and Messmer, K. (1975). *Bibliotheca Haematologica*, **41,** 16
20. Michenfelder, J. D. and Theye, R. A. (1969). *Anesthesiology*, **31,** 449
21. Race, D., Dedichen, H. and Schenk, W. G. (1967). *J. Thoracic Cardiovasc. Surg.*, **53,** 578
22. Mares, E. (1892). *C.R. Soc. Bull.*, **44,** 313
23. Hegnauer, A. H. and Angelakos, E. T. (1959). *Ann. N. Y. Acad. Sci.*, **80,** 336
24. Boylan, J. W. and Hong, S. K. (1966). *Am. J. Physiol.*, **211,** 1371
25. Scribner, B. H. and Burnell, J. M. (1956). *Metabolism*, **5,** 468
26. Kanter, G. S. (1963). *Am. J. Physiol.*, **205,** 1285
27. Kanter, G. S. (1963). *Am. J. Physiol.*, **204,** 953
28. Roberts, K. E., Magida, M. G. and Pitts, R. F. (1953). *Am. J. Physiol.*, **172,** 47
29. Morales, P., Carbery, W., Morello, A. and Morales, G. (1957). *Ann. Surg.*, **145,** 488
30. Irvine, R. O. H. and Dow, J. W. (1966). *Clin. Sci.*, **31,** 317

31. Irvine, R. O. H. and Dow, J. W. (1968). *Metabolism*, **21**, 563
32. Irvine, R. O. H. and Dow, J. W. (1968). *Aust. Ann. Med.*, **17**, 206
33. Clancy, R. L. and Brown, E. B. (1966). *Am. J. Physiol.*, **211**, 1309
34. Bernsmeier, A. and Rudolph, W. (1961). *Verhandl. Deutch. Ges. Kreislauff.*, **27**, 59

26
'Which priming fluids?'

M. A. TOBIAS AND J. M. FRYER

It is 16 years since the South Central Association of Blood Banks met in Oklahoma City under the chairmanship of Dr Zuhdi and discussed which priming fluids were most suitable for cardiopulmonary bypass[1]. The title was 'Blood, mannitol, dextran, sugar, water and confusion', and in spite of the many papers published on the subject since then, agreement as to what constitutes the ideal prime has still not been reached. It is the purpose of this chapter to outline the changes which have taken place over the years and review some aspects of physiology relevant to the subject.

During the early period of open-heart surgery, the heart–lung machines were primed with fresh heparinized homologous blood of the same group. These film oxygenators had large priming volumes (3–5 litres), and the problem of providing an adequate supply of fresh donor blood soon forced clinicians to switch to routinely collected banked blood[2]. It is instructive to recall that in those early days of open-heart surgery, it was considered a fundamental error to administer more than the barest minimum of clear fluid during these operations. Even the volume of heparinized saline required to flush the pressure catheter was suspected of causing the pulmonary oedema sometimes observed[3].

The disadvantages of perfusing patients with large volumes of genetically different blood soon became manifest and are still present today. These include the 'homologous blood syndrome'[4,5] where plasma migrates from the intravascular compartment in an unpredictable fashion following perfusion with large amounts of homologous blood. The cause is unexplained but probably involves immunological mechanisms.

Transfusion hepatitis remains a serious problem which has not been eliminated even after carefully screening donors for the presence of Australia antigen. The reported incidence following transfusion varies[6] from 0.16 % to 6 % and has not been reduced by the introduction of frozen washed cells[7].

Post-operative pulmonary hypoxia and congestion ('pump lung') was often seen after whole-blood perfusion, possibly caused by obstruction of the

Table 1 Disadvantages of whole blood perfusion

Homologous blood syndrome
Transfusion hepatitis
'Perfusion lung'
Iso-antibody formation
Incompatibility reactions
Allergic reactions
Damage from oxygenator and roller pumps
(a) to red blood corpuscles (haemolysis)
(b) to plasma proteins (denaturation)
Extravagant demands on blood transfusion services

pulmonary vascular bed with platelet aggregates[8] or immunologically-triggered opening of pulmonary shunts[9]. Other problems with whole-blood primes[6] are listed in Table 1.

Stored blood becomes a progressively more unphysiological fluid with age, as shown in Table 2. The reduction in erythrocyte levels of 2,3-diphosphoglyceric acid shifts the oxyhaemoglobin dissociation curve to the left, impeding oxygen delivery from blood to the tissues[10] and it may take at least 4 hours in the circulation before stored erythrocytes recover normal function[11]. Since 1959[12], various centres have experimented with haemodiluted primes in order to conserve blood. Long and co-workers[13] used dextran and albumin to improve the flow characteristics of blood and avoid the capillary blockage produced by intravascular aggregates (sludging)[14]. Zuhdi's group[15] used low volume primes of 5% dextrose in water and perfused at low flow rates (20 ml/kg per min). More recently higher volume primes utilizing more physiological flow-rates have been introduced. Some authors advocate electrolyte solutions only[16, 17] and others crystalloid–colloid mixtures[18, 19] sometimes supplementing with autologous blood transfusion post-bypass[20]. Universal agreement exists that high-volume dilution reduces intra-operative and post-operative blood requirements. Verska *et al.*[21] were able to show a total peri-

Table 2 Changes in citrated blood during storage at 4 ± 1°C

Blood constituent	*Storage period* (days) 0	7	14	21
Haemoglobin mg/100 ml	0–10	25	50	100
pH	7.00	6.85	6.77	6.68
Glucose mg/100 ml	350	300	245	210
Lactic acid mg/100 ml	20	70	120	140
Inorganic phosphate mg/100 ml	1.8	4.5	6.6	9.0
Sodium mmol/l	150	148	145	142
Potassium mmol/l	3–4	12	24	32
Ammonia μg/100 ml	50	260	470	680

From Strumia, Crosby *et al.*, reference 106

operative blood requirement of 1500 ml using non-blood prime compared with 3500 ml using partial blood prime. It has been shown by Hallowell *et al.*[22] that a further reduction averaging 860 ml per case can be achieved by employing autologous blood transfusion. Platelet counts are consistently higher and there is less post-operative bleeding in patients treated with total haemodilution and autologous blood transfusion compared with patients receiving part-blood primes[23].

Before scrutinizing the plethora of claims advanced in support of the various different recipes, it is worth reviewing some of the relevant physiology pertaining to haemodilution.

BLOOD RHEOLOGY

The flow pattern and deformability of blood depend upon two factors; its viscosity function and its yield stress[24].

Viscosity function

This term refers to the fact that the viscosity of non-Newtonian fluids (like blood), varies with the flow-rate. Fluid viscosity depends upon two factors:

(1) SHEAR STRESS – the force applied to the liquid per unit area; this represents a measure of how difficult it is to deform a particular fluid at a fixed speed. The more viscous the material, the greater the shear stress.

(2) SHEAR RATE – this represents the rate at which different planes of the fluid slide past one another, i.e. the velocity gradient. The higher the shear rate for any particular fluid, the greater the shear stress required to move it.

For simple Newtonian fluids there is a linear relationship between shear stress and shear rate which can be represented mathematically by the formula:

$$\tau = \eta \cdot \dot{y}$$

where τ = shear stress η = viscosity value for that particular fluid $\dot{y}$ = shear rate, as shown in Figure 1.
When blood flows slowly, aggregation and rouleaux formation occurs between erythrocytes and this creates a fluid of high viscosity. As velocity increases, the aggregates are broken up and the blood becomes 'thinner'. Once all aggregates are dispersed, a critical value is reached above which viscosity remains unchanged at higher velocities.

Yield stress

At very low flow rates the viscosity of blood increases enormously, so that when blood stops flowing, a very high force is required to restart it. This is because, at rest, erythrocytes are interconnected by negatively-charged

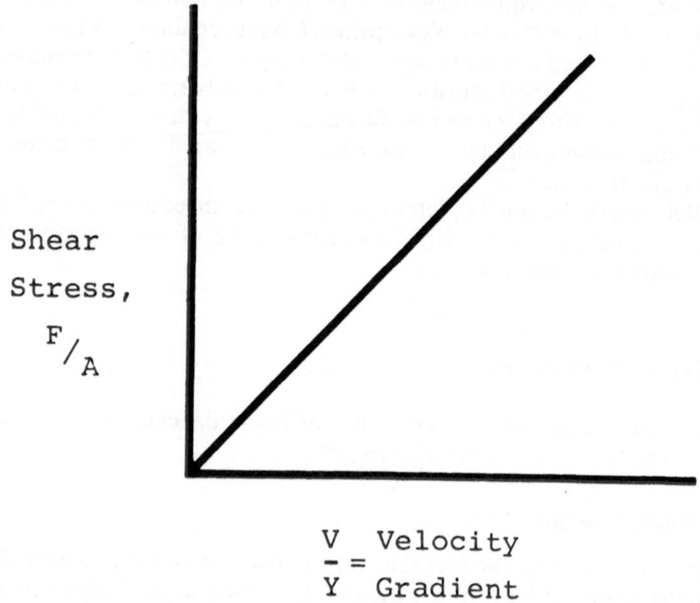

Figure 1 The linear relationship for Newtonian fluids between shear stress (force/area) and shear rate (velocity/separation). Redrawn with permission from R. J. Gordon and M. B. Ravin, 1978, reference 24

fibrinogen molecules. The initial high force required to overcome these charges and set the system in motion is called the yield stress, as shown in Figure 2.

Viscosity function and yield stress have important practical consequences for the management of cardio-pulmonary bypass. Let us consider some of these.

Haematocrit and systemic vascular resistance

The viscosity of blood depends mainly upon its haematocrit, and the latter drops markedly when using clear primes during cardio-pulmonary bypass. Systemic vascular resistance depends upon two factors, arteriolar vasodilation and viscosity[25] as shown in Table 3. Calculations for changes in systemic vascular resistance usually ignore the effect of viscosity on the assumption that this remains constant. However the fall in blood pressure frequently seen when going on bypass using crystalloid primes has been shown by Gordon *et al.*[26] to be due substantially to the acute reduction in viscosity produced by haemodilution, as illustrated in Figure 3. Other factors contributing to the occurrence of hypotension at the commencement of cardiopulmonary bypass include:

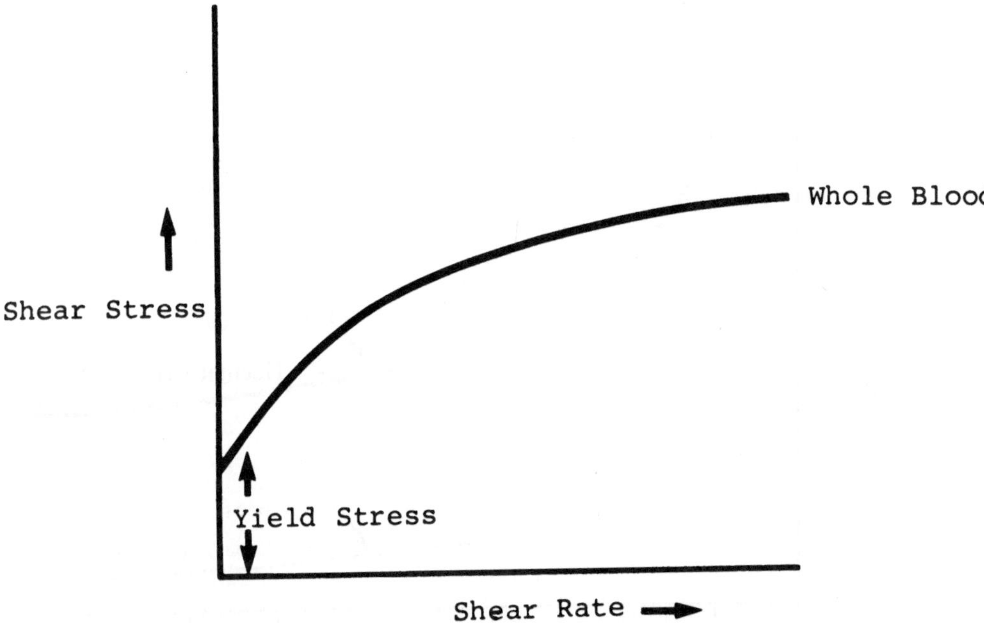

Figure 2 Shear stress plotted against shear rate for whole blood. A minimum stress, the yield stress, is required to initiate flow. Redrawn with permission from R. J. Gordon and M. B. Ravin, 1978, reference 24

(1) Reflex vasodilation of resistance and capacitance vessels during partial bypass, possibly caused by triggering of the baroreceptor system due to pulse generation by the beating heart during continuous fluid infusion from the arterial line[27].

(2) Alteration in baroreceptor perception as blood flow changes from a pulsatile to a non-pulsatile mode[28].

(3) Dilution of circulating catecholamines by the extracorporeal priming volume[29].

Table 3 Systemic vascular resistance and viscosity

$$\text{SVR} = \frac{\overline{\text{AP}} - \overline{\text{RAP}}}{\text{CO}} \times \frac{\eta_1}{\eta}$$

SVR = systemic vascular resistance
$\overline{\text{AP}}$ = mean arterial pressure
$\overline{\text{RAP}}$ = mean right atrial pressure
CO = cardiac output
η = normal blood viscosity at high flow at 37°C (3·8 centipoise)
η_1 = viscosity of haemodiluted blood at measured temperature

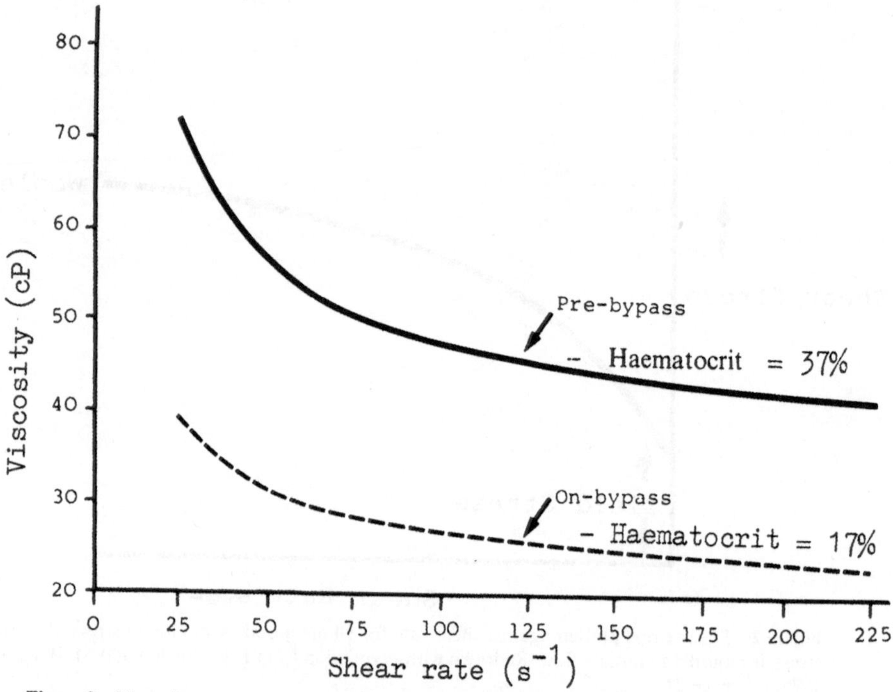

Figure 3 Viscosity versus shear rate measured before and after the initiation of cardiopulmonary bypass. Redrawn with permission from R. J. Gordon *et al.*, 1975, reference 26

Optimal haematocrit

Patients not on bypass respond to acute normovolaemic haemodilution, such as produced by autologous blood removal, by increasing cardiac output by two mechanisms.

(a) Augmentation of venous return (increased preload)[30]
(b) Smaller end-systolic volume (reduced afterload)[31].

Blood pressure and heart-rate remain stable. Because cardiac output rises faster than oxygen content falls, oxygen availability actually increases as haematocrit is reduced[32] from 45 % to 30 % as shown in Figure 4.

Oxygen availability falls steeply below a haematocrit of 20 % and two other compensatory mechanisms are brought into play[33].

(i) Enhanced oxygen extraction by lowering the venous PO_2 at tissue level.
(ii) Displacement of the oxygen dissociation curve to the right.

During cardio-pulmonary bypass, induced hypothermia is an important protective mechanism during haemodilution. Gott *et al.*[34] have shown that oxygen consumption is reduced to 50 % of normal at 30 °C and 20 % at 20 °C.

Table 4 Change in viscosity with temperature at a velocity gradient of $213\,s^{-1}$

	Viscosity, cP		
Fluid	37 °C	32 °C	27 °C
Plasma	1.4	1.7	2.0
Blood – haematocrit = 20%	2.5	2.8	3.1
haematocrit = 40%	3.8	4.3	4.8
haematocrit = 60%	6.5	7.1	7.9

In addition more oxygen can be dissolved in the plasma as temperature decreases. Viscosity also increases with drop in temperature[35], (Table 4) and helps to compensate for the initial viscosity change produced by clear perfusion primes. Clowes[36] has shown that oxygen consumption falls and base deficit rises at perfusion flows below $2\,l\,m^{-2}\,min^{-1}$ but flow rates above this value do not incur any further benefit.

It can be concluded that the employment of high flow rates and moderate hypothermia (30 °C) will ensure adequate tissue oxygen delivery down to a haematocrit of 20 % or even less for short periods. Evidence in support comes from Kessler and Messmers' work[37] demonstrating adequate tissue PO_2 values in haemodiluted dogs.

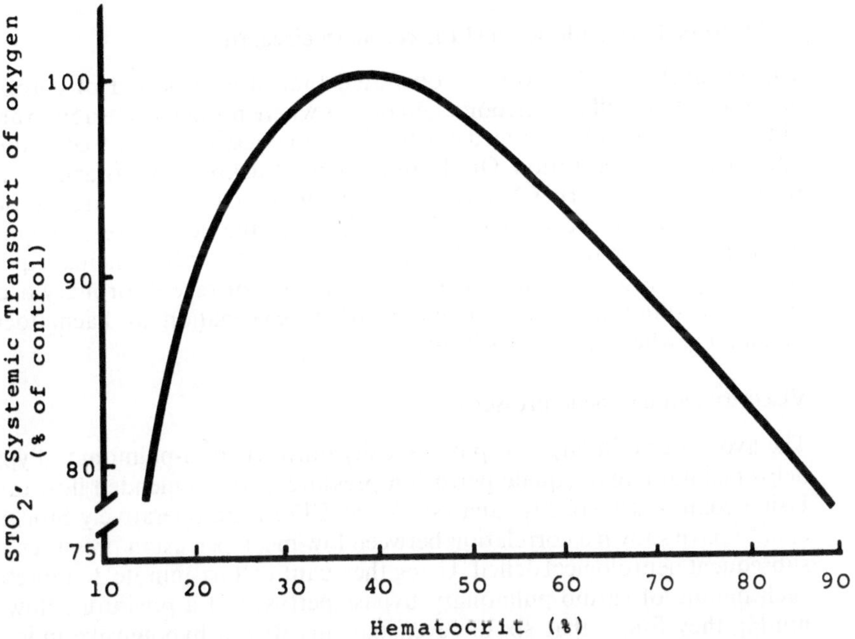

Figure 4 Total systemic transport of O_2 versus haematocrit. Values are relative to a control haematocrit of 45 %

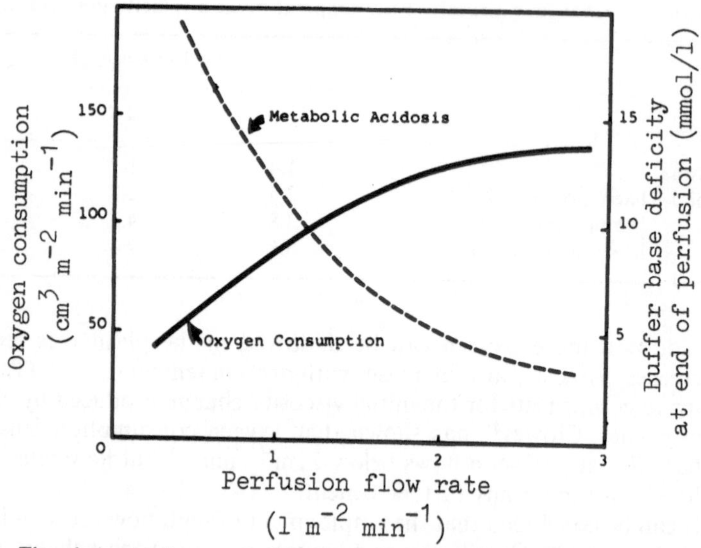

Figure 5 The relationship between perfusion flow rate, total body oxygen consumption and the development of metabolic acidosis during normothermic (34–37 °C) cardiopulmonary bypass. Both oxygen consumption and base deficit reach an asymptotic level at about 2 l/m²/min. Note the reciprocal relationship between the two. From G. H. A. Clowes, 1972, reference 36, with permission

Yield stress, haemodilution and the coronary circulation

Various authors[39, 39] have demonstrated that after a period of coronary occlusion, a 'no reflow' phenomenon occurs where normal perfusion to areas of the heart cannot be resumed due to a local increase in viscosity consequent upon haemoconcentration. On the other hand, Buckberg and Brazier[40], and Kleinman and co-workers[41] have shown in dogs that under certain conditions of normothermia and moderate haemodilution, the flow increase required to maintain normal oxygen delivery to the subendocardium is inadequate, suggesting that some patients with aortic stenosis or severe coronary occlusion may suffer impaired sub-endocardial oxygenation at haematocrits below 30 % when the heart is beating.

Viscosity and perfusion pressure

The avoidance of a large drop in viscosity during cardio-pulmonary bypass helps maintain an adequate perfusion pressure at recommended flow rates. Using compressed spectral analysis of the EEG intra-operatively Stockard *et al.*[42] have shown a correlation between low mean perfusion pressures and subsequent neurological deficit. Using the quantity 'torr-minute' to represent each minute of cardio-pulmonary bypass perfused at a pressure below 50 mmHg they found that six of seven patients with a hypotensive index in excess of 100 torr-minutes sustained post-operative neurological deficits, in contrast to only three patients out of sixteen who had an index less than 100

Table 5 Postoperative neurological complications versus intraoperative hypotension in a series of 23 patients requiring cardiopulmonary bypass studied prospectively

		No deficit	*Temporary deficit*	*Organic brain syndrome*	*Permanent deficit*	*Irreversible coma*
Hypotension as tm^{50} / (50 mm Hg-MAP) δt in torr-minutes	>600				①	①
	350–600			③	③	
	100–350	•	⑥ ⑤ ④	⑤ ④	②	②
	0–100	• • • • • • • • • • • • •	• •	•		

(Reproduced from Stockard, J. J., Bickford, R. G. and Schauble, J. F.: Pressure-dependant cerebral ischemia during cardiopulmonary bypass. *Neurology* 23: 521, 1973), with permission.

torr-minutes. It would seem advisable therefore to maintain mean arterial pressures greater than 50 mmHg during bypass. An interesting finding is that administration of methoxamine as a pressor agent during bypass has been shown to selectively increase subendocardial blood flow as well as increasing total coronary flow[43].

OSMOMETRY

The osmotic pressure is that pressure which must be exerted on a solution to prevent the net passage of solvent molecules across a semi-permeable membrane. When a solute is dissolved in a solvent, the osmotic pressure increases and this can be measured by measuring the depression produced upon the freezing point of the solvent. Osmolality refers to the particle concentration per kilogram of water, whereas osmolarity refers to particle concentration per litre of solution. In clinical practice, these terms can be regarded as synonymous.

Tonicity

A fluid is isotonic if it causes neither expansion nor contraction of red blood cells in it. Normal serum osmolality is 285 ± 5 mosmol/kg and solutions of such dissimilar chemical composition as 5% dextrose and Ringer-lactate have the same particle concentration and are said to be isotonic[44]. The osmolality of body fluids is primarily dependent on the high concentration of small ions and can be considered as 'crystalloid osmolality'. Body fluids also contain a small number of large (MW = 30000) particles, mainly proteins, which contribute only about 0.5% to the total osmolality of plasma. However, this colloid component is important in the distribution of water between the body fluid spaces because of the limited colloid permeability of capillary membranes. Consequently osmotic forces influencing the movement of water are generated wherever colloid concentration gradients exist.

Crystalloid osmotic pressure

The maintenance of osmolar constancy is regulated primarily by the hypothalamus which adjusts the secretion of anti-diuretic hormone to modify renal excretion of water[45]. Maximal dilution and concentration of urine produce urine osmolalities ranging from 50 to 1400 mosmol/kg. Hyperosmolality in the conscious patient produces thirst, cerebral dehydration and coma,

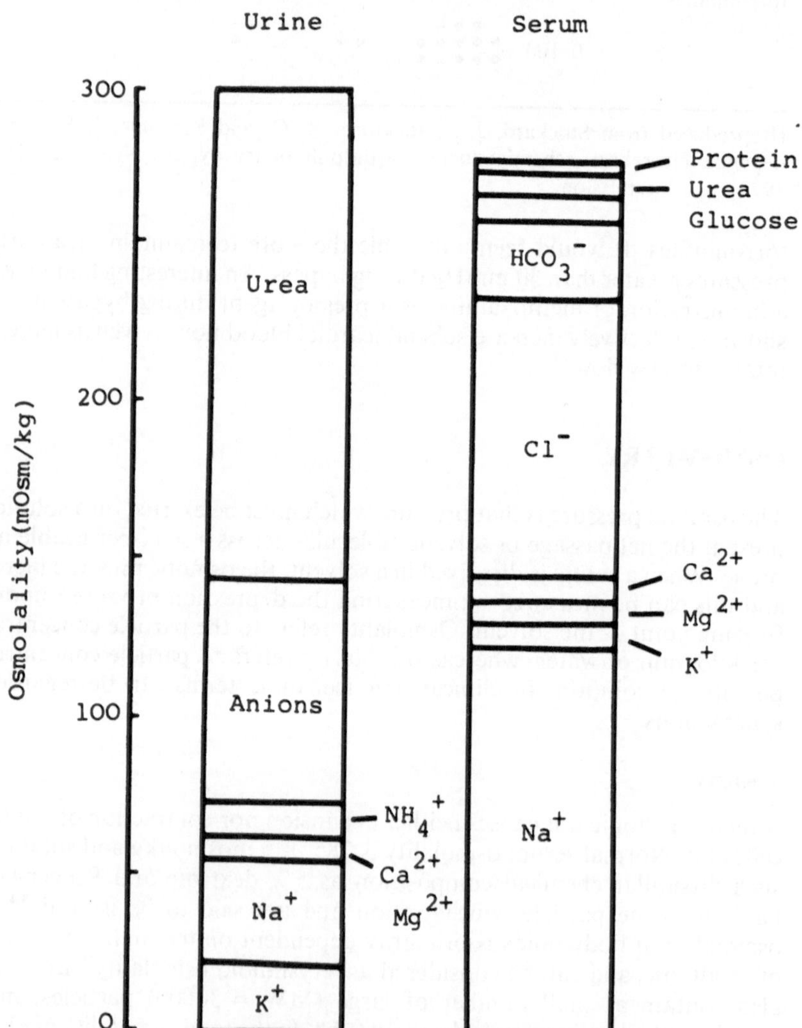

Figure 6 The osmotic constituents of urine and normal serum of a healthy subject

whereas hypo-osmolality produces brain swelling, nausea and muscle weakness[46]. In conditions of both water depletion, and water overload, increasing the solute load presented to the kidney results in the production of urine isotonic with plasma.

Deverall *et al.*[47] have commented on the occurrence of plasma hypotonicity post-operatively in children receiving crystalloid haemodilution, which was not altered by adjusting the osmolal concentration of the prime nor by severely restricting water intake post-operatively. During the first forty-eight hours, a water diuresis did not occur and this may be related to the inappropriately high anti-diuretic hormone (ADH) levels commented upon by

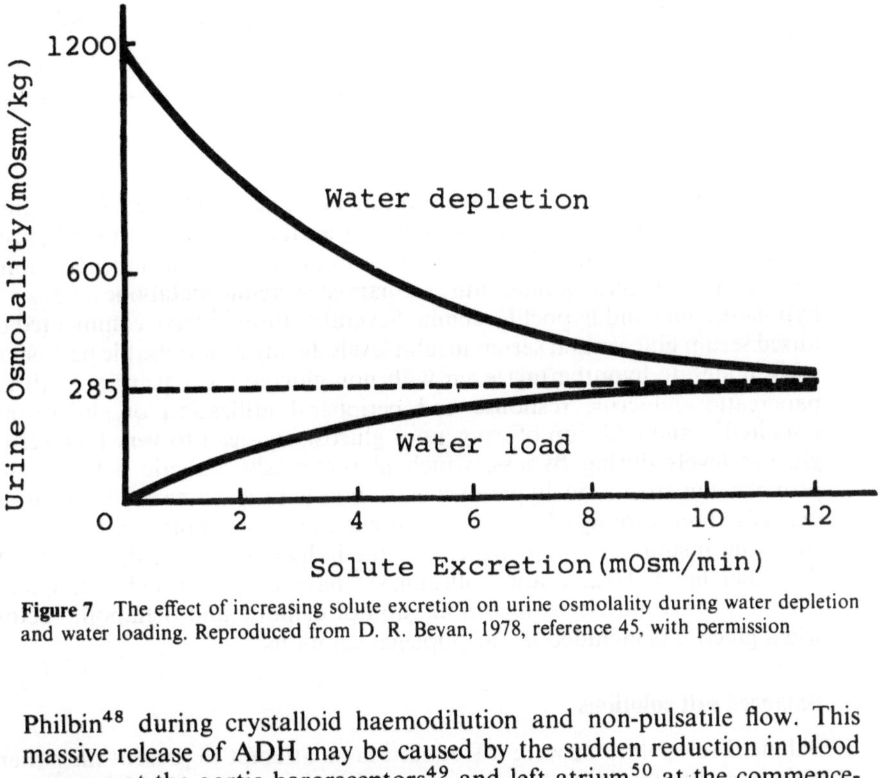

Figure 7 The effect of increasing solute excretion on urine osmolality during water depletion and water loading. Reproduced from D. R. Bevan, 1978, reference 45, with permission

Philbin[48] during crystalloid haemodilution and non-pulsatile flow. This massive release of ADH may be caused by the sudden reduction in blood pressure at the aortic baroreceptors[49] and left atrium[50] at the commencement of bypass using low-viscosity primes.

Crystalloids

At this stage it is worth reviewing the three crystalloids most commonly employed in the cardio-pulmonary bypass circuit in the United Kingdom, namely 5% dextrose, Hartman's Ringer-lactate and mannitol.

Table 6 Comparison of crystalloid fluids used for priming in the UK

	5% *Dextrose*	*Hartmans'*	*'Plasmolyte 148'*	10% *Mannitol*
Cations (mmol/l)				
Na^+	0	131	140	0
K^+	0	5	5	0
Ca^{++}	0	2	0	0
Mg^{++}	0	0	1.5	0
Anions (mmol/l)				
Cl^-	0	111	98	0
Lactate	0	29	0	0
Acetate	0	0	27	0
Gluconate	0	0	23	0
Osmolality (mosmol/kg)	278	278	294	549
pH	4	5–7	4–6	4.5–7
NHS Cost/Litre	88p	91p	£1.33p	£2.90p

5% Dextrose

5% Dextrose is cheap, readily available and extensively studied. It is slightly hypotonic and becomes steadily more so, as the dextrose is metabolized, leaving the patient with a large water load to excrete, and the large dilutional effect on plasma bicarbonate causes a marked systemic metabolic acidosis[51], hyponatraemia and hypochloraemia. Several authors[52] have commented on raised serum glucose and serum insulin levels during non-pulsatile perfusions with moderate hypothermia even with non-glucose clear primes. Both the pancreatic endocrine response and peripheral utilization of glucose are impaired[53] and addition of exogenous glucose can lead to very high serum glucose levels during bypass, which in previously diabetic patients may provoke hyperosmotic hyperglycaemic non-ketotic coma[54]. There is an extensive literature which suggests that glucose, in combination with potassium and insulin may be beneficial to the ischaemic myocardium[55,56]. On the other hand, Hearse and colleagues[57] have demonstrated a damaging effect on heart muscle by a combination of osmotic and metabolic factors when glucose is included in cardioplegic solutions.

Balanced salt solutions

Balanced salt solutions were introduced in an attempt to present the patient with a perfusate similar in ion concentration to his or her own serum. Lactate-containing solutions are initially slightly acid, but the liver converts lactate to bicarbonate, eventually producing a metabolic alkalosis. 'Plasmolyte 148' has a slight advantage over Ringer-lactate in that it contains 1.5 mmol/l magnesium, and presents alternative pathways for bicarbonate production, using acetate and gluconate.

Large volumes of crystalloid prime resulting in low colloid oncotic pressures lead to diffusion of perfusate into the interstitial fluid during bypass with subsequent re-entry into the intra-vascular space post-operatively. Neville *et al.*[58] have demonstrated that low haematocrits occurring after the third post-operative day were due to dilutional hypervolaemia and not to a decreased red cell mass, which was best treated with fluid restriction and diuretics, rather than blood transfusion. Beattie *et al.*[59] have shown during crystalloid haemodilution that albumin enters the intravascular compartment at the rate of 0.2 g per minute. This represents a transfer of 16 g albumin during an average pump run, or approximately, 40 % of the rapidly exchangeable body albumin pool. With a Ringer-lactate prime, several authors have observed no significant change in sodium or chloride but a decrease of potassium during extracorporeal circulation[60].

Aetiological factors provoking hypokalaemia include hyperglycaemia[61], noradrenaline release during acidosis[62], previous diuretic therapy[63] and changes in phosphate metabolism[64]. Administration of extra potassium into the extracorporeal circuit results in improved vascular tone with increases in both arterial and venous pressures. High potassium replacement to achieve serum K^+ levels in the range 5–5.5 mmol/l have been shown by Babka and Pifarré[65] to promote spontaneous defibrillation and reduce the incidence of ventricular arrythmias post-operatively. Westhorpe *et al.*[66] have shown that calcium supplementation is unnecessary when using clear primes, and immediately after bypass the intravenous administration of calcium chloride should not exceed 10 mg/kg if gross hypercalcaemia is to be avoided. Holden[67] and Kahn[68] have stressed the importance of magnesium supplementation during cardio-pulmonary bypass.

Mannitol

Mannitol is an inert non-metabolizable 6-carbon polyhydric alcohol. Intravenous infusion of this hypertonic low-molecular weight crystalloid withdraws fluid initially across the capillary into the plasma. It rapidly diffuses into interstitial fluid, and increases the volume of the whole extra-cellular phase by withdrawing water from body cells. Mannitol is readily filtered into the tubular lumen and this strongly hygroscopic solute produces a brisk water diuresis[69] even in the presence of high levels of ADH.

Mannitol is only a very transient plasma expander, and Das *et al.*[70] have shown that osmolal equilibration between prime and patients extracellular fluid occurs within 10 minutes of commencing perfusion. A prime adjusted to 340–360 mosmol usually gives a final patient/prime value of approximately 300–310 mosmol. Renal plasma flow is linearly related with serum osmolality[71] and urine flow on bypass is greater than with isotonic primes. Total urine and solute excretion over the next twenty-four hours diminishes however and the final output is similar to patients receiving isotonic primes.

Initially transfer of fluid from the intracellular to extracellular fluid space with mannitol may cause interstitial pulmonary oedema and impair oxygenation[72], and rapid infusion produces hypotension by vasodilation in skeletal muscles[73]. Mannitol's influence on the heart is controversial. Willerson *et al.*[74] reported improved ventricular performance and increased coronary flow in patients in whom serum osmolality was increased to a mean of 309 ± 3 mosmol. On the other hand, using cardioplegia solution containing mannitol with a much higher osmolality, Hearse[57] reported a deleterious effect caused by excessive cellular dehydration.

COLLOID OSMOTIC PRESSURE

Colloid osmotic pressure is derived almost entirely from the plasma proteins especially albumin and fibrinogen. Starling[75] formulated an equation which relates the transcapillary movement of water to the balance of hydrostatic and osmotic forces as shown in Table 7. For practical purposes the occurrence of pulmonary oedema can be regarded as depending primarily on the difference between colloid osmotic pressure and pulmonary capillary wedge pressure (COP–PCWP gradient)[76].

Guyten and Lindsey[77] have shown that the critical left atrial pressure for transudation of plasma into the pulmonary parenchyma is 24 mmHg when protein concentration is normal. Schüpbach *et al.*[78] have shown in rabbits

Table 7 Transcapillary movement of water

$$V = Kf((Pc - P_{If}) - (\pi_p - \pi_{If}))$$

V = rate of liquid movement
Kf = capillary filtration coefficient
Pc = pulmonary capillary wedge pressure ($\simeq +7$ mmHg)
P_{If} = interstitial fluid hydrostatic pressure ($\simeq -6$ mmHg)
π_p = plasma colloid osmotic pressure ($\simeq +22$ mmHg)
π_{If} = interstitial fluid colloid osmotic pressure ($\simeq +1$ mmHg)

that reduction of colloid osmotic pressure below the normal level of 24 mmHg is compensated for by increased tissue lymph flow which removes interstitial protein and limits interstitial oedema down to a critical pressure of 16 mmHg on cardio-pulmonary bypass, this representing a plasma protein concentration of 42 g/l (30 g/l albumin). Reduction of colloid osmotic pressures below this level cause progressive increases in myocardial[79], pulmonary[80], and intestinal wall[81] accumulation of extracellular water, capable of interfering with ventricular function, respiration, wound healing and intestinal motility during the post-operative period. (Figure 8)

Laver and Buckley[16] could detect no sign of pulmonary oedema or deterioration in A–aD_{O_2} gradients despite extreme haemodilution in patients to a total protein level of 24 g/l. On the other hand, Hewson[81] has demonstrated a significant correlation between increasing hydrostatic pressure on bypass and deteriorating A-aD_{O_2} in patients with low colloid oncotic pressures. A high plasma oncotic pressure inhibits renal ultrafiltration during hypotension, and urine flow is diminished[82]. Metabolic acidosis during cardiopulmonary bypass has little connection with measured lactate levels but varies inversely with the buffering capacity of the perfusate as representated by its protein content[78].

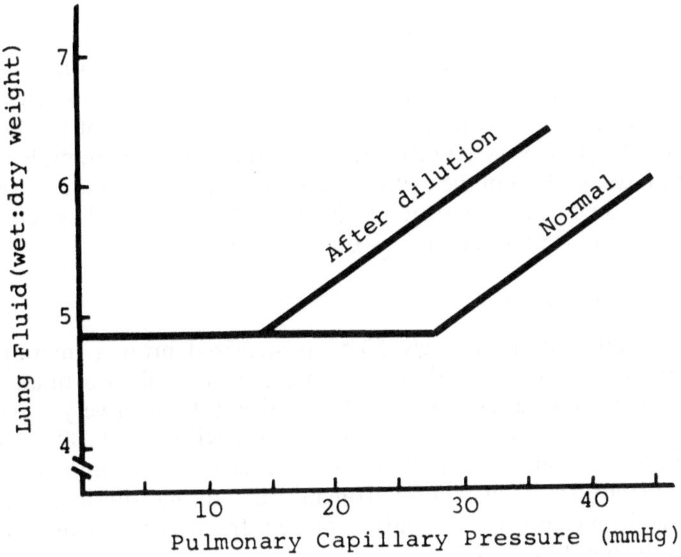

Figure 8 The effect of increasing pulmonary capillary pressure on the appearance of pulmonary oedema (wet/dry lung ratio) in the isolated sheep's lung, perfused with whole blood and blood diluted 50 % with isotonic saline. Reproduced from D. R. Bevan, 1980, reference 76, with permission

Plasma preparations

The use of fresh plasma, human dried plasma and stored, pooled plasma for the maintenance of colloid osmotic pressure on bypass cannot be justified because of the risk of hepatitis transfer. Table 8 shows some physical properties of some colloid solutions presently available in the United Kingdom.

Table 8 Comparison of colloid fluids used for priming

	pH	*Colloid osmotic pressure*	*Osmolality* (mosmol/kg)	*Viscosity* (blood = 3.8 cP)	*Half-life in circulation* (hours)	*NHS cost per litre*
Plasma protein fraction	6.7–7.3 (buffering capacity)	iso-oncotic	285	1.3	15	up to £60
Haemaccel	7.2–7.3 (buffering capacity)	iso-oncotic	302	1.8	1.5	£5.56
Dextran 70	5.1–5.7	hyperoncotic	308	3.4	> 12	£4.60
Dextran 40	4.5–5.6	markedly hyperoncotic	308	5.4	4.5	£7.44

A prerequisite for the selection of an appropriate synthetic colloid-substitute is that it should be metabolized or excreted completely in the body after fulfilling its function. A balance is achieved between the intravascular and extravascular compartments following colloid infusion, which is shown as an increase of circulating plasma volume, diffusion of smaller particles beyond the blood vessels and excretion of fractions with low molecular weight by the kidneys. Part of the colloid solution returns to the blood stream via the lymphatics while part is stored in the reticulo-endothelial system, mainly in the liver, and is gradually released and excreted[83].

Plasma protein fraction

This contains approximately 50 g/l pasteurized protein (mainly albumin) and requires four blood donors to provide one unit. Fortunately, plasma collected from time-expired blood is used but it is still very expensive. The commercial equivalent, 5 % albumin, costs the NHS about £40 per bottle. 20 % ('salt-poor') albumin is even more expensive. 1 g albumin retains 18 ml water in the intravascular compartment[84], and the half-life in the circulation[85] is 15 h. Rapid infusion of plasma protein fraction may cause vasodilation and a drop in blood pressure[86]

Dextrans

Dextrans are high molecular polysaccharides constructed of glucose molecules. The colloid-osmotic effectivity is based on the fact that each gram of dextran binds 20–25 ml water. The volume effect of dextran 70 (Macrodex) is initially slightly greater than the amount infused, whereas dextran 40 (Rheomacrodex) has a more pronounced effect, drawing in almost twice the amount infused, but its action is less sustained because of more rapid renal excretion[87]. The renal tubular concentration of Rheomacrodex may rise so quickly that the urine becomes very viscous and of low-volume, an effect that can be completely reversed in patients with normal renal function, by adequate hydration and concurrent administration of mannitol[88]. However, very high dosage can be followed by tubular blockage and acute renal failure in some patients with pre-existing renal insufficiency[89]. At doses exceeding 1.5 g/kg dextrans can cause impairment of haemostasis by the formation of a dextran film on the surfaces of platelets and vascular endothelium[90]. This dose should be reduced further in the presence of heparin because of its synergism with dextran[91]. Anaphylactoid reactions to dextrans have been reported and usually are apparent within ten minutes of starting infusion. Ring and Messmer[92] found an incidence of reactions of 0.008 % for dextran compared with 0.038 % for gelatin solutions in 200906 infusions carried out in a multicentre prospective trial. (Figure 9)

Gelatins

Gelatins are manufactured from bovine collagen and possess a molecular weight of approximately 35000. The main portion of a gelatin solution is therefore excreted within a few hours. This accounts for the relatively short half-life for gelatins of 1.5 hours[93]. The commonest gelatin studied during cardio-pulmonary bypass is Haemaccel[94,95]. De Vries and associates[96] found in dogs that potassium and calcium levels rose to dangerously high values using Haemaccel as the sole diluting agent and metabolic changes occurred suggestive of impaired tissue oxygenation. Haemaccel also has a poorer colloid osmotic effect than Macrodex because of its rapid excretion.

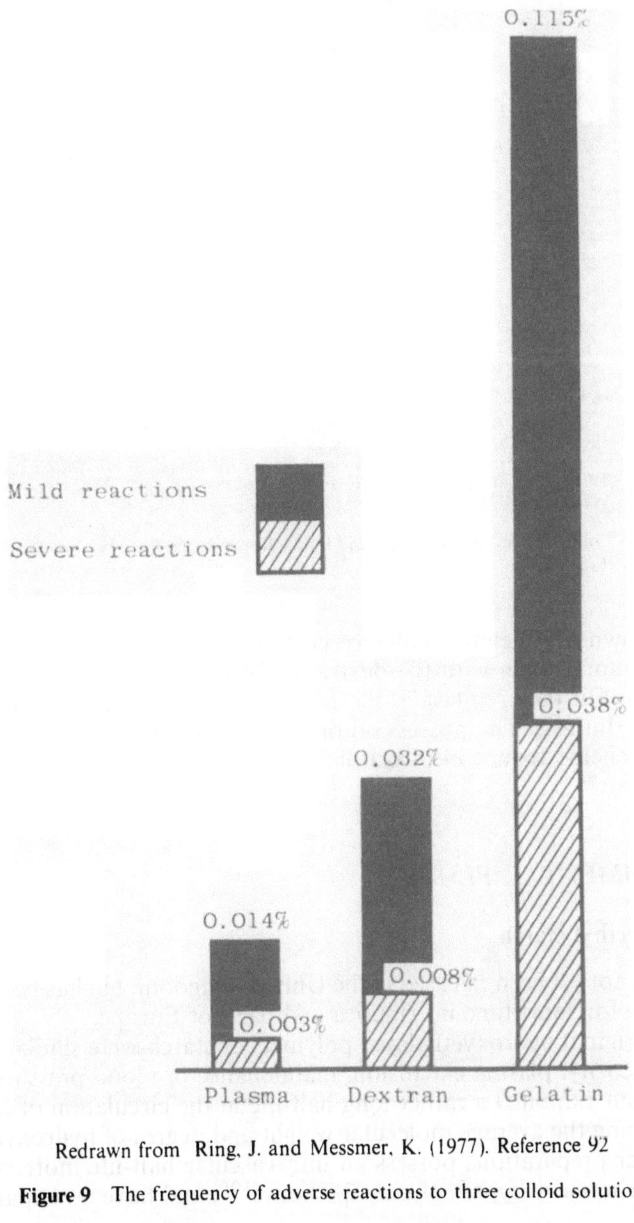

Redrawn from Ring, J. and Messmer, K. (1977). Reference 92

Figure 9 The frequency of adverse reactions to three colloid solutions

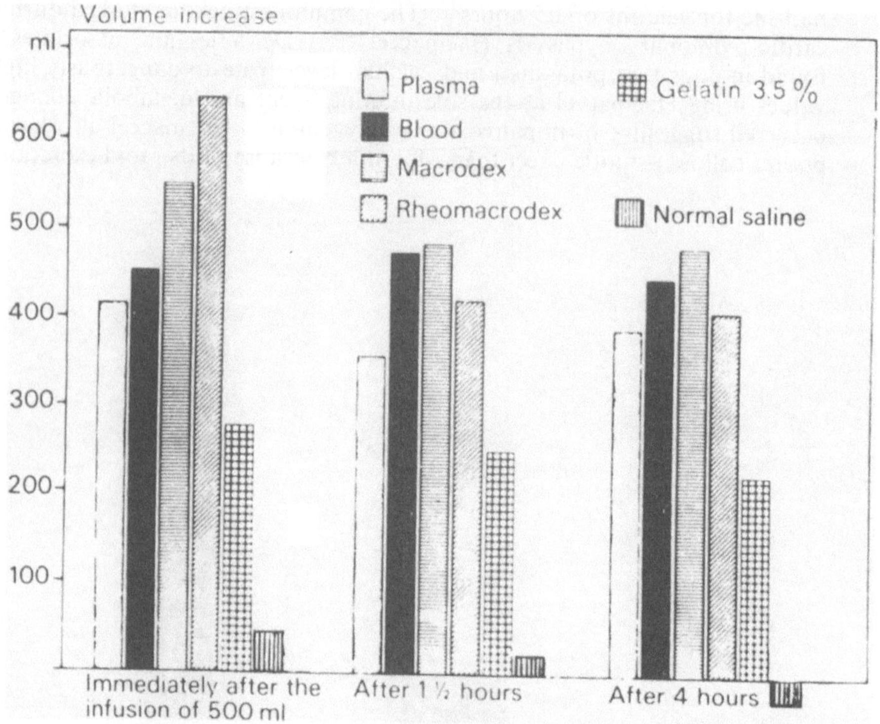

Figure 10 Volume effect of various colloid fluids. Reproduced from booklet 98–256, courtesy of Pharmacia (G.B.) Ltd

It is known that gelatins enhance erythrocyte aggregation[97] and reactions are commoner than with the dextrans, histamine release being a particular problem. On the credit side, the gelatins are pharmacologically inert and enhance diuresis. The possession of a neutral pH (7.3) plus some buffering capacity helps reduce electrostatic forces on erythrocytes hence reducing haemolysis[98].

EXPERIMENTAL FLUIDS

Hydroxyethyl starch

This has not yet been released in the United Kingdom, but has been generally available for some time in America and parts of Europe.

The original hydroxyethylated polymers of starch were similar to dextran 70 in viscosity, plasma expansion, maintenance of blood-pressure and side-effects, but exhibited a rather long half-life in the circulation of 26 hours[99]. By reducing the average molecular weight and degree of hydroxyethylation, the newer preparations possess an intravascular half-life more suitable for cardiopulmonary bypass of only 2.7 hours[100], and have no apparent effects on renal and hepatic biochemical indices. Reports of the use of low-molecular weight hydroxyethyl starch in the extracorporeal circulation have not yet appeared.

Heterologous stroma-free haemoglobin (SFHS)

Holdefer and Dowling[101] have studied the oxygenating characteristics of SFHS in puppies undergoing bypass. The substance underwent rapid renal clearance so anaemia and hypoxaemia developed quickly. Further progress awaits the development of a non-toxic inert molecular carrier to prolong half-life in the circulation.

Poloxalkol (Pluronic-F68)

This is a copolymer with both hydrophobic and hydrophilic properties. Vasko *et al.*[102] investigated dogs receiving Poloxalkol as a constituent of the bypass priming fluid, and demonstrated that it had excellent O_2 and CO_2 carrying properties, was non-toxic even in large doses (6 g/kg) and was totally excreted, unchanged. However, it prolonged the clotting time and had a negative inotropic effect on the heart. Human studies have not been carried out to date.

Fluorocarbon

Fluorocarbons are efficient carriers of respiratory gases but have a detrimental effect on the vascular tree in mammals[103]. Wallace *et al.*[104] devised a technique to avoid carry-over of fluorocarbon into the circulation by encapsulating oxygen bubbles in an oxygenator with a layer of fluorocarbon and recovering the latter by gravity, for recycling. *In vitro* experiments with human blood brought into contact with fluorocarbon revealed no biochemical alterations, however, the use of fluorocarbons remains experimental.

CONCLUSIONS

Despite the enormous literature on extracorporeal circulation, it would be rash to assert that we have any true understanding of what constitutes the optimal biochemical state under these conditions. Logic rebels at the notion that the 'normal' blood values necessarily have any relevance to a patient who is anaesthetized, paralysed, cooled and artificially perfused. The main criterion of adequacy should be the clinical and chemical state of the patient after the operation[105]

By this standard, haemodilution utilizing mainly crystalloid primes, with little regard to the preservation of normal levels of colloid oncotic pressure or plasma viscosity have stood the test of time in most British cardiac surgical units. Cheapness and absence of toxicity of balanced salt solutions have to date proscribed large-scale colloid supplementation, either on the grounds of cost (plasma protein fraction) or possible side-effects (dextrans, gelatins). A mass of theoretical and clinical evidence, however, indicates some solid

Table 9 Survey of 23 UK cardiac surgery units (1980) Adults – maintenance haematocrit during bypass

Maintenance haematocrit (%)	*No. of centres*
Under 23	13
23–27	6
Over 27	4

Table 10 Survey of 28 cardiac surgery units (1980) in UK. Priming fluids used during cardiopulmonary bypass

Primary fluids	*No. of centres*
Crystalloid primes only	12
Crystalloids, including mannitol	7
Crystalloids plus blood	4
Non-blood colloids plus crystalloids, including mannitol	5

advantages accruing to the partial replacement of crystalloids by cheap colloid-substitutes, and most of the requirements outlined earlier might be satisfied by the adoption of a regime as suggested in Table 11, provided patients have pre-existing normal renal function, are well hydrated pre- and post-operatively, and that the heparin dosage is carefully controlled by serial measurement of activated clotting times.

Table 11 Provisional regime for priming fluid composition for use during cardiopulmonary bypass for adults

Bypass-Prime (2500 ml)	
500 ml	Rheomacrodex/saline
500 ml	Haemacel
1000 ml	'Plasmolyte 148'
50–100 ml	Sodium bicarbonate (pH 7–8)
400 ml	Ringer-lactate
Add slowly during perfusion:	
	10% Mannitol 250–350 ml
	$MgCl_2 + KCl$

Any fluid additions on bypass might comprise Ringer-lactate or whole blood to keep the haematocrit above 20%. It would seem prudent to choose plasma protein fraction as the non-blood colloid component of priming fluid for children, because they possess a much smaller pool of readily exchangeable albumin than adults. Finally, it must be emphasized that the above hypothesis requires to be tested, that there still remains no consensus upon what constitutes an optimal prime, and that the whole area merits further scientific investigation.

References

1. Zuhdi, N., Carey, J. and Greer, A. (1964). Blood, mannitol, dextran, sugar, water and confusion. Presented at the *6th Annual meeting of the South Central Association of Blood Banks*, March 27, Oklahoma City, USA
2. Zuhdi, N., McCollough, B., Carey, J. and Greer, A. (1960). The use of citrated banked blood for open heart surgery. *Anesthesiology*, **21,** 496
3. Trede, M. (1969). Experimental investigations into the behaviour of coagulation and renal function during high dilution perfusions with glucose, Haemaccel and Rheomacrodex. In P. Lundsgaard-Hansen, A. Hässig and H. Nitschmann (eds.) *Modified Gelatins as Plasma Substitutes: Bibliotheca Haematologica*, **33,** p. 553. (Basel: Karger)
4. Dow, J. W., Dickson III, J. F., Hamer, N. A. and Gadboys, H. L. (1960). Anaphylactoid shock due to homologous blood exchange in the dog. *J. Thor. Surg.*, **39,** 449
5. Gadboys, H. L., Slonim, R. and Litwak, R. S. (1962). Homologous blood syndrome: 1. Preliminary observations on its relationship to cardio-pulmonary bypass. *Ann. Surg.*, **156,** 793
6. Doenicke, A., Grote, B. and Lorenz, W. (1977). Blood and blood substitutes. *Br. J. Anaesth.*, **49,** 681
7. Götz, E., Thoma, H. and Schäfer, A. (1975). Hepatitis in Abhangigkeit von der transfundierten Konservenzahl. *Anesthesiol. Wiederb.*, **90,** 346
8. McNamara, J. J., Burran, E. L., Larson, E., Omiya, G., Suchiro, G. and Yamase, H. (1972). Effects of debris in stored blood on pulmonary microvasculature. *Ann. Thor. Surg.*, **14,** 133
9. Melrose, D. G., Nahas, R., Alvarez, D., Todd, I. A. D. and Dempster, W. J. (1965). Post-operative hypoxia after extracorporeal circulation – a possible graft against host reaction. *Experienta*, **21,** 47
10. Benesch, R. and Benesch, R. E. (1967). The effect of organic phosphates from the human erythrocyte on the allosteric properties of haemoglobin. *Biochem. Biophys. Res. Commun.*, **26,** 162
11. Bentler, E. and Wood, L. (1969). The *in-vivo* regeneration of red cell 2,3-diphosphoglyceric acid (DPG) after transfusion of stored blood. *J. Lab. Clin. Med.*, **74,** 300
12. Panico, F. and Neptune, W. (1959). Mechanism to eliminate donor blood prime from pump oxygenator. *Surg. Forum.*, **10,** 65
13. Long, D. M., Sanchez, L., Varco, R. L. and Lillehei, C. W. (1961). The use of low molecular weight dextran and serum albumin as plasma expanders in extracorporeal circulation. *Surgery*, **50,** 12
14. Gelin, L. E. (1956). Studies in anaemia of injury. *Acta Chir. Scand.*, Suppl 210
15. Zuhdi, M., McCollough, B., Carey, J., Krieger, C. and Greer, A. (1961). Hypothermic perfusion for open-heart surgical procedures: report on the use of a heart-lung machine primed with 5% dextrose in water inducing haemodilution. *J. Int. Coll. Surg.*, **35,** 319.
16. Laver, M. B. and Buckley, M. J. (1972). Extreme hemodilution in the surgical patient. In K. Messmer and H. Schmid-Schönbein (eds.) *Hemodilution. Theoretical Basis and Clinical Application*, p. 215. (Basel: Karger)
17. Lilleasen, P., Frøysaker, T. and Stokke, O. (1978). Cardiac surgery in extreme haemodilution without donor blood, blood products or artificial macromolecules. *Scand. J. Thor. Cardiovasc. Surg.*, **12,** 249
18. Lee, W. H., Rubin, J. W. and Huggins, M. P. (1975). Clinical evaluation of priming solutions for pump oxygenator perfusion. *Ann. Thor. Surg.*, **19,** 529

19. Zubiate, P., Kay, J. H., Mendez, A. M., Krohn, B. G., Hockman, R. and Dunne, E. F. (1974). Coronary artery surgery. A new technique with use of little blood, if any. *J. Thor. Cardiovasc. Surg.*, **68,** 263
20. Hardesty, R. L., Bayer, W. L. and Bahnson, H. T. (1968). A technique for the use of autologous fresh blood during open-heart surgery. *J. Thor. Cardiovasc.*, **56,** 683
21. Verska, J. J., Ludington, L. G. and Brewer, L. A. (1974). A comparative study of cardiopulmonary bypass with non-blood and blood prime. *Ann. Thor. Surg.*, **18,** 72
22. Hallowell, P., Bland, J. H. L., Buckley, M. J. and Lowenstein, E. (1972). Transfusion of fresh autologous blood in open heart surgery. *J. Thor. Cardiovasc.*, **64,** 941
23. Lilleaasen, P. (1977). Moderate and extreme haemodilution in open-heart surgery. *Scand. J. Thor. Cardiovasc. Surg.*, **11,** 97
24. Gordon, R. J. and Ravin, M. (1978). Rheology and anesthesiology *Anesth. Analg.*, **52,** 252
25. Smith, E. E. and Crowell, J. W. (1967). Role of an increased haematocrit in altitude acclimatization. *Aerosp. Med.*, **38,** 39
26. Gordon, R. J., Ravin, M., Rawitscher, R. E. and Daicoff, G. R. (1975). Changes in arterial pressure, viscosity and resistance during cardiopulmonary bypass. *J. Thor. Cardiovasc. Surg.*, **69,** 552
27. Boulanger, M. (1977). Levels of circulating norepinephrine and epinephrine before, during and after cardiopulmonary bypass in man. *Survey Anesthesiol.*, **21,** 48
28. Dunn, J., Kirsch, M. M., Harness, J., Carroll, M., Straker, J. and Sloan, H. (1974). Hemodynamic, metabolic, and hematologic effects of pulsatile cardiopulmonary bypass. *J. Thor. Cardiovasc. Surg.*, **68,** 138
29. Balasaraswathi, K., Glisson, S. N., El-Etr, A. A. and Azad, C. (1980). Effect of priming volume on serum catecholamines during cardiopulmonary bypass. *Canad. Anaesth. Soc. J.*, **27,** 135
30. Guyton, A. C. and Richardson, T. Q. (1961). Effect of hematocrit on venous return. *Circulat. Res.*, **9,** 157
31. Murray, J. F., Escobar, E. and Rapaport, E. (1969). Effects of blood viscosity on haemodynamic responses in acute normovolaemic anemia. *Am. J. Physiol.*, **216,** 638
32. Thorén, L. (1977). Shock-principles of fluid therapy. In D. H. Lewis (ed.) *Dextran – 30 years. Acta Univ. Ups. Symp. Univ. Ups.* **3,** 83 (Stockholm: Almqvist and Wiksell)
33. Messmer, K. (1977). Acute pre-operative hemodilution: an alternative to transfusion of donor blood. In D. H. Lewis (ed.) *Dextran – 30 years. Acta Univ. Ups. Symp. Univ. Ups.*, **3,** 93 (Stockholm: Almqvist and Wiksell)
34. Gott, V. L., Bartlett, M., Long, D. M., Lillehei, C. W. and Johnson, J. A. (1962). Myocardial energy substances in the dog heart during potassium and hypothermic arrest. *J. Appl. Physiol.*, **17,** 815
35. Lowenstein, E. (1976). *Anaesthesia for cardiac surgery*, p. 36. Massachusetts General Hospital. Harvard Medical School. (unpublished)
36. Clowes, G. H. A., Jr. (1972). The physiological basis of cardiac surgery. In J. C. Norman (ed.) *Cardiac Surgery*. 2nd Edn., p. 13. (New York: Appleton-Century-Crofts).
37. Kessler, M. and Messmer, K. (1975). Tissue oxygenation during hemodilution. In K. Messmer and H. Schmid-Schönbein (eds.) *Intentional Hemodilution. Bibliotheca Haematologica* **41,** 16 (Basel: Karger)
38. Leaf, A. (1973). Cell swelling: a factor in ischemic tissue injury. *Circulation*, **48,** 455

39. Kloner, R. A., Ganote, C. E. and Jennings, R. B. (1974). The 'no-reflow' phenomenon after temporary coronary occlusion in the dog. *J. Clin. Invest.*, **44,** 1496
40. Buckberg, G. D. and Brazier, J. (1975). Coronary blood flow and cardiac function during haemodilution. In K. Messmer and H. Schmid-Schönbein (eds.) *Intentional Hemodilution. Bibliotheca Haematologica*, **41,** 173 (Basel: Karger)
41. Kleinman, L. H., Yarbrough, J. W., Symmonds, J. B. and Wechsler, A. S. (1978). Pressure-flow characteristics of the coronary collateral circulation during cardiopulmonary bypass. Effects of hemodilution. *J. Thor. Cardiovasc. Surg.*, **75,** 17
42. Stockard, J. J., Bickford, R. G. and Schauble, J. F. (1973). Pressure-dependent cerebral ischemia during cardiopulmonary bypass. *Neurology*, **23,** 521
43. Symmonds, J. B., Kleinman, L. H. and Wechsler, A. S. (1977). Effects of methoxamine on the coronary circulation during cardiopulmonary bypass. *J. Thor. Cardiovasc. Surg.*, **74,** 577
44. Bevan, D. R. (1978). Osmometry. 1. Terminology and principles of measurement. *Anaesth.*, **33,** 794
45. Bevan, D. R. (1978). Osmometry. 2. Osmoregulation. *Anaesth.*, **33,** 801
46. Bevan, D. R. (1978). Osmometry. 3. Clinical applications. *Anaesth.*, **33,** 809
47. Deverall, P. B., Muss, D. C., Macartney, F. J. and Settle, J. D. (1973). Osmolal balance after open intracardiac operations in children. *Thorax*, **28,** 756.
48. Philbin, D. M., Coggins, C. H., Emerson, C. W., Levine, F. H. and Buckley, M. J. (1979). Plasma vasopressin levels and urinary sodium excretion during cardiopulmonary bypass. Comparison of halothane and morphine anaesthesia. *J. Thor. Cardiovasc. Surg.*, **77,** 582
49. Kleeman, C. R. and Cutler. R. (1963). The neuro-hypophysis. *Ann. Rev. Physiol.*, **25,** 385
50. Goetz, K. K., Bond, G. C. and Bloxham, D. D. (1975). Atrial receptors and renal function. *Physiol. Rev.*, **55,** 157.
51. Ing, T. S., Wu, C., Rosenberg, J. C., Ng, P. S. Y., Su, W-S., Bernard, A. A. and Wilson, R. F. (1977). Cerebrospinal fluid changes in experimental cardiopulmonary bypass using haemodilution with glucose water. *Neurology*, **27,** 85
52. Hewitt, R. L., Woo, R. D., Ryan, J. R. and Drapanas, T. (1972). Plasma insulin and glucose relationships during cardiopulmonary bypass. *Surgery*, **71**, 905.
53. Landymore, R. W., Murphy, D. A. and Langley, W. J. (1979). Effect of cardiopulmonary bypass and hypothermia on pancreatic endocrine function and peripheral utilisation of glucose. *Canad. J. Surg.*, **22,** 248
54. Mills, N. L., Beaudet, R. L., Isom, O. W. and Spencer, F. C. (1973). Hyperglycemia during cardiopulmonary bypass. *Ann. Surg.*, **177,** 203.
55. Kones, R. (1975). Glucose, insulin and potassium therapy for heart disease. *N.Y. State J. Med.*, **1,** 1463
56. Brachfield, N. (1973). The glucose–insulin–potassium regime in the treatment of myocardial ischaemia. *Circulation*, **48,** 459
57. Hearse, D. J., Stewart, D. A. and Braimbridge, M. V. (1978). Myocardial protection during ischemic cardiac arrest. Possible deleterious effects of glucose and mannitol in coronary infusates. *J. Thor. Cardiovasc. Surg.*, **76,** 16
58. Neville, W. E., Thomason, R. D. and Hirsch, D. M. (1966). Postperfusion hypervolemia after hemodilution cardiopulmonary bypass. *Arch.* Surg., **93,** 715
59. Beattie, H. W., Evans, G., Garnett, E. S., Regoeczi, E., Webber, C. E. and Wong, K-L. (1974). Albumin and water fluxes during cardiopulmonary bypass. *J. Thor. Cardiovasc. Surg.*, **67,** 926
60. Dieter, R. A. Jr., Neville, W. E. and Pifarré, R. (1970). Serum electrolyte changes after cardiopulmonary by-pass with Ringer's lactate solution used for hemodilution. *J. Thor. Cardiovasc. Surg.*, **59,** 168

61. Barnard, C. N., DeWall, R. A., Varco, R. L. and Lillehei, C. W. (1959). Pre and postoperative care for patients undergoing open cardiac surgery. *Dis. Chest*., **35,** 194
62. DeWall, R. A., Warden, H. E., Gott, V. L., Read, R. C. and Lillehei, C. W. (1956). Total body perfusion for open cardiotomy utilizing the bubble oxygenator. *J. Thor. Surg*., **32,** 591
63. Lockey, E., Longmore, D. B., Ross, D. N. and Sturbridge, M. F. (1966). Potassium and open heart surgery. *Lancet*, **1,** 673
64. Vasko, K. A., DeWall, R. A. and Riley, A. M. (1973). Hypokalaemia: Physiological abnormalities during cardiopulmonary bypass. *Ann. Thor. Surg*., **15,** 347
65. Babka, R. and Pifarré, R. (1976). Potassium replacement during cardiopulmonary bypass. *J. Thor. Cardiovasc. Surg*., **73,** 212.
66. Westhorpe, R. N., Varghese, Z., Petrie, A., Wills, M. R. and Lumley, J. (1978). Changes in ionized calcium and other plasma constituents associated with cardiopulmonary bypass. *Br. J. Anaesth*., **50,** 951.
67. Holden, M. P., Ionescu, M. I. and Wooler, G. H. (1972). Magnesium in patients undergoing open-heart surgery. *Thorax*, **27,** 212.
68. Khan, R. M. S., Hodge, J. S. and Bassett, H. F. M. (1973). Magnesium in open-heart surgery. *J. Thor. Cardiovasc. Surg*., **66,** 185
69. Dagher, F. J., Lyons, J. H., Ball, M. R. and Moore, F. D. (1966). Hemorrhage in normal man: II. Effects of mannitol on plasma volume and body water dynamics following acute blood loss. *Ann. Surg*., **163,** 505
70. Das, J. B., Eraklis, A. J. and Jones, J. E. (1969). Water and solute excretion following cardiopulmonary bypass with hemodilution. The effects of the osmolarity of the perfusion prime. *J. Thor. Cardiovasc. Surg*., **58,** 789.
71. Navar, L. G., Guyton, A. C. and Langston, J. B. (1966). Effect of alterations in plasma osmolarity on renal blood flow autoregulation. *Amer J. Physiol*., **211,** 1387
72. Edde, R. R. and Smalley, S. (1979). Defect in oxygenation associated with mannitol. *Anesth. Analg*., **58,** 145
73. Coté, C. J., Greenhow, D. E. and Marshall, B. E. (1979). The hypotensive response to rapid intravenous administration of hypertonic solutions in man and in the rabbit. *Anesthiol*., **50,** 30
74. Willerson, J. T., Curry, G. C., Atkins, J. M., Parkey, R. and Horwitz, L. D. (1975). Influence of hypertonic mannitol on ventricular performance and coronary blood flow in patients. *Circulation*, **51,** 1095
75. Starling, E. H. (1896). On the absorption of fluids from the connective tissue spaces. *J. Physiol. (London)*, **19,** 312
76. Bevan, D. R. (1980). Colloid osmotic pressure. *Anaesth*., **35,** 263
77. Guyton, A. C. and Lindsey, A. W. (1959). Effect of elevated left atrial pressure and decreased plasma protein concentration on the development of pulmonary oedema. *Circ. Res*., **7,** 649
78. Schüpbach, P., Pappova, E., Schilt, W., Kollar, J., Kollar, M., Sipos, P. and Vucic, D. (1978). Perfusate oncotic pressure during cardiopulmonary bypass. Optimum level as determined by metabolic acidosis, tissue oedema, and renal function. *Vox Sang*., **35,** 332
79. Laks, H., Standeven, J., Blair, O., Hahn, J., Jellinek, M. and Willman, V. L. (1977). The effects of cardiopulmonary bypass with crystalloid and colloid hemodilution on myocardial extravascular water. *J. Thor. Cardiovasc. Surg*., **73,** 129
80. Lowenstein, E., Cooper, J. D., Erdman III, A. J., Geffin, G., Laver, M. B. and Yoshikawa, H. (1975). Lung and heart water accummulation associated with hemodilution. In K. Messmer and H. Schmid-Schönbein (eds.) *Intentional Hemodilution Bibliotheca Hematologica*, **41,** 190 (Basel: Karger)

81. Hewson, J. R. (1978). Perfusion characteristics during cardiopulmonary bypass and subsequent changes in alveolar–arterial oxygen tension gradients. *Anesth. Analg.*, **57**, 298.
82. Brenner, B. M. and Humes, H. D. (1977). Mechanics of glomerular ultrafiltration. *N. Engl. J. Med.*, **297**, 148
83. Rudowski, W. J. (1980). Evaluation of modern plasma expanders and blood substitutes. *Br. J. Hosp. Med.*, **23**, 389
84. Gruber, U. F. (1969). *Blood Replacement*, p. 48 (Berlin: Springer–Verlag)
85. Farrow, S. P. (1967). *MSc Thesis*, University of Birmingham, England
86. Bland, J. H. L., Laver, M. B. and Lowenstein, E. (1973). Vasodilator effect of 5% plasma protein fraction. *J. Am. Med. Assoc.*, **224**, 1721
87. Gruber, U. F. (1969). *Blood Replacement*, p. 103 (Berlin: Springer–Verlag)
88. Bergentz, S-E., Falkheden, T. and Olsson, S. (1965). Diuresis and urinary viscosity in dehydrated patients: influence of dextran 40 000, with and without mannitol. *Ann. Surg.*, **161**, 582
89. Matheson, N. A. (1966). Renal failure with low-molecular weight dextran. *Br. Med. J.*, **2**, 1198
90. Hässig, A. and Stampfli, K. (1969). Plasma substitutes, past and present. In P. Lundsgaard-Hansen, A. Hässig and H. Nitschmann (eds.) *Modified Gelatins as Plasma Substitutes. Bibliotheca Haematologica*, **33**, 4 (Basel: Karger)
91. Åberg, M., Hedner, U. and Bergentz, S-E. (1977). The effect of dextran on hemostasis and coagulation with special regard to factor VIII. In D. H. Lewis (ed.) *Dextran – 30 years. Acta. Univ. Ups. Symp. Univ. Ups.*, **3**, 23 (Stockholm: Almqvist and Wiksell)
92. Ring, J. and Messmer, K. (1977). Incidence and severity of anaphylactoid reactions to colloid volume substitutes. *Lancet*, **1**, 466
93. Gruber, U. F. (1969). *Blood Replacement*, p. 133 (Berlin: Springer–Verlag).
94. Moyes, D. G. (1974). Haemodilution with a plasma expander as priming solution in cardiopulmonary bypass. *S-A Mediese Tydskrif*, 1615
95. Merikallio, E. (1976). Haemodilution in cardiopulmonary bypass using a gelatine derivative for priming. *Ann. Chir. Gynaecol.*, **65**, 138.
96. De Vries, H. W., Zimmerman, A. N. E. and Goslinga, H. (1978). Haemodynamic and metabolic consequences of haemodilution with different diluents. *Tijdschr. Diergeneesk.*, **103**, 1057
97. Werner, F. M. (1974). Dextranen of gelatines. *Ned. T. Geneesk.*, **118**, 1121
98. Mullerworth, M. H., Currie, T. T., Cockbill, M. T. and Stubbs, A. E. (1973). Repolymerized gelatin as a priming solution for extracorporeal circulation: An experimental study in dogs. *Surgery*, **74**, 666.
99. Metcalf, W., Papadopoulos, A., Tufaro, R. and Barth, A. (1970). A clinical physiologic study of hydroxyethyl starch. *Surg. Gynecol. Obstet.*, **131**, 255.
100. Mishler, J. M., Parry, E. S., Sutherland, B. A. and Bushrod, J. R. (1979). A clinical study of low molecular weight hydroxyethyl starch, a new plasma expander. *Br. J. Clin. Pharmacol.*, **7**, 619.
101. Holdefer, W. F. and Dowling, E. A. (1974). Experimental use of heterologous stroma-free hemoglobin solution (SHFS) as a whole blood substitute. *J. Surg. Oncol.*, 451
102. Vasko, K. A., Riley, A. M. and DeWall, R. A. (1972). Poloxalkol (Pluronic-F68): A priming solution for cardiopulmonary bypass. *Trans. Am. Soc. Artif. Organs*, **18**, 526
103. Sloviter, H. A. and Kamimoto, T. (1967). Erythrocyte substitute for perfusion of brain. *Nature*, **216**, 458
104. Wallace, H. W., Asher, W. J. and Li, N. L. (1973). Liquid-Liquid oxygen: a new approach. *Trans. Am. Soc. Artif. Organs*, **19**, 80

105. Harris, E. A., Seelye, E. R. and Barratt-Boyes, B. G. (1970). Respiratory and metabolic acid–base changes during cardiopulmonary bypass in man. *Br. J. Anaesth.*, **42,** 912
106. Strumia, M. M., Crosby, W. H., Gibson, J. G., Greenwalt, T. J. and Krevans, J. R. (1963). General principles of blood transfusion. *Transfusion*, **3,** 306

27
Can cardiopulmonary bypass be a safe procedure?

D. R. WHEELDON

INTRODUCTION

'Safe' is a difficult word when applied to the many-faceted procedure of cardiopulmonary bypass. The dictionary definition is 'without risk' and risk itself is very much a subjective matter. For instance most of us think of the home as an acceptably safe place in which to live, and we accept most modern forms of public transport to be 'safe'. However figures published by the Royal Society for the Prevention of Accidents (RoSPA)[1] show that in 1977 there were 7076 deaths (42% of the total) due to transport accidents and 6407 (37%) deaths resulting from accidents in the home in Great Britain. There were 110 reported deaths (0.5%) due to surgical and medical misadventure, but this is undoubtedly a gross underestimate.

In the same year there were 9868 patients who underwent open cardiac surgery in the UK, of whom 1012 (10.2%) died within 30 days of operation[2]. The figures for closed cardiac operations were 129 (7.4%) deaths following operation. A recent UK survey revealed that a fatal perfusion accident occurred once per 1500 procedures, and that a serious incident occurred once per 300 procedures. Similar figures were obtained by a recent American survey[3].

During the past two decades cardiac surgery has developed rapidly and much interest and endeavour has been directed towards the solution of technical problems and to the crude survival statistics. As can be seen from Figure 1, the results in terms of hospital mortality at Papworth reflect this worldwide trend and on this basis cardiac surgery itself must be regarded as now being relatively 'safe'. However what *we* now mean by 'safe' is that a patient should leave our care able to enjoy a better quality of life than he did before he came into our care. After all, if he has had the right operation carried out with the correct technical expertise and we have adequately preserved the functional integrity of his organs whilst surgical intervention has taken place, there is no good reason why this should not be so.

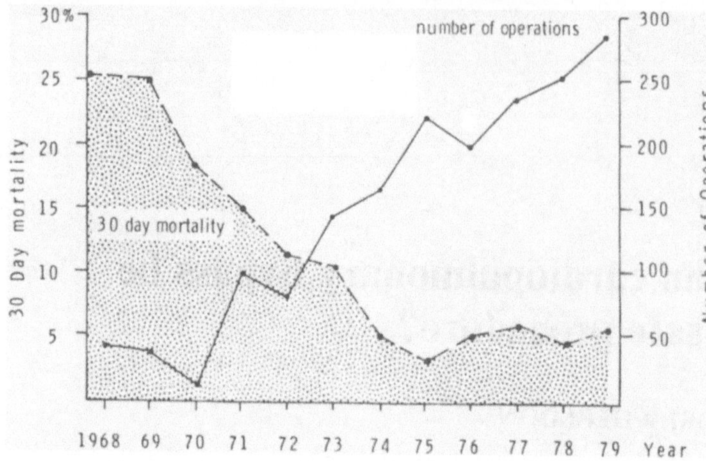

Figure 1 Mortality and number of open heart operations (Papworth)

The degree to which this goal is being achieved is very difficult to assess due to the paucity of literature on the subject (it is difficult enough to obtain reliable information on mortalities and accidents). However a recent study by a Regional Cardiothoracic Unit[4] into the quality of life after operation showed that 20 months after operation 68% of the survivors denied limitation of normal activity compared with a preoperative figure of 12%, and there had been a corresponding pattern in the return to useful employment. There was no analysis of those patients who did not benefit or who were worse as a result of the treatment.

The incidence of postoperative organ dysfunction is very difficult to ascertain due to the disparate reports from different centres and the lack of truly quantitative means of measuring these complications. Cerebral complications have been reported to vary from an incidence of 0.5%[5] to 44%[6], and significant renal dysfunction has been recently reported as varying from an incidence of 0.5% (Bethune *et al.*, personal communication) to 3.6%[7]. Complications resulting from inadequate myocardial preservation probably represent the most significant category but information relating to the incidence of this complication is difficult to come by. The incidence of postoperative respiratory complications has all but disappeared, having once been one of the major complications following open heart surgery.

Improving the mortality and morbidity resulting from open heart surgery results in a positive feedback mechanism whereby improved results give rise to earlier referral, which in turn should give rise to further improvements in the results. However it is all too easy to become complacent and I would now like to expand on a philosophy geared towards improving the quality of perfusion in an evolving way.

Cardiopulmonary bypass as a system involves an assembly of components in an organized way. The components themselves are affected by being in the system (they may have different characteristics out of the system or in another system) and the system itself is influenced by the variable inputs to which it is subjected (the patient and the operator(s)). This may, at first sight, look like an unnecessarily complex way of examining a bypass circuit, but it represents a new and growing technology known as 'systems performance'[8] which is used by agencies such as NASA and the Atomic Energy Commission.

The basis of systems thinking is first of all to break the system down into a series of subsystems with the individual components being represented as a series of 'black boxes' having particular characteristics and being interconnected in a particular way. The 'black boxes' are then individually studied and analysed so that representations of their characteristics may be mapped out. Using this methodology it soon becomes apparent just what the relationships between the various components are; it enables a closer inspection of possible failure modes and even a prediction of the relative probabilities of failure; and it also enables one to examine the effects of replacing the various components with substitutes, in an objective manner.

Because cardiopulmonary bypass involves people it becomes what is known as 'a human activity system' and hence the people involved, that is patient, surgeon, anaesthetist, and perfusionist, become part of the system – in other words 'black boxes' and herein lies the major problem. A complete systematic study of cardiopulmonary bypass would necessarily entail much more time and space than is available to me at the moment so I propose to illustrate the point with a look at two common systems and to detail some of the more important features of some of the major components.

SYSTEMS

The characteristics of different circuits are probably more influenced by the type of oxygenator used than any other single component. A system incorporating a membrane oxygenator, for instance, will impose very different relationships and hence failure modes on the other components from a system employing either a disc or bubble oxygenator. I have illustrated just two possible circuits (Figures 2 and 3), one employing a hard-shell bubble oxygenator and the other a low-pressure membrane oxygenator. Even the most cursory glance shows how different these two systems are, and the very different relationships between the various components. The substitution of other components, such as filters or cardiotomy reservoirs, will obviously have a less profound effect on the circuit, but it is precisely because this is less obvious that potential hazards may be overlooked if a systematic approach is not used. Many perfusionists have, through experience, developed such an approach without formalizing it, but with the variety of equipment now available and the increase in the number of staff in any one department involved in perfusion I feel that it is well worth the effort to develop a more formal approach. It may well be that the discipline of this approach, and the development of systems thinking within a unit, may be enough to minimize hazards without the detailed analysis of every subsystem; however the analysis is a necessary prerequisite to establish the discipline!

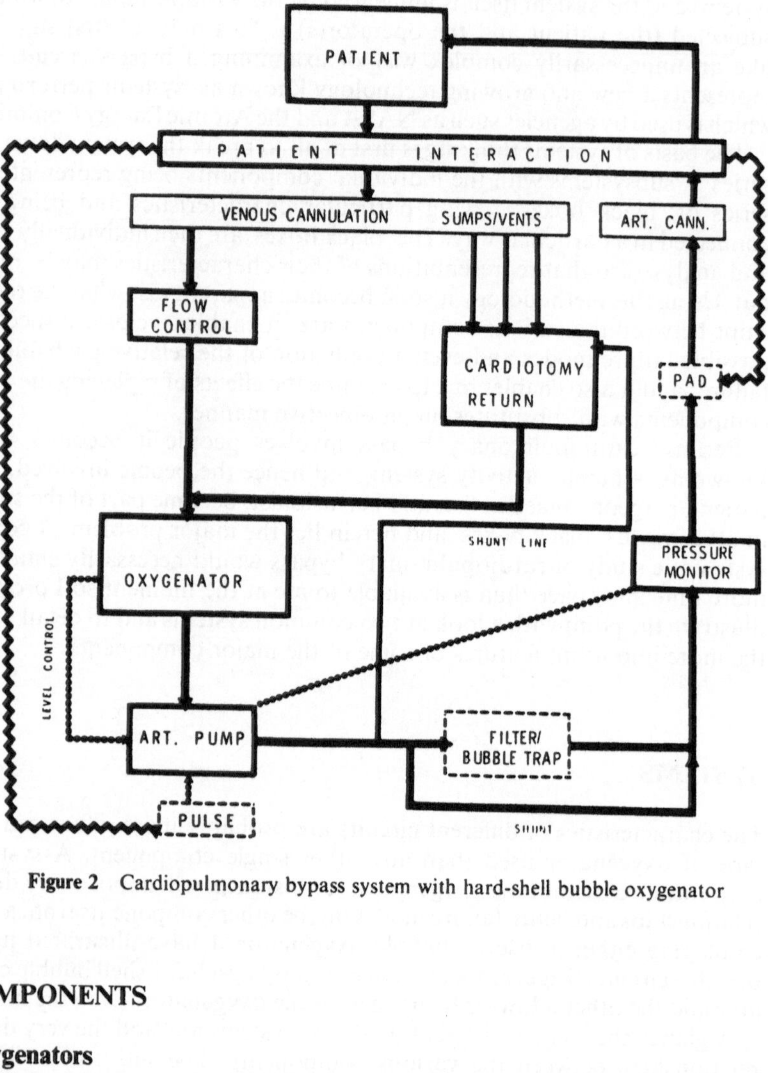

Figure 2 Cardiopulmonary bypass system with hard-shell bubble oxygenator

COMPONENTS

Oxygenators

Performance data on oxygenators are usually either provided in a non-standard manner by the manufacturer or not provided at all. It is therefore frequently necessary for the perfusionist to evaluate a new device so as to obtain data which is meaningful to him. It is hoped that this situation will soon be resolved with the adoption of international standards.

Features which are useful to know from a safety point of view include:

(1) Performance – gas transfer – rated blood flow. Operating range.
(2) Pressure drops – blood and gas – especially with membranes.
(3) Venous return function curve. Rated operating level (R vi – MOL).
(4) Volumes – min. and max. Dynamic priming. Non-recoverable prime.

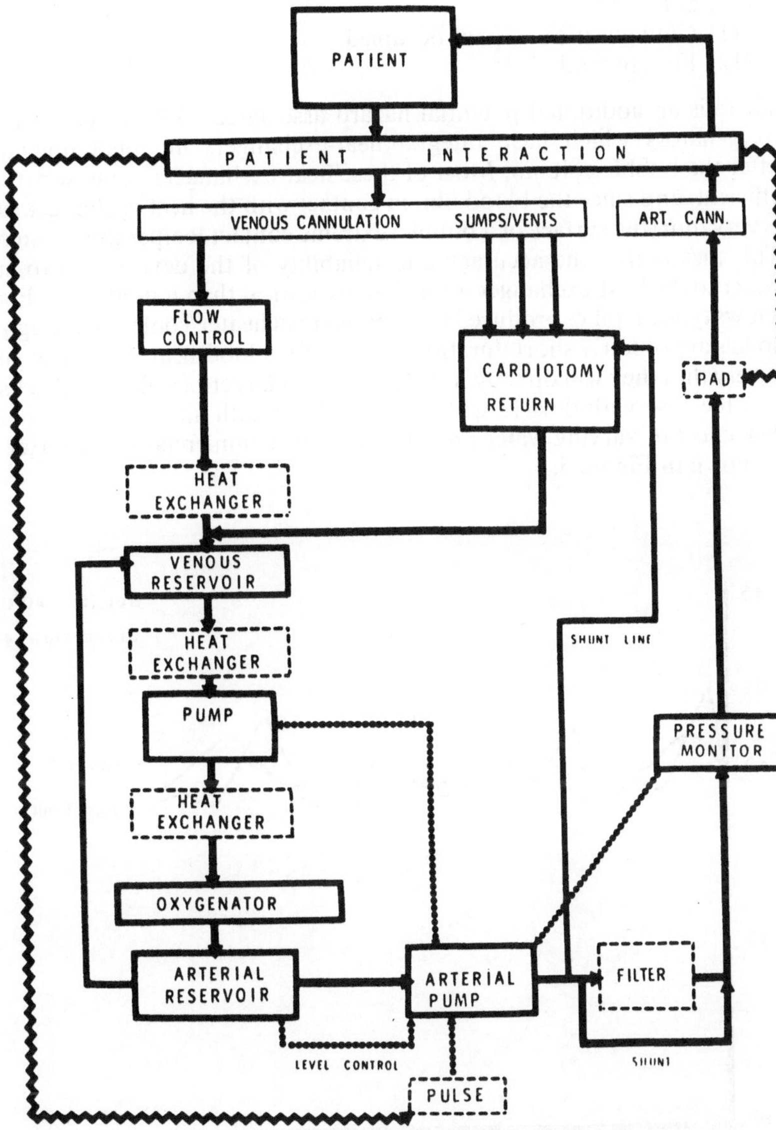

Figure 3 Cardiopulmonary bypass system with low-pressure membrane oxygenator

(5) Microbubble generation. Defoaming capacity. Flows/levels.
(6) Heat-exchanger. Position. Resistance.
(7) Sparger bubble point flow.
(8) Particulate contamination.
(9) Connectors/failure modes.
(10) Set-up time.
(11) Configuration – space occupied.
(12) Failure modes[9-12].

There is an additional potential hazard associated with modern hard-shell oxygenators which have integral heat-exchangers mounted immediately after the bubble column. Most of these heat-exchangers are now extremely efficient, and since the blood film in contact with the heat-exchanger surface is very thin (the surface of a bubble) extreme contact temperatures can occur. This means that the accuracy and reliability of the device used to supply water to the heat-exchanger is much more critical than it used to be. Figure 4 shows typical spikes produced by a commercial heater/cooler. Although these spikes are of fairly short duration because the blood/heat-exchanger surface is very thin they will directly influence a much larger population of cells than was the case with devices with a wider blood path and of lower efficiency. The effect of varying water pressure on some commercial water mixer units is shown in Figure 5.

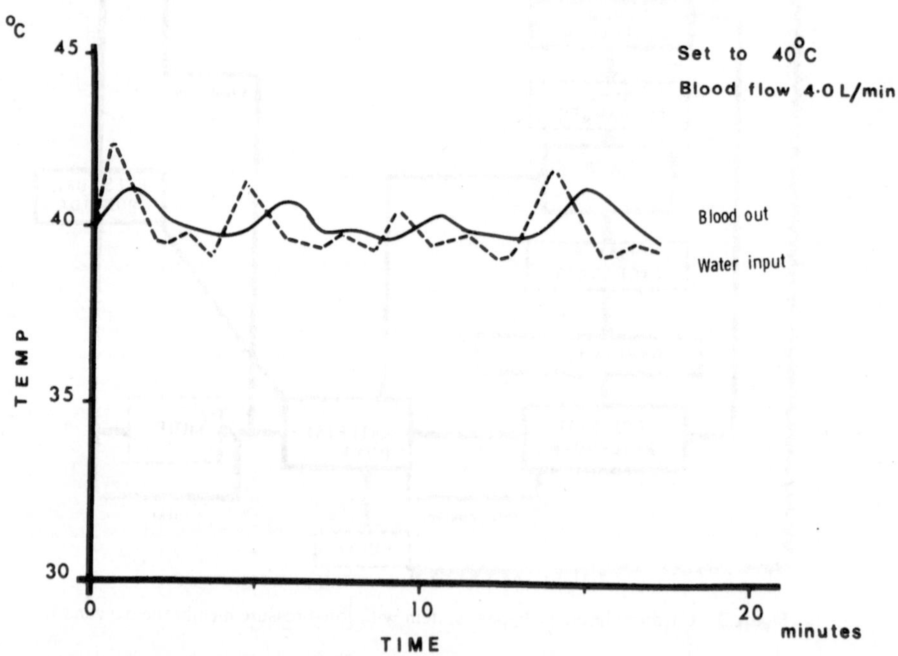

Figure 4 Temperature variations produced by commercial thermocirculator connected to Shiley S100 heat-exchanger

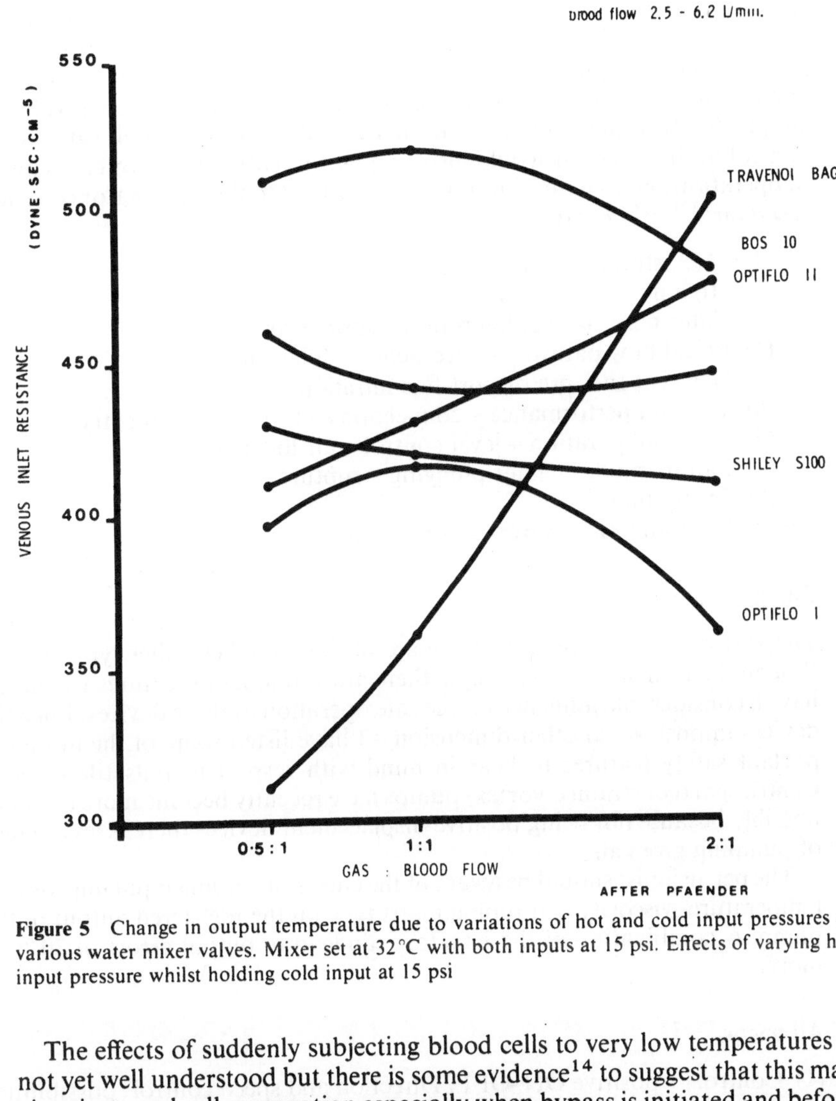

Figure 5 Change in output temperature due to variations of hot and cold input pressures of various water mixer valves. Mixer set at 32°C with both inputs at 15 psi. Effects of varying hot input pressure whilst holding cold input at 15 psi

The effects of suddenly subjecting blood cells to very low temperatures is not yet well understood but there is some evidence[14] to suggest that this may give rise to red cell aggregation especially when bypass is initiated and before the prime is well mixed with the patient's blood. This may mean that we should be more cautious with early body cooling – especially when using high efficiency integral venous heat-exchangers.

Cardiotomy reservoirs

Cardiotomy reservoirs can exert an important influence on the rest of the system, especially in those procedures where large volumes of suctioned blood, together with air and debris, require to be handled. There is now a tendency for reservoirs with integral fine filters (20–40 μm) to be offered by the manufacturers. These reservoirs can pose a potential hazard if they are constructed in such a way that obstruction of the filters causes an increase in pressure on the input side of the reservoir with no visible indication to the perfusionist. No manufacturer offers a positive pressure relief valve – a simple device which would render hard-shell reservoirs much safer. Level control in the reservoir would also be a useful feature both for convenience of operation and to reduce the microbubble load to the oxygenator or venous reservoir[13,15,16]. Features which are useful to know include:

(1) Max. storage capacity.
(2) High flow filtration rate.
(3) Filter pore size/configuration – surface area.
(4) Blood flow pathway – turbulence – splashing.
(5) Gas vent site–pre or post-fine filtration.
(6) Vacuum performance – connections – top or bottom entry.
(7) Exit configuration – level control – air locking.
(8) Failure modes – filter plugging – rupture pressure.
(9) Set-up time.
(10) Microbubble removal – flow/levels.

Pumps

The vast majority of pumps in use are of the DeBakey roller type, and although the principle is very simple there are a number of features which can have a considerable influence on the safe operation of these devices. Pulsatile devices impose yet another dimension – I have listed some of the more important safety features to bear in mind with respect to pulsatile devices. Centrifugal (constrained vortex) pumps have recently become more popular, possibly because not being positive displacement devices there is less chance of pumping gross air.

The perfusionist should be aware of the effects of varying input impedance, temperature, viscosity and tubing insert type on the registered output of the pump. A combination of these factors can lead to output errors of 30 % or more.

All pumps[18–22]

(1) Controls – positive ON–OFF. Direction and speed control; possibilities of accidental operation.
(2) Calibration – accuracy under all operational conditions.
(3) Failure modes – speed control – runaway failure. Electrical failure – fusing. Mechanical failure – head drive – roller assembly – ease of hand operation.
(4) Failure indicators.

Roller pumps

(1) Tubing location in pump head.
(2) Occlusion setting – accuracy – security.

(3) Torque – head slippage.
(4) Head–back plate tolerances.
(5) Ease of maintenance.

Centrifugal (constrained vortex)

(1) Flow control – inline flowmeter imperative.
(2) Energy transfer – heat transfer at zero forward flow for various rev/min.
(3) Alternatives in the event of power failure.

Pulsatile

(1) Roller pump – control devices – manual override – maximum negative pressure – calibration.
(2) PAD devices – those employing negative pressure not recommended.
(3) Centrifugal – combination of those problems associated with centrifugal pumps (much more load-dependent) and control devices.
(4) Valved diaphragm – reliable diaphragm – hand operation – valves.

The above lists are not by any means exhaustive but can serve as useful checklists. Time and space do not permit similar treatment of all the circuit components – however I do feel that it is worthwhile for each perfusionist to construct such lists for each component and to keep it updated.

ORGANIZATION

Medical devices

Despite the recent explosive proliferation in the number and variety of medical devices (over 5000 are now in use in the average modern hospital)[23] there has been little regulation or standardization and this has been reflected in the number of reports on malfunctioning apparatus. Although moves towards implementing standards for perfusion equipment are now advancing quite rapidly there is as yet no statutory protection available to us. It therefore rests on the individual technician to determine that the devices which he uses meet *his* standards and are maintained so that they continue to do so.

A recent publication in Health Devices[24] contains an excellent overview of perfusion problems together with a very useful checklist for inspection and preventative maintenance. It is suggested that this procedure is carried out every 100 hours or once every 3 months – whichever is the sooner.

Organization – protocols

The Health and Safety at Work Act, built upon the recommendations of the Robens Committee, came into being in July 1974. Although it will still be some time before the Act is fully effective in the Health Service, I feel that we as perfusionists should put our own house in order before regulations are imposed upon us. The following list is intended as a general guide towards implementing organizational safety features into a perfusion department.

General

(1) Establishment of equipment records:

(a) Identification of each individual device.
(b) Record of maintenance or repairs to each device.
(c) Establishment of suitable preventative inspection and maintenance checks; ensure that these are carried out when due.
(d) Faults book – record of all equipment failures – malfunctions.

(2) Establish agreed protocols to be followed by all personnel in the following procedures:

(a) Basis for the selection of equipment to be deployed in all the various clinical situations likely to be encountered.
(b) Preoperative machine checks.
(c) Priming solutions and techniques for all circuits used.
(d) Case records – patients' statistics – equipment used – fluids – drugs – measured parameters – frequency of entries.
(e) Basic guidelines for perfusion management – flow – pressures – volumes – electrolytes – acid/base – anticoagulation – gas tensions – temperatures.
(f) Procedures to be followed in the event of equipment failures: electrical power – mechanical pump failure – oxygenator failure – reservoir failure – gas supply failure – temperature control – circuit rupture.

Ensure that all perfusionists are capable of effecting emergency action in the event of any of the above equipment failures, in the minimum time and using a method which has been established as representing the minimum risk to the patient. All perfusionists should be required to demonstrate this ability once every 3 months.

(3) Team responsibility and communications. Establish agreed areas of responsibility and systems of communication. Establish a procedure in the event of failure situations.
(4) Establish a protocol for cleaning and decontamination of all non-disposable equipment – especially with respect to contamination with specific pathogens.

Perfusion – specific

(1) Identification of patient.
(2) Patient statistics – diagnosis – preoperative haematology, biochemistry, drug therapy. Proposed surgical procedure.
(3) Selection of equipment according to protocol.
(4) Machine checks – availability of alternative systems. Calibration checks, occlusion checks.
(5) Circuit components. Sterility. Visual checks for defects. Availability of alternatives.

(6) Prime according to protocol.
(7) Institute case record. Double check (two people) (a) intravenous fluids; (b) drugs; (c) donor blood.
(8) Management of perfusion according to protocol. Record any non-standard events.
(9) Ensure a record of identification data on equipment and fluids used.
(10) Follow protocol for cleaning and decontamination.

ACCIDENTS

RoSPA describes an accident as being the consequence of a sequence of random events, always involving multiple causal factors, with chance alone often determining the resultant severity. Where clear causations are involved it is difficult to define the event as an accident. Human failure, rather than environmental and mechanical defects, is a factor in 80% of accidents. RoSPA also gives a list of causations for accidents which occur in the general community at work and play (Table 1). Some of these factors are very relevant to cardiopulmonary bypass if rather more difficult to proportionate.

Table 1 Accident causations (RoSPA)

Non-human elements
Mechanical defects
Environmental factors
Lighting conditions
Human factors
Adventurous spirit
Inadequate training
Negligence and irresponsibility
Fatigue
Stress
Impatience
Carelessness
The ageing process.

The results of two recent surveys of perfusion related accidents, one in the UK and one in the USA, are presented in Table 2. The UK survey included about 70% of the perfusions conducted during the 6 years 1974–9, and the American survey included about 90% of the perfusions conducted during 1972–7. This means that the American survey looked at about ten times as many perfusions; however the findings were very similar apart from the reported incidence of disseminated intravascular coagulation (DIC). In America DIC was thought to be second only to arterial line gas embolism as a serious incident. In the UK this problem seems to be much less prevalent, or is not as well recognized. Alternatively it could be that the recent advances in heparin therapy management have brought about a marked reduction in

Table 2 Perfusion accidents (numbers per 1000 perfusion)

	Incidents			Permanent injury			Deaths		
	UK		USA	UK		USA	UK		USA
Arterial line embolism	26	(0.79)	(1.14)	4	(0.12)	(0.16)	2	(0.07)	(0.28)
Vent air embolism	4	(0.12)	(0.05)	1	(0.01)	(—)	2	(0.07)	(—)
Electrical failure	33	(1.00)	(0.67)	1	(0.01)	(—)	1	(0.01)	(0.01)
Mechanical failure	9	(0.27)	(0.38)	0	(—)	(0.01)	0	(—)	(0.01)
Oxygenator failure	16	(0.59)	(0.33)	0	(—)	(0.02)	0	(—)	(0.01)
Inadequate perfusion	10	(0.30)	(—)	2	(0.07)	(—)	4	(0.15)	(—)
Donor blood	3	(0.11)	(—)	0	(—)	(—)	2	(0.07)	(—)
DIC	9	(0.27)	(1.26)	0	(—)	(0.07)	3	(0.11)	(0.43)
TOTAL	113	(3.42)	(3.30)	8	(0.24)	(0.27)	14	(0.42)	(0.70)

USA, 1972–7: approx. 375 000 perfusions
UK, 1974–9: approx. 33 000 perfusions
These figures show that there was a serious incident every 300 perfusions. There was an accident resulting in death once every 1500 perfusions

the incidence of this complication over the last few years. Heparin monitoring was employed by 63% of the respondents in both surveys.

Serious incidents were shown to occur about once every 300 perfusions and an accident resulting in death about once every 1000 perfusions. The UK 30-day mortality for open heart surgery in 1978 was 10.52% so that perfusion accidents accounted for about 0.4% of these mortalities. It is difficult to put these statistics into perspective, firstly because we know that the numbers are incomplete and secondly because they represent only the tip of the iceberg as far as morbidity is concerned.

What is not shown by any of these statistics, but which should command our utmost attention, is the quality of life which our patients enjoy as a result of the many things which we do or do not do. Looking at the frequency of incidents (Table 3) we can see that electrical failure, air embolism and oxygenation failure feature most prominently. However when these problems

Table 3 UK accident survey

Frequency of incidents	Numbers/1000 perfusions
1. Electrical failure	1.00
2. Arterial line embolism	0.79
3. Oxygenator failure	0.59
4. Inadequate perfusion	0.30
5. DIC 6. Mechanical failure	0.27
7. Vent air embolism	0.12
8. Donor blood	0.11

are rearranged according to the frequency of resultant mortalities, inadequate perfusion, DIC and air embolism represent the major problems (Table 4).

Adequate perfusion

Even after 25 years of cardiopulmonary bypass we still do not have a reliable means of monitoring the adequacy of whole body preservation during perfusion. Many guidelines have been proposed from the monitoring of A-V saturation differences and developing acidosis to the use of oxygen consumption plateauing[26–28]. However none of these methods is reliable and the

Table 4 UK accident survey

Frequency of mortalities	*Numbers/1000 perfusions*
1. Inadequate perfusion	0.15
2. DIC	0.11
3. Arterial line embolism 4. Vent air embolism 5. Donor blood	0.07
6. Electrical failure	0
7. Oxygenator failure	0
8. Mechanical failure	0

present situation can be summed up in the words of Edward Berger in his recent book *The Physiology of Adequate Perfusion*[29] where he states that 'adequate perfusion is yet an art rather than an exact science'.

Anticoagulation

Although heparin has been used as an anticoagulant since 1935 its structure and metabolism are still poorly understood. Like many other aspects of perfusion a sense of security has developed from the use of set protocols since the serious errors in control which can occur as a result of this practice can occur without any immediate clinical evidence. In 1975 Brian Bull *et al.*[30] brought to our attention the fact that some monitoring of heparin therapy was required, and it has since been shown by a number of workers that patients have a wide range of sensitivity to heparin as well as displaying an unpredictable rate of heparin metabolism[31,32]. In addition, methods available for heparin assay are not very accurate, so that there may be quite wide variations in batch strength. The criteria for adequate anticoagulation includes the prevention of consumptive coagulopathies and the formation of fibrin monomers without the use of excessive amounts of heparin. The use of the activated clotting time has proved to be a reliable and uncomplicated method. I suspect that complications resulting from inadequate anticoagulation have been much more common than is generally recognized.

Alarms

The most sudden and distressing incident which occurs during cardiopulmonary bypass is gross air embolism, yet the attitude of perfusionists towards the use of devices designed to minimize this hazard varies enormously. A personal survey by Daniel Doyle[33] in the USA in early 1977 found 25 perfusionists who had pumped air. By the end of the year the number had risen to 48. Mr Doyle's concluding remark was that we should beware of thinking 'it can't happen to me'. It has happened to many excellent perfusionists.

Another widely held opinion is that perfusionists fall into two groups – those who have pumped air, and those who are about to. Yet perfusionists do violently disagree about the use of alarms. There are those, who are typified by one respondent to my questionnaire who entered across the section on alarms the words 'NONE – perfusionist in attendance at all times!' and those who believe in a variety of devices, with or without servoregulation, of the arterial pump.

It is interesting to note from the UK survey that the two deaths reported from air embolism occurred in units where no alarms of any kind are used, as did almost all the incidents reported. My own feeling is that a level alarm can be a useful aid, as long as it is used as such and does not become a substitute for proper vigilance. The perfusionist should also be aware of the particular characteristics of the system in use with respect to protection from this hazard. Figure 6 demonstrates the varying consequences of total venous obstruction on systems employing different oxygenators with and without an arterial line filter and the effect of a shut-off valve on the arterial outlet. (These traces were obtained using an ultrasonic bubble detector (TM8) placed on the arterial line.) It can be seen that the valve closes positively after allowing a small volume of air through, whilst the arterial reservoir on the VT 5000 collapses without letting any air through although foam is formed in the line. The inclusion of an arterial line filter extends the time delay by 30–80 %, depending on the oxygenator. Although there is a natural emotional resistance amongst most perfusionists to include mechanical valves in an arterial line, it is difficult to escape the conclusion that the use of the ASO–100* valve offers considerable protection against gross air embolism (especially if a hard-shell oxygenator is employed) without introducing any measurable disadvantages.

Should gross air embolism occur it does not necessarily mean that death or even permanent injury is inevitable, provided that swift action is taken. The arterial pump should be stopped immediately, the patient placed in a steep head-down position, as much air as possible aspirated from the heart and great vessels (flooding the entire chest cavity can help), the arterial circuit re-primed and bypass slowly re-instituted whilst applying carotid compression. Intravenous steroids should be administered and rapid core cooling to about 28 °C instituted, whilst the remaining intracardiac surgery is completed as quickly as possible. Bypass should be discontinued with the patient temperature at about 32 °C and the patient moved to a hyperbaric chamber if

* Delta Medical.

available. Hyperbaric treatment at 6 atm. for 12 hours has resulted in complete recovery in patients who have suffered a massive air embolism[34,35].

Vent air embolism

There are a number of predisposing factors responsible for this hazard which would seem to be on the increase. The major reason is probably the recent introduction of hard-shell cardiotomy reservoirs which if not vented or provided with a positive pressure relief valve can very easily cause air to

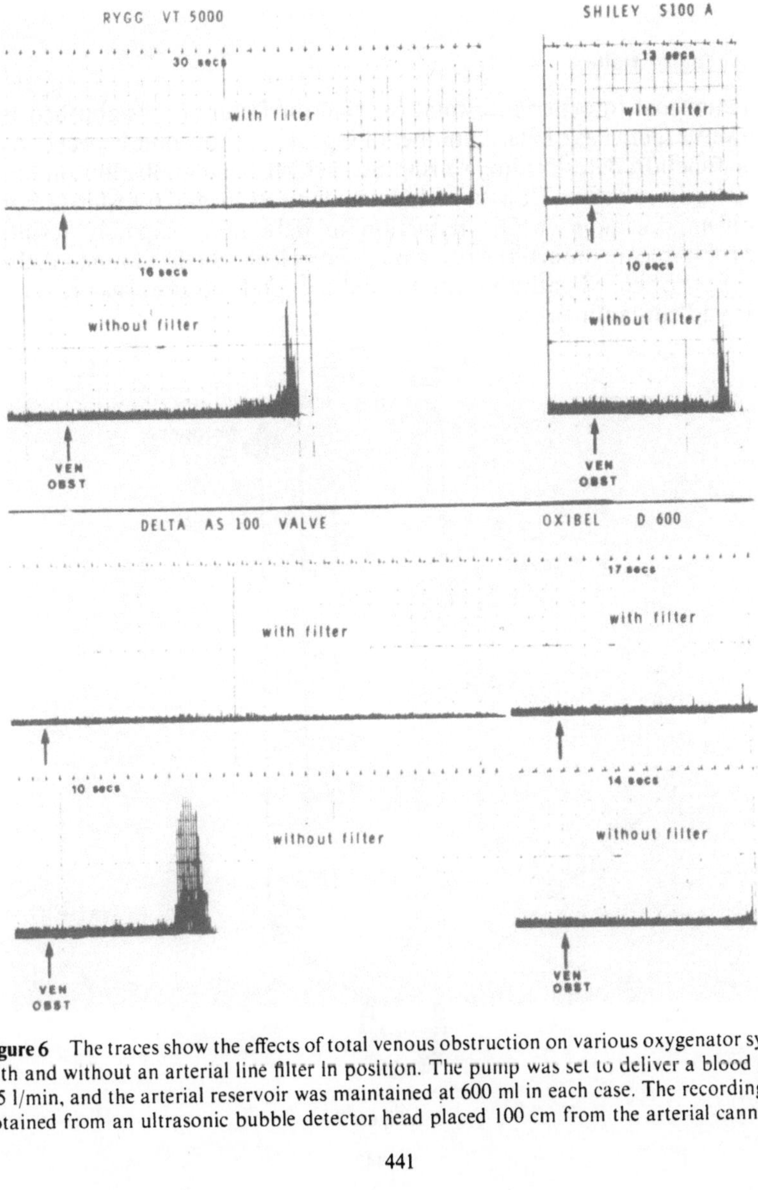

Figure 6 The traces show the effects of total venous obstruction on various oxygenator systems, with and without an arterial line filter in position. The pump was set to deliver a blood flow of 4.5 l/min, and the arterial reservoir was maintained at 600 ml in each case. The recordings were obtained from an ultrasonic bubble detector head placed 100 cm from the arterial cannula

travel back up a gravity vent line or through a non-occlusive vent pump. The other major cause of this problem is a vent pump which is set to run in reverse. This is a section of the perfusion system in which systems analysis can be very helpful. A detailed analysis (which should not be very complicated) can illuminate the potential hazards. Particular care should be exercised when substituting a different cardiotomy reservoir. Our own system consists of controlled low-pressure vacuum applied to the cardiotomy reservoir, together with a manometer T-piece in the vent line (Figure 7). It is also important to visually monitor the vent line for air, especially during surgical manoeuvres when the heart is beating.

Oxygenator failure

It is unusual to experience total oxygenator failure on established bypass. However there have been a number of reports[36,37] of some aspect of oxygenator function deteriorating during use, which makes substitution desirable or even imperative. Causes include: reduction in gas transfer (a common problem during ECMO); reduction in defoaming capacity resulting in microbubbles in the arterial reservoir; a large leak which cannot be contained; blockage of blood pathway with thrombus; total rupture – gas vent obstructed; and contamination.

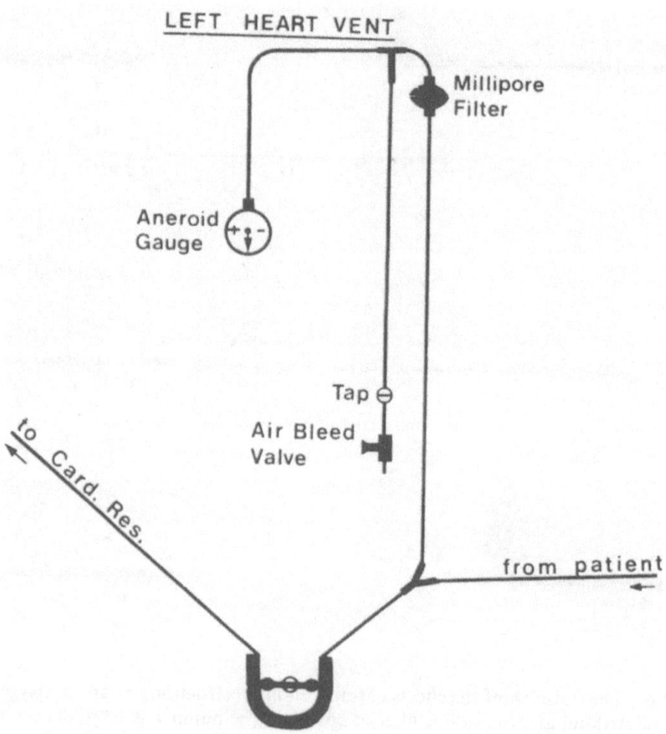

Figure 7

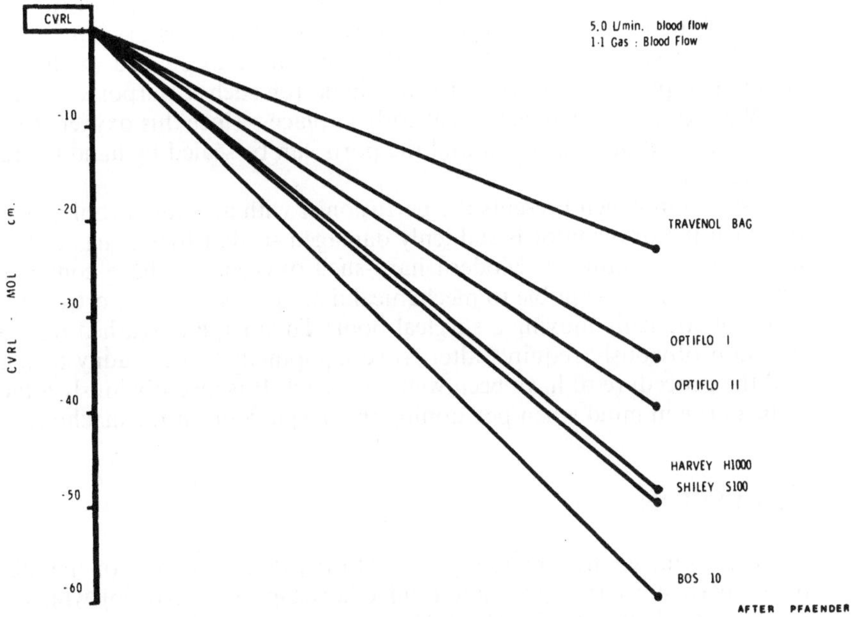

Figure 8 Height of minimum operating level (MOL) below simulated central venous reservoir level (CVRL) 5.0 l/min blood flow; 1:1 gas:blood flow (after Pfaender[9])

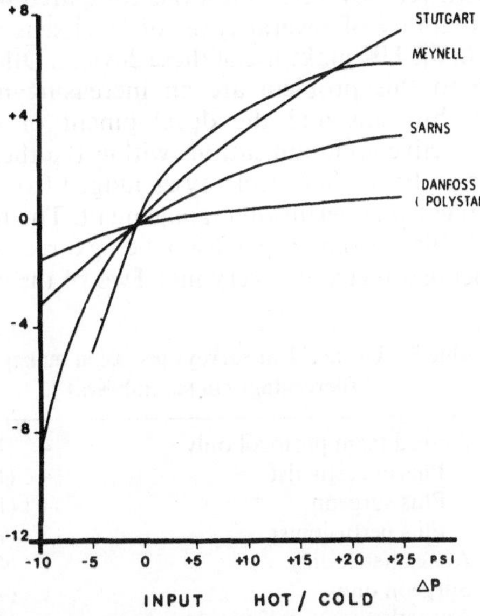

Figure 9 The effect of gas : blood flow on bubble oxygenator venous resistance. Blood flow 2.5–6.2 l/min. Mixer set at 32°C with both inputs at 15 psi. Effects of varying hot input pressure whilst holding cold input at 15 psi

Emergency changing of oxygenators is not difficult if the perfusionist has practised the procedure at regular intervals and the necessary equipment is available at short notice. There is also something to be said for having a standard replacement oxygenator available for such a purpose. We use a VT 5000 which has connections already in place – since this oxygenator can be primed without a gas flow and the ports can be sealed by hand for rapid connection.

A situation which presents the perfusionist with an acute problem is that in which the oxygenator is suddenly damaged so that bypass has to be immediately discontinued. Modern hard-shell oxygenators have connections which are very susceptible to mechanical damage – such as a bored surgical assistant suddenly moving a surgical boot! To emerge unscathed from this situation obviously requires alternative equipment to be readily available and the procedure to have been well rehearsed. It is also obviously a factor to be borne in mind when positioning the oxygenator on the machine.

DISCUSSION

The preceding remarks obviously do not form a definitive work on the subject of safe perfusions. It is difficult to think of any aspect of perfusion which does not have a safety factor involved. However a number of developing features are evident and are perhaps worthy of further comment.

It would seem that the incidence of arterial line embolism is on the increase and that the most likely cause of this is the advent of hard-shell oxygenators which are run with very low reservoir levels compared with previous devices. Despite the availability of several types of level-sensing alarms only 48% of perfusionists in the UK make use of these devices. Other factors which may be contributing to this problem are an increasing number of relatively inexperienced technicians and the development of stress and resultant breakdown of effective communications within the theatre. The concept of teamwork seems to be in some disarray as judged from the replies received to the question regarding perfusion management. The replies showed a very wide variation (Table 5) from the perfusion being directed by a single member of the team to being directed by everyone! Two of the major manufacturers

Table 5 UK accident survey: perfusion management (percentages in parentheses)

Agreed team protocol only	4	(15)
Plus anaesthetist	4	(15)
Plus surgeon	4	(15)
Plus perfusionist	2	(7)
Anaesthetist only	1	(4)
Surgeon only	1	(4)
Anaesthetist + perfusionist	1	(4)
Anaesthetist + surgeon	2	(7)
Everyone!	4	(15)

of perfusion equipment now include a low-level alarm and shut-off system as mandatory equipment for consoles purchased.

Only 37% of the respondents to the UK survey reported undertaking any form of regular emergency drill. In the event of a major systems failure the chances of recovering the situation without the benefit of proper preparation are very slim. A secondary benefit of regular emergency training is a psychological one – the perfusionist is forced to regularly consider the possible hazards, and develops confidence in his ability to meet almost any problem which he may be confronted with.

Although about 60% of the respondents to the survey reported anticoagulation monitoring, it would seem to me that the importance of this aspect of perfusion management is yet to be fully appreciated. Perhaps when full confidence has been gained in the monitoring technique universal acceptance will follow.

By far the most important aspect of perfusion safety is, I believe, the development of a critical systematic approach, the constant attention to detail, and the relentless pursuit of quality.

References

1. RoSPA (1979). *The Facts About Accidents* (SE 62). (Birmingham: The Royal Society for the Prevention of Accidents)
2. *Cardiac Surgical Register.* (Administered by the Society of Thoracic and Cardiovascular Surgeons of Great Britain)
2. Stoney, W. S. *et al.* (1979). Air embolism and other accidents using pump oxygenators. Paper presented at the annual meeting of the Southern Thoracic Surgical Association, San Antonio, Texas, USA, 1 November, 1979
4. Ross, J. K. *et al.* (1978). Wessex cardiac surgery follow-up survey: the quality of life after operation. *Thorax*, **33,** 3
5. Aberg, T. and Khilgren, M. (1977). Cerebral protection during open heart surgery. *Thorax*, **32,** 525
6. Tufo, H. M. *et al.* (1970). Central nervous system dysfunction following open heart surgery. *J. Am. Med. Assoc.*, **212,** 1333
7. Abel, R. M. *et al.* (1976). Acute postoperative renal failure in cardiac surgical patients. *J. Surg. Res.*, **20,** 341
8. *Systems Performance*. The Open University Technology 3rd level course, TD 3421
9. Pfaender, L. M. and Riley, J. B. (1979). An in vitro comparison of the venous return dynamics of elven bubbler oxygenators and four venous reservoirs for extracorporeal circulation. *J.E.C.T.*, **11 : 4**
10. Pastoriz-Pinol, J. V. *et al.* (1969). An analysis of micro-embolic particles originating in the extra-corporeal circuit before bypass. *J.E.C.T.*, **11 : 6**
11. Brooks, J. D. *et al.* (1979). Efficacy of particulate removal by a pre-bypass filter with different oxygenation systems. *AmS.E.C.T. Proceedings – Houston*, **11,** 175
12. Filters, filtration and sources of filterable emboli. *Polystan News and Information*, September 1979
13. Pearson, D. T. *et al.* (1978). An ultrasonic analysis of the comparative efficiency of various cardiotomy reservoirs and micropore blood filters. *Thorax*, **33,** 352
14. Green, C. G. (1978). Can the use of heat exchangers in the cooling phase cause platelet aggregation. Paper presented at the Meeting of the Cercle D'Etude De La Circulation Extracorporelle, Paris, June, 1978

15. Miller, S. S. *et al.* (1977). Comparison of the effectiveness of various extracorporeal filters at reducing gaseous emboli. *AmS.E.C.T. Proc.*, 55
16. Duvall, R. M. *et al.* (1978). Unrecognized plugging of Bentley cardiotomy reservoir with internal 3 stage microporous filter. *J.E.C.T.*, **10 : 2**
17. Pfaender, L. M. *et al.* (1979). An in vitro comparison of the effects of temperature on the stroke volume and occlusion setting of various tubing types in a roller pump. *J. extracorp. Tech.*, **11,** 78
18. Landis, G. H. *et al.* (1979). Pump flow dynamics of the roller pump and constrained vortex pump. *AmS.E.C.T. Proceedings – Houston,* **11,** 201
19. Mandl, J. P. (1977). Comparison of emboli production between a constrained force vortex pump and a roller pump. *AmS.E.C.T. Proc.*, 27
20. Kurusz, M. *et al.* (1979). Runaway pump head: new cause of gas embolism during cardiopulmonary bypass. *J. Thorac. Cardiovasc. Surg.*, **77,** 792
21. Wise, E. A. *et al.* (1978). Gaseous emboli generation by a pulsatile assist device. *J.E.C.T.*, **10:2**
22. Kurusz, M. *et al.* (1979). Runaway pump head: new cause of gas embolism during cardiopulmonary bypass. *J. Thorac. Cardiovasc. Surg.*, **77,** 792
23. Brown, J. H. U. (1976). Medical devices as medical problems: the regulation of devices for clinical use. *Biomd. Eng.*, (October), 337
24. *Health Devices.* (ECRI)
25. *Report on Confidential Enquiries into Maternal Deaths in England and Wales,* 1973–1975. (London: HMSO)
26. Cieslak, F. C. *et al.* (1977). Adequate tissue oxygenation during cardiopulmonary bypass. *AmS.E.C.T. Proc.*, **V**
27. Streczyn, M. V. (1977). The oxygen available to tissues during perfusion. *AmS.E.C.T. Proc.*, **V**
28. Mandl, J. P. and Motley, J. R. (1979). Oxygen consumption plateauing: a better method of achieving optimum perfusion. *J. E.C.T.*, **11 : 2**
29. Berger, E. C. (1979). *The Physiology of Adequate Perfusion.* (St. Louis: C. V. Mosby)
30. Bull, B. S. *et al.* (1975). The use of a dose response curve to individualize heparin and protamine dosage. *J. Thorac Cardiovasc. Surg.*, **69,** 685
31. Mabry, C. D. *et al.* (1979). Identification of heparin resistance during cardiac and vascular surgery. *Arch. Surg.*, **114,** 129
32. Berg, E. *et al.* (1979). Monitoring heparin and protamine therapy during cardiopulmonary bypass by activated clotting time. *AmS.E.C.T. Proceedings,* **11,** 229
33. Doyle, D. L. (1978). The prevalence of gross air embolism during cardiopulmonary bypass. *AmS.E.C.T. Proc.*, **VI**
34. Winter, P. M. *et al.* (1971). Hyperbaric treatment of cerebral air embolism during cardiopulmonary bypass. *J. Am. Med. Assoc.*, **215,** 1786
35. Steward, D. *et al.* (1977). Hypothermia in conjunction with hyperbaric oxygenation in the treatment of massive air embolism during cardiopulmonary bypass. *Ann. Thorac. Surg.*, **24,** 591
36. McMillan, J. *et al.* (1979). Case report – emergency changing of an oxygenator during total cardiopulmonary bypass. *Anaesth. Intensive Care,* **VII : 3**
37. Adachi, H. (1976). Interchangeable circuit for membrane and bubble oxygenator. *Jpn. J. Thorac. Surg.*, **29,** 100
38. Page, P. A. (1977). Clinical evaluation of a new non-invasive electromagnetic oxygenator blood level sensor. *AmS.E.C.T. Proc.*, 1977
39. Burgess, F. M. (1977). A new anti-air embolism device. Burgess F. M. *AmS.E.C.T. Proc.*, 1977

28
Toxins in open heart surgery

D. B. LONGMORE AND MERILYN SMITH

INTRODUCTION

From the beginning of open heart surgery, there have been sporadic cases in which patients and sometimes groups of patients, have shown signs and symptoms of toxicity. Patients who undergo heart surgery with cardiopulmonary bypass do less well than those who have a similar operation without the use of bypass apparatus. It is common for the patient who has had open heart surgery performed with the use of heart/lung machines to be on the ventilator for 12 hours and to be in the intensive care ward for 24 hours. Postoperative cerebral complications, postoperative bleeding and some degree of multi-organ impairment are all common sequelae of open heart surgery. These complications are not commonly seen in patients operated on without bypass support nor in cases operated on using surface cooling and so-called closed operations, e.g. closed mitral valvotomy. Some of these problems are known to be associated with microemboli[1] but others appear to relate to materials liberated from the bypass apparatus or to some chemical change which occurs in the blood during operation. Blood travels about 20 miles through the tubing during an open heart operation and is thereby in contact with a vast area of potentially bio-incompatibile material. In addition to this, the various circulating and suction pumps will release particulate matter into the circulation from wear of the tubing. The opportunities for toxic materials to be leeched from the extracorporeal apparatus and for the occurrence of mechanical trauma, both to the formed elements of the blood and to the plasma proteins[2] are considerable. The tubing of the extracorporeal apparatus is commonly made of polyvinyl chloride (PVC). This heterogenous material consists of pellets of the polymer separated by plasticizers and various fillers. The plasticizers are often complex mixtures. Many of the components of these are themselves highly toxic and some have a significant solubility in an aqueous electrolyte solution. The roughness of the interior wall of a PVC tube is illustrated in Figure 1 in which the size of a red cell is compared with surface irregularities of various materials commonly used in bypass circuits. Because PVC and many of the other plastics used are

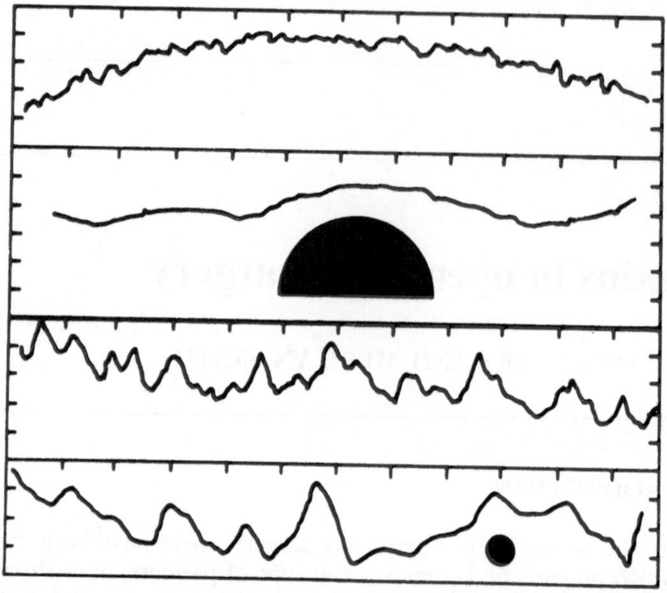

Figure 1 In the lower part of this illustration a red cell is compared with the surface of a natural blood vessel and with an electro-polished stainless steel surface. The upper part of the illustration shows a red cell on a different scale related to the surface of PVC and silicone rubber tubes

heat labile they have to be sterilized by methods other than steam autoclaving. The pathologists in charge of sterilization would prefer us to use steam sterilization although we have reservations about this technique as well, since water softeners and other materials are added to the boilers which allow solid materials to pass into the hospital steam rather than furring up the boilers. Deposits of calcium and other materials are shown in Figure 2 on the inside of a heat exchanger viewed under ultra violet light.

Apart from steam sterilization two other methods are commonly used.

1. ETHYLENE OXIDE (ETO)

When in the late fifties, ETO came into general use as a sterilizing agent for heart lung equipment, it was usually prepared as a mixture of 8% ETO in 92% carbon dioxide. This mixture was safe because it contained sufficient CO_2 to eliminate the risk of explosion and to dilute the powerful oxidizing effect of the ETO. There was a problem, however, in that unless steps were actively taken to mix the gases before use, there was a tendency for the CO_2 to separate, leaving an ETO-rich layer at the top of the cylinder. Because of this, there were occasional failures of sterilization. After this experience, the major manufacturer of sterilizing gas mixtures changed to a composition of 12% ETO in 88% assorted freons. Around 1964, and coincident with this change, the incidence of apparent chemical toxicity increased and it looked as if there was a relationship between these two events. Some patients even

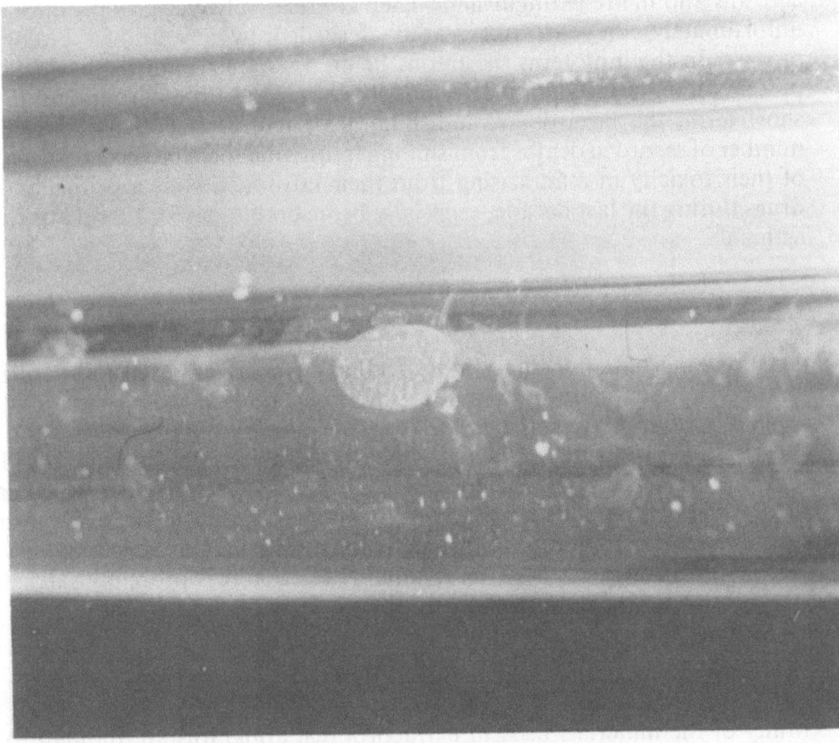

Figure 2 Shows the inside of a heat exchanger viewed under ultra violet light. It shows heavy deposits of calcium and other materials which are invisible under normal light

exhibited gross pulmonary oedema with pink froth exuding from their lungs looking as if they had been poisoned with phosgene or some other extremely irritant material.

It is known that when blood or saline passes over materials containing ETO, highly toxic ethylene chlorhydrin will be formed. ETO itself, in addition to its powerful oxidizing capabilities, is highly damaging to all the constituents of blood, causing, amongst its many harmful effects, changes in the chemical nature of the blood proteins. The previously accepted practice of leaving tubing on the shelf for a week before use, developed when using ETO in CO_2, was no longer adequate. Investigation in 1971 by Thomas and Longmore[3] of a batch of oxygenators which had been airfreighted from the USA and kept in store for several weeks revealed ETO in loose combination with the plastics used, present in concentrations sufficient to cause severe cerebral and multiorgan damage. The investigation also showed that there were much larger volumes of residues of the freon dilutents in the tubing. At that time the possible dangers of freons were not appreciated. Freons were first produced in 1928 as a safe substitute for ammonia in refrigerators. Their stability, low boiling point, apparent non-toxicity and inability to support combustion have meant that they have been widely used as a propellant in aerosols and in fire extinguishers. They are relatively cheap to produce, but unfortunately, they are not readily degraded by any known biological process. In the long term the freons being discharged into the atmosphere present an unknown, cumulative possible hazard to the environment. In the short term, the hazards are indisputable. There have been an increasing number of recorded deaths from sniffing freons and there has been a suspicion of their toxicity in man arising from their introduction as a propellant for drugs during the last decade, especially bronchodilators for the treatment of asthma[4].

2. GAMMA IRRADIATION

This ionizing radiation can readily and conveniently be used for sterilizing extracorporeal apparatus. Usually a dose of 2 million rads is chosen. This level of radiation is sufficient to degrade some of the plastics and the plasticisers, producing acid and other toxic materials. Whereas residual ETO and freons are difficult to remove with a simple flushing of the heart/lung apparatus, it is a straightforward matter to flush out the acids formed during gamma irradiation. Although the tubing may appear a somewhat unpleasant brown colour after gamma irradiation it is probably safer than the clear colourless tubing which is obtained after using ETO.

BIOCOMPATABILITY OF PLASTICS

Many of the materials used in extracorporeal apparatus are thought to be bioincompatible in that apart from releasing known and obvious toxins like residual ETO and ethylene chlorhydrin they appear to irritate tissues by contact.

A BIO-ASSAY TECHNIQUE FOR DETECTING HAZARDOUS MATERIALS IN EXTRACORPOREAL APPARATUS

A method was needed to aid the search for toxic residues and intrinsic bioincompatibility. Although it is possible using complex equipment to detect free ETO and freons when they are present in large quantities[5], it is much more difficult to detect these materials and other less obvious contaminants when they are present in extremely small quantities. A method was required to detect, and to quantify, any toxic materials in extracorporeal apparatus and to solve the more difficult problem of assessing the biocompatibility of its components. Ideally this method should use effects on vascular or heart tissue to measure possible harmful effects.

The fetal heart organ culture method was originally described by Dame Honor Fell of Strangeways Laboratory, Cambridge, and established by Dr K. Wildenthal[6,7]. The method has been under development in the laboratories of the National Heart and Chest Hospitals since 1972 using mouse hearts. It appeared to provide a suitable, stable bio-assay method for our purposes. Heart tissue has long been stored as single beating cells in tissue culture[8].

The advantages of the organ culture technique over single cell cultures are that muscle differentiation and beating characteristics in single cells are rapidly lost over a few days[9], whereas the fetal heart can be stored in a functional, although catabolic state, for periods up to 4 weeks. During this period it will beat spontaneously with a rate which gradually falls. Before death there is often a transient increase in rate, sometimes associated with arrhythmias and atrioventricular dissociation. For the first 20 days the hearts respond to neutrotransmitters and most cardioactive drugs, develop bradycardia when given acetylcholine or propanolol or when they become hypothermic and tachycardic when given catecholamines or when made hyperthermic[10]. The rate of beating and survival time is linked to its stage of development; the younger hearts beating faster and living longer than the near term hearts[11]. Figure 3 shows the gestation days and stage of development of the fetal mouse heart. Fetal heart tissue is less sensitive to hypoxia than adult tissue and has a relatively large store of glycogen enabling glycolytic metabolism to produce ATP for muscle contraction. The tissue is not completely differentiated and possesses a high mitotic index. Figure 4 shows histology sections of a fetal mouse heart before and after culture.

Initially the organ culture technique was used in our laboratories to study the effect of implanting fetal material in adult animals to study the mitogenic effect[12].

The extreme sensitivity of the fetal heart to changes in its environment suggested to us that it would be an ideal sensitive bio-assay preparation for the detection of toxicity in many aspects of heart/lung bypass work.

Gestation (days)	*Stages of development of the fetal mouse heart*
9	Heart starts pulsating regularly giving a circulatory flow of blood.
10	The atrium and ventricular chamber start to be divided by the development of the endocardial cushion and interventricular septum.
11	The interatrial foramen is constricted and the endocardial cushion fused. Sinusoids commence development.
12	The ventricles of the heart appear almost occluded by expanding trabeculae. The intraventricular foramen persists as the intraventricular septum grows cephalad. Development of the capillary rudiments.
13	The aortic, pulmonary and interventricular septa and the atrioventricular valves are complete. The sinusoids and capillary rudiments start to anastomose.
14	The heart is essentially complete. The foramen ovale persists and the aortic and pulmonary semilunar valves appear.
15	Nucleated red cells make up only 5 % of the blood cells. Coronary arteries start to develop.
16–17	Sinusoids are transformed into the thebesian veins. Enlargement of the myofibrils and further differentiation of the myocardium.
17–22	The final completion of the vasculature of the heart takes place after parturition.

Figure 3

The potential for variability in this model is considerable.

(1) The culture fluid can be changed and essential materials added or subtracted or the relative concentrations can be changed.
(2) Drugs can be added to the culture fluid to evaluate their cardioactivity and potential toxicity.
(3) The same can be done for the metabolites of drugs which are undergoing investigation. Substances can be exhibited to the hearts at an early stage of development, e.g. before β receptors are developed and at a later stage of development after the β-receptors are present.
(4) The protein phase in the culture medium can also be varied. If human protein is being used it can be taken from the blood from patients who exhibit various clinical situations or from the bypass apparatus at the beginning of bypass after the blood and prime have mixed and at the end of the perfusion. It is essential if blood is being taken at the end to take this from the extracorporeal apparatus before various catacholamines are added.
(5) To test for biocompatibility of materials, both before and after sterilization. It is possible to place the fetal heart in apposition with small pledgelets of the plastic. This test will detect either incompatibility or toxic materials which leach out of the solutions from the plastic, including the products of sterilization.
(6) It is also possible to alter the gas phase of the culture chamber and to add various gases up to 50% concentration. When this is done the control hearts are placed in an identical chamber with nitrogen up to 50%.
(7) It is also possible to place the chamber in an environment in which various forms of radiation are present. Strong magnetic fields and gamma irradiation from a cobalt source are 2 examples which have been studied. It is also possible to use combined fields as in nuclear magnetic resonance (NMR).

Fetal hearts from Theier's (TO) pure strain mice which had been mated 13–16 days previously are usually used. The gestation period for this strain is 22 days. Figure 5 shows the relationship between the stage of development to the expected survival time of the hearts in organ culture.

Method of dissection

The mice are killed by luxation of the neck. This enables the fetal hearts to be dissected without being subjected to depressant or anaesthetic drugs. Dissection takes place in a Pathfinder sterile air cabinet. Careful surgical dissection removing the heart and preparing it for explanation is essential for successful cultivation of the organ. It is very important to avoid injury and yet to ensure complete removal of surrounding tissue. The technique which is described below has been found to be the quickest method of obtaining a very high percentage of successful cultures.

The mouse is dipped in alcohol to sterilize the skin. The skin of the abdomen is everted to expose the uterus. Using fine sterile stainless steel watch-

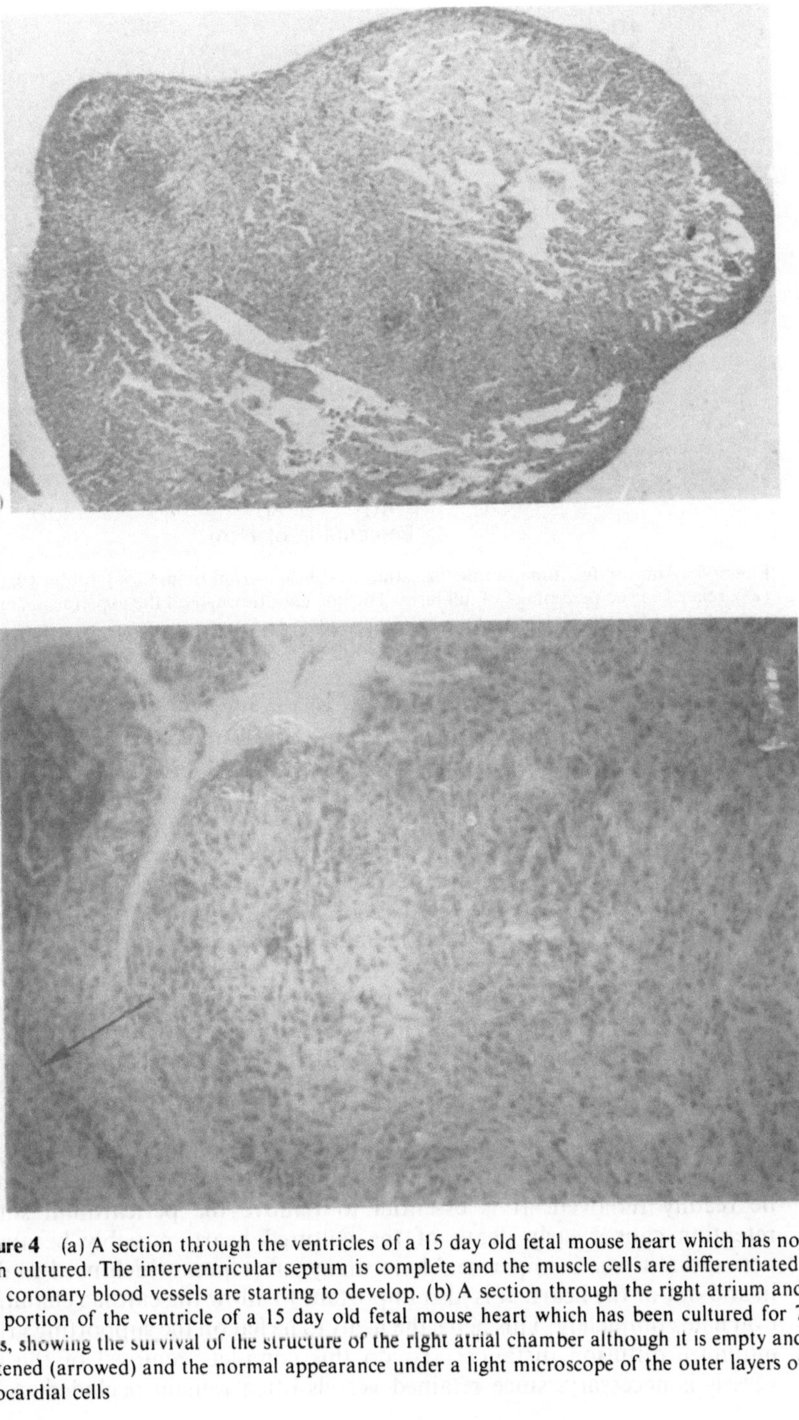

(a)

(b)

Figure 4 (a) A section through the ventricles of a 15 day old fetal mouse heart which has not been cultured. The interventricular septum is complete and the muscle cells are differentiated. The coronary blood vessels are starting to develop. (b) A section through the right atrium and top portion of the ventricle of a 15 day old fetal mouse heart which has been cultured for 7 days, showing the survival of the structure of the right atrial chamber although it is empty and flattened (arrowed) and the normal appearance under a light microscope of the outer layers of myocardial cells

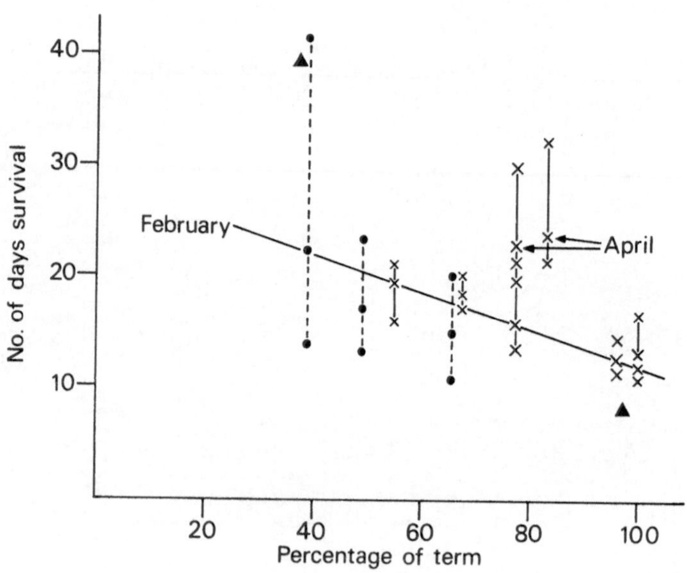

Figure 5 The survival time of intact beating fetal hearts from mouse (×), rabbit (●) and cat (▲), related to the percentage of full term. The line goes through all the experiments except for two conducted in April, which show atypical results.

maker scissors and forceps both horns of the uterus is aseptically removed from the pregnant mouse and placed in a sterile 90 mm petri dish. Figure 6a & b shows stages of removal. The fetuses are removed, still in their amniotic sac and transferred to another petri dish. The remaining membranes are removed and each fetus decapitated. The lower part of the trunk is cut off below the diaphragm, the forelimbs removed at the shoulders and the remaining top part of the trunk is placed in a petri dish. All further dissection takes place under a Wild Heerbrugg 79775 dissecting binocular microscope. The tip of one blade of the scissors is slipped up under the sternum (care being taken not to damage the heart which lies just beneath) and the sternum cut open. The rib cage on either side is then cut back giving a clear view of the heart and great vessels. The prominent thymus lobes are carefully removed, the aorta and pulmonary veins cut and the heart lifted out, cutting connective tissue as necessary (with hearts below 14 days term the lungs are also removed and dissected at the next stage). The heart is then placed in a sterile petri dish containing Wellcome 199 medium (stored at 4 °C and warmed prior to use to 37 °C). Any connective tissue still adhering to the heart will float up and can be readily removed. It is essential to remove the pericardium since its retention causes early death of the cultured heart, possibly because the pericardial tissue is impermeable to many substances which need to diffuse in and out of the heart. It is also important to allow the cardiac chambers to evacuate completely. This helps the heart to lie flat on the supporting grid and minimize diffusion distances. To do this complete removal of the major vessels is necessary, since retained vessels often remain occluded. A small sterile square of Whatman's filter paper (No. 1) is slipped under the isolated heart which is then removed to a prepared stainless steel grid (mesh size 0.1 mm) in a 30 mm petri dish containing culture medium. The smaller petri dish is placed in a 90 mm dish lined with filter paper soaked in sterile water to

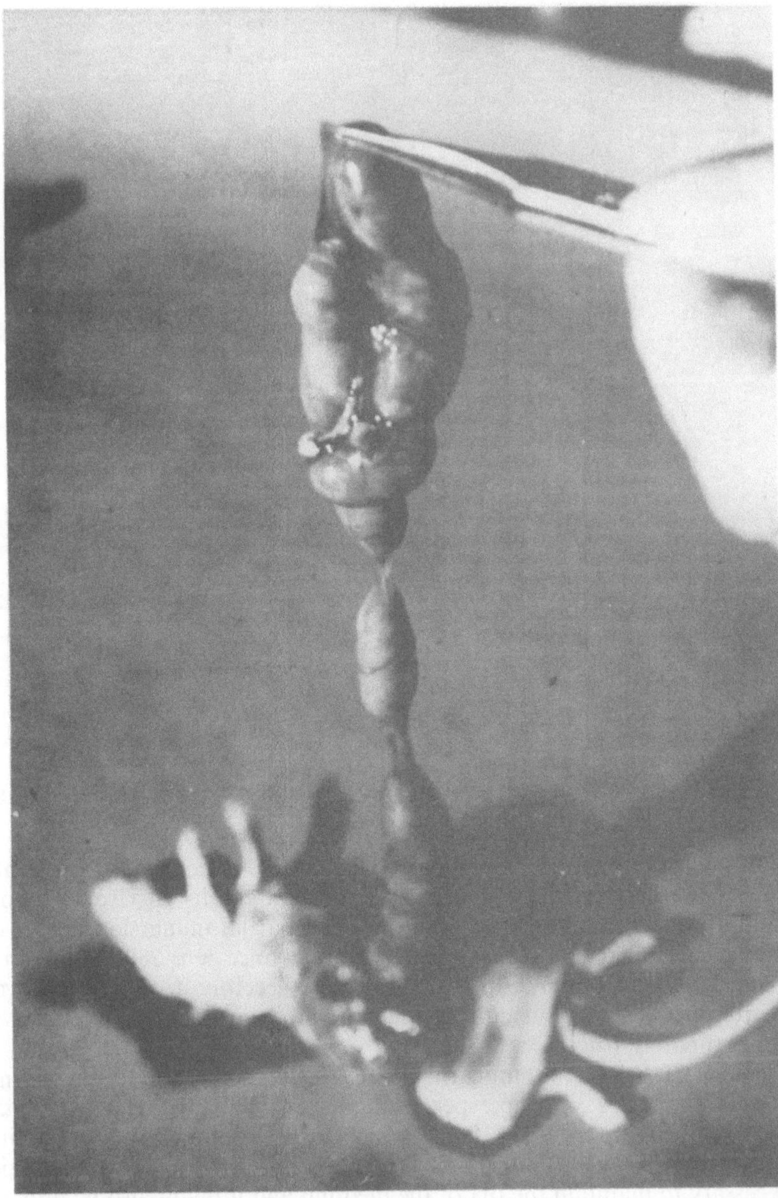

Figure 6 (a) Fetuses being aseptically removed from the abdomen of the mouse

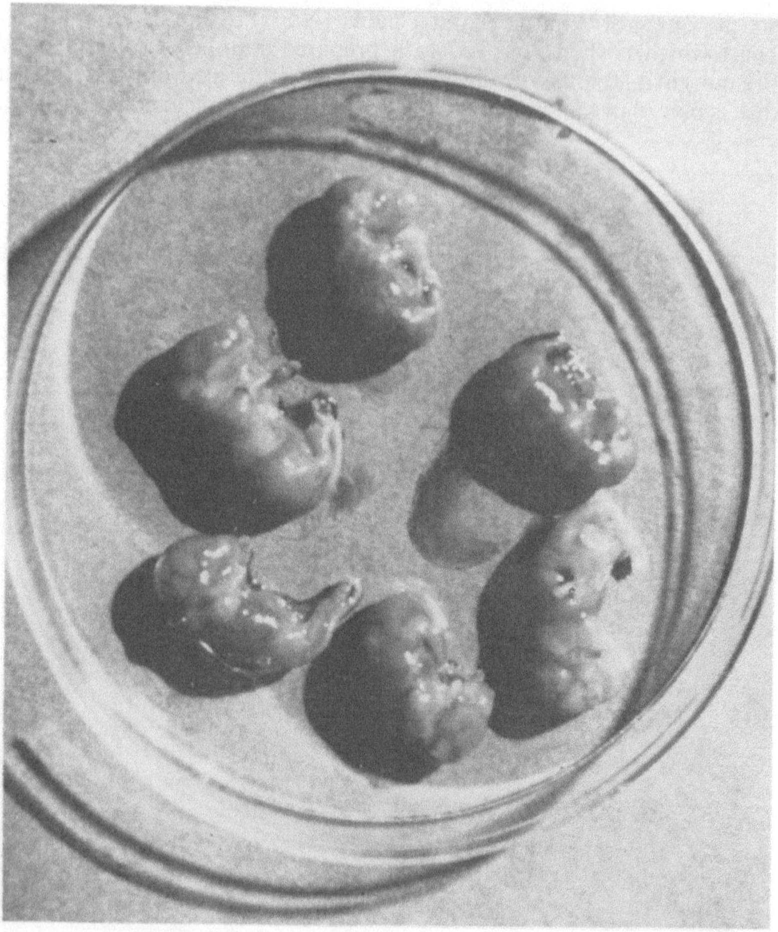

Figure 6 (b) Isolated fetuses in a sterile petri dish after removal from the amniotic sac

maintain humidity, as in Figure 7. The exact position of the heart at the liquid/air interface in the culture is important for its survival. The organ should not be submerged in liquid as even partial immersion causes early death. The heart commences to deteriorate once it is removed from the maternal O_2 supply and nutrients and it is therefore necessary to have the hearts dissected and in culture medium in an incubator at 37 °C within approximately 1 hour.

The petri dishes containing the hearts are stacked in an airtight McIntosh or specially made 3 litre perspex container and filled with 95 % O_2 and 5 % CO_2 as in Figure 8. Wildenthal[6] found that 95 % oxygen was the optimum concentration for the fetal hearts in organ culture. The 5 % carbon dioxide is necessary to maintain the pH of the medium and it might also be utilized by the fetal hearts in the priming of the tricarboxylic acid cycle as it can be taken up and condensed with pyruvic acid to form oxaloacetic acid. Often the hearts remain beating through the dissection but where beating ceases, providing the tissue has not been damaged, it will usually recommence within 24 hours. Only hearts which are beating strongly at a constant rate after 24 hours are used in an experiment. Care is taken to use hearts of litter mates of the same size. Any abnormal hearts are discarded.

Method of observation

The beating rate is sensitive to temperature, beating usually stops completely if the temperature falls below 25 °C. To avoid cooling during observation a photographic reflector lamp is positioned in the sterile air cabinet to maintain a temperature at 37 °C. The petri dishes are removed from the incubator and the hearts examined under a dissecting microscope. Observation is carried out at 24 or 48 hour intervals. The cultures are sensitive to disturbance of atmosphere and temperature and doubling the frequency of observation doubles the death rate. A necrotic centre usually appears after 2–4 days in the centre of the ventricular mass. Such degeneration is usual in differentiated

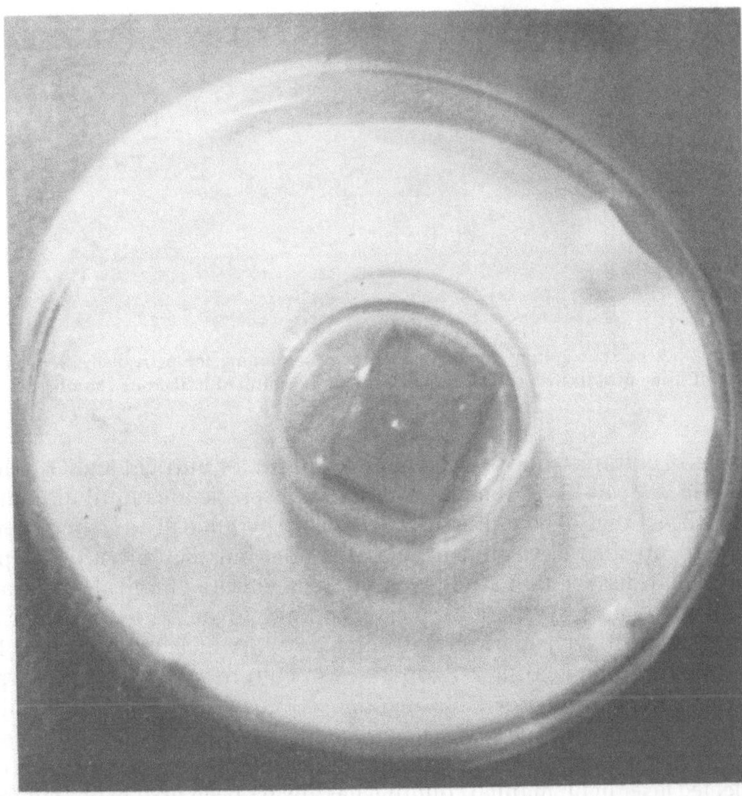

Figure 7 Two fetal hearts are seen resting on stainless steel grids which are bent so that the fetal heart is lifted at the level of the surface of the culture medium

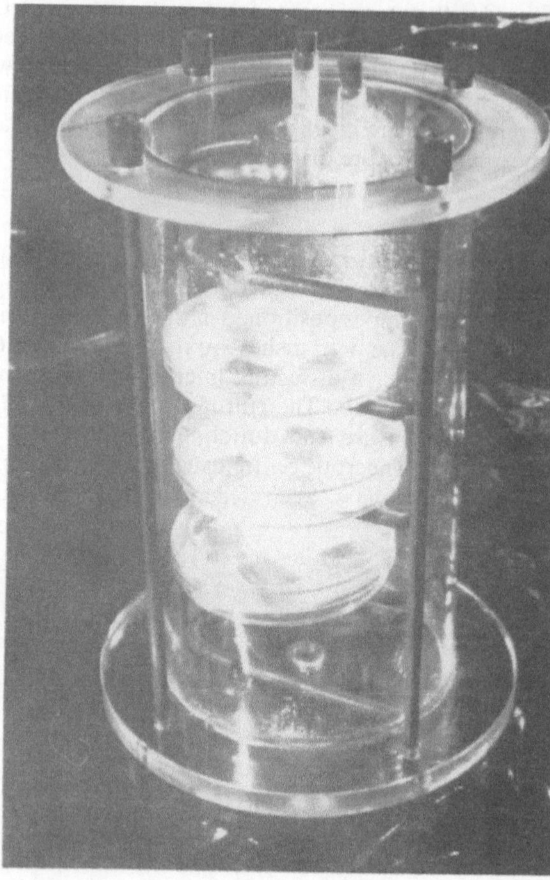

Figure 8 A perspex culture chamber with racks containing the petri dishes showing the gas ports. If using a McIntosh chamber 21 hearts can be cultured in the one chamber

organs in culture[13] due to inadequate diffusion of nutrient and O_2, although a viable layer of fibres remains around the necrotic area until ultimately the entire heart dies. The cultured hearts beat rhythmically and spontaneously in the controlled environment until they die but they often develop atrio-ventricular dissociation after several days in culture. Surgical denervation of the heart causes sympathetic nerve endings to die and to release stored noradrenalin over a period of several days[14] which may account for the initial increase in beating rate observed in culture. After the beating pattern of each heart is recorded the medium is renewed to replace metabolized compounds and to remove accumulated waste products. Although it is possible to use automatic counting[15] either with a proximity device or with reflected laser light, manual counting has always been used in our laboratories because it gives the additional opportunity of assessing the physical state of the heart. Towards the end of their life the hearts may become quiescent, but, if viable, can be stimulated to beat by touching lightly with a fine sterile needle. When a heart ceases to beat even with stimulation for longer than 24 hours it is removed before the products of decomposition affect the remaining hearts.

The cultured hearts have their own innate circadian rhythm making it desirable for observation to be carried out at the same time of the day. It has also been observed in our laboratories that the beating and survival pattern are sex-linked; the male hearts beat faster and live for a shorter time[16] than the female hearts. There is no sign of growth in fetal hearts in organ culture. Usually they lose up to 4% of their original weight.

Preparation of the culture medium

Components:

(1) Tissue culture medium, Wellcome 199, TC20 with the addition of streptomycin and penicillin.
(2) Uninactivated colostrum-deprived fetal calf serum (Wellcome or Gibco-Biocult). If human protein is to be used serum is obtained from blood samples taken from the extracorporeal apparatus at the appropriate time for the study.
(3) Hydrocortisone sodium succinate injection B.P. (Organon Laboratories). 100 mg vials diluted with sterile physiological saline to a concentration of 0.1 μg/ml.
(4) Insulin 80 i.u./ml (Weddel Pharmaceuticals).

For the preparation of 100 ml of culture fluid 63.5 ml of medium 199 is mixed with 35 mls of calf serum, 1 ml of the diluted hydrocortisone solution is added together with 0.5 ml of insulin. Insulin is used in other organ cultures. It improves the growth and synthetic activity of cultured fat pads[17] and under some conditions the growth of cultured cartilage. The addition of the combination of insulin and cortisol prolongs the life and function of many cultures *in vitro*[18].

Establishing the baselines for survival and beating performance

Detailed statistical analyses of the beating rates and survival times suggested to our hospital statistician, Miss M. Rehahn, that we were not dealing with a homogenous population but that there were two or more sub groups. We decided to see if the sex of the fetuses had any influence on the survival times. In the human there is a changing sex ratio throughout life. In early fetal life there are two males for every female[19]. By age 55 the sexes are equal[20]. Over the age of 75 there are two females for every male. This suggests an underlying mechanism making the female more durable than the male in man even when excessive male deaths from accidents etc. are taken into consideration. If the life span of each organ or cell is preordained then the fate of transplanted cells or organs may also be dictated by their intrinsic biological time clock.

We set out to examine this thesis by culturing 100 fetal hearts at 19 day term. The fetuses were sexed by visual inspection at dissection; 53 were found to be male, 44 female and 3 were indeterminate. The results shown graphically in Figure 9 shows that the male hearts beat faster but have a shorter survival time than the female hearts. The effect of this variation is relatively small and because we are able to overcome any effect by using larger control and experimental groups we have not explored this sex difference further.

The fetal hearts also have a circadian rhythm. Hearts counted at 12 noon beat at a significantly faster rate than those counted at midnight. We are unable to explain why isolated fetal hearts, cultured in an artificial medium in a light free chamber and taken from fetuses not yet at term should have a diurnal rhythm. The variation is sufficient to make it desirable to examine the hearts at the same time of day. If groups of 30 or more hearts are used in the control and experimental groups, sex and diurnal variations are not sufficient to invalidate the results.

Once we had established baselines we used the fetal heart preparation as a bioassay in order to study cardiopulmonary bypass with a view to increasing its safety. However, before doing this the technique was used in several practical applications.

Dr A. Nathan of the Royal Free Hospital had observed that patients with cardiomyopathy, particularly hypertrophic, often have a higher than expected history of thyrotoxicosis. He wishes to establish whether thyroid stimulating immunoglobulins caused myocarditis in addition to thyrotoxicosis. In association with our group he studied plasma from patients with high levels of thyroid stimulating immunoglobulins in the organ culture medium and compared these with plasma samples with low TSI levels after plasmaphoresis. The TSI appeared to impair the performance of the fetal hearts, causing premature death as well as causing an increase in mean heart rate compared to the controls[21].

The common constituents of the contraceptive pill, ethinyl oestradiol (1 μg and 10 μg), norgestrol (1 μg and 10 μg), norethisterone acetate (1 μg and 10 μg), were added to the culture medium and the results showed that norethisterone acetate had a profound depressant effect on the beating rate with a reduction in survival time[22].

Fentanyl 5 ng/ml and 50 ng/ml and Omnopon (papaveretum) 10 μg/ml were studied and it was found that fentanyl had a slight depressant effect on the beating rate of the fetal hearts whereas Omnopon significantly caused a reduction in survival time as well as depression of beating rate.

The effects of various cardioactive drugs on the fetal hearts[23] showed the sensitivity of this preparation and in studies involving the patient's blood it was obviously important to take a sample when either no cardioactive drugs had been administered or as long as possible after administration of drugs.

Damage to the blood during extracorporeal bypass

One of the limiting factors to the duration of a heart/lung bypass operation appears to be the cumulative blood damage. Obvious blood damage which can be readily measured is due to mechanical destruction of the formed elements of the blood, red cell destruction with the release of constituents of the red blood cells releasing free haemoglobin and other more toxic materials. Red cell destruction has always been the more obvious of the two forms of

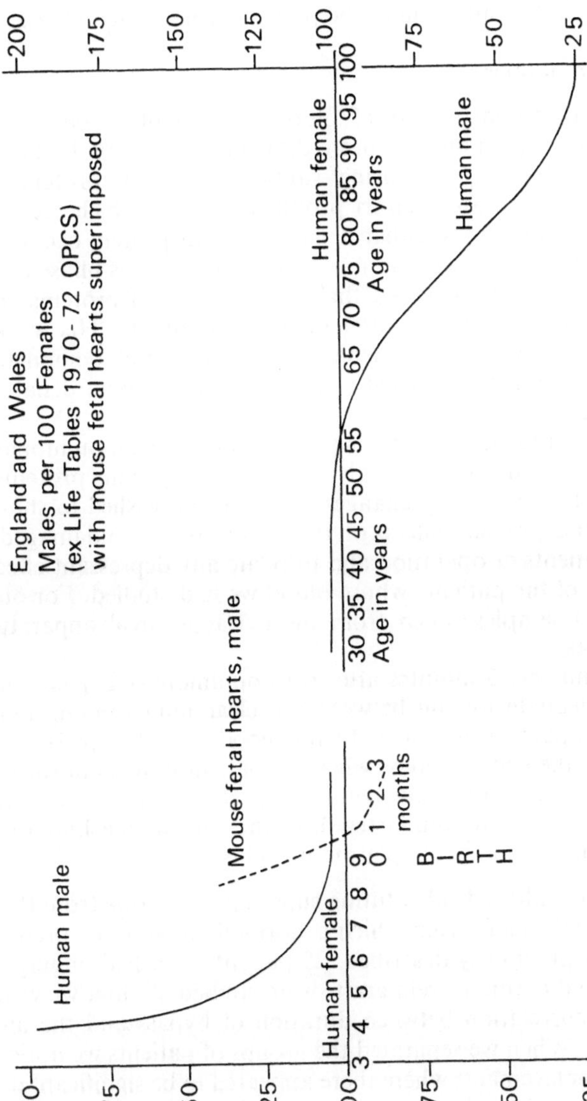

Figure 9 The sex ratio of human males to females from conception to age 100 is compared to the sex ratio of fetal hearts in organ culture suggesting an innate biological difference in survival of an organ as well as in intact man. The horizontal line represents 100 live females and is derived from a decaying exponential curve

blood damage, as plasma from patients who have been on bypass will be pink and the patient will pass port wine urine. Haemolysis on its own does not appear to be particularly harmful. Platelet counts fall during extracorporeal bypass[24]. When platelets which normally have a survival time of about 4 days are prematurely destroyed the granular elements are released and these probably contribute to the patient's generalized illness.

Denaturation of proteins

Damage to other constituents of blood is probably a far more serious complication of bypass but it is more difficult to quantify. Unlike counting red cells and platelets, measuring subtle changes in protein chemistry requires a major laboratory effort producing results which are not readily interpreted. It is well known that denaturation of protein occurs when the molecules are in contact with an interface between a gas phase and a water phase[25,26]. Lee *et al.*[2] suggested that denaturation of proteins could be a cause of morbidity and death after open heart surgery. His work did not show any direct evidence of denatured proteins but demonstrated the physical, chemical and biological changes attendant upon denaturation of plasma proteins.

We wished to study the changes in protein during cardiopulmonary bypass in a way which would detect not only changes in the plasma proteins but also point to the relevence of any changes detected. We wished to show if there were any direct depressant effects on the fetal hearts from damaged proteins taken from patients at operation and to relate any depressant effects to the clinical course of the patients whose blood we had studied. For our studies we used blood samples taken from the extracorporeal apparatus at the following stages:

(1) Approximately 5 minutes after cardiopulmonary bypass commences when adequate mixing between the clear fluid priming fluid of the bypass apparatus and the patient's blood has taken place.
(2) Towards the end of bypass when the patient is again normothermic if hypothermia is used, but before Isoprel or other cardioactive compounds have been administered, to prevent the masking of any true effects due to changes in plasma proteins.

The hearts are cultured substituting supernatant plasma from the patients under study for the calf serum which is normally used in the preparation of culture fluid as previously described. 25 patients who had undergone valve replacements and coronary vein grafts were studied. At first we were unable to establish a correlation between duration of bypass and the amount of protein change. When we separated the groups of patients we noticed that it was the valve replacements where there appeared to be significant damage to the proteins as compared to the coronary vein grafts. Figure 10 shows the effect on the fetal hearts of plasma taken pre and post-operatively from 12 patients who had undergone mitral and aortic valve replacements. This led us to study the relationship between protein damage detected and measured by our test and the amount of suction used during the operations. Discussions were held with the surgeons concerned, Mr D. N. Ross and Mr M. Yacoub

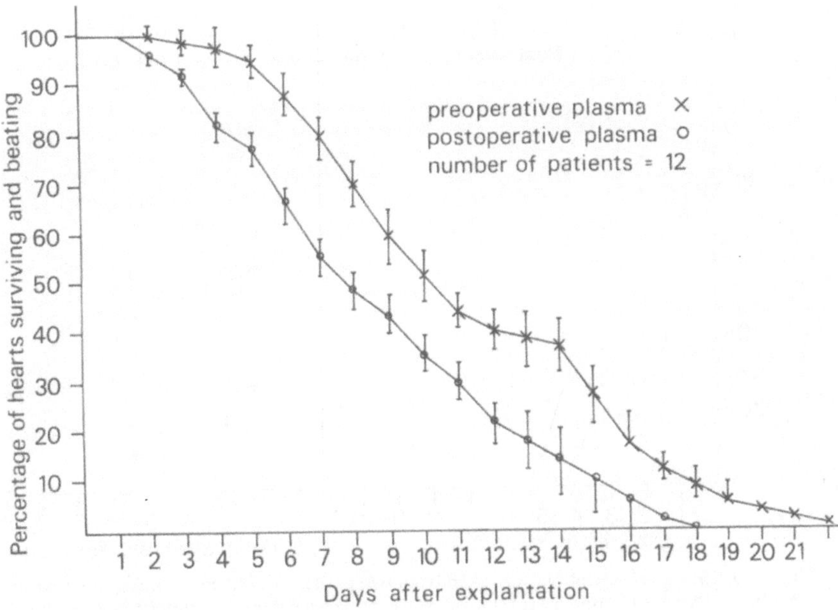

Figure 10 Survival curves of mouse hearts exposed to plasma from patients at the beginning and the end of cardiopulmonary bypass in valve replacement operations before a concerted effort was made to reduce suction

and with their co-operation efforts were made to reduce the amount of pump suction. The results were dramatic. These findings were, in retrospect, not surprising for the suction system is widely recognised as a site of massive blood trauma[27,28].

We studied five patients from another hospital where early pattern TMO oxygenators were being used and the change in plasma protein appeared to be greater than studies where bubble oxygenators had been used. We felt the difference was related more to the amount of suction used than to the oxygenator and if this test is to be used to compare oxygenators it will be necessary to quantify the amount of suction used.

Interesting results came from specific patients. In our series there were only two deaths. In both of these patients the plasma proteins taken at the beginning of bypass were lethal to the fetal hearts as shown in Figure 11, a fact which was to become important to us later when we used the method to investigate unexplained bypass deaths and complications at another hospital (See Figure 13).

The other interesting observation was from one patient in our series who had a complicated postoperative period. This patient had undergone mitral and tricuspid valve replacement with a bypass time of 95 minutes. The postoperative course was unremarkable initially but 6 days postoperatively he became oliguric. The registrar in charge of the patient was sufficiently concerned about this to give him massive doses of frusemide and spironolactone. The patient became acutely ill, jaundiced, confused and drowsy.

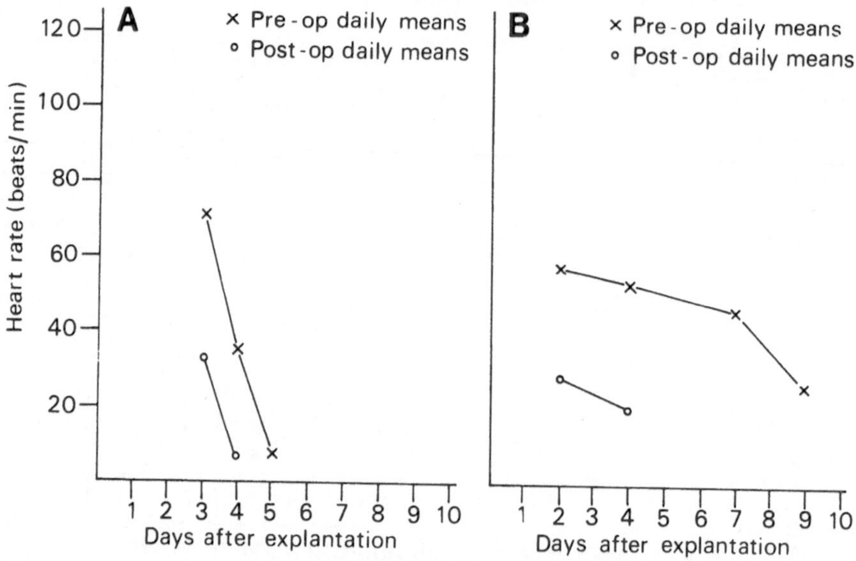

Figure 11 Shows effects of plasma taken from two patients who died within 24 hours of bypass operation. Patient (a) underwent mitral valve replacement and coronary vein graft with a bypass time of 132 minutes. Patient (b) underwent correction left transposition, right ventricular reconstruction with a bypass time of 115 minutes. We now know that neither patient would be expected to survive with plasma which is toxic to this degree to fetal hearts

Whether this was related to this therapy or whether the oliguria had a common causitive factor we were not sure. We took a further blood sample at this stage and his plasma proteins as shown in Figure 12 showed a severe inhibitory effect on the fetal hearts with early death as seen previous in patients who were unlikely to survive. The diuretic combination was withdrawn and the patient made a gradual recovery with the loss of toxic effects. We took a further sample 13 days postoperatively and the result is shown in Figure 12 suggesting that whatever plasma protein changes were associated with the acute illness had now clearly recovered. In Intensive Care at the same time were two other patients, not included in our original series, who also developed toxic effects. Blood samples were taken when they became ill and their plasma proteins had the same impairing effect on the fetal hearts as the patient described above. They had also been given massive doses of frusemide and spironolactone and recovered when these were withdrawn. We cannot explain the relationship between these drugs and the clinical course of the patients which was mirrored by the performance of the fetal heart cultures.

We were consulted by another hospital that had been experiencing some unexplained complications during and after bypass, including sporadic outbreaks of haematuria. We took a series of blood samples starting after the induction of anaesthesia and at intervals throughout the operation. We were able to identify the origin of the protein damage which was a constituent in the pump prime. The results of two patients studied in this way are shown to illustrate this point in Figure 13a and b. It is not known whether this toxicity in the prime was due to residual ETO or to other toxic products of sterilization or to some contaminant. The surgeons concerned immediately set about changing every possible source of contamination and toxicity in the prime with elimination of the haematuria.

We have also used the fetal heart test on protein damage in an attempt to assess the value of prostacyclin as an agent to protect the plasma proteins

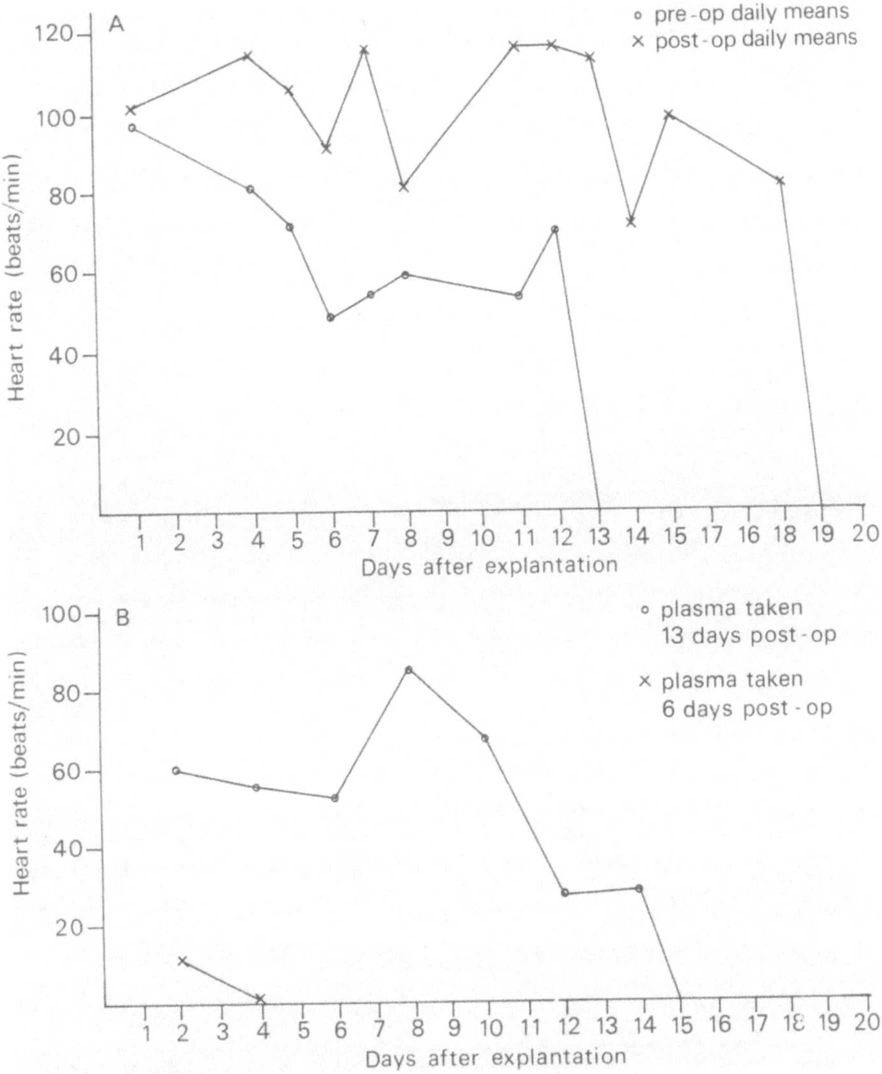

Figure 12 (a) Shows the beating rate and survival time of the fetal hearts exposed to plasma taken from the patient at the beginning and the end of a 95 minute bypass. (b) Shows the extreme inhibition of the beating rate and the reduced survival time from the same patient 6 days post-operatively with partial recovery reflected in the performance of the hearts exposed to plasma 13 days postoperatively

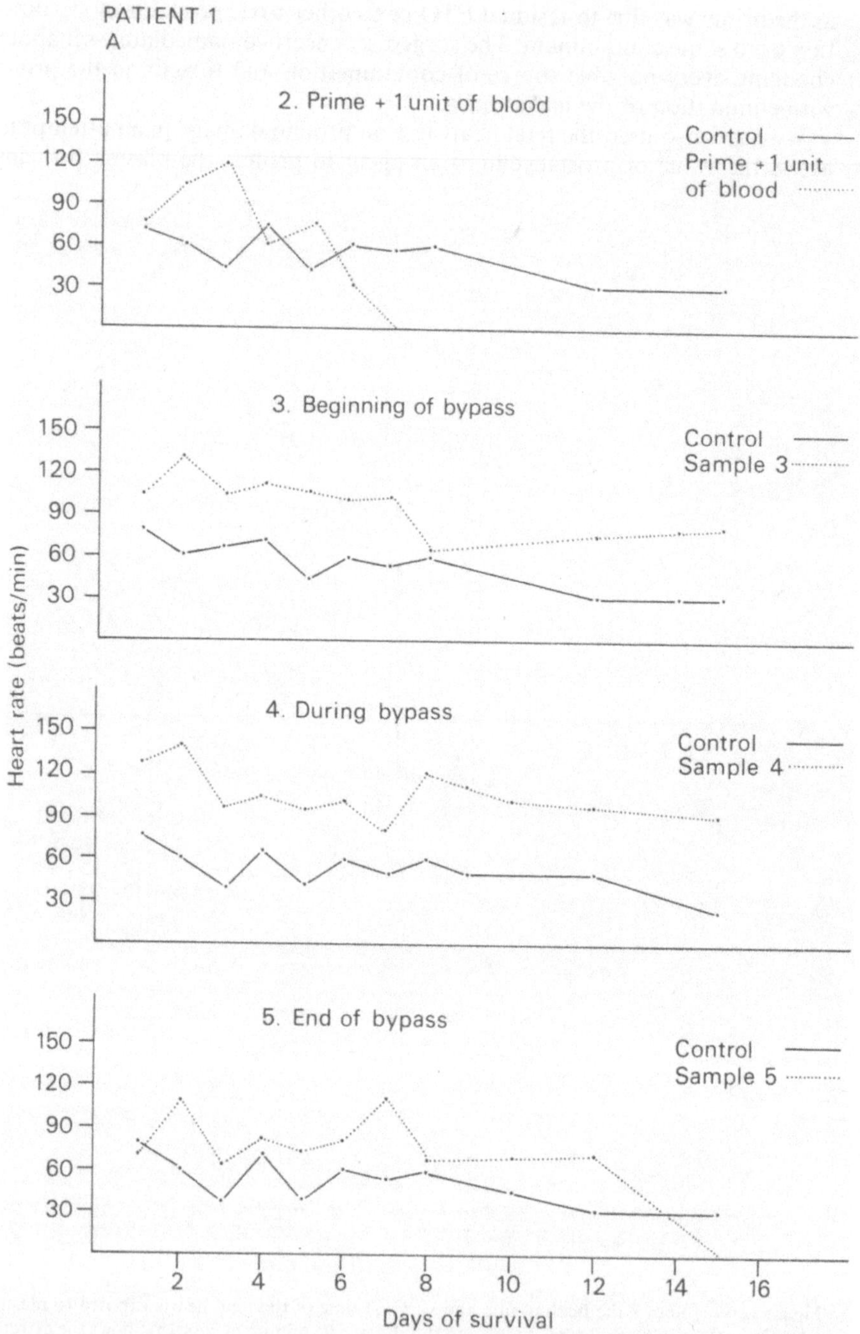

Figure 13 (a) and (b) In both of these patients it may be seen that the contents of the oxygenator prime which were added to the fetal hearts along with colostrum-deprived calf serum were toxic. This corresponded with haematuria when the patient went on to bypass

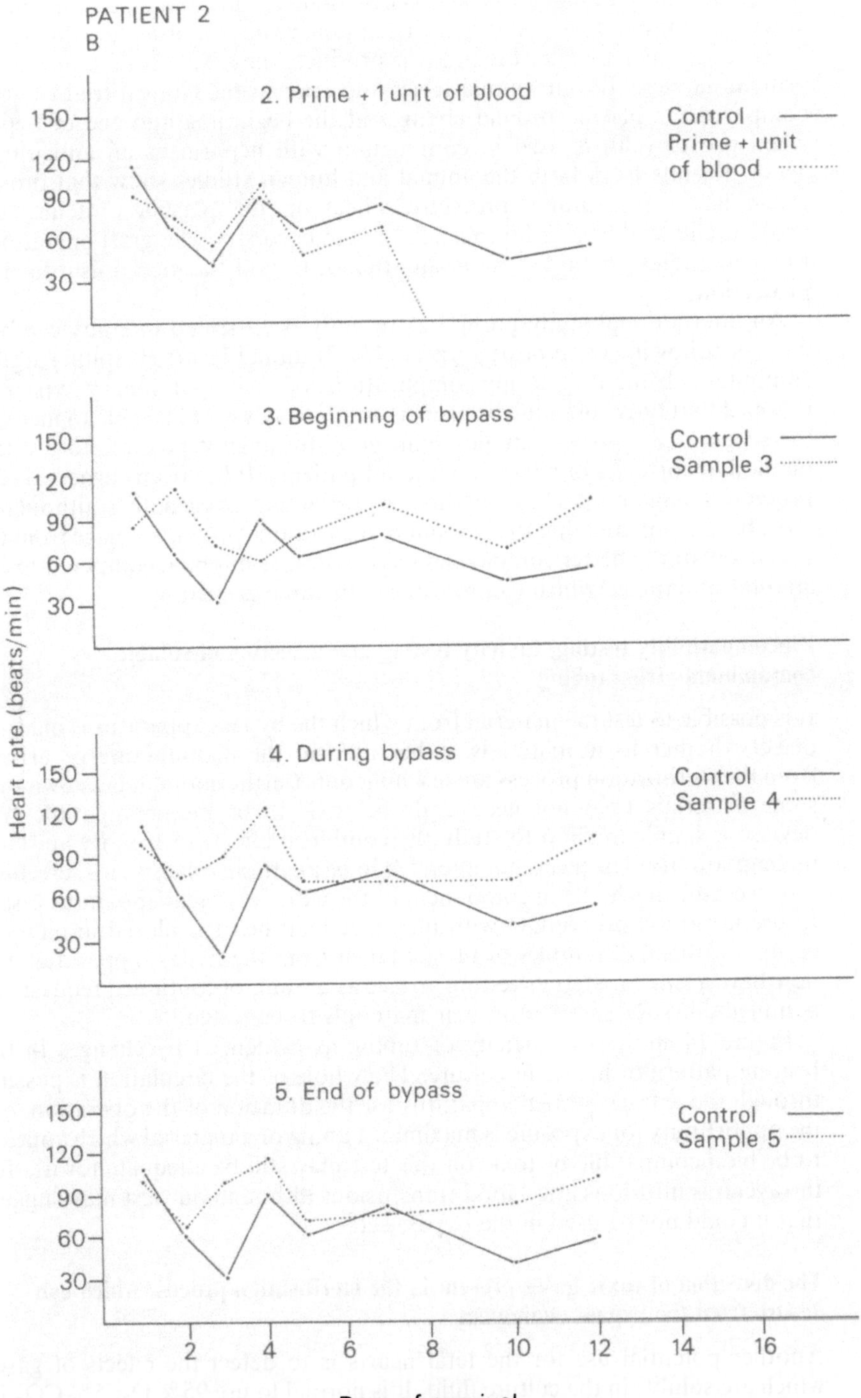
PATIENT 2
B
2. Prime + 1 unit of blood
Control
Prime + unit of blood
3. Beginning of bypass
Control
Sample 3
4. During bypass
Control
Sample 4
5. End of bypass
Control
Sample 5
Heart rate (beats/min)
150
120
90
60
30
2
4
6
8
10
12
14
16
Days of survival

during cardiopulmonary bypass. When platelets are damaged and break down the granular elements which contain toxic materials are liberated. These and other platelet breakdown products may be a source of plasma protein damage. In our animal series and later in the clinical trial we have compared the plasma protein changes at the beginning and end of bypass when prostacyclin is used in conjunction with heparin as an anticlotting agent. Results from both the animal and human studies show that prostacyclin has a measurable protective effect on the plasma proteins. The prostacyclin trial has, so far, been limited to coronary vein graft operations. Further studies are underway in an attempt to find the mechanism for this protection.

An international study group has recently been set up to study cerebral damage following open heart surgery. The National Heart Hospital surgical computer is being used to log complications of cardiopulmonary bypass. It is hoped that once this study is properly underway we will be able to increase the scope of the protein studies sufficiently to make it possible to use this method to correlate of a large number of patients. It has been suggested that protein damage might be a method of evaluating oxygenators although it must be remembered that the amount of measurable protein damage from the use of any of the better commercial oxygenators is minimal compared to the amount of damage which can be done with careless suction.

Biocompatibility testing, toxicity testing and detection of soluble contaminants from tubing

It is possible to test the material from which the bypass apparatus is made to detect whether toxic materials, either used in the manufacture or arising from the sterilization process are leaching out. Furthermore, it is known that some materials need not necessarily be toxic to be bioincompatible. We devised a simple method to study the combined effects of toxicity and bioincompatibility. The test is not intended to be anything other than a screening test to establish whether a component of the extracorporeal apparatus is safe to use in prolonged contact with blood. A fetal heart is placed in physical contact with small samples of plastic taken from the bypass apparatus. We now have a small materials testing service as a result of continued requests by manufacturers for samples of their materials to be tested.

Figure 14 shows the toxicity of tubing as evidenced by changes in the beating pattern of hearts in culture. The whole of the circulation is passing through the extracorporeal apparatus for the duration of the operation and the opportunity for exposure is maximal. Tubing or a material which appears to be bioincompatible or toxic on this test may still be adequate for use for intravenous infusions and blood transfusions although our test may suggest that it could not be used in the bypass set.

The detection of toxic gases present in the sterilisation process which can desorb from the bypass equipment

Another potential use for the fetal hearts is to detect the effects of gases which are soluble in the culture fluid. It is normal to use 95% O_2, 5% CO_2 in

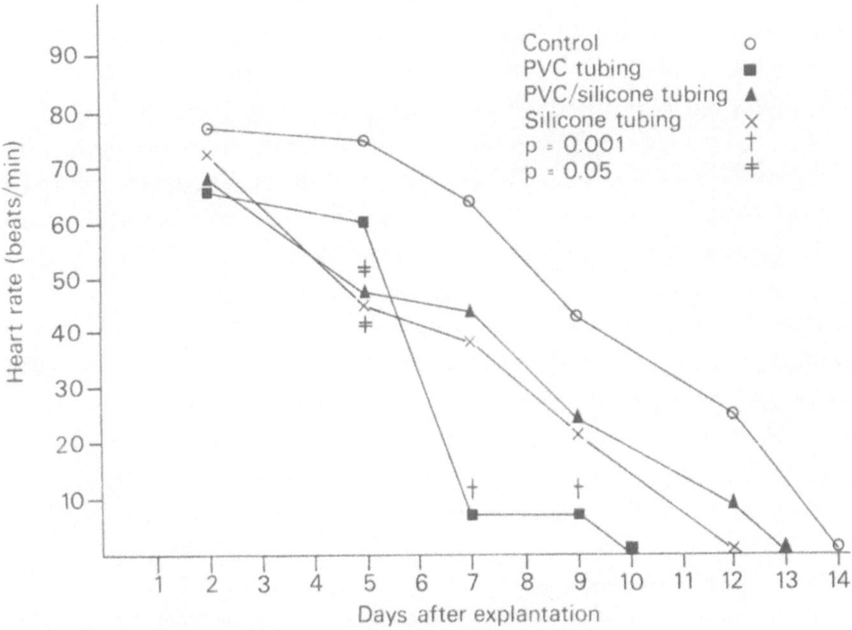

Figure 14 Shows the effect on the inhibition of beating rate and survival time of PVC tubing compared with the control and acceptable PVC/silicone and silicone tubes

the culture chamber as this gives the optimum survival time, but concentrations of O_2 as low as that in air do not cause enough reduction in overall performance to make a study invalid. Because of this it is relatively easy to test gas mixtures of O_2 and test gas in concentrations of up to 75% test gas.

The hearts were subjected to varying concentrations of nitrous oxide and it was shown that this gas had a cardiodepressant effect on the beating rate and reduced the survival time of the cultures, thus demonstrating that it is possible to quantify the effect of gasses on the fetal hearts. This finding is paralleled by clinical experience.

It was therefore decided to study freons as a mixture of this gas, usually from 11, 12 and 13, is used as a propellent for the ETO in sterilizing plastic apparatus. Any residual gasses from the sterilizing process are left in solution or weakly combined with the plastics used in the extracorporeal apparatus, although freons will be present in much greater concentrations than ETO residues because normally 88% freon and 12% ETO are used. This discrépancy in gas concentrations is increased after flushing the tubing when the highly reactive ETO will form ethylene chlorhydrins leaving freons in the plastic. We have been able to desorb several grams of freons from commercially sterilized apparently clinically safe bubble oxygenators. Although freons are classed as a group 6 gas by the FDA and are, therefore, considered to be non-toxic there are records of people becoming unconscious in the presence of freons and young addicts who sniff freons have been known to

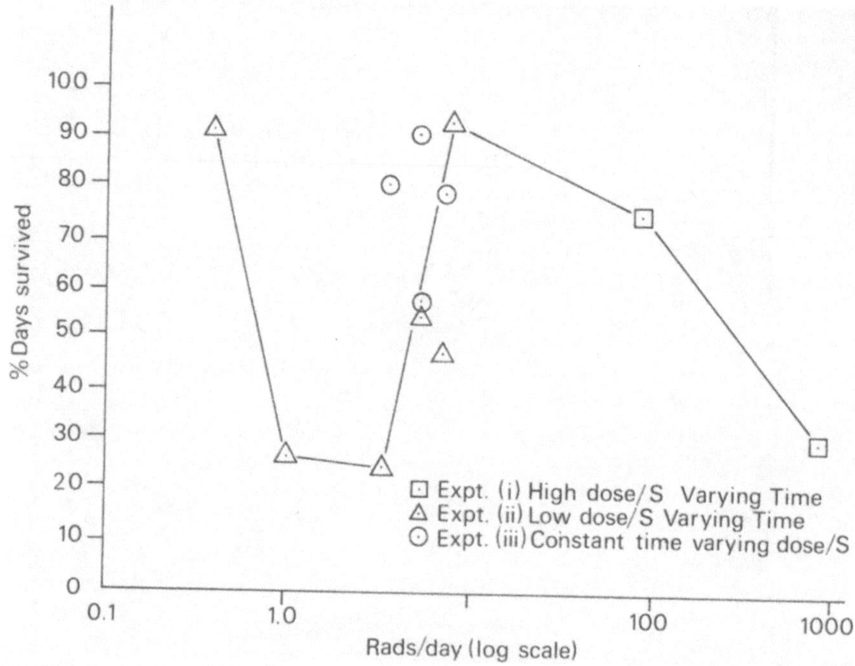

Figure 15 This illustrates the relationship between increasing concentrations of freon-12 in the gas phase of the culture chamber on the beating rate and survival time of fetal hearts

die. For these reasons we wondered if some of the unexplained cerebral and multiorgan complications could be related to residual freons.

We tested three concentrations – 20 %, 50 % and 80 %. With each increasing concentration there was an increasing deleterious effect on both the beating rate and the survival time of the fetal hearts as demonstrated in Figure 15.

An assay of the biological effects of ionizing radiation

The chamber as shown in Figure 8 can be exposed to various forms of radiation. The effect of nuclear magnetic resonance on the cultured hearts is currently being explored. In association with Professor G. N. Walton at Imperial College the effect of gamma irradiation using a Cobalt-60 source has been studied in detail. We set out to demonstrate whether in this non-repairing biological system there was a threshold of radiation necessary before biological damage occurred or whether in fact there was a tailing off effect with very small doses of radiation still causing minimal damage. This was studied in two ways. Firstly, using a constant time exposure at different dose rates and secondly at a constant dose rate with varying time exposures. Our initial results were so remarkable that we repeated the experiments in order to convince ourselves that we were not seeing an artefact. Our findings as shown in Figure 16 suggest that there are two thresholds of radiation damage. The fetal heart preparation shows extreme sensitivity to radiation

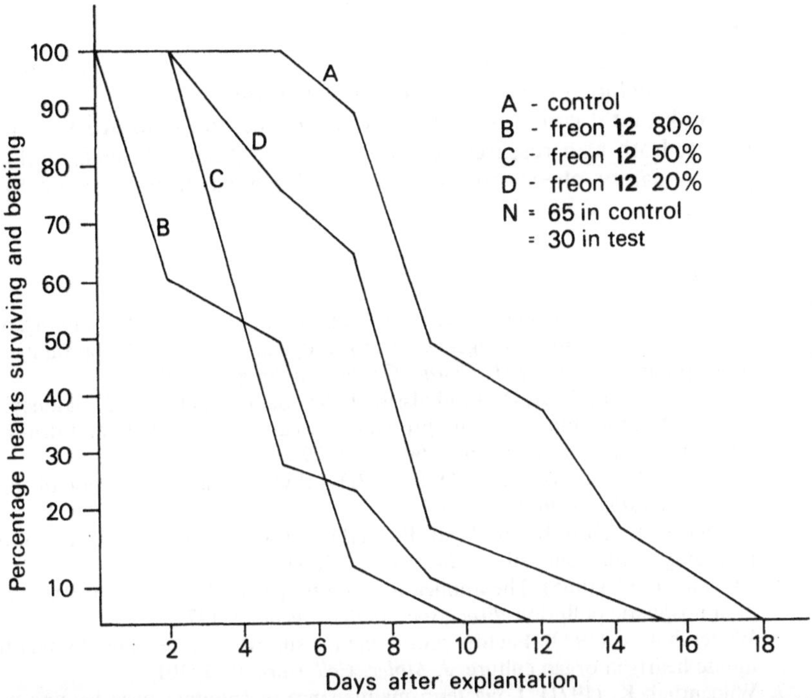

Figure 16 In this study we have shown the reduction in survival time to between 20 and 30 % of the control survival time at dose levels of between 0.5 and 4 rads per day, suggesting that there is extreme sensitivity in this non-repairing biological system to radiation at these levels

between 0.5 and 4 rads, becoming less sensitive again at 6 rads before showing a linear increase in sensitivity. At the moment we can offer no definite reason for this anomaly and further work is planned.

CONCLUSION

The use of the fetal heart preparation is in its early stages as a method of analysing *in vitro* potentially dangerous aspects of cardiopulmonary bypass. However, the baselines of performance are now well known and although cultured fetal hearts are not normal growing organs and undergo some central degeneration and necrosis, a major part of the organ continues to function well enough to beat as an integrated unit for several weeks, and as such we feel it may be a vital bioassay method of detecting at what stage damage and toxicity in the plasma protein occurs, thereby providing a method of reducing postoperative morbidity. It is also useful in measuring and evaluating the biocompatibility and toxicity of the materials used in bypass apparatus, both before and after sterilization by various methods.

However, if meaningful results are to be obtained it is necessary to perform this technique accurately and carefully. Sterile technique is essential otherwise important groups of hearts may have their performance modified by the effect of contamination. To eliminate variables due to the two populations which can be found in the cultured hearts we recommend that a minimum of 30 hearts is included in each control and test group.

We think that it would be valuable to have a central laboratory using this technique, both as a research tool and, more importantly, as a method of keeping a safety check on all aspects of the cardiopulmonary bypass procedure.

References

1. Allardyce, D. B., Yoshida, S. H. and Ashmore, P. G. (1966). The importance of microembolism in the pathogenesis of organ dysfunction caused by prolonged use of the pump oxygenator. *J. Thorac. Cardiovasc. Surg.*, **52,** 706
2. Lee, W. H., Krumhaar, D., Fonkalsrud, E. W., Schjeide, O. A. and Maloney, J. V. (1961). Denaturation of plasma proteins as a cause of morbidity and death after intracardiac operations. *Surgery*, **50,** No. 1, 29
3. Thomas L. C. and Longmore, D. B. (1971). Ethylene oxide sterilization of surgical stores. *Anaesthesia*, **26,** No. 3, 304
4. Speizer, F. E., Doll, R. and Heaf, P. J. (1968). Investigation into the use of drugs preceding death from asthma. *Br. Med. J.*, **1,** 339
5. Thomas, L. C. (1965). The application of long-path (40) gas cells to the analysis of atmospheric pollution. *Proc. Soc. Analyt. Chem.*, **2,** 147
6. Wildenthal, K. (1970). Factors promoting the survival and beating of intact foetal mouse hearts in organ culture. *J. Molec. Cell. Cardiol.*, **1,** 101
7. Wildenthal, K. (1971). Long term maintenance of spontaneously beating mouse hearts in organ culture. *J. Appl. Physiol.*, **30,** No. 1, 153
8. Burrows, M. T. (1912). Rhythmical activity of isolated heart muscle cells *in vitro. Science, N.S.*, **36,** 90
9. Harary, I. (1964). Studies on individual heart cells. *Circ. Res.*, **19,** (Suppl. II), 120
10. Ingwall, Y. S. and Wildenthal, K. (1978). Foetal mouse hearts in organ culture: Studies in cardiac metabolism. *Recent Adv. Stud. Card. Struct. Metab.*, **12,** 21
11. Hughes, D. M. and Longmore, D. B. (1972). Relationship between the stage of development of foetal hearts and their survival in organ culture. *Nature*, **235,** 334
12. Hughes, D. M. (1974). An investigation into the possible use of implanted fetal tissue in the repair of cardiac infarcts. Ph.D. University of London
13. Moscona, A. O. A., Trowell, O. A. and Willmer, E. N. (1965). *Methods: Cell and Tissues in Culture. Methods: Biology and Physiology*. Vol. 1, p. 19. (London and New York: Academic Press)
14. Cooper, T., Gilbert, J. W., Bloodwell, R. D. and Crout, J. R. (1961). Chronic extrinsic cardiac denervation by regional neural ablation. *Circ. Res.*, **9,** 275
15. Wildenthal, K., Harrison, D. R., Templeton, G. H. and Reardon, W. C. (1973). Method for measuring the contractions of small hearts in organ culture. *Cardiovasc. Res.*, **7,** 139
16. Rehahn, M. and Longmore, D. B. (1976). The intrinsic life span of cells. Unpublished data
17. Sidman, R. L. (1956). The direct effect of insulin on organ culture of brown fat. *Anatom. Rec.*, **124,** 723
18. Wildenthal, K. (1969). The influence of insulin in promoting the survival and beating of intact foetal mouse hearts in organ culture. *J. Physiol.*, **207,** 33
19. Ciocco, A. (1938). *Hum. Biol.*, **10,** 36
20. Registrar General's Statistical Review of England and Wales, 1972

21. Nathan, A. W., Dandona, P., Williams, S., Smith, M. and Longmore, D. B. (1980). Cardiac effects of thyroid stimulating immunoglobulins. (Submitted for publication)
22. Hassan, M. M. and Longmore, D. B. (1973). Effects of contraceptive pill constituents on foetal mouse hearts. *Nature*, **244**, No. 5415, 349
23. Armstrong, S. R. and Longmore, D. B. (1973). The effects of cardioactive drugs on the performance of cultured fetal hearts. *Nature*, **243**, No. 5406, 350
24. Longmore, D. B., Bennett, J. G., Gueirrara, D., Smith, M., Bunting, S., Moncada, S., Reed, P., Read, N. and Vane, J. R. (1979). Prostacyclin: a solution to some problems of extracorporeal circulation. *Lancet*, **1**, No. 8124, 1002
25. Bull, H. B. and Neurath, H. (1937). The denaturation and hydration of proteins. II. Surface denaturation of egg albumen. *J. Biol. Chem.*, **118**, 163
26. Neurath, H., Greenstein, J. P., Putnam, F. W. and Erickson, J. O., (1944). The chemistry of protein denaturation. *Chem. Rev.*, **34**, 157
27. Solis, R. T., Kennedy, P. S., Beall, A. C., Noon, G. P. and DeBakey, M. E. (1975). Cardiotomy bypass: microembolisation and platelet aggregation. *Circulation*, **52**, 103
28. Solis, R. T., Noon, G. P., Beall, A. C. and DeBakey, M. E. (1974). Particulate microembolism during cardiac operation. *Ann. Thorac. Surg.*, **17**, 332

29
Long term extracorporeal membrane oxygenation (ECMO)

R. WYATT

Credit for the concept of an artificial lung belongs to Robert Hooke (1635–1703) who in 1667, at the conclusion of a paper on lung function read to the Royal Society, wrote: 'I propose to expose the blood of an animal to fresh air in a vessel, and return the blood, to see if this will not suffice for the life of the animal . . . and determine what benefit this may be to mankinde'. It is not known whether or not this experiment was actually performed but we now know that the direct blood–gas interface of such a system would have been the limiting factor, the benefits of artificial oxygenation being outweighed after a few hours by blood damage and by gaseous microembolism.

Thus while surgical operations involving bypass of the heart and lungs were rendered feasible by disc, screen and bubble oxygenators, life support systems capable of running more than a few hours were impractical until the introduction of a more physiological means of artificial blood–gas exchange, namely the membrane oxygenator. As Gallietti[1] has pointed out, this technological advance was not brought about in response to medical demand, but as a 'spin-off' from the semiconductor industry's requirements for large quantities of ultra-thin, pinhole free sheets of various kinds of plastic which had been subjected to stringent quality control.

Given a suitable membrane (silica-filler-free silicone and, latterly, the polyurethanes, have been amongst the most biocompatible) two aspects have predominantly occupied the minds of manufacturers: firstly, safety and ease of use; in these respects the Lande–Edwards device, the first commercially available in the UK, was a failure, despite the technical brilliance and detail of the design. Secondly, one must consider the CO_2-eliminating properties of a given membrane as well as the oxygen transfer capability. The former is limited by the trans-membrane gradient, while the latter is limited by the amount of blood-path mixing. As a consequence, the current generation of membrane oxygenators requires the use of methods to generate secondary blood-phase mixing which are necessarily associated with a high resistance, such as the 'shim' required with the TMO, or the spiral coil used by the Kolobow oxygenator.

The high resistance of these currently available devices has had an important sequel: either the oxygenator acts as a depulsator; or twin, powerful, pumps of the roller type must be employed. Such pumps generate considerable amounts of plastic debris[2], whilst, as we have shown, non-rubbing pumps of the centrifugal type are unable to cope with relatively small changes in input resistance (Figure 1). One awaits eagerly the introduction of low-resistance devices utilizing, perhaps, pulsatile flow to generate mixing at low resistance[3].

Encouraged by the results obtained during surgical bypass with membrane oxygenators – better immunocompetence, psychoneurological function,

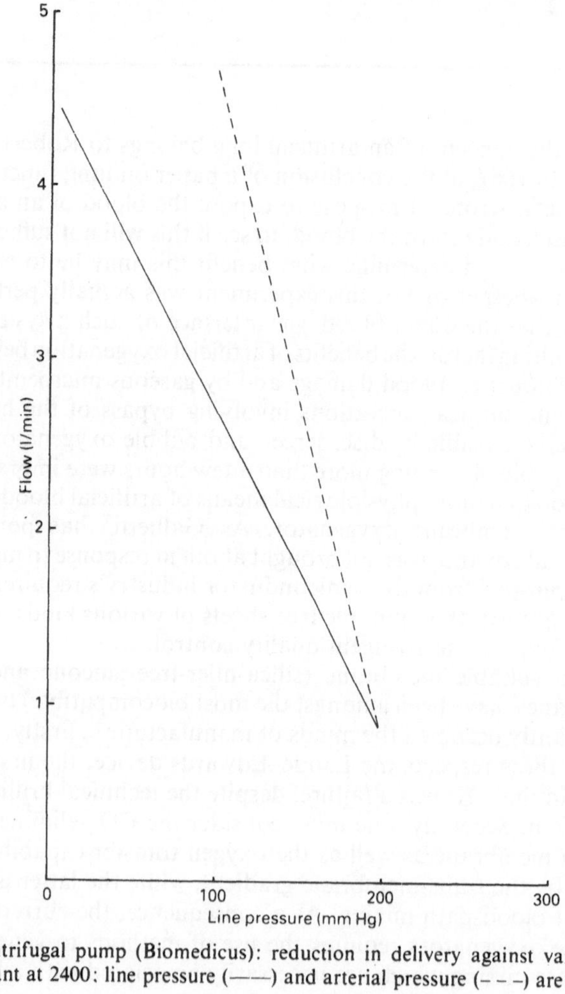

Figure 1 Centrifugal pump (Biomedicus): reduction in delivery against variable resistance (rpm = constant at 2400: line pressure (——) and arterial pressure (- - -) are variable

haematological and circulatory response being amongst the improvements noted – our unit in 1976 contemplated the extension of the use of membrane oxygenators from the operating theatre to the intensive care unit (where we estimated from past records that approximately one patient per million population per annum would present with a potentially reversible pulmonary failure with hypoxia not responding to maximal intensive therapy). Being a regional cardiothoracic unit, this would bring us 10–20 patients per annum. At that time our facilities for performing procedures of proven value would have been severely reduced by this case-load so we opted initially for a 'have pump, will travel' service. Latterly we obtained more facilities, and had also learnt that the extracorporeal gas exchange system was but a part of the highly intensive therapy required, and which units other than ours were in practical terms unable to provide. Also, we found after-hours visits to units up to 70 miles away to be exhausting to personnel and prone to cause blinkering of the mind.

Our criteria for acceptance for extracorporeal membrane oxygenation (ECMO) were:

(1) A potentially reversible acute pulmonary failure not responding to optimal, maximum, conventional intensive therapy.

(2) Arterial PO_2 less than 6.6 kPa (50 mmHg) on ventilator therapy plus PEEP, either:
   (a) on 100% inspired oxygen (leading to immediate acceptance)
   (b) on 60% oxygen for 24 h.

   In practise only one patient referred had a PaO_2 greater than 5 kPa at the time of institution of ECMO.

   During our clinical series, we felt obliged to adopt more stringent criteria in the light of our experiences:

(3) (a) Pathology confined to the lungs.
   (b) Patients under 50 years of age.
   (c) Viral infections excluded (usually excluded under 2(a) anyway).

Our choice of circuitry was dictated by two major considerations:

(1) The circuit should be simple, safe, and easy to connect via peripheral access cannulae.

(2) The patients' oxygen debt would be relatively small compared to the total available oxygen (otherwise death would have occurred too rapidly for ECMO to be contemplated).

Thus, we chose the veno-venous route, hoping to obtain the advantages of low-pressure connections, partial autoregulation of the patient–circuit complex by the patient's own capacitance system, and a wider choice of peripheral access sites with less risk of doing harm. By contrast, choice of veno-arterial bypass would, we felt, expose the patient to the hazards of systemic embolism, reduce pulmonary blood flow, increase left ventricular after-load and, the oxygenated return being from the periphery, it would not be distributed in a physiological manner to priority organs such as the brain by the left heart (see Table 1). However, a veno-venous bypass is not without deficiencies:

Table 1 Comparison of veno-venous and veno-atrial bypass systems

VENO-VENOUS BYPASS

Advantages

Autoregulation by patient's capacitance.
Low-pressure system.
Physiological distribution of blood by left heart.
More sites available, ? percutaneous?

Disadvantages

Ultimately limited by RA mixing.
No direct cardiac assistance.
Noxious effects, if any, go direct to PA.

VENO-ARTERIAL BYPASS

Advantages

RV unloading

Disadvantages

Retrograde perfusion.
Poor carotid and coronary oxygenation.
Vascular damage potential.
Systemic embolism hazard.
High-pressure system.

ultimately artificial oxygenating ability is limited by right atrial mixing, adequate pumping ability of the right ventricle is essential to success, and any noxious effects of the bypass arrive, via the pulmonary artery, at the critical organ, namely the lung itself. Amongst the worrying noxious effects are the particles generated by double roller-pumps – of the order of 10^6 particles >5 μm in size per hour (see Figure 1). A centrifugal pump such as the 'Biomedicus', with no rubbing surfaces, generates no particles but its output falls unacceptably when confronted with the aforementioned high resistance of present oxygenators (see Figure 1). The plastic particles are potentially harmful in that being non-deformable they may not pass a capillary bed even though of comparable size to an erythrocyte (and a proportion is larger). They may also, not being truly inert, act as foci for micro-aggregate formation or for tissue reaction[2].

From March 1976 to October 1978 we performed 10 veno-venous ECMOs, originally transferring the pump-oxygenator device to the referring unit; for the last two cases transferring the patient to our own centre. There were no long-term survivors, five patients dying while on the bypass and five dying later. The results are summarized in Tables 2 and 3.

Of the deaths during ECMO, two are attributable to our failure to appreciate the huge cardiac output a young trauma victim can generate in response to hypoxia. Prior to our acquiring the ability to measure cardiac output directly in these cases, we assumed that our 2–3 l bypass flow was a major contribution. This assumption was confounded when, with the introduction of the thermodilution technique, we were able to demonstrate outputs of 10–15 l/min (with a veno-venous bypass, steal from the right atrium might be expected to produce inaccuracies in measurement, but comparison between right atrial and right ventricular injection sites shows that, in our hands at least, the difference is insufficient to influence clinical management). Use of a small heat-exchanger to induce normal or mildly hypothermic (35 °C) core temperature enabled us indirectly to reduce cardiac output to within normal range. Heavy sedation, usually with morphine $1\,mg\,kg^{-1}\,h^{-1}$, was used.

One case – a 54-year-old obese barmaid, with psittacotic pneumonia – died due to migration of the return cannula into a pelvic vein; this case was treated 75 miles away from our unit. Two other patients died during ECMO, both from an inability of the heart to continue pumping; certainly in one case, and probably in the other, due to a viral myocarditis.

Five of the ten patients were successfully weaned off ECMO in the sense that, at the least, adequate oxygenation could be maintained simply by artificial ventilation and less than 50% inspired oxygen; these deaths are more disturbing and, one hopes, of more value for the analyst. In three of these cases it became clear that cerebral death, probably due to hypoxia, had occurred prior to ECMO and supportive therapy was withdrawn. In one case an intracerebral haematoma was found at autopsy, but although it

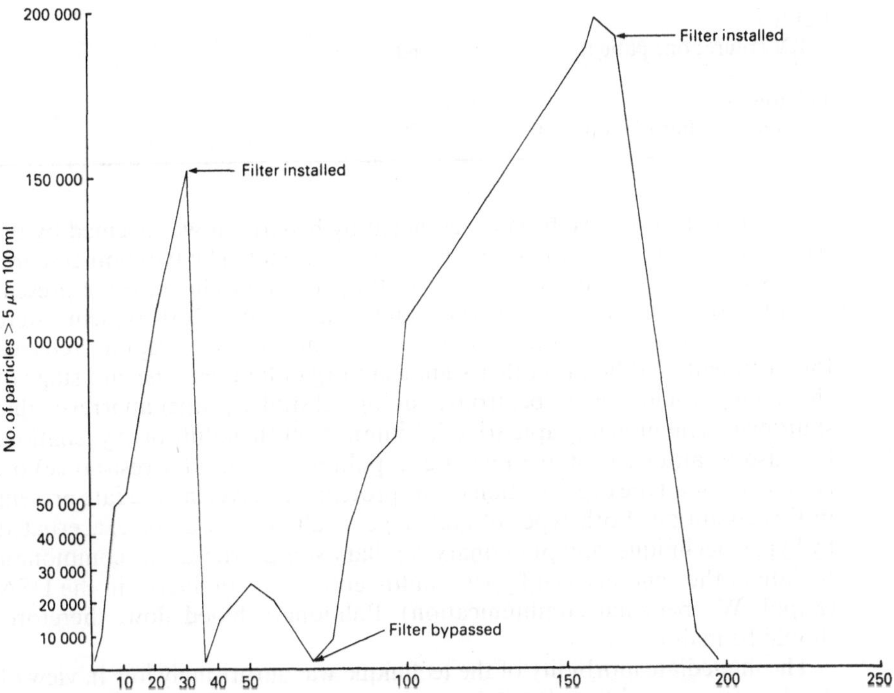

Figure 2 Particle generation in dummy circuit after preliminary cleaning up with experimental 3 μm filter (Pall)

Table 2 Deaths on veno-venous ECMO

Cause	*Time on ECMO* (h)
Inadequate oxygenation	
high-output VECMO; two patients	48
	79
badly placed return cannula; one patient	54
Circulatory failure	
viral myocarditis; one patient	120
V.F. × 3 pre-ECMO	2

Table 3 Deaths after veno-venous ECMO

Cause	*Time on ECMO* (h)	*Survival time after ECMO* (days)
Cerebral		
late referral; two patients	70	10
	125	4
head injury; one patient	52	3
Cardiac		
RV failure; one patient	60	2
Pulmonary		
pulmonary fibrosis; one patient	130	26

could theoretically have been exacerbated by heparin, it was deemed by the pathologist to have arisen at the time of the accident. The two non-cerebral deaths were chronologically the last in the series and illustrate the present dilemma with the mode of therapy under discussion. Both patients were victims of a post-traumatic, 'shock lung' syndrome, were rapidly referred for treatment, and had no other significant organ failures. The end-stage of shock lung would seem to be, from histological studies, either an irreversible shutdown of pulmonary capillaries (leading not only to failure of oxygenation, but also to an unacceptable increase in pulmonary vascular resistance) or, later, a fibrotic-type organization of the protein-rich alveolar exudate present in this condition. Both types of end-stage result could well be exacerbated by bypass technique, and pulmonary capillary shutdown was the commonest finding in the veno-arterial bypass multi-centre trial conducted in the USA (Zapol, W., personal communication). Pulmonary blood flow, therefore, should be maintained.

The immediate morbidity of the technique was surprisingly low in view of its invasiveness and the often adverse circumstances under which it was set up; no patients suffered coagulation or anticoagulation problems, thanks to the availability of bedside tests based on activated clotting time (Bart,

'Haemochron'). No platelet transfusions were required. Two patients displayed a curious digital ischaemia unresponsive to vasodilator drugs but which cleared dramatically after Dextran 70 infusion. This substance was subsequently added to the regime as a routine and the problem did not reoccur. While running at low flow, during weaning, fibrin deposition did occur in one case; as with all extracorporeal devices, the ability to get away with light anticoagulation does depend upon a high flow. All staff concerned found the system surprisingly simple and trouble-free.

In conclusion, it is eminently possible to maintain life during acute pulmonary failure using ECMO, given prompt referral; under these circumstances one is now able to offer a simple, morbidity-free system in terms of bleeding, clotting, plumbing and ancillary expertise. However, the time bought by ECMO is not being used to achieve recovery of the original condition, and indeed this may not be possible, given the natural history of 'shock lung'. The possibility also exists that an ECMO system such as we have used could exacerbate both pulmonary microcirculatory shutdown and the fibrotic-type syndrome. One cannot avoid analogies with other well-recognized forms of extra-corporeal technology:

(a) Intra-aortic balloon: if instituted early, using good predictive criteria, and perioperatively, prior to 2° organ failures, results are very good.
(b) Haemodialysis: organ failure may be permanent, requiring permanent replacement.

The few currently reported successes, in Europe, of ECMO techniques are related to perioperative cases of right ventricular failure, where a veno-arterial bypass has been used[5]. This is analogous to the current status of left heart assist systems.

In terms of ECMO therapy for severe acute pulmonary failure, we should look for:

(a) A prognostic index.
(b) Rapid referral and transport.
(c) Low-resistance oxygenators.
(d) Non-particle-generating pumps.
(e) Percutaneous access sites.
(f) Permanent replacement, by transplant or prosthesis, in the event of irreversible failure.

Meanwhile, parallel developments have taken place in conventional therapy, particularly the use of wedge pressure monitoring, early administration of high-dose steroid, and the use of albumen to maintain plasma oncotic pressure, such that, in our hands, the incidence of cases where ECMO would be considered is currently falling. However, we have established the basis of a support system pending permanent replacement.

The author believes that the problems of transplantation, namely donor availability and immunosuppression, are such that in the foreseeable future bioprostheses will be the more practical and economical solution.

References

1. Gallietti, P. M. (1977). Membrane oxygenation – An overview. In *Artificial Organs*. 1st Ed., p. 11. (London: Macmillan)
2. Wyatt, R. and Arnold, A. (1979). *The Perfusionist*, Vol. 16
3. Bellhouse, B. J. (1977). A high performance membrane lung. In *Artificial Organs*. 1st Ed., p. 61. (London: Macmillan)
4. Weiss, M., Bruniaux, J., Daniel, J. P., Nicolas, F., Safar, D., Planche, C., Hvass, U. and Binet, J. P. (1979). Successful treatment of uncontrollable post operative cardiac failure in young children by extracorporeal membrane oxygenation. *Proc. ESAO*, **VI,** 227

30
Why pulsatile flow during cardiopulmonary bypass?

K. M. TAYLOR

The use of pulsatile perfusion during cardiopulmonary bypass is not a new concept. Early studies by Parsons and by McMaster[1,2] had indicated the physiological importance of arterial pulsatility many years before the introduction of clinical perfusion. Some pioneer workers in the field of perfusion attempted to develop pulsatile bypass pumps, but were hampered by inadequate technology and fears of increased haemolysis with pulsatile perfusion. Over the past two decades, non-pulsatile perfusion has become accepted as the conventional, if fundamentally unphysiological, mode of total-body perfusion during open heart surgical procedures.

Interest in the clinical applicability of pulsatile perfusion has recently been reawakened, both as a result of the development of reliable, commercially available pump systems, and also in view of the results of recent clinical research, indicating the clear physiological superiority of pulsatile perfusion, and the hitherto largely unrecognized pathological effects of non-pulsatile perfusion.

In advocating the adoption of pulsatile cardiopulmonary bypass as the routine method of perfusion in cardiac surgical practice, the following aspects will be considered:

(1) The physiological concept of pulsatile arterial flow.
(2) Metabolic and haemodynamic superiority of pulsatile perfusion.
(3) Safety and practicability of pulsatile perfusion in clinical practice.

THE PHYSIOLOGICAL CONCEPT OF PULSATILE ARTERIAL FLOW

The precise mechanism by which pulsatility exerts its physiological effects has not yet been established. There are, however, at least three principal theories:

The concept of 'energy equivalent pressure'

This theoretical advantage of pulsatile over non-pulsatile flow was proposed by Shepard *et al.*, in 1966[3]. He suggested that the production of blood flow depends not on a pressure gradient, but on an energy gradient. He defined an 'energy equivalent pressure', to represent the energy content within pulsatile and non-pulsatile flow. He has demonstrated, in dogs, that the 'energy equivalent pressure' in the systemic circulation is up to 2.3 times the mean pressure for a pulsatile arterial wave-form. His theory gains some support from the finding that a pulsatile arterial wave dissipates significantly more utilizable energy to the tissues than does a non-pulsatile wave of the same mean pressure[4]. It has been postulated that this increased energy content of pulsatile flow may oscillate cell boundary layers with resultant improved diffusion characteristics and an increase in available energy for cell metabolism in general[5,6]. Shepard's theory predicts higher mean flow rates for pulsatile flow compared with non-pulsatile flow at equal perfusion pressures, and while this is the case in clinical practice[7,8] the significant reduction in peripheral vascular resistance associated with pulsatile perfusion[6,7,9] could be an alternative explanation.

Effects of pulsatility on the microcirculation

There is little doubt that non-pulsatile perfusion is associated with a reduction in the flow of lymph and interstitial fluid[1,2] and of capillary blood flow[10]. It has been suggested by Burton[11] that as the arterial pressure begins to fall at the end of systole, blood flow in the microcirculation will continue until the 'critical closing pressure' of the precapillary arterioles is reached, when capillary perfusion ceases. Burton suggests that the peak of pulsatile systolic pressure will ensure an effectively greater period of microcirculatory 'patency' for equivalent levels of mean arterial pressure. This theory gains support from the observations of Takeda[12] who demonstrated the presence of microcirculatory shunting and widespread capillary collapse during non-pulsatile perfusion. Matsumoto *et al.*[10] reported widespread capillary stasis and cell sludging during non-pulsatile flow, with prevention of these abnormalities when pulsatility was restored. Similar effects have recently been demonstrated in cerebral capillary beds by De Paepe *et al.*[13].

Neuro-endocrine reflex mechanisms triggered by baroreceptor discharge

It is well known that baroreceptors do respond to both static and pulsatile aspects of the arterial pressure wave[14–18]. The change from pulsatile to non-pulsatile perfusion has been shown to result in a marked increase in the discharge frequency of carotid sinus baroreceptors[19–23].

This central baroreceptor stimulus may possibly initiate reflex neuro-endocrine responses which remain operative throughout the period of non-pulsatile perfusion. Previous authors have suggested that this baroreceptor mechanism may induce reflex vasoconstriction in the peripheral circulation, either by direct neural reflexes or by stimulating the release of humoral vasoconstrictive substances (e.g. angiotensin or catecholamines) by neuro-humoral release mechanisms[24,25].

METABOLIC AND HAEMODYNAMIC SUPERIORITY OF PULSATILE PERFUSION

Metabolic effects of pulsatile perfusion

It is increasingly recognized that non-pulsatile perfusion is associated with a progressive disturbance in the basic processes of cell metabolism. Many authors have reported progressive reduction in cellular oxygen consumption[6,26,27], and increase in lactic acidosis[26,28]. Reduced cellular uptake of glucose has also been demonstrated[29]. These disturbances in cellular metabolism may simply reflect a reduction in capillary perfusion from the capillary closure effect of non-pulsatile perfusion previously described[11].

There are many comparative studies of oxygen consumption and lactic acid build-up during pulsatile and non-pulsatile perfusion. The overwhelming weight of evidence from these studies indicates that pulsatile perfusion is associated with significantly higher levels of oxygen consumption[6,7,30,31], and lower levels of lactic acidosis[7,28,30,31]. Though some studies[30,32] have been unable to demonstrate significant differences at high flow rates (above 100 ml kg^{-1} min^{-1}, most authors indicate that the metabolic superiority of pulsatile perfusion is evident whatever the flow rate.

The results of these studies of cellular metabolism agree with similar studies of organ metabolism during non-pulsatile perfusion.

Kidney function

Several authors have described defects in renal excretory function during non-pulsatile perfusion[24,33,34]. Many *et al.*[24,34,35] in a comprehensive programme of studies into renal function, have demonstrated a reduction in tubular sodium excretion, and a rise in renal secretion of renin, during non-pulsatile perfusion[36]. Other studies have shown that renin release is stimulated by a decrease in arterial pulse pressure, rather than by reduced mean arterial pressure[25,37]. Clinical studies by Taylor *et al.*[38] and Favre *et al.*[39] have also indicated increased production of the vasoconstrictive substance angiotensin II, during non-pulsatile perfusion.

In comparative studies, preservation of renal cortical blood flow[32,40], renal venous return[41], and renal tubular histology[42] has been reported with pulsatile perfusion. Pulsatile perfusion has also been shown to produce significantly lower plasma levels of angiotensin II[43] and renin[44] compared with the markedly elevated levels found during non-pulsatile perfusion.

The value of the pulse in renal physiology has also been attested to by the widespread adoption of pulsatile perfusion in renal homograft preservation[40,45].

Brain function

Diffuse cerebral cellular changes have been described after non-pulsatile perfusion by Sanderson and Wright[5]. These changes were not seen after pulsatile perfusion. Significant constriction in cerebral capillaries has also been reported during non-pulsatile perfusion[10,13].

The author and his colleagues have studied the pituitary–adrenal stress response during pulsatile and non-pulsatile perfusion. During non-pulsatile perfusion, the pituitary fails to respond to the trophic stimulus of thyrotrophin-releasing-hormone (TRH), in contrast to the normal response seen during major non-bypass surgery[46]. Anterior pituitary release of ACTH falls to sub-stress levels during perfusion[47], and adrenal secretion of cortisol is reduced[48]. Within the first hour after the end of the non-pulsatile perfusion, the pituitary TRH response returns to normal, ACTH secretion is restored, and adrenal secretion of cortisol resumes.

This syndrome of pituitary–adrenal axis 'switch-off' during the period of non-pulsatile perfusion is prevented by the use of pulsatile perfusion[49–51]. Figure 1 illustrates the difference in TRH response patterns during pulsatile and non-pulsatile perfusions. In Figure 2, the differences in cortisol secretion are seen.

Cerebral dysfunction is frequently encountered following open heart surgery. It may be that the brain is more susceptible to the unphysiological characteristics of non-pulsatile perfusion that was thought previously. Recent

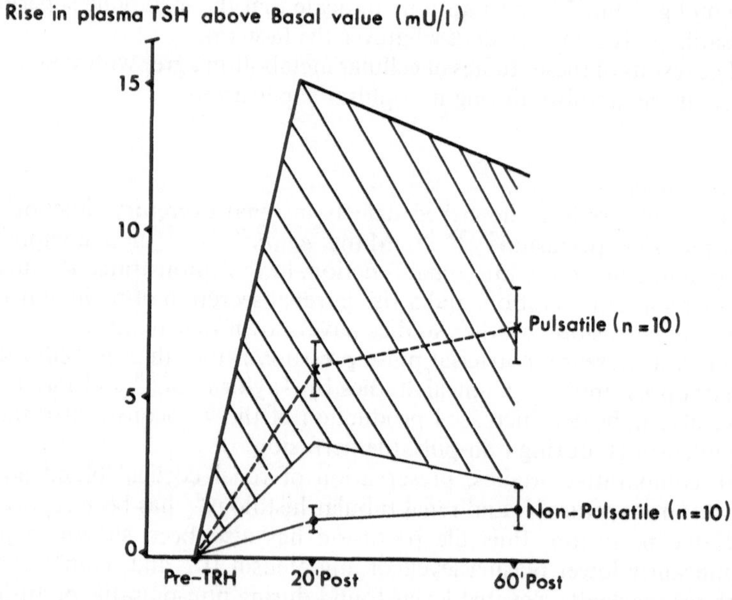

Figure 1 Anterior pituitary response to TRH injection during pulsatile and non-pulsatile perfusion (means ± SEM). Normal response range shown in cross-hatched area. *Key:* Pre-TRH = plasma TSH before TRH injection: 20′ Post = plasma TSH 20 min after TRH injection: 60′ Post = plasma TSH 60 min after TRH injection

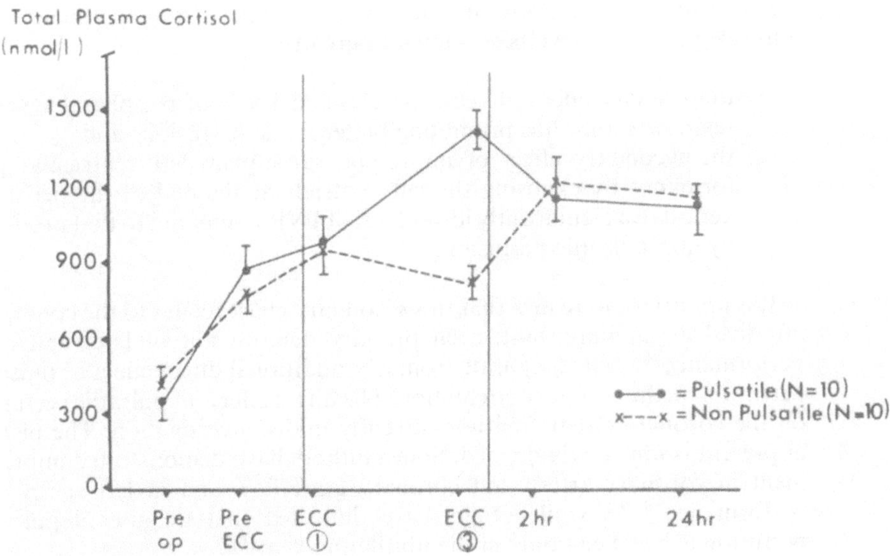

Figure 2 Plasma cortisol levels (corrected for dilution) in 10 patients perfused with pulsatile flow and 10 patients perfused with non-pulsatile flow. There were no significant differences in mean pump flow and mean perfusion pressure between the groups. *Key:* ECC1 = 2 min after start of perfusion: ECC3 = 2 min before end of perfusion

development of a study model for brain cell damage based on iso-enzyme release into the cerebrospinal fluid has demonstrated very high levels of isoenzyme release during non-pulsatile perfusion[52].

Pancreatic function

Increased plasma amylase levels have been reported after non-pulsatile perfusion[53] and Feiner has reported a 16% incidence of ischaemic pancreatitis in patients dying after open heart surgery[54]. Recent studies have demonstrated that pulsatile perfusion is associated with significantly lower levels of serum amylase [55] and a significantly lower incidence of elevated amylase creatinine clearance ratio (ACCR)[56]. The possibility that the frequent but relatively ignored gastrointestinal upsets in the early postoperative period may reflect mild pancreatic damage is worthy of further detailed investigation.

Haemodynamic effects of pulsatile perfusion

There is general agreement among previous investigators that non-pulsatile perfusion is associated with an increase in peripheral vascular resistance (PVR) during the period of perfusion, and that pulsatile perfusion is accompanied by significantly lower PVR levels[7,28,31,57].

The relatively recent emphasis on the potentially hazardous haemodynamic consequences of increased vascular resistance has resulted in numerous investigations into the patterns of change in PVR, possible aetiological mechanisms, and appropriate therapy. The haemodynamic benefits of pulsatile perfusion have been shown to involve:

(1) the primary effect of reducing elevated levels of peripheral vascular resistance and thus promoting better tissue perfusion; and
(2) the secondary effect of improving subsequent left ventricular performance by exposing the left ventricle at the end of the perfusion period to a significantly lower level of PVR compared to that produced by non-pulsatile perfusion.

It is important to realize that this secondary effect relates to the concept of afterload as an important, even primary determinant of left ventricular performance[58], and is separate from any additional direct effect of pulsatile perfusion on the coronary circulation. The direct effects of pulsatile perfusion on the coronary circulation are currently under investigation. The picture at present is not clearly defined. Some authors have demonstrated improvement in coronary artery and coronary graft flow and in left ventricular performance[59-61], while others have indicated that the use of pulsatile perfusion is beneficial only in the fibrillating heart[62].

It is of crucial importance in the design and interpretation of such studies concerned with the effects of perfusion on the heart and coronary circulation, that these two separate but interrelating mechanisms be identified and considered – the effect of the peripheral resistance on left ventricular performance, and the direct effect of the perfusion itself on the coronary circulation.

In confining ourselves at present to the effects on the peripheral circulation the studies of Estafanous *et al.* in Cleveland have drawn attention to the post-bypass hypertension–vasoconstriction phenomenon[63,64]. Other investigators have confirmed that the elevation in PVR levels during non-pulsatile perfusion persists and may increase further in the early post-operative period[7,65,66]. The use of vasodilator techniques, such as epidural anaesthesia[66], or drug therapy with sodium nitroprusside[67,68] has been shown to produce a significant improvement in cardiac performance as the PVR falls.

The use of pulsatile perfusion during cardiopulmonary bypass offers the possibility of prevention or minimizing the elevation in PVR during perfusion. In Figure 3, the pattern of change in PVR is shown for 10 dogs submitted to a 60 min period of non-pulsatile perfusion. The progressive rise in PVR is clearly seen. In Figure 4, using an identical protocol but substituting pulsatile flow at the same mean arterial pressure, there is no rise in PVR during the period of perfusion. The dogs perfused with pulsatile flow also show a significantly higher cardiac index value in the immediate post-bypass period (Figure 5).

The results of these experimental studies have been confirmed in parallel clinical studies, indicating that pulsatile perfusion maintains a significantly lower level of PVR during perfusion and in the immediate post-perfusion period[43,44] and that this reduced vascular resistance level is associated with improved left ventricular performance[69].

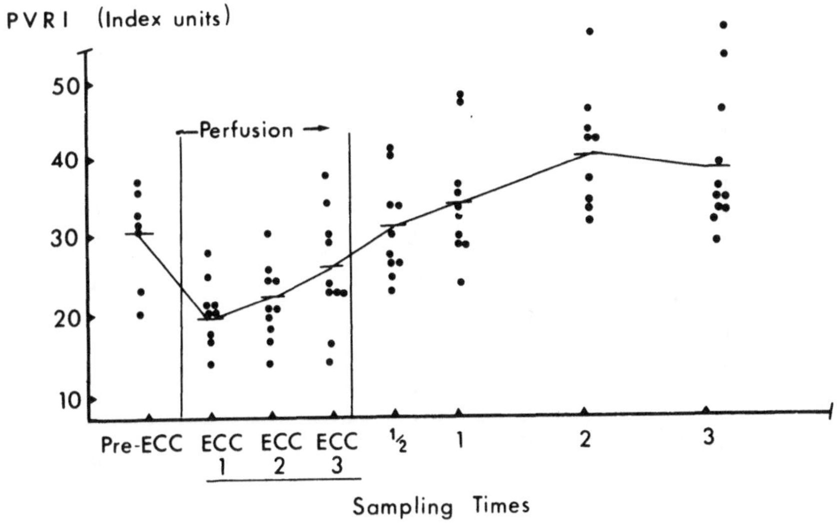

Figure 3 Peripheral vascular resistance index (PVRI) in 10 dogs submitted to 60 min non-pulsatile perfusion at a mean perfusion pressure = 50 mmHg. *Key:* ECC1, 2, 3 = start, mid-point, end of perfusion period

These studies clearly suggest a significant haemodynamic superiority with pulsatile perfusion and this is reflected in an increasing number of clinical reports[44,60,61,70].

The aetiological mechanism by which pulsatile perfusion exerts its haemodynamic effects remains controversial. Baroreceptor reflex mechanisms have been postulated[64], increased catecholamine activity has been suggested[44,65] though several studies have been unable to correlate catecholamine activity with the haemodynamic changes[44,65,71,72].

The author and his colleagues have studied the role of the renin–angiotensin system in the generation of increased levels of PVR during perfusion. Non-pulsatile perfusion is associated with marked elevation of plasma angiotensin II (AII) levels with persistence of these elevated levels in the early postoperative period[38]. A subsequent study has demonstrated a highly significant correlation between the rise in AII levels and the rise in PVR levels during non-pulsatile perfusion[73]. Renin–angiotensin activation during non-pulsatile perfusion has now been demonstrated by several other authors[44,65,74,75].

The use of specific AII inhibitor substances after non-pulsatile perfusion has been shown by Taylor *et al.*[76] and by Roberts *et al.*[77] to be associated with significant reduction in elevated PVR and significant increase in cardiac performance, thus strengthening the thesis that angiotensin II is a major factor in the development of increased PVR during and after non-pulsatile perfusion. Pulsatile perfusion has been shown to be associated with significantly lower levels of renin[44], and of angiotensin II[43] in recent studies.

Whatever the relative importance of the effect of pulsatile perfusion in reducing renin–angiotensin activation, it is clear that pulsatile perfusion

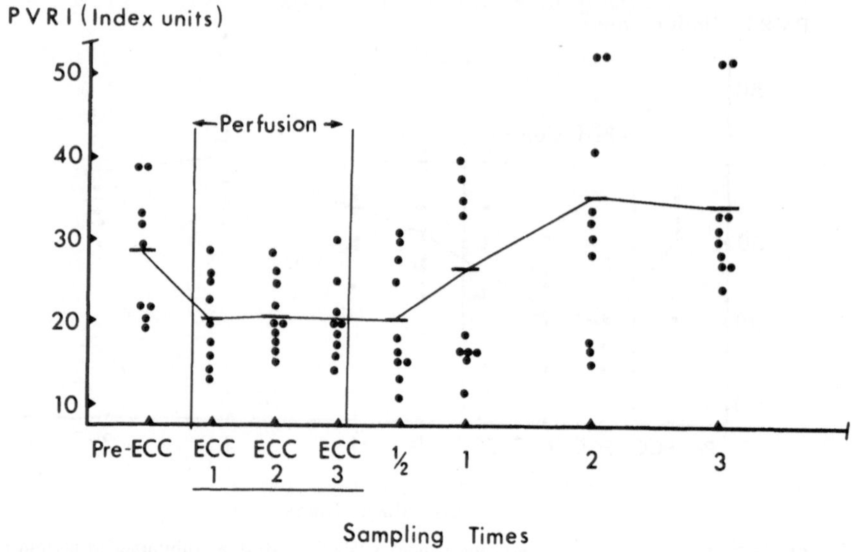

Figure 4 Peripheral vascular resistance index (PVRI) in 10 dogs submitted to 60 min pulsatile perfusion at a mean perfusion pressure = 50 mmHg. *Key:* ECC1, 2, 3 = start, midpoint, end of perfusion period

prevents or significantly reduces the progressive rise in PVR associated with non-pulsatile perfusion. Lower levels of PVR have been shown to be associated with improved tissue perfusion, and with a secondary improvement in left ventricular performance.

SAFETY AND PRACTICABILITY OF PULSATILE PERFUSION IN CLINICAL PRACTICE

Though the weight of evidence in the literature indicates that pulsatile perfusion is physiologically superior to conventional non-pulsatile perfusion, the clinical acceptance of pulsatile perfusion has been hampered by various factors.

(1) The lack of acceptably reliable and simple pulsatile pump systems.
(2) Fears that pulsatile perfusion would significantly increase haemolysis in clinical perfusions.
(3) The paucity of clinical studies describing experience with routine pulsatile perfusion in open heart surgical practice.

In view of the continuous expansion in industrial technology in recent years, one might have anticipated the development of pumps able to deliver adjustable and reliable pulsatile flow. In the past few years, two principal types of pulsatile systems have been used in clinical practice – the first based on balloon inflation chambers (a development of the intra-aortic balloon pump) and the second type based on modified roller pumps. Though newer

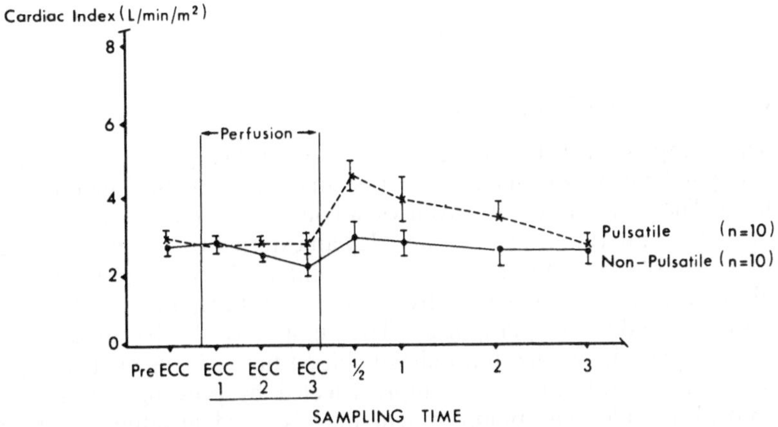

Figure 5 Cardiac index values in 10 pulsatile and 10 non-pulsatile dogs submitted to a 60 min period of perfusion at a mean perfusion pressure = 50 mmHg. *Key:* ECC1, 2, 3 = start, mid-point, end of perfusion period

systems are currently being introduced or reintroduced, the subsequent discussion will focus on those systems which have been fairly widely used in clinical practice.

Clinical experience with the balloon inflation systems (pulsatile assist devices, or PAD) has indicated that they are capable of producing acceptable arterial pulsatility at conventional flow rates in the majority of patients. Studies by Bregman *et al.*[59,60] have reported increased coronary flow, increased urine output during bypass, and the indication that pulsatile perfusion decreases both the incidence of perioperative myocardial infarction and the need for postoperative intra-aortic balloon pumping. Similar results with a PAD system have been reported by Pappas *et al.*[61,78]. There are, however, possible negative factors relevant to this type of pump system. It is to some extent more complex than the modified roller-pump system described below. In addition, its use as a synchronized counterpulsation device in the cardiac recovery period after release of the aortic cross-clamp has been questioned. Steed and co-workers[62] have shown that though pulsatile flow with a PAD (Avco system) increased mean coronary flow in the fibrillating heart, it caused a net decrease in mean coronary flow in the empty beating heart. They attributed this effect to the prominent retrograde flow which accompanied balloon deflation during ventricular systole. Despite this feature, the authors confirmed the beneficial reduction in PVR during pulsatile perfusion. While further studies are required to substantiate this reversal of flow in systole with balloon deflation, there may be no such problem inherent in the modified roller-pump systems which can maintain a small but significant constant forward blood flow through the system.

The author and his colleagues have used a modified roller-pump system (the Cobe–Stockert system) in both experimental studies and clinical practice. Since its introduction to the unit in 1977, around 1000 patients have had pulsatile perfusion during their open heart procedure. This considerable clinical experience has allowed a comprehensive programme of evaluation of this particular system, and of routine clinical pulsatile perfusion in general.

Cobe–Stockert pulsatile system

The pump, seen in Figure 6, is a modified roller pump based on a large 'stepping' motor, which can accelerate and decelerate the low-intertia pump head. The pump motor is driven via a control module (Figure 7) which can provide an internal trigger or can relay an external trigger from the patient's ECG and thereby allow synchronized counterpulsation. The control module allows the operator to set the frequency, amplitude, and duration of pulsation delivered by the pump head. The pump may also be run as a standard roller pump, delivering non-pulsatile blood flow. Change between pulsatile and non-pulsatile modes is simply effected by pressing a button on the control module. The pump system may be used in adult and paediatric practice, using aortic return cannulae from 22F to 10 or 12F gauge, and at conventional flow rates, a satisfactory pulse pressure in excess of 25–30 mmHg has consistently been achieved (Figure 8).

Haemolysis studies

There is no doubt that some early experimental pulsatile systems were associated with a high haemolysis index[7,79,80]. More recently, however, haemolysis studies have suggested that pulsatile perfusion does not increase haemolysis significantly[28,60,81]. Zumbro *et al.*[82] have, however, recently reported a significant increase in haemolysis using the PAD (Datascope system).

Extensive studies of our own patients have consistently shown an acceptably low index of haemolysis with pulsatile perfusion using the Cobe–Stockert system[69,83] and the results of Soyer's group in Rouen are identical (R. Soyer; unpublished data). Table 1 shows haemolysis figures in a study of 80 consecutive pulsatile patients from the Glasgow series.

Table 1 Haematological study in 80 consecutive pulsatile perfusions (mean values)

Pre-bypass free haemoglobin	3.84 mg/100 ml	(range 1.2–4.8)
End-bypass free haemoglobin	43.62 mg/100 ml	(range 18–64)
Δ bypass free haemoglobin	39.78 mg/100 ml	(range 15–63)
24 h postoperative platelet count	122.8×10^3	(range 68–327)
Volume of homologous blood used	2.87 units/case	
Reopened for postoperative bleeding	four cases (5 %)	

Clinical studies of mortality and morbidity using pulsatile and non-pulsatile perfusion

The ultimate argument for the use of pulsatile perfusion in clinical practice is in relation to demonstrable improvement in morbidity and even mortality. The present paucity of such clinical data is reflected in the uncertainty in

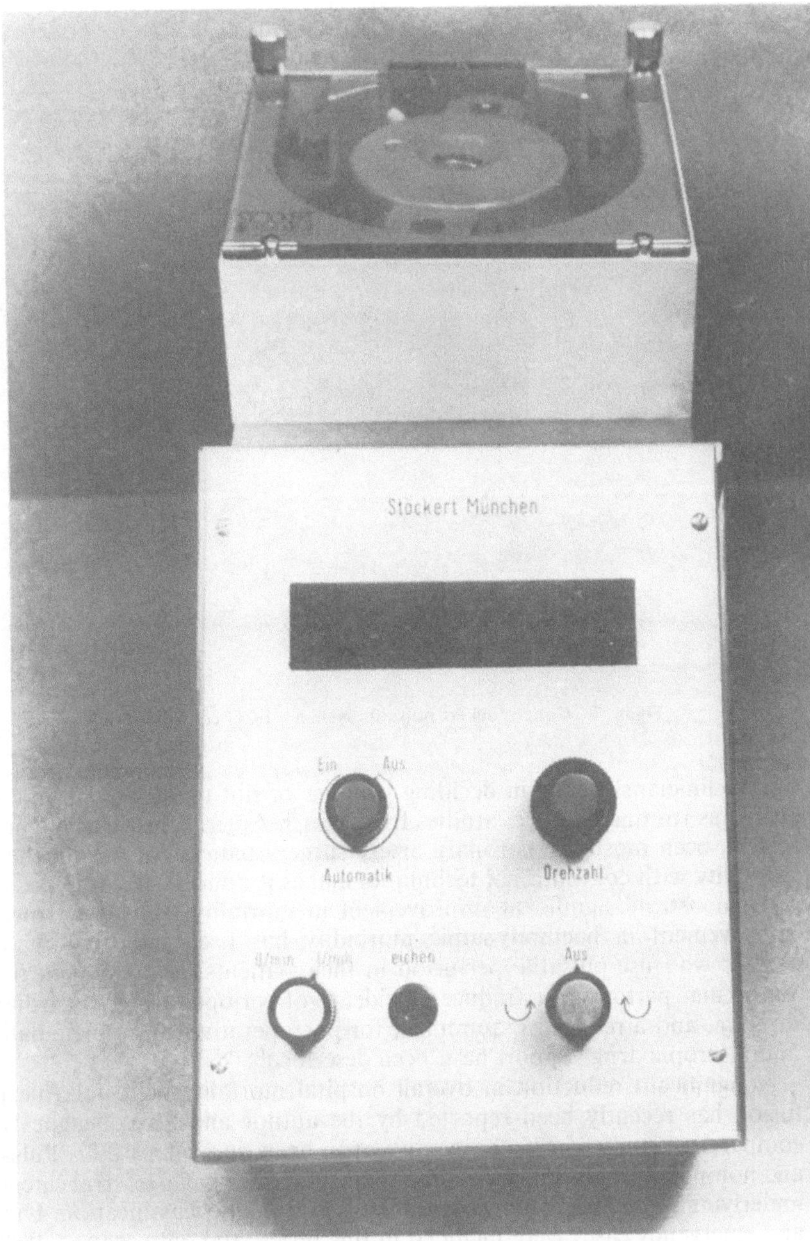

Figure 6 Cobe–Stockert pulsatile system – pump

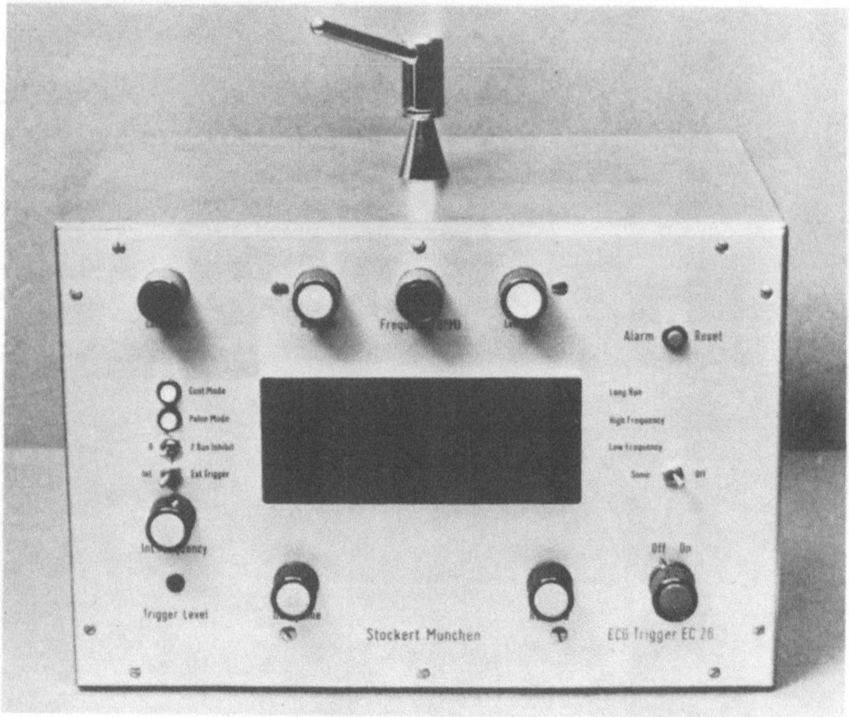

Figure 7 Cobe–stockert pulsatile system – ECG control module

many clinicians' minds in deciding whether or not to adopt pulsatile perfusion as routine practice. Studies from North America have, as one might expect, been mostly in coronary artery surgery patients, in whom the low mortality with conventional techniques makes it difficult, if not impossible, to demonstrate significant improvement in mortality statistics. However, improvement in haemodynamic morbidity has been reported by those centres who use pulsatile perfusion in their patients. Improvement in left ventricular performance, reduced incidence of perioperative myocardial infarction, and a reduced requirement for postoperative intra-aortic balloon and inotropic drug support have been described[60,61,84].

A significant reduction in overall hospital mortality with pulsatile perfusion has recently been reported by the author and his colleagues in a comparative study of 325 consecutive open heart surgical cases[69]. Pulsatile and non-pulsatile groups were comparable in terms of age, referral category, underlying pathology, and preoperative symptomatic classification. Urgent and emergency cases were included in this series, and only around 45 % of the cases in each group were coronary surgery procedures. The mortality figures are shown in Table 2. The total mortality in the pulsatile group (5.3 %) was significantly lower than that in the non-pulsatile group (10.3 %).

Table 2 Mortality figures for pulsatile and non-pulsatile groups

	Pulsatile	*Non-pulsatile*	*p*
Number of cases	150	175	
Total deaths	8 (5.3%)	18 (10.3%)	<0.05
Percentage Mortality			
Elective cases	3.8%	8.4%	<0.05
Urgent cases	18.2%	27.2%	N.S.
Emergency cases	14.3%	22.2%	N.S.

Elective mortality was also significantly lower (3.8% compared to 8.4%), though the smaller numbers of urgent and emergency cases showed a small but not significant difference. In addition to mortality figures, the results were assessed in terms of the incidence of low-output syndromes and the need for circulatory support by intra-aortic balloon pump (IABP) or inotropic infusion. The results are shown in Table 3.

Table 3 Occurrence of low cardiac output syndromes in pulsatile and non-pulsatile groups

	Pulsatile	*Non-pulsatile*	*p*
Total deaths	8	18	<0.05
Intraoperative deaths*	1 (12.5%)	7 (39%)	<0.01
Total low-output deaths*	2 (25%)	11 (61%)	<0.01
Use of IABP†	1 (0.67%)	6 (3.43%)	<0.01
Use of inotrope infusion†	7 (4.67%)	19 (10.86%)	<0.01

* = expressed as percentage of total deaths
† = expressed as percentage of total cases
IABP = intra-aortic balloon pump

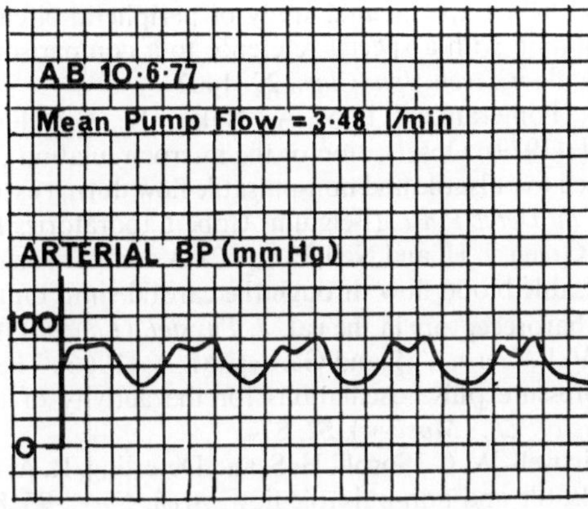

Figure 8 Typical radial artery pressure wave-form of patient on pulsatile bypass using the modified roller-pump system (Cobe–Stockert)

These results are in agreement with the reduced haemodynamic morbidity described by Bregman *et al.*[60,84], particularly in respect of the reduced requirement for IABP and inotropes. These results are also in keeping with the experimental studies concerning the haemodynamic superiority of pulsatile perfusion, previously discussed.

References

1. Parsons, R. J. and McMaster, P. D. (1938). The effect of the pulse upon the formation and flow of lymph. *J. Exp. Med.*, **68**, 353
2. McMaster, P. D. and Parsons, R. J. (1938). The effect of the pulse on the spread of substances through tissues. *J. Exp. Med.*, **68**, 377
3. Shepard, R. B., Simpson, D. C. and Sharp, J. F. (1966). Energy equivalent pressure. *Arch. Surg.*, **93**, 730
4. Wilcox, B. R., Coulter, N. A., Peters, R. M. and Stacey, R. W. (1967). Power dissipation in the systemic and pulmonary vasculature of dogs. *Surgery*, **62**, 25
5. Sanderson J. M., Wright, G. and Sims, F. W. (1972). Brain damage in dogs immediately following pulsatile and non-pulsatile blood flows in extracorporeal circulation. *Thorax*, **27**, 275
6. Shepard, R. B. and Kirklin, J. W. (1969). Relation of pulsatile flow to oxygen consumption and other variables during cardiopulmonary bypass. *J. Thorac. Cardiovasc. Surg.*, **58**, 694
7. Dunn, J., Kirsh, M. M., Harness, J., Carroll, M., Straker, J. and Sloan, H. (1974). Haemodynamic, metabolic, and hematologic effects of pulsatile cardiopulmonary bypass. *J. Thorac. Cardiovasc. Surg.*, **68**, 138
8. Mandelbaum, I. and Burns, W. H. (1965). Pulsatile and non-pulsatile blood flow. *J. Amer. Med. Assoc.*, **191**, 657
9. Taylor, K. M., Morton, J. J., Brown, J. J., Bain, W. H. and Caves, P. K. (1977). Plasma angiotensin II levels during open-heart surgery. *Br. J. Surg.*, **64**, 827
10. Matsumoto, T., Wolferth, C. C. and Perlman, M. H. (1971). Effects of pulsatile and non-pulsatile perfusion upon cerebral and conjunctival microcirculation in dogs. *Am. Surg.*, **37**, 61
11. Burton, A. C. (1954). Relationof structure to function of the tissues of the wall of blood vessels. *Physiol. Rev.*, **34**, 618
12. Takeda, J. (1960). Experimental study of peripheral circulation during extracorporeal circulation with a special reference to a comparison of pulsatile flow with non-pulsatile flow. *Arch. Jpn. Chir.*, **29**, 1407
13. De Paepe, J., Pomerantzeff, P. M. A., Nakiri, K., Armelin, E., Verginelli, G. and Zerbini, E. J. (1979). Observation of the microcirculation of the cerebral cortex of dogs subjected to pulsatile and non-pulsatile flow during extracorporeal circulation. In *A Propos du Debit Pulse*. (Belgium: Cobe Laboratories Inc.)
14. Ead, H. W., Green, J. H. and Neil, E. (1952). A comparison of the effects of pulsatile and non-pulsatile blood flow through the carotid sinus on the reflexogenic activity of the sinus baroreceptors in the cat. *J. Physiol.* (*London*), **118**, 509
15. Filistovich, V. I., Gero, Y. I. and Gerova, M. A. (1966). The significance of the amplitude of pressure pulse oscillations for the activity of the carotid sinus baroreceptors. *Fiziol. Zh.* (*Moscow*), **52**, 874
16. Giron, F., Birtwell, W. C., Soroff, H. S. and Deterling, R. A. (1966). Haemodynamic effects of pulsatile and non-pulsatile flow. *Arch. Surg.*, **93**, 802
17. Koushanpour, E. and McGee, J. P. (1969). Effect of mean pressure on carotid sinus baroreceptor response to pulsatile pressure. *Am. J. Physiol.*, **216**, 599

18. Soroff, H. S., Many, M., Birtwell, W. C., Giron, F. and Deterling, R. A. (1969). Haemodynamic effects of pulsatile and non-pulsatile blood flow. II. Selective depulsation of the aortic arch and brachiocephalic trunk. *Arch. Surg.*, **98,** 321
19. Angell-James, J. E. (1971). The effects of altering mean pressure, pulse pressure and pulse frequency on the impulse activity in baroreceptor fibres from the aortic arch and right subclavian artery in the rabbit. *J. Physiol.*, **214,** 65
20. Angell-James, J. E. and deBurgh Daly, M. (1970). Comparison of the reflex vasomotor responses to separate and combined stimulation of the carotid sinus and aortic arch baroreceptors by pulsatile and non-pulsatile pressure in the dog. *J. Physiol.*, **207,** 257
21. Angell-James, J. E. and de Burgh Daly, M. (1971). Effects of graded pulsatile pressure on the reflex vasomotor responses elicited by changes of mean pressure in the perfused carotid sinus–aortic arch regions of the dog. *J. Physiol.*, **214,** 51
22. Harrison, T. S., Chawla, R. C., Seaton, G. F. and Robinson, B. H. (1970). Carotid sinus origin of adrenergic responses comprising the effectiveness of artificial circulatory support. *Surgery*, **68,** 20
23. Harrison, T. S. and Seaton, G. F. (1973). An analysis of pulse frequency as an adrenergic excitant in pulsatile circulatory support. *Surgery*, **73,** 868
24. Many, M., Soroff, H. S., Birtwell, W. C. and Deterling, R. A. (1968). Effects of bilateral renal artery depulsation on renin levels. *Surg. Forum*, **19,** 387
25. Kohlstaedt, K. G. and Page, I. H. (1940). The liberation of renin by perfusion of kidneys following reduction of pulse pressure. *J. Exp. Med.*, **72,** 201
26. Cheng, H., Kusonoki, T., Bosher, L. H., McElvein, R. B. and Blake, D. A. (1959). A study of oxygen consumption during extracorporeal circulation. *Trans. Am. Soc. Artif. Internal Organs*, **5,** 273
27. Clowes, G. H. A., Neville, W. E., Sabga, G. and Shibota, Y. (1958). The relationship of oxygen consumption, perfusion rates and temperature to the acidosis associated with cardiopulmonary circulatory bypass. *Surgery*, **44,** 220
28. Trinkle, J. K., Helton, N. E. and Bryant, L. R. (1969). Metabolic comparison of a new pulsatile pump and a roller pump for cardiopulmonary bypass. *J. Thorac. Cardiovasc. Surg.*, **58,** 562
29. Brennan, R. W., Patterson, R. H. and Kessler, J. (1972). Cerebral blood flow and metabolism during cardiopulmonary bypass: evidence of microembolic encephalopathy. *Proc. Am. Acad. Neurol.*, (G56), **374**
30. Ogata, T., Ida, Y., Nonayama, A., Takeda, J. and Sasaki, H. (1960). A comparative study on the effectiveness of pulsatile and non-pulsatile blood flow in extracorporeal circulation. *Arch. Jpn. Chir.*, **29,** 59
31. Jacobs, L. A., Klopp, E. H., Seamone, W., Topaz, S. R. and Gott, V. L. (1969). Improved organ function during cardiac bypass with a roller pump modified to deliver pulsatile flow. *J. Thorac. Cardiovasc. Surg.*, **58,** 703
32. Boucher, J. K., Rudy, L. W. Jr. and Edmunds, L. H. Jr. (1974). Organ blood flow during pulsatile cardiopulmonary bypass. *J. Appl. Physiol.*, **36,** 86
33. Judson, W. E. and Rausch, N. H. (1957). The effects of acute reduction of renal artery blood pressure on renal haemodynamics and excretion of electrolytes and water. *J. Lab. Clin. Med.*, **50,** 923
34. Many, M., Giron, F., Birtwell, W. C., Deterling, R. A. and Soroff, H. S. (1969). Effects of depulsation of renal blood flow upon renal function and renin secretion. *Surgery*, **66,** 242
35. Many, M., Soroff, H. S., Birtwell, W. C., Giron, F., Wise, H. and Deterling, R. A. (1967). The physiologic role of pulsatile and non-pulsatile blood flow: II. Effects on renal function. *Arch. Surg.*, **95,** 762
36. Many, M., Soroff, H. S., Birtwell, W. C., Wise, H. M. and Deterling, R. A. (1968).

The physiologic role of pulsatile and non-pulsatile blood flow. III. Effects of unilateral renal artery depulsation. *Arch. Surg.*, **97,** 917
37. Corcoran, A. C. and Page, I. H. (1938). Observations on relation of experimental hypertension to renal clearance and renal ischemia. *Am. J. Physiol.*, **123,** 43
38. Taylor, K. M., Morton, J. J., Brown, J. J., Bain, W. H. and Caves, P. K. (1977). Hypertension and the renin–angiotensin system following open-heart surgery. *J. Thorac. Cardiovasc. Surg.*, **74,** 840
39. Favre, L., Vallotton, M. B. and Muller, A. F. (1976). Relationship between plasma concentrations of angiotensin I, angiotensin II and plasma renin activity during cardiopulmonary bypass in man. *Eur. J. Clin. Invest.*, **4,** 135
40. Belzer, F. O., Ashby, B. S., Huang, J. S. *et al.* (1968). Etiology of rising perfusion pressure in isolated organ perfusion. *Ann. Surg.*, **168,** 382
41. Nakayana, K., Tamiya, T., Yamamoto, K., *et al.* (1963). High amplitude pulsatile pump in extracorporeal circulation with particular reference to hemodynamics. *Surgery*, **54,** 798
42. Dalton, M. L., McCarty, R. T., Woodward, K. E. and Barila, T. G. (1965). The army artificial heart pump. II. Comparison of pulsatile and non-pulsatile flow. *Surgery*, **58,** 840
43. Taylor, K. M., Bain, W. H., Russell, Margaret, Brannan, J. J. and Morton, I. J. (1979). Peripheral vascular resistance and angiotensin II levels during pulsatile and non-pulsatile cardiopulmonary bypass. *Thorax*, **34,** 594
44. Landymore, R. W., Murphy, D. A., Kinley, C. E., Parrott, J. C., Moffitt, E. A., Longley, W. J. and Qirbi, A. A. (1979). Does pulsatile flow influence the incidence of postoperative hypertension? *Ann. Thorac. Surg.*, **28,** 261
45. Agishi, T., Peirce, E. C. III and Kent, B. B. (1969). A comparison of pulsatile and non-pulsatile pumping for ex vivo renal perfusion. *J. Surg. Res.*, **9,** 623
46. Taylor, K. M., Wright, G. S., Bremner, W. F., Bain, W. H., Caves, P. K. and Beastall, G. H. (1978). Anterior pituitary response to thyrotrophin-releasing-hormone during open-heart surgery. *Cardiovasc. Res.*, **12,** 114
47. Taylor, K. M., Jones, J. V., Walker, M. S., Rao, L. G. S. and Gray, C. E. (1975). Plasma levels of cortisol, free cortisol and corticotrophin during cardiopulmonary bypass. *J. Endocrinol.*, **67,** 29
48. Taylor, K. M., Jones, J. V., Walker, M. S., Rao, L. G. S. and Bain, W. H. (1976). The cortisol response during open-heart surgery. *Circulation*, **54,** 20
49. Taylor, K. M., Wright, G. S., Reid, J. S., Bain, W. H., Caves, P. K., Walker, M. S. and Grant, J. K. (1978). Comparative studies of pulsatile and non-pulsatile flow during cardiopulmonary bypass. II. The effects on adrenal secretion of cortisol. *J. Thorac. Cardiovasc. Surg.*, **75,** 574
50. Taylor, K. M., Wright, G. S., Bain, W. H., Caves, P. K. and Beastall, G. H. (1978). Comparative studies of pulsatile and non-pulsatile flow during cardiopulmonary bypass. III. Anterior pituitary response to thryotrophin-releasing-hormone. *J. Thor. Cardiovasc. Surg.*, **75,** 579
51. Taylor, K. M., McIntyre, H. B., Grant, J. K. and Ratcliffe, J. G. (1979). Pituiatry–adrenal response patterns during open-heart surgery. *J. Endocrinol.*, **81,** 127
52. Taylor, K. M., Devlin, B. J., Mittra, S., Gillan, J. G., Brannan, J. J. and McKenna, J. M. (1980). Assessment of cerebral damage during open-heart surgery: a new experimental model. *Scand. J. Thor. Cardiovas. Res.* (In press)
53. Malingrey, L., Buisine, J. P., Bleser, F., Marchal, C. and Benichoux, R. (1975). Low cardiac output associated with increased amylasaemia following open-heart surgery. *Proc. X Congress European Society for Experimental Surgery. Paris*, European Surgical Research
54. Feiner, H. (1976). Pancreatitis after cardiac surgery. *Am. J. Surg.*, **131,** 684

55. Moores, W. Y., Gago, O., Morris, J. D. and Peck, C. C. (1977). Serum and urinary amylase levels following pulsatile and continuous cardiopulmonary bypass. *J. Thorac. Cardiovasc. Surg.*, **74**, 73
56. Murray, W. R., Mittra, S., Mittra, D., Roberts, L. B. and Taylor, K. M. (1980): The amylase creatinine clearance ratio following cardiopulmonary bypass. *Br. J. Surg.* (In press)
57. Wright, G. and Sanderson, J. M. (1972). Brain damage and mortality in dogs following pulsatile and non-pulsatile blood flows in extracorporeal circulation. *Thorax*, **27**, 738
58. Sonnenblick, E. H. and Downing, S. E. (1963). After load as a primary determinant of ventricular performance. *Am. J. Physiol.*, **204**, 604
59. Bregman, D., Bailin, M., Bowman, F. O., Parodi, E. N. Haubert, S. M., Edie, R. N., Spotnize, H. M., Reetsma, K. and Malm, J. R. (1977). A pulsatile assist device (PAD) for use during cardiopulmonary bypass. *Ann. Thorac. Surg.*, **24**, 574
60. Bregman, D., Bowman, F. O., Parodi, E. N., Haubert, S. M., Edie, R. N., Spotnize, H. M., Reetsma, K. and Malm, J. R. (1977). An improved method of myocardial protection with pulsation during cardiopulmonary bypass. *Circulation* (*Suppl.* 11), **56**, 157
61. Maddoux, G., Pappas, G., Jenkins, M., Battock, D., Trow, R., Smith, S. C. and Steele, P. (1976). Effect of pulsatile and non-pulsatile flow during cardiopulmonary bypass on left ventricular ejection fraction early after aortocoronary bypass surgery. *Am. J. Cardiol.*, **37**, 1000
62. Steed, D. L., Follette, D. M., Foglia, R., Maloney, J. V. and Buckborg, G. D. (1978). Effects of pulsatile assistance and non-pulsatile flow on subendocardial perfusion during cardiopulmonary bypass. *Ann. Thorac. Surg.*, **26**, 133
63. Estafanous, F. G., Tarazi, R. C., Viljoen, J. F. and El Tanil, M. Y. (1973). Systemic hypertension following myocardial revascularisation. *Am. Heart. J.*, **85**, 732
64. Estafanous, F. G., Tarazi, R. C., Buckley, S. and Taylor, P. C. (1978). Arterial hypertension in immediate post-operative period after valve replacement. *Br. Heart J.*, **40**, 718
65. Roberts, A. J., Niarchos, A. P., Subramanian, V. A., Abel, R. M., Herman, S. D., Sealey, J. E., Case, D. B., White, R. P., Johnson, G. A., Laragh, J. H. and Gay, W. A. (1977). Systemic hypertension associated with coronary artery bypass surgery. *J. Thorac. Cardiovasc. Surg.*, **74**, 846
66. Hoar, P. F., Hickey, R. F. and Ullyot, D. J. (1976). Systemic hypertension following myocardial revascularisation. *J. Thorac. Cardiovasc. Surg.*, **71**, 859
67. Stinson, E. B., Holloway, E. L., Derby, G. C., Copeland, J. G., Oyer, P. E., Beuhler, D. L. and Griepp, R. B. (1977). Control of myocardial performance early after open-heart operations by vasodilator treatment. *J. Thorac. Cardiovasc. Surg.*, **73**, 523
68. Kaplan, J. A. and Jones, E. L. (1979). Vasodilator therapy during coronary artery surgery. *J. Thorac. Cardiovasc. Surg.*, **77**, 301
69. Taylor, K. M., Bain, W. H., Davidson, K. G., Turner, M. A., Mittra, S. and Russell, Margaret. (1979). A comparative study of pulsatile and non-pulsatile cardiopulmonary bypass in 325 patients. *Proc. Eur. Soc. Artif. Org.* **VI**, 238
70. Moores, W. Y., Hannon, J. P., Crum, J. *et al.* (1977). Coronary flow distribution and dynamics during continuous and pulsatile extracorporeal circulation in the pig. *Ann. Thorac. Surg.*, **24**, 582
71. Turton, M. B. and Matthews, H. R. (1974). Catecholamines and peripheral vasoconstriction after open-heart surgery. *Clin. Chim. Acta*, **50**, 419
72. Hine, I. P., Wood, W. G., Mainwaring-Burton, R. W., Butler, M. J., Irving, M. H. and Booker, B. (1976). The adrenergic response involving cardiopulmonary bypass,

as measured by plasma and urinary catecholamine concentrations. *Br. J. Anaesth.*, **48,** 355

73. Taylor, K. M., Brannan, J. J., Bain, W. H., Caves, P. K. and Morton, J. J. (1979). The role of angiotensin II in the development of peripheral vasoconstriction during cardiopulmonary bypass. *Cardiovasc. Res.*, **8,** 269
74. Favre, L., Vallotton, M. B. and Muller, A. F. (1976). Relationship between plasma concentrations of angiotensin I, angiotensin II and plasma renin activity during cardiopulmonary bypass in man. *Eur. J. Clin. Invest.*, **4,** 135
75. Dudley, H. L. Plasma renin levels during open-heart surgery. (Unpublished data)
76. Taylor, K. M., Casals, J., Morton, J. J., Mittra, S., Brannan, J. J. and Bain, W. H. (1979). The haemodynamic effects of angiotensin blockade after cardiopulmonary bypass. *Br. Heart J.*, **41,** 380
77. Roberts, A. J., Niarchos, A. P., Subramanian, V. A., Abel, R. M., Hoover, E. L., McCabe, J. C., Case, D. B., Laragh, J. H. and Gray, W. A. (1978). Hypertension following coronary artery bypass graft surgery. Comparison of haemodynamic responses to nitroprusside, phentolamine, and converting enzyme inhibitor. *Circulation, Suppl.* 1, **58,** 43
78. Pappas, G. (1974). A simple method of producing pulsatile flow during clinical cardiopulmonary bypass. *Ann. Thorac. Surg.*, **17,** 405
79. Wemple, R. R., Mockros, L. F. and Lewis, F. J. (1969). Pulmonary function during pulsatile and non-pulsatile right heart bypass. *J. Thorac. Cardiovasc. Surg.*, **57,** 190
80. Wesolowski, S. A., Fisher, J. H. and Welch, C. S. (1953). Perfusion of the pulmonary circulation by non-pulsatile flow. *Surgery*, **33,** 370
81. Sanderson, J. M., Morton, P. G., Tolloczko, T., Vennart, T. and Wright, G. (1972). The Morton–Keele pump: a new hydraulically activated pulsatile pump for use in extracorporeal circulation. *Med. Biol. Eng.*,
82. Zumbro, G. L., Shearer, G., Fishback, M. E. and Galloway, R. F. (1978). A prospective evaluation of the pulsatile assist device. *Ann. Thorac. Surg.*, **28,** 269
83. Taylor, K. M., Bain, W. H., Maxted, K. J., Hutton, M. H., McNab, W. Y. and Caves, P. K. (1978). Comparative studies of pulsatile and non-pulsatile flow during cardiopulmonary bypass. I. Pulsatile system employed and its haematological effects. *J. Thorac. Cardiovasc. Surg.*, **75,** 569
84. Bregman, D. in discussion of paper: Zumbro, G. L., Shearer, G., Fishback, M. E. and Galloway, R. F. (1978). A prospective evaluation of the pulsatile assist device. *Ann. Thorac. Surg.*, **28,** 269

SECTION III

Aspects of Postoperative Care (I)

31
Introduction: emphasis of clinical assessment

D. J. WHEATLEY

Competent postoperative care is essential in ensuring the safety of cardiac surgery. Skilled postoperative management can salvage critically ill post-operative patients but can never substitute for accurate surgery performed under optimal conditions. While neglect in the postoperative phase can result in death or complications, it is true that the major determinant of success in cardiac surgery is the conduct of the operation. With effective surgery appropriate to the pathology and skill in minimizing injury to the myocardium and to the viscera of the body, postoperative care becomes a relatively simple matter and in these circumstances is primarily orientated towards patient monitoring in order to detect and correct deviations from the normal postoperative course, thus avoiding complications.

One of the most striking changes that has occurred in the experience of many cardiac surgical units in recent years has been the increased awareness of the hazard of myocardial injury associated with myocardial ischaemia. The use of cardioplegic techniques has resulted in considerably better myo-cardial performance following surgery, with a corresponding reduction in the problems of low cardiac output and the need for inotrope support. This is a clear example of improved operative techniques resulting in considerable reduction in postoperative problems and enhanced patient safety.

It is of interest to review 500 consecutive adult patients undergoing open heart surgery in Glasgow during 1979. This review gives some indication of the importance of postoperative care and its role in ensuring the safety of cardiac surgery today. Forty-five per cent of these patients were operated on for ischaemic heart disease, 51% for valvular heart disease and the remainder for various conditions including cardiac trauma.

MORTALITY

There were 32 hospital deaths in this group, giving an overall mortality rate of 6.4%. It is of interest to note that only seven of the 32 deaths occurred in the operating room, the remaining 25 deaths occurring in the intensive care ward between 1 day and 6 weeks following surgery. All seven operating room deaths were caused by low cardiac output with presumed myocardial infarction. Low cardiac output not reversed by inotropes or intra-aortic balloon pumping was the cause of death in 19 of the 25 intensive care ward deaths, and in these patients the problem was clearly established at the time the patient was returned to the intensive care ward. The remaining six deaths were due to unexpected myocardial infarction occurring during an apparently uneventful postoperative course.

Although inotrope support and intra-aortic balloon pumping have been used in Glasgow in patients other than those dying in the postoperative period, the use of inotrope support is now relatively uncommon, being used in fewer than 10 % of patients. However, approximately 30 % of patients are given nitroprusside for hypertension in the postoperative phase and it is believed that this change in postoperative drug therapy reflects improvements in myocardial protection due to cardioplegic solutions. The selection of patients and surgical techniques appear to have altered little in the past decade but the introduction of cardioplegia (using St Thomas' solution) is a relatively recent modification.

BLEEDING

The next commonest problem in the postoperative period has been bleeding. Twenty-two patients, or 4.4 % of the group, required reopening of the chest in the early postoperative phase for excessive bleeding. Nine per cent of the group required blood transfusion of more than 10 units during their hospital stay. The majority of these were patients undergoing repeat cardiac surgery, or with thoracic injury involving the heart and great vessels, or dissecting aneurysm. Blood loss is still a problem in cardiac surgery. This is further reflected by the fact that only 46 % of the group required transfusion of 4 units or less. Careful attention to haemostasis at the time of surgery greatly influences the blood loss and avoidance of unnecessary mobilization of pericardial adhesions over the left ventricle has been of considerable help in reducing blood loss in patients undergoing repeat surgery. The introduction of left-sided vents into the left atrium makes it unnecessary to mobilize the left ventricle, but considerable care is required to ensure efficient myocardial cooling, either by use of increased volumes of cardioplegic solution or by topical cooling over the surface of the left heart by opening the left pleural cavity, and cooling pericardium and the adherent underlying left ventricular muscle. It is also essential to take particular care in removing air from the aortic root prior to unclamping the aorta.

PULMONARY COMPLICATIONS

Ventilatory insufficiency was less of a problem. Twenty-six patients, or 5.2 % of the group, required postoperative ventilation of more than 24 h duration.

Chest infection or atelectasis was a serious problem in 5.2% of the group and, commonly, these were patients who had had prolonged postoperative ventilation.

CEREBRAL COMPLICATIONS

Cerebral complications, which included postoperative confusion and evidence of cerebral embolism occurring during cardiopulmonary bypass, were present in 13 patients or 2.6% of the group. It is well recognized that assessment of cerebral complications by most cardiac surgical teams misses very many patients with less overt cerebral injury, and it would seem likely that a major improvement in ensuring the safety of cardiac surgery would follow from a more critical assessment of cerebral status in the postoperative phase, together with attempts to link cerebral injury with surgical events in order to assist prevention of injury.

RENAL FAILURE

Renal failure, often with hepatic dysfunction, was commonly a feature of end stages of illness in those patients succumbing to low cardiac output conditions. Renal failure as an isolated problem requiring peritoneal dialysis occurred in four of the 500 patients.

FLUID AND ELECTROLYTE PROBLEMS

By North American standards, Glasgow has an extremely high incidence of valvular heart disease (52% of the group). The majority of these patients had long-standing valvular heart disease and had almost invariably been on long-term digoxin and diuretic therapy with potassium supplements. The practice of using clear fluid primes in Glasgow, as is common practice elsewhere, has been associated with large volumes of urine output in the early postoperative hours. Low potassium values in the postoperative period have been observed commonly in spite of potassium replacement therapy and have been the cause of cardiac arrest in at least five patients of the group, and undoubtedly the cause of ventricular irritability in a greater number still. Frequent measurement of serum potassium levels to allow safe potassium replacement therapy clearly has a major role in ensuring the safe recovery of patients after cardiac surgery. Serious dysrhythmias requiring lignocaine or mexiletine were not unduly common, being seen in 16 of the patients (3.2% of the group).

WOUND INFECTION

Wound infection was a problem in 25 patients, that is 5.2% of the group. This varied from delayed areas of healing with discharge of fluid from areas of the wound, to wound disruption and instability of the sternum. Meticulous attention to surgical techniques is likely to influence the incidence of wound infection considerably. Extensive use of diathermy and bone wax may well devitalize sufficient tissue to inhibit wound healing and create accumulations of necrotic tissue under the skin surface.

It is a salutary observation that only 67.4% of the group (that is about two-thirds of all patients undergoing heart surgery in Glasgow) were discharged well, without complications, within 2 weeks of their surgery. The remainder included the hospital deaths as well as 25% of the total group who required more than 2 weeks in the postoperative phase before discharge. Many of these required merely a slightly longer recovery period; some for 'social' reasons.

These figures, coming from a relatively large British centre over the past year, indicate clearly that although the crude hospital mortality rate was below the national average, as quoted in the United Kingdom Cardiac Surgical Register for 1978, there remains a significant hazard to cardiac surgery and many of the problems require to be dealt with during the postoperative period.

To look only at the problems further obscures the fact that many of our uneventful patients are uneventful precisely because the postoperative care is now largely a well-established routine matter. Much of the knowledge of postoperative changes is derived from observation of the postoperative course of patients from many centres in the past. The ability to anticipate electrolyte and metabolic changes in our patients has largely been built up by the wealth of experience from units which have pioneered cardiac surgery.

One of the most important aspects of postoperative care is the observation of patients and the early detection of changes in haemodynamic and biochemical parameters, so that complications can be avoided or reduced. It is important to record these changes in a simple way to give ready indication of changes in parameters; here the possibility of using computers to display trends in patient parameters and derived indices of haemodynamic performance has great promise. However, one reservation about the use of computers is the risk that over-emphasis on sophisticated equipment tends to supplant clinical skills and there is a danger of treating a computer or a biochemical profile, rather than looking at the patient. Clinical experience and common sense can rarely be replaced by computers but, with intelligent use, this facility should result in considerable benefit.

ROUTINE FOR POSTOPERATIVE CARE OF CARDIAC SURGICAL PATIENTS

On return from the operating theatre, most patients will be connected to a mechanical ventilator, blood pressure monitors, and chest drains. Intravenous fluids and/or blood transfusion will be running and a bladder catheter is usually in place.

There is usually considerable activity in moving the patient from the operating theatre into the intensive care ward and in transferring the patient into his bed. This period is one which carries a degree of hazard in that continuous monitoring is not easy at this stage and the patient is probably still in a relatively unstable cardiovascular status. It is important that someone accompanying the patient from the operating theatre keeps a close watch on an ECG or blood pressure display from a portable monitor or has a finger on a pulse. Ventilation is usually maintained temporarily by hand during transfer to the intensive care ward. It is important not to clamp chest drains at this time, as their function is to allow easy and rapid drainage of any accumulated blood around the heart. Clamping of the drains during movement runs the risk of developing tamponade and although it is frequently standard nursing teaching that chest drains should be clamped whenever the patient is moved, this commonly results in unduly prolonged periods of interruption of chest drainage. If blood loss is relatively high, this may result in severe degrees of tamponade.

Once the patient has been transferred to the intensive care ward bed, the arterial cannula is connected to the pressure monitor and the electrocardiogram is connected. Patients are frequently still quite cold and peripherally constricted, particularly when hypothermia is used in cardiopulmonary bypass. The patient should be covered to avoid heat loss and should be nursed flat until vital functions are stable, when the head may be elevated a little for comfort.

Monitoring of parameters of cardiac output

It is frequently possible nowadays to measure cardiac output by dye dilution or thermodilution catheters in the intensive care ward. Although this is done for most patients in Glasgow, it is important not to rely on this measurement alone but to use clinical judgment. Assessment of skin temperature and the state of venous filling, assessment of cerebral state, and assessment of urine output all give important information regarding the adequacy of perfusion of these regions. There are clear difficulties with a patient who is cold, vasoconstricted, and still unconscious from anaesthesia, but, by and large, considerable reliance can be placed on the assumption that a patient who is conscious, responsive to commands, passing adequate volumes of urine and who has warm, dry skin with good capillary filling and visible veins on the dorsa of hands and feet, has an adequate cardiac output. Measurements are made and recordings are kept of heart rate, blood pressure, central venous or left atrial pressure, and skin temperature. Although blood pressure can be measured from monitors, it is wise to check these periodically by the cuff method to confirm the accuracy of the monitor. Should a left atrial pressure line be present, considerable care must be taken to avoid the introduction of air bubbles or clot. Urine volume is measured hourly and should exceed 0.5 ml kg^{-1} h^{-1}, although frequently with a fluid prime the volumes of urine vastly exceed this level for the first few hours.

Chest drains and blood balance

Collection of blood in underwater seal drains without suction is entirely satisfactory and any accumulating blood that remains in the tubes should be gently milked down toward the bottle to prevent clot forming in the tubes. The volume of blood is measured initially every quarter of an hour until it is clear that blood loss is not excessive, and thereafter hourly. A blood loss of more than 200 ml in an hour suggests that excessive bleeding is occurring and usually is an indication to reopen the chest to check haemostasis. Judgment regarding blood transfusion should be based on the observation of adequacy of cardiac output and evidence of blood pressure, heart rate and venous pressure. It is reasonable to replace blood loss in approximately the same volume as recorded in the chest drainage bottles, but attention to the state of cardiac output and clinical perfusion will avoid the occasional error which can occur if a large amount of blood accumulates within the pleural space and is not detected in the chest drains. Similarly, the unthinking maintenance of a pre-set central venous pressure can result in illogical blood replacement practice. Venous pressure changes are more important than the absolute values. The venous pressure gives evidence of venous filling and the state of overall cardiac contraction but, as an isolated value, is not a good parameter for deciding the need for blood transfusion.

Artificial ventilation

Patients are usually returned to the intensive care ward attached to a ventilator. It is important to check that chest movements are visibly adequate and that there is audible air entry in both lungs. A portable chest X-ray made with the patient supine should be obtained within the first hour of the patient's return as a check that both lungs are fully expanded, that there is not an excess of blood or air in a pleural space, that there are no retained foreign bodies of unintentional nature such as swabs or instruments, and that the endotracheal tube has not engaged the right main bronchus. Inflation pressure should be measured from the ventilator and the arterial blood gases monitored to confirm the adequacy of ventilation. Once the patient has recovered consciousness and is haemodynamically stable, he can be disconnected from the ventilator and a short trial of breathing with an oxygen mask over the end of the endotracheal tube can be assessed. The ability to move an adequate volume of ventilatory gas without undue clinical distress is the important criterion for removing the endotracheal tube and allowing normal ventilation with an oxygen mask. While the endotracheal tube is in place, regular suction with careful sterile precautions is required to clear the tube and bronchial tree. After most cardiac surgery it is perfectly feasible to discontinue mechanical ventilation within 2–3 h of surgery, and routine prolonged ventilation contributes little to patient safety but does expose him to the risk of chest infection. However, those patients who remain haemodynamically unstable, or who clearly have to use a considerable amount of muscular effort to move an adequate tidal volume, will require ventilation possibly for 12–24 h. Blood gas assessments are required to confirm the adequacy of ventilation but should not form the sole basis for deciding whether to remove the patient from the ventilator. Clinical assessment is of considerable importance in this regard. Those patients suspected preoperatively of having poor ventilatory function should have arterial blood gases measured to allow reasonable judgment postoperatively in ventilatory management. It is not uncommon to find patients who have quite severely abnormal blood gases prior to cardiac surgery being left on a ventilator postoperatively because their blood gases are abnormal, without the realization that the same patients lived with these abnormal blood gases preoperatively.

Intravenous fluids

Maintenance of 5% dextrose water at a rate of 80 cc/h is common practice in the postoperative phase. Potassium chloride (80 mmol KCl) over 12 h is given to maintain adequate serum potassium levels, but it is important both to check the serum potassium levels and to monitor urine volumes. Oliguria should act as a warning against giving intravenous potassium until serum levels are measured, and very high urine output suggests that potassium will be required in large dosage. Again, serum potassium levels should be measured and a level in the region of 4–5 mmol/l should be aimed for.

It is important to record the volumes of intravenous fluids that are given.

Antibiotics

The use of prophylactic antibiotics to cover the period of surgery and the early postoperative phase is standard, although the type of antibiotic varies from unit to unit. The important principle is to give the antibiotic immediately prior to surgery so that high blood levels are attained during the period that the patient is at greatest risk from bacteraemia, that is during the time that his chest is open and his blood exposed to the atmosphere during cardiopulmonary bypass. It is usual practice to give the antibiotic for 48 h.

Drugs

Inotrope support drugs are indicated where the cardiac output is clinically inadequate. Isoprenaline is used where heart rate is slow. If bradycardia is the sole source of concern, the use of intravenous atropine is often a better alternative. Dopamine or adrenaline are less commonly required than in the past and unless these drugs rapidly improve cardiac output, the use of intra-aortic balloon pumping should be instituted to improve myocardial and renal perfusion.

Relief of pain and return to activity

It is important to use adequate analgesia for patients in the postoperative phase. Small doses of opiates intravenously should be given until the patient is comfortable. It is of considerable importance to talk to the patients and reassure them that all is well – this is particularly easy to omit in the early stages when the patient is still on a ventilator and may appear to be still anaesthetized. It is important to consider the possibility that the patient may be largely paralysed but aware of his surroundings, and communication with the patient at this stage is of considerable importance. A quiet, efficient, and orderly atmosphere in the intensive care ward adds greatly to the reassurance of the patients, who should be able to get some sleep during the first postoperative night. Unnecessary and frequent intervention for monitoring carries a risk of depriving the patients of sleep so that they become unwell, irritable, and exhausted by the first postoperative day. It is important to bear in mind that patients may not remember what is said to them in the early postoperative period and they commonly need reassurance and explanation later on in the postoperative phase.

It is of considerable help to the patients to be out of bed in a chair on the first postoperative day and to start walking on the second postoperative day, with graded and rapid return to full activity. The assistance and moral support of skilful physiotherapy is very important in this regard.

MANAGEMENT OF COMPLICATIONS

Low cardiac output

Low cardiac output may occur as a result of myocardial injury sustained during surgery, or it may occur from postoperative myocardial infarction (cardiogenic shock), from blood loss (oligaemic shock), or from cardiac tamponade. Diagnosis of the cause is usually relatively simple from observation of the measured parameters and a knowledge of the events in the operating room. A patient who has difficulty in maintaining circulation immediately after discontinuation of cardiopulmonary bypass, who has a persistently low blood pressure, poor urine output and high central venous pressure, will be readily recognized as suffering from cardiogenic shock and requires inotrope support. The patient who has a high blood loss in the early postoperative phase, but who had no difficulty in maintaining a circulation when cardiopulmonary bypass was discontinued, clearly is at risk of tamponade. A rise in central venous pressure with tachycardia and hypertension then make this diagnosis so likely that rapid and early reopening of the chest is essential. This procedure should be done without delay and this usually requires reopening of the chest in the intensive care ward, unless there is very rapid and easy access to an operating theatre. Doubt about the diagnosis usually arises in those patients who have poor cardiac output from a combination of cardiogenic causes and tamponade, and it is frequently necessary to reopen the chest simply to exclude the presence of tamponade. Low cardiac output due to oligaemia is usually manifested by a low central venous pressure or low left atrial pressure, tachycardia and hypotension, with obvious disparity between blood loss and blood replacement. Occasional difficulties arise where considerable blood loss occurs into a pleural space, unknown to the intensive care ward staff. This can usually be anticipated by early chest X-ray and the treatment, of course, is rapid blood transfusion.

Ventricular dysrhythmias

Ventricular ectopic beats or ventricular fibrillation may result from low serum potassium levels. This should usually be prevented by monitoring serum potassium regularly and giving replacement. The occurrence of coupling or frequent ventricular ectopic beats should prompt immediate serum potassium measurement. If the level is below 4 mmol/l, a bolus of 5–10 mmol of potassium given fairly rapidly intravenously, followed by an increased maintenance dose and repeated estimates of serum potassium, should resolve the problem. The occurrence of ventricular fibrillation requires immediate external cardiac massage and countershock with urgent potassium replacement. A bolus of 100 mg of intravenous lignocaine followed by a drip of lignocaine, 1 mg/min, may be used to suppress ventricular ectopics not due to low serum potassium. Episodes of atrioventricular dissociation or extreme bradycardia may be treated by artificial pacemaking if temporary epicardial pacing wires have been left at the time of surgery. Alternatively, the use of isoprenaline will increase the heart rate.

Ventilatory insufficiency

Prolonged ventilatory support may be necessary, particularly where lung function has been previously compromised by long-standing mitral valve disease, chronic bronchitis, or pulmonary vascular disease due to high flow resulting from left to right shunts. It is usually possible to leave an endotracheal tube in place for up to a week, but if it is obvious that prolonged ventilation is necessary after the first few days, it is wise to perform tracheostomy which allows more adequate bronchial aspiration. It is important to ensure adequate humidification of the ventilatory gases and strict asepsis in bronchial aspiration aids considerably in reducing the infective complications of prolonged ventilation. Chest infections and atelectasis require antibiotics, physiotherapy, and occasionally endobronchial suction through a bronchoscope.

Renal failure

Oliguria is a common problem which may be due to dehydration, excessive use of diuretics without adequate fluid replacement, or may be due to renal failure where poor cardiac output is prolonged. Low urine urea in an oliguric patient suggests renal failure; high urine urea levels with oliguria indicate dehydration. Where dialysis is indicated, haemodialysis is the most effective method and requires help from nephrologists. Peritoneal dialysis is less efficient but may be necessary if haemodynamic instability precludes haemodialysis.

Neurological complications

Unconsciousness, fits, paralysis, or weakness of limbs usually indicates embolism, either of air or calcium at the time of cardiac surgery, but may also be due to insufficient cerebral perfusion due to inadequate perfusion pressure, the presence of unsuspected cerebral arterial disease, or may occasionally be due to cerebral bleeding. Maintenance of adequate cardiac output, reduction of general metabolic requirements by ventilation and sedation or paralysis, and adequate oxygenation, together with the use of intravenous steroids, all have an important role in reducing established cerebral injury. Avoidance of pressure ulceration, hypostatic pneumonia, and nutritional problems, requires the skills of nursing staff, physiotherapists and physicians.

Wound infection

Most wound infections settle with local dressings, but more extensive infections may require drainage of pus, removal of infected suture material, and the administration of systemic antibiotics based on the results of bacteriological culture and sensitivity tests.

Urinary tract infections

The routine use of bladder catheterization is occasionally followed by urinary tract infection. The tip of the catheter should be routinely cultured on its removal, as this may give early warning of infective problems. Where symptoms arise postoperatively urine culture is important, to identify the organism and its sensitivity, and the appropriate antibiotics should then be administered systemically.

Details of the management of specific problems are well beyond the scope of this chapter. However, improved cardiac surgical techniques, careful monitoring and early intervention for haemodynamic and biochemical abnormalities, have considerably reduced the incidence of postoperative infections following cardiac surgery, and attention to details in postoperative care plays an important role in improving the safety of cardiac surgery.

32
Is inotropic stimulation outdated?

P. A. POOLE-WILSON

Several years ago inotropic drugs, particularly catecholomines, were widely used by clinicians for the treatment of patients with low cardiac output and heart failure associated with hypotension[1-7]. A satisfactory response was frequently observed in that blood pressure rose, urine flow increased and peripheral perfusion improved. However, these apparently advantageous effects were often transient and long-term survival of patients was largely unaffected[1,4-6]. Experimental work on animals and clinical studies in man[5,6] indicated that catecholamines could under some circumstances increase myocardial damage[8-10]. The transient clinical improvement in patients was achieved at the expense of further compromising the potential recovery and long-term function of the very organ, namely the heart, which had been the original cause of the low cardiac output[11].

In the 1970s vasodilators were advocated as an alternative form of therapy[12-17]. Intravenous nitroglycerin, nitroprusside, and α-receptor blocking drugs were used in many different clinical conditions. The role and mechanism of action of such drugs have since been extensively investigated both in man and animals. More recently the value of inotropic drugs has been re-examined and their use is enjoying a modest revival[18-20]. This has been brought about by the development of new drugs with selective effects on the heart and peripheral circulation, by the possibility of therapy with a combination of an inotrope and a vasodilator, by improved definition of therapeutic objectives, and above all by a better understanding of the pathophysiology of myocardial failure, especially when it is the result of myocardial ischaemia.

Inotropic drugs are used in the treatment of patients with widely differing clinical syndromes such as acute heart failure, chronic heart failure, cardiogenic shock, septic shock and after cardiac surgery. The definitions of these syndromes are imprecise and often ill patients have several clinical problems at the same time. The difficulties of obtaining groups of patients with the same disease, makes trials of therapy almost impossible. The use of inotropes in acute myocardial infarction and in patients after cardiac surgery can be more readily assessed. In these situations the primary problem is myocardial failure and groups of patients with similar haemodynamic problems can be obtained.

The general objectives of treatment with inotropic drugs are to prolong life; maintain adequate perfusion of the body organs, particularly the brain, kidneys, myocardium, and liver; prevent pulmonary oedema; and avoid increase of myocardial damage. To this end physicians assess peripheral perfusion by clinical observation and measure left ventricular end-diastolic pressure (either directly or estimated from the pulmonary capillary wedge pressure or pulmonary artery end-diastolic pressure), central venous pressure, blood pressure, urine flow and sometimes cardiac output. Current methods for assessing cardiac output do not allow continuous measurement. The most commonly used method is the thermodilution technique; it is expensive and values for cardiac output can only be obtained at a single moment of time on a limited number of occasions. Thus the variables which are monitored in the intensive care unit are not directly related to the objectives of treatment. It is important to recall the objectives of treatment when these measurements are being used to determine treatment.

In the absence of coronary artery disease the primary therapeutic objective is to maintain or increase perfusion of the body tissues including the myocardium itself. The level of the blood pressure is of little importance in itself, if tissue perfusion is adequate, although systolic pressures below 80 mmHg are likely to be associated with reduced tissue perfusion. Blood flow through an organ is dependent on the driving force, that is the perfusion pressure, and the vascular resistance. Increase of blood pressure by a drug which increases vascular resistance due to constriction of arterioles is therefore illogical since tissue perfusion is not increased while myocardial oxygen consumption rises. Drugs acting in this manner may also be harmful since blood flow to vital organs may be diminished and blood flow to non-vital organs such as skeletal muscle may be increased[17]. The overall result is a disadvantageous redistribution of blood flow. Drugs which increase tissue perfusion by reduction of vascular resistance (vasodilators) or by a positive inotropic effect on the heart to increase cardiac output and thus tissue perfusion pressure, are to be preferred. The major problem with the use of inotropes is that the increased workload on the myocardium due to increased contractility and afterload may exceed the advantage of better perfusion of body tissues and particularly the myocardium[4–10]. In most situations myocardial disease is the primary problem and further damage to the myocardium is likely to be lethal. An additional difficulty is that little is known of the distribution of the increased blood flow to the body organs.

ENERGY CONSUMPTION AND PRODUCTION IN MYOCARDIUM

Ischaemia of the myocardium has traditionally been considered to alter contractility as a result of an imbalance between oxygen supply and demand[21]. This concept is misleading. The myocardium does not demand oxygen nor is it clearly established that supply of oxygen is the limiting or direct cause of diminished cardiac contractility, particularly if the ischaemic episode is acute. Indeed, the reduced contractility may act as a protective mechanism to diminish the need for oxygen[11]. Oxygen is, under extreme conditions, almost certainly the limiting substrate for the myocardium since the concentration of glucose, lactate and free fatty acids, the metabolic substrates, are not low in the coronary sinus. However, an additional purpose of blood flow is to remove the products of metabolism. During ischaemia a key metabolite is the hydrogen ion which accumulates within seconds, is a powerful negative inotropic agent, and inhibits glycolysis and other metabolic pathways[22]. The concept of supply and demand of oxygen is represented at cellular level as an imbalance between the consumption of ATP and blood flow (Figure 1). Coronary blood flow has a dual purpose: it is necessary to provide substrates for ATP production and to prevent the retention of metabolic products which inhibit metabolic pathways and directly affect myocardial contractility.

ATP CONSUMPTION——ISCHAEMIA——BLOOD FLOW—substrate supply, product removal

ATP consumption		Blood flow
major	heart rate	duration of diastole
	wall tension	diastolic blood pressure
	contractility	diastolic ventricular pressure
minor	external work	

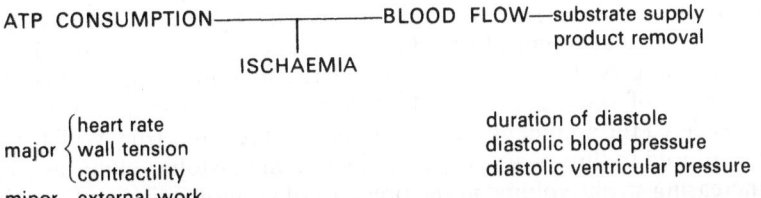

Figure 1 Myocardial ischaemia

The major determinants of ATP consumption are heart rate, contractility and muscle tension in the wall of the myocardium[21]. The major determinants of blood flow to the myocardium are perfusion pressure (often assumed to be the difference between aortic and left ventricular diastolic pressures), and the duration of diastole[23-25] since it is in this period that coronary flow to the left ventricle is greatest.

Heart rate has two major effects. Not only does it increase ATP consumption but it is also reduces myocardial perfusion (Figure 1). At a rate of 86 beats/min systole occupies 0.23 s and diastole 0.47 s. As heart rate increases diastole shortens in relation to systole so that the proportion of a minute during which the heart is in diastole and during which coronary flow to the left ventricle occurs, is diminished. For this reason the maintenance of heart rate above 100 beats/min is to be avoided. Isoprenaline is a strong chronotropic drug and its use in man in several clinical situations is associated with increased lactate production and myocardial oxygen consumption. At least a part of these effects is due to increase of heart rate. The clinical use of isoprenaline should be limited to increasing ventricular rate when a low cardiac output is associated with bradycardia or heart block.

The second major determinant of ATP consumption is wall tension. It is determined by the ventricular pressure and is also, directly proportional to the radius of the ventricular chamber (Laplace relationship, tension = 2 ×

pressure × radius). If blood pressure is reduced by vasodilator treatment then wall tension will be reduced at the moment the aortic valve opens. It is a property of cardiac muscle that reduction of afterload is associated with a greater degree of muscle shortening[26]. Cardiac output is dependent on muscle shortening so that under some circumstances a lowering of blood pressure can have the apparently paradoxical result of increasing cardiac output, reducing wall tension and thus reducing ATP consumption by the myocardium. An additional reason for reduced ATP consumption is the well-known phenomenon that external work performed by the heart against a high pressure consumes more ATP than an equal amount of external work against a low pressure[21].

A similar reduction of ATP consumption can also occur even if blood pressure does not change at a constant heart rate and left ventricular end-diastolic pressure[25]. There are three important mechanisms which are illustrated in Figure 2 and 3. Suppose that end-diastolic blood pressure is 80 mmHg and that the aortic valve closes when pressure is 120 mmHg. Between these points there is a complex relationship between pressure and flow out of the ventricle which determines the amount of blood ejected and thus ventricular volume. By the Laplace relationship wall tension, the variable determining ATP consumption, is related to ventricular volume. For the purposes of the argument wall thickness is ignored; if wall thickness is considered the argument is more complex but remains true. Wall tension can be reduced in three ways. First a reduction in diastolic volume as a result of increasing stroke volume in the presence of an inotropic agent (i.e. decrease in heart size) will decrease wall tension. Second, the increment of wall tension

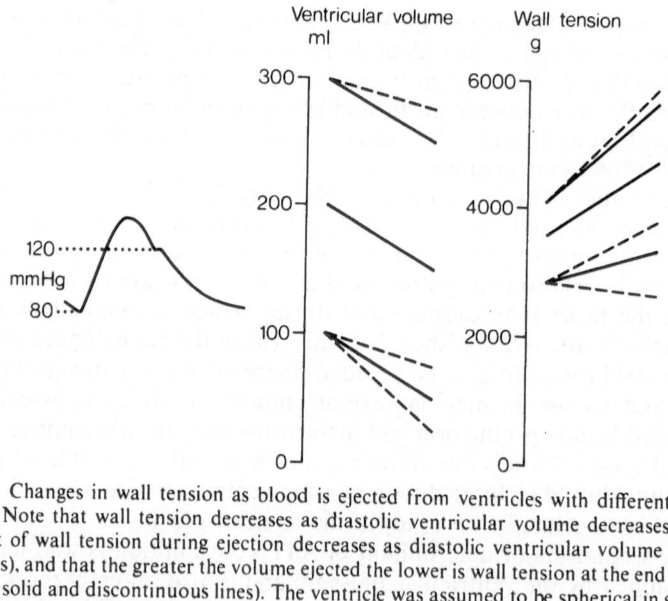

Figure 2 Changes in wall tension as blood is ejected from ventricles with different diastolic volumes. Note that wall tension decreases as diastolic ventricular volume decreases, that the increment of wall tension during ejection decreases as diastolic ventricular volume decreases (solid lines), and that the greater the volume ejected the lower is wall tension at the end of systole (compare solid and discontinuous lines). The ventricle was assumed to be spherical in shape and wall thickness was ignored

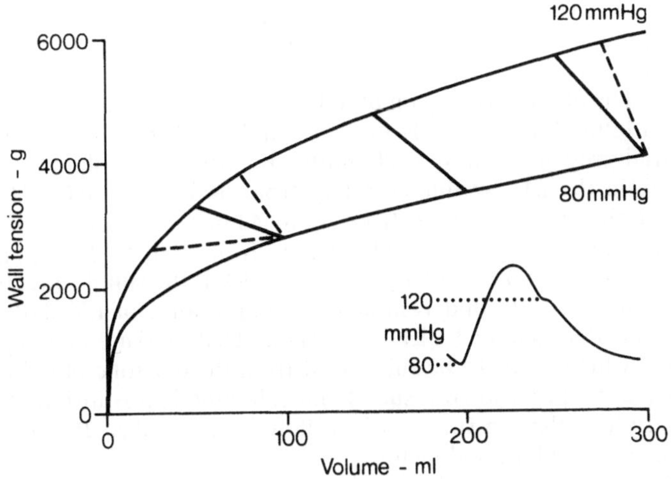

Figure 3 As for Figure 1. Wall tension, a major determinant of ATP consumption by heart muscle, is plotted against ventricular volume

during the ejection phase decreases as diastolic ventricular volume decreases. In Figure 3 the slopes of the lines representing ejection of the same volume of blood, 50 ml, are steeper the higher the initial diastolic volume. Third, the greater the stroke volume the smaller will be the ventricular volume at the end of systole. Wall tension in a heart with an initial volume of 100 ml is decreased at the end of systole as the stroke volume increases from 25 to 75 ml (Figure 3).

MYOCARDIAL PERFUSION

The determinants of myocardial perfusion have been characterized by the diastolic pressure time index[23–25], and are represented by the equation:

$$\text{Myocardial perfusion} = \frac{\text{DBP} - \text{LVEDP}}{\text{HR}}$$

where DBP is the diastolic blood pressure; LVEDP is the left ventricular end-diastolic pressure and HR is the heart rate.

Some difficulties with the concept have recently been discussed[24,25,28]. Though undoubtedly this simple relationship has clinical applicability at least three important problems arise. First, the equation implies that the pressure gradient for perfusion is determined by the LVEDP. While such an assumption is often valid, it may not be justified in the presence of a low LVEDP and high right atrial pressures. Under these circumstances, which are associated with right ventricular failure and occur after cardiac surgery and inferior myocardial infarction, right atrial pressure may be an important determinant of myocardial perfusion pressure. Second, the above equation suggests that LVEDP is relatively unimportant. For example if the diastolic blood pressure were 75 mmHg, a 100% increase of LVEDP from 15 to 30 mmHg would reduce perfusion pressure from 60 to 45 mmHg, a reduction of 25%. The observed effect on blood flow may be greater, particularly in the endocardium. A recent study in dogs[29] indicated that an increase of mean left atrial pressure from 6 to 20 mmHg by infusion of blood increased the pressure in the left circumflex artery from 54 to 63 mmHg. The pressure gradient changed, therefore, from 48 to 43 mmHg (decrease of 10%) but caused a fall in endocardial blood flow from 1.40 to 1.10 ml min^{-1} g^{-1} (decrease of 21%). Particularly at high LVEDP the simple equation shown above may seriously underestimate the importance of LVEDP. The third problem is that neither LVEDP nor right atrial pressure may represent the pressure which needs to be subtracted from the diastolic blood pressure to obtain the true perfusion pressure. If diastolic blood pressure is plotted against coronary flow the pressure at which flow is zero (called P_{zf}) appears to be determined by additional factors[28-31].

Coronary perfusion in the presence of coronary artery disease is even more complex. The effects of drugs are not yet fully understood[19,24,25]. The major problems are the distribution of coronary flow between endocardium and epicardium, the determinants of perfusion pressure, the importance of collateral circulation and the possible existence of 'coronary steal' between endo- and epicardium and between adjacent tissue perfused by normal and diseased vessels. The state of vessel tone regulated by the autonomic nervous system and by circulating catecholamines[31] appears to be more important than previously supposed from experiments on anaesthetized animals. An important consequence of appreciating the complexities in assessing the effect of an inotropic agent on myocardial blood flow and ATP consumption is that the use of inotropes can and should be reconsidered. Recent experiments[19] show that if heart rate is unchanged the use of cardiac glycosides reduces the area of ischaemia in dogs, provided LVEDP and ventricular diastolic volume were large. That is, the harmful effect of an inotropic stimulant in increasing myocardial contractility and ATP consumption is far outweighed by the benefits of reduced wall tension (due to reduced diastolic ventricular volume and increased stroke volume) and increased myocardial perfusion (due to a greater perfusion pressure as a result of a reduction of LVEDP and increased diastolic blood pressure).

The inotropic drugs currently available are the catecholamines (Table 1 and Figures 4 and 5), the cardiac glycosides, and calcium. The newer sympathomimetic amines for use after cardiac surgery include dobutamine, dopamine, and salbutamol.

DOBUTAMINE

Dobutamine is a synthetic catecholamine[32] in which a hydrogen of the terminal amine group of dopamine has been substituted (Figure 5). The major action of dobutamine is on β1-receptors in the myocardium but it is also a weak stimulant of β2- and α-receptors in the peripheral vasculature (Table

Table 1 Sympathomimetic amines – actions on receptors

	β1	*β2*	*α*	*Dopaminergic*	*Dosage* ($\mu g\ kg^{-1}\ min^{-1}$)
Isoprenaline	+++	+++	0	0	0.02–0.20
Adrenaline	+++	++	++	0	0.06–0.18
Noradrenaline	+	0	+++	0	0.001–0.08
Dopamine	+++	0	+ → +++	+++	1–30
Dobutamine	+++	+	+	0	2–40
Salbutamol	?+	+++	0	0	4 mg t.d.s. oral 0.1–0.4 i.v.

1)[33]. Low doses cause a small degree of peripheral vasoconstriction and higher doses cause vasodilation.

In isolated muscle dobutamine has chronotropic and inotropic effects similar to other catecholamines[34,35]. When infused into anaesthetized dogs cardiac output increases and left ventricular end-diastolic pressure decreases. Systemic vascular resistance is slightly diminished and arterial pressure may either increase or decrease[32,36,37]. In comparison to isoprenaline, dobutamine exerts a greater inotropic than chronotropic effect[32]. The difference appears to be a direct effect on the sino-arterial node since the same differences are present after vagotomy and in the presence of sympatholytic drugs.

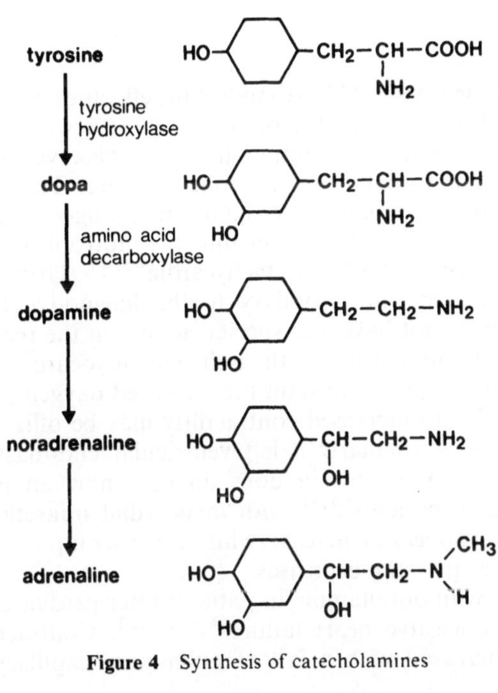

Figure 4 Synthesis of catecholamines

Adrenaline

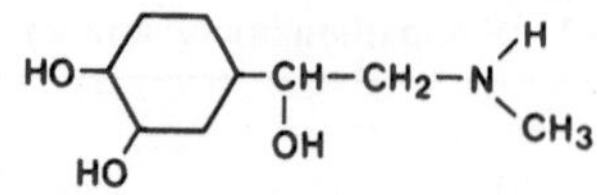

Noradrenaline

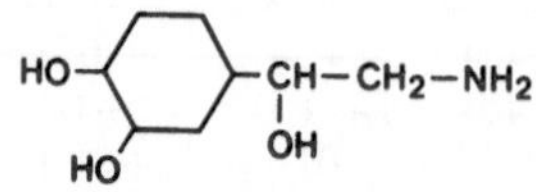

Isoprenaline

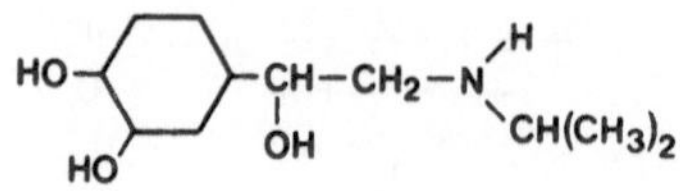

Dopamine

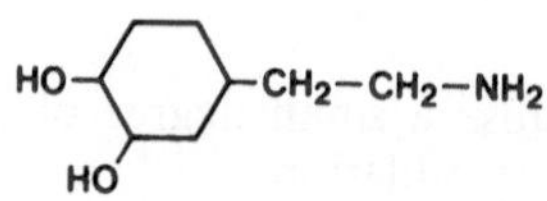

Dobutamine

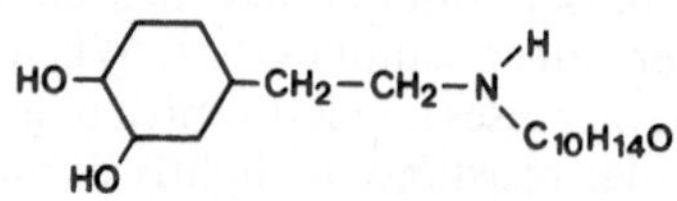

Salbutamol

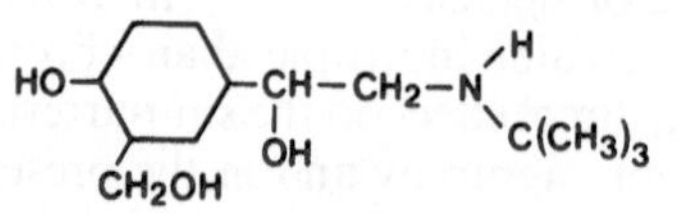

Figure 5 Sympathomimetic amines

Many investigators[38–43] have studied the effects of dobutamine in patients with heart failure; the drug has been recently reviewed[44]. In general a dose-related increase of cardiac output has been observed with an associated decline of left ventricular end-diastolic pressure. The increase of cardiac output was not accompanied by significant changes of heart rate or blood pressure. In comparison to isoprenaline the inotropic effect of dobutamine in man is associated with less tachycardia[45–47]. Urine flow and sodium excretion increased but secondary to the haemodynamic improvement; dobutamine does not have any specific action on the renal vasculature.

The effect of dobutamine on the ischaemic myocardium is complex. Provided heart rate remains constant the increased oxygen consumption of the myocardium due to increased contractility may be offset by a reduction in ventricular size, particularly if left ventricular end-diastolic pressure was high initially. Experiments in dogs do not show an increase in infarct size[48,49], and in patients[50,51] with myocardial infarction the size of the infarct does not appear to increase, whilst cardiac output rises and pulmonary capillary wedge pressure decreases.

The results with dobutamine in patients after cardiac surgery are similar to those in congestive heart failure[46,47,52,53]. Contractility of the myocardium is increased with a fall of pulmonary capillary wedge pressure.

Tachycardia is less than with isoprenaline. Dobutamine appears, therefore, to be a relatively specific $\beta 1$ agent (Table 1) and its clinical use in the context of cardiac surgery should be greatest when an inotropic effect and no other effect is desired. If the depression of cardiac failure is caused by ischaemia then the value of dobutamine will be subject to the same problems as other catecholamines[8-10,19].

DOPAMINE

Dopamine is a naturally occurring catecholamine (Table 1; Figures 4 and 5) whose clinical use has become apparent in the last decade[42,54,55]. Dopamine has a direct $\beta 1$-stimulating effect on cardiac muscle[35,55,56] and also reacts with dopaminergic and α-receptors in the vascular system. Stimulation of dopaminergic receptors in the renal, mesenteric, coronary, and intracerebral arterial vascular beds causes vasodilation. The effect is not antagonized by propranol but is by haloperidol and phenothiazines. A specific receptor distinct from α- and β-receptors appears to exist. Increase of renal blood flow occurs at low concentrations of dopamine (in man 0.5–3 $\mu g\ kg^{-1}\ min^{-1}$) whilst α-stimulation resulting in an increase of peripheral vascular constriction occurs at high doses ($>10\,\mu g\,kg^{-1}\,min^{-1}$). The increase in renal blood flow in normal subjects is accompanied by an increase of glomerular filtration rate and sodium excretion[54,57,58]. Other effects such as redistribution of intracortical renal blood flow may also result[59].

The haemodynamic response to dopamine in man depends on the rate of infusion. At a rate of 1–10 $\mu g\ kg^{-1}\ min^{-1}$ there is a dose-dependent increase in cardiac contractility. Heart rate and blood pressure are usually unchanged. Renal blood flow increases. At higher rates of infusion blood pressure increases.

Dopamine has been widely used for the treatment of congestive cardiac failure[41,43,57,60-63], cardiogenic shock[67], and septic shock[42,64-67].

In dogs dopamine increases coronary blood flow[54,68,69]. The increase is partially a consequence of the increase in contractility but may also be a result of a reduction of coronary vascular resistance by stimulation of dopaminergic receptors[70]. However, dopamine can increase myocardial ischaemia in dogs, and in patients with myocardial infarction variable results have been obtained. Coronary sinus oxygen tension and the extraction of lactate have been shown to be unchanged[71] or to be increased[72]. The difference is important since the patients of Crexells *et al.*[71] had higher arterial pressures and less severe ischaemia than those of Mueller *et al.*[72]. Thus in patients with cardiogenic shock resulting from acute myocardial infarction the beneficial haemodynamic changes brought about by dopamine, namely increase of blood pressure and cardiac output, may be offset by the increase of myocardial contractility compromising the already threatened myocardium. This problem seems to be common to all catecholamines.

SALBUTAMOL

Salbutamol is a $\beta 2$ agonist used for the treatment of asthma (Table 1; Figure 5). In isolated heart muscle the drug can also be shown to have $\beta 1$ agonist properties[76]. The increase in heart rate observed with its use in normal man[73] and occasionally in heart failure[74] may also be partially due to direct $\beta 1$ stimulation rather than a reflex response to peripheral vascular dilatation from $\beta 2$ stimulation.

Salbutamol has been used in the treatment of congestive heart failure[75–77]. Cardiac output is increased, heart rate and blood pressure unchanged, and pulmonary capillary wedge pressure slightly reduced. These effects might be the consequence of an inotropic ($\beta 1$) stimulation[75] but can more probably be accounted for by the vasodilator properties ($\beta 2$) of salbutamol[76,77]. The plasma concentration, which is observed in man, is too small to cause an inotropic effect in isolated muscle[76].

Salbutamol has also been used in acute myocardial infarction[78–80] and after cardiac surgery[74,81,82]. Though the haemodynamic changes are beneficial, whether these prolong life or are achieved without an increase in myocardial oxygen consumption or alteration of coronary blood flow is unknown.

COMPARISONS BETWEEN DRUGS

There have been several direct comparisons between sympathomimetic inotropic drugs. Because dobutamine has less chronotropic effect it is preferable to isoprenaline after cardiac surgery[46,47]. During emergence from cardiopulmonary bypass, when presumably the inotropic properties of drugs are of greatest import, dopamine, dobutamine, and epinephrine are equally effective[53]. In chronic heart failure dobutamine has been favoured in comparison to dopamine[41,43,62]. Dopamine at high doses in these patients increases afterload by causing vasoconstriction due to its α effect. As a result cardiac output increases less and LVEDP may be unchanged or even rise. The result of comparisons between these drugs depends, therefore, on the dose used and the pre-existing haemodynamics. One study claims that dopamine is superior to dobutamine[83].

Perhaps surprisingly vasodilators such as nitroglycerin cause almost identical haemodynamic changes[19,20] as positive inotropic drugs such as dobutamine (Tables 1 and 2)[18]. The major difference between the two is a small increase of blood pressure with dobutamine and decrease with nitroglycerin[18]. Vasodilators increase cardiac output secondarily to the reduction of systemic vascular resistance, whereas myocardial stimulants cause reflex vasodilation as a result of an increased cardiac output[18]. A synergistic effect of the two types of drug is predictable and has been shown to be of potential clinical value. Dopamine has been combined with nitroprusside[84–86], nitroglycerin[87], and chlorpromazine[89]. Salbutamol has been combined with isosorbide dinitrate[77] and nitroglycerin[78]. Dobutamine has additive effects with nitroglycerin[18].

Table 2

	Inotropic stimulant	*Vasodilator*
CO	↑	↑
LVEDP	↓	↓
SVR	↓	↓
HR	↑ or →	↑ or →
BP	→ or ↑	→ or ↓
MVO_2	↑	↓
CBF	↑ or ↓	↑ or ↓
Ischaemia	↑ or ↓	↑ or ↓

POSITIVE INOTROPIC DRUGS AND CARDIAC SURGERY

Under what circumstances should an inotropic drug be used in patients after cardiac surgery? Which drug should be chosen? There is at present no simple answer to either of these questions. Both vasodilators and inotropic drugs have been and are used (Table 3). Most information pertains to patients after they have returned to the intensive care unit, and there are few reports on the use of inotropic drugs in the operating theatre where there is a major indication for inotropic drugs to augment myocardial contractility as the patient comes off cardiopulmonary bypass[53]. The use of drugs under these circumstances is usually transient.

Increased haemodynamic monitoring has offered a more logical approach to therapy. A raised left atrial pressure >18 mmHg in the presence of adequate tissue perfusion is treated in order to avoid pulmonary oedema with an intravenous vasodilator such as nitroglycerin or nitroprusside. Often cardiac output increases and blood pressure remains unchanged. If blood

Table 3 A basis for treatment

LVEDP (mmHg)	*BP*	*Tissue perfusion*	*Treatment*
>18	N	N	vasodilator
	N	L	vasodilator
	L	N	vasodilator + inotrope
	L	L	inotrope + vasodilator
<18	N	N	eureka
	N	L	vasodilator
	L	N	leave ? or inotrope
	L	L	inotrope + ? vasodilator
<10	L	N or L	volume expansion
	N	N or L	volume expansion

N = normal: L = low

pressure does fall and tissue perfusion is inadequate, an inotropic agent can be added. Either dopamine[53,87,90–92] or dobutamine[46,47,52,53] are appropriate. Adrenaline is also used[53,90]. Dopamine has the advantage of improving blood flow to the myocardium, brain, and kidney by stimulating dopaminergic receptors[55]. A low left atrial pressure should be treated by expansion of the blood volume until left atrial pressure is approximately 15 mmHg. If blood pressure is still low, treatment is not indicated unless cardiac output is much reduced or more importantly tissue perfusion is inadequate. A low blood pressure (70 mmHg) with underperfusion of tissue is treated with an inotropic drug. Excessive increases in heart rate must be avoided. Isoprenaline has a marked chronotropic effect and should not be used[46,47,92]. If no improvement is achieved with catecholamines an infusion of calcium can be tried. A reduction of plasma calcium activity is not a cause of reduced contractility after cardiac surgery unless very large blood transfusions have been given (unpublished observation), but additions of calcium can be used to increase myocardial contractility.

Recent work has suggested that the combination of a vasodilator and positive inotropic agent may be particularly beneficial, after cardiac surgery[34,87] and in heart failure[18,20,85,86,88,89]. Tissue perfusion and the metabolic state of the myocardium may be optimized if the increased contraction of the myocardium delivers the increased cardiac output into an unconstricted circulation and if normal and collateral flow in the coronary arteries are maximized. At the same time left atrial pressure can be maintained at a level to prevent pulmonary oedema. New drugs may emerge in which both these two attributes are present. Salbutamol is a vasodilator with a small inotropic effect and has a useful role after cardiac surgery[74,82]; greater inotropic and venodilator effects by manipulation of the structure of the drug would result in greater utility. A drug with the combination of $\beta 1$- and $\beta 2$-stimulating properties without a chronotropic effect is not yet available. Even then not all clinical difficulties could be resolved. The mechanisms which control the proportion of the cardiac output delivered to the different body organs, and the determinants of the distribution of coronary blood flow to the myocardium, are not fully understood. These problems limit our approach to treatment.

References

1. Gunnar, R. M., Loeb, H. S., Pietras, R. J. and Tobin, Jr. (1967). Ineffectiveness of isoproterenol in shock due to acute myocardial infarction. *J. Am. Med. Assoc.*, **202,** 1124
2. Smith, H. J., Oriol, A., Morch, J. and McGregor, M. (1967). Haemodynamic studies in cardiogenic shock: treatment with isoproterenol and metaraminol. *Circulation*, **35,** 1084
3. Goldberg, L. I. (1968). Use of sympathomimetic amines in heart failure. *Am. J. Cardiol.*, **22,** 177
4. Kuhn, L. A., Kilne, H. J., Goodman, P., Johnson, C. D. and Marano, A. J. (1969). Effects of isoproterenol on haemodynamic alterations myocardial metabolism, and coronary flow in experimental acute myocardial infarction with shock. *Am. Heart. J.*, **77,** 772

5. Mueller, H., Ayres, S. M., Gregory, J. J., Giannelli, S. and Grace, W. J. (1970). Haemodynamics, coronary blood flow, and myocardial metabolism in coronary shock; response to 1-norepinephrine and isoproterenol. *J. Clin. Invest.* **49,** 1885
6. Mueller, H., Ayres, S. M., Giannelli, S., Conklin, E. F., Mazzara, J. T. and Grace, W. J. (1972). Effect of isoproterenol, 1-norepinephrine, and intraaortic counterpulsation on haemodynamics and myocardial metabolism in shock following acute myocardial infarction. *Circulation,* **45,** 335
7. Misra, S. N. and Kezdi, P. (1973). Haemodynamic effects of adrenergic stimulating and blocking agents in cardiogenic shock and low output state after myocardial infarction. *Am. J. Cardiol.,* **31,** 724
8. Maroko, P. R., Kjekshus, J. K., Sobel, B. E., Watanabe, T., Covell, J. W., Ross, I. and Braunwald, E. (1971). Factors influencing infarct size following experimental coronary artery occlusions. *Circulation,* **43,** 67
9. Maroko, P. R., Libby, P. and Braunwald, E. (1973). Effect of pharmacologic agents on the function of the ischemic heart. *Am. J. Cardiol.,* **32,** 930
10. Vatner, S. F., McRitchie, R. J., Maroko, P. R., Patrick, T. A. and Braunwald, E. (1974). Effects of catecholamines, exercise, and nitroglycerin on the normal and ischemic myocardium in conscious dogs. *J. Clin. Invest.,* **54,** 563
11. Katz, A. M. (1973). Biochemical "defect" in the hypertrophied and failing heart. Deleterious or compensatory. *Circulation,* **47,** 1076
12. Awan, N. A., Miller, R. R., Vera, Z., Demaria, A. N., Amsterdam, E. A. and Mason, D. T. (1976). Reduction of S-T segment elevation with infusion of nitroprusside in patients with acute myocardial infarction. *Am. J. Cardiol.,* **38,** 435
13. Chatterjee, K. and Parmley, W. (1977). Vasodilator treatment for acute and chronic heart failure. *Br. Heart. J.,* **39,** 706
14. Cohn, J. N. and Franciosa, J. A. (1977). Vasodilator therapy of heart failure. *N. Engl. J. Med.,* **297,** 27–31, 254–257
15. Braunwald, E. (1977). Vasodilator therapy – a physiologic approach to the treatment of heart failure. *N. Engl. J. Med.,* **297,** 331
16. Mason, D. T. (1978). Afterload reduction and cardiac performance. Physiologic basis of systemic vasodilators as a new approach in treatment of congestive heart failure. *Am. J. Med.,* **65,** 106
17. Zelis, R., Flaim, S. F., Moskowitz, R. M. and Nellis, S. H. (1979). How much can we expect from vasodilator therapy in congestive heart failure? *Circulation,* **59,** 1092
18. Mikulic, E., Cohn, J. N. and Franciosa, J. A. (1977). Comparative haemodynamic effects of intropic and vasodilator drugs in severe heart failure. *Circulation,* **56,** 528
19. Kirk, E. S., Le Jemtel, T. H., Nelson, G. R. and Sonnenblick, E. H. (1978). Mechanisms of beneficial effects of vasodilators and inotropic stimulation in the experimental failing ischemic heart. *Am. J. Med.,* **65,** 189
20. Cohn, J. N. and Franciosa, J. A. (1978). Selection of vasodilator, inotropic or combined therapy for the management of heart failure. *Am. J. Med.* **65,** 181
21. Braunwald, E. (1971). Control of myocardial oxygen consumption. Physiologic and clinical considerations. *Am. J. Cardiol.,* **27,** 416
22. Cobbe, S. M. and Poole-Wilson, P. A. The time of onset and severity of acidosis in myocardial ischaemia. *J. Mol. Cell. Cardiol.,* (in press)
23. Buckberg, G. D., Fixler, D. E., Archie, J. P. and Hoffman, J. I. E. (1972). Experimental subendocardial ischaemia in dogs with normal coronary arteries. *Cir. Res.,* **30,** 67
24. Kirk, E. S., Urschel, C. W. and Sonnenblick, E. H. (1974). Problems in cardiac performance: regulation of coronary blood flow and the physiology of heart failure. In Guyton, A. C. and Jones, C. E. (eds.) *Cardiovascular Physiology*. Physiology Series One Vol. 1. MTP International review of science. (London: Butterworth)
25. Hoffman, J. I. E. and Buckberg, G. D. (1976). Transmural variations in myocardial

perfusion. In Yu, P. N. and Goodwin, J. F. (eds.) *Progress in Cardiology*, pp. 37–89. (Philadelphia: Lea and Febiger)

26. Sonnenblick, E. H. (1966). The mechanics of myocardial contraction. In Briller, S. A. and Conn, H. L. (eds.) *The Myocardial Cell: Structure, Function and Modification by Cardiac Drugs*, pp. 173. (Philadelphia: University of Pennsylvania Press)
27. Weber, K. T. and Janicki, J. S. (1979). The heart as a muscle-pump system and the concept of heart failure. *Am. Heart J.*, **98,** 371
28. Snyder, R., Downey, J. M. and Kirk, E. S. (1975). The active and passive components of extravascular coronary resistance. *Cardiovasc. Res.*, **9,** 161
29. Ellis, A. K. and Klocke, F. J. (1980). Effects of preload on the transmural distribution of perfusion and pressure-flow relationships in the canine coronary vascular bed. *Circ. Res.* **46,** 68
30. Panerai, R. B., Chamberlain, J. H. and Sayers, B. McA. (1979. Characterization of the extravascular component of coronary resistance by instantaneous pressure-flow relationships in the dog. *Circ. Res.* **45,** 378
31. Klocke, F. J., Ellis, A. K. and Orlick, A. E. (1980). Sympathetic influences on coronary perfusion and evolving concepts of driving pressure, resistance, and transmural flow regulation. *Anesthesiology*, **52,** 1
32. Tuttle, R. R. and Mills, J. (1975). Dobutamine – development of a new catecholamine to selectively increase cardiac contractility. *Circ. Res.*, **36,** 185
33. Robie, N. W., Nutter, D. O., Moody, C. and McNay, J. L. (1974). In vivo analysis of adrenergic receptor activity of dobutamine. *Circ. Res.*, **34,** 663
34. Bodem, R., Skelton, C. L. and Sonnenblick, E. H. (1974). Inotropic and chromotropic effects of dobutamine on isolated cardiac muscle. *Eur. J. Cardiol.*, **2,** 181
35. Lumley, P., Broadley, K. J. and Levy, G. P. (1977). Analysis of the inotropic: chromotropic selectivity of dobutamine and dopamine in anaethetised dogs and guinea-pig isolated atria. *Cardiovas. Res.* **11,** 17
36. Robie, N. W. and Goldberg, L. I. (1975). Comparative systemic and regional haemodynamic effects of dopamine and dobutamine. *Am. Heart. J.*, **90,** 340
37. Vatner, S. F., McRitchie, R. J. and Braunwald, E. (1974). Effects of dobutamine on left ventricular performance, coronary dynamics, and distribution of cardiac output in conscious dogs. *J. Clin. Invest.*, **53,** 1265
38. Beregovich, J., Bianchi, C. D'Angelo, R., Diaz, R. and Rubler, S. (1975). Haemodynamic effects of a new inotropic agent (dobutamine) in chronic cardiac failure. *Br. Heart J.*, **37,** 629
39. Akhtar, N., Mikulic, E., Cohn, J. N. and Chaudhry, M. H. (1975). Haemodynamic effect of dobutamine in patients with severe heart failure. *Am. J. Cardiol.*, **36,** 202
40. Leier, C. V., Webel, J. and Bush, C. A. (1977). The cardiovascular effects of the continuous infusion of dobutamine in patients with severe cardiac failure. *Circulation*, **56,** 468
41. Loeb, H. S., Bredakis, J. and Gunnar, R. M. (1977). Superiority of dobutamine over dopamine for augmentation of cardiac output in patients with chronic low output cardiac failure. *Circulation*, **55,** 375
42. Goldberg, L. I., Hsieh, Y. and Resnekov, L. (1977). Newer catecholamines for treatment of heart failure and shock: An update on dopamine and a first look at dobutamine. *Prog. Cardiovasc. Dis.*, **19,** 327
43. Leier, C. V., Heban, P. T., Huss, P., Bush, C. A. and Lewis, R. P. (1978). Comparative systemic and regional hemodynamic effects of dopamine and dobutamine in patients with cardiomyopathic heart failure. *Circulation*, **58,** 466
44. Sonnenblick, E. H., Frishman, W. H. and Lejemtel, T. H. (1979). Dobutamine: a new synthetic cardioactive sympathetic amine. *N. Engl. J. Med.*, **330,** 17

45. Jewitt, D., Birkhead, J., Mitchell, A. and Dollery, C. (1974). Clinical cardiovascular pharmacology of dobutamine; a selective inotropic catecholamine. *Lancet*, **2**, 363
46. Kersting, F., Follath, F., Moulds, R., Mucklow, J., McCloy, R., Sheares, J. and Dollery, C. (1976). A comparison of cardiovascular effects of dobutamine and isoprenaline after open heart surgery. *Br. Heart J.*, **38**, 622
47. Lewis, G. R. J., Poole-Wilson, P. A., Angerpointer, T. A. Farnsworth, A. E., Williams, B. T. and Coltart, D. J. (1978). Measurement of the circulatory effects of dobutamine, a new inotropic agent, in patients following cardiac surgery. *Am. Heart J.*, **95**, 301
48. Willerson, J. T., Hutton, I., Watson, J. T., Platt, M. R. and Templeton, G. H. (1976). Influences of dobutamine on regional myocardial blood flow and ventricular performances during acute and chronic myocardial ischemia in dogs. *Circulation*, **53**, 828
49. Tuttle, R. R. Pollock, G. D., Todd, G., MacDonald, B., Tust, R. and Dusenberry, W. (1977). The effect of dobutamine on cardiac oxygen balance, regional blood flow, and infarction severity after coronary artery narrowing in dogs. *Circ. Res.* **41**, 357
50. Meyer, S. L., Curry, G. C., Donsky, M. S., Twieg, D. B., Parkey, R. W. and Willerson, J. T. (1976). Influence of dobutamine on hemodynamics and coronary blood flow in patients with and without coronary artery disease. *Am. J. Cardiol.* **38**, 103
51. Gillespie, T. A., Ambos, H. D., Sobel, B. E. and Roberts, R. (1977). Effects of dobutamine in patients with acute myocardial infarction. *Am. J. Cardiol.*, **39**, 588
52. Sakamoto, T., Yamada, T. (1972). Hemodynamic effects of dobutamine in patients following open heart surgery. *Circulation*, **55**, 525
53. Steen, P. A., Tinker, J. H., Pluth, J. R., Barnhorst, D. A. and Tarhan, S. (1978). Efficiency of dopamine, dobutamine and epinephrine during emergence from cardiopulmonary bypass in man. *Circulation*, **57**, 378
54. Goldberg, L. I. (1972). Cardiovascular and renal actions of dopamine: potential clinical applications. *Pharmacol. Rev.*, **24**, 1
55. Goldberg, L. I. (1974). Dopamine: clinical uses of an endogenous catecholamine. *N. Eng. J. Med.*, **291**, 707
56. Schmidt, H. D., Hoppe, H. and Heidenreich, L. (1979). Direct effects of dopamine, orciprenaline and norepinephrine on the right and left ventricle of isolated canine hearts. *Cardiology*, **64**, 133
57. McDonald, R. H., Goldberg, L. I., McNay, J. L. Tuttle, E. P. (1964). Effects of dopamine in man: augmentation of sodium excretion, glomerular filtration rate, and renal plasma flow. *J. Clin. Invest.*, **43**, 1116
58. Hollenberg, N. K. and Adams, D. F., Mendell, P., Abrams, H. L. and Merrill, J. P. (1973). Renal vascular responses to dopamine: haemodynamic and angiogrophic observations in normal man. *Clin. Sci. Mol. Med.*, **45**, 733
59. Hardaker, W. T. and Wechsler, A. S. (1973). Redistribution of renal intracortical blood flow during dopamine infusion in dogs. *Circ. Res.*, **33**, 437
60. Goldberg, L. I., McDonald, R. H. Jr. and Zimmerman, A. M. (1963). Sodium diuresis produced by dopamine in patients with congestive heart failure. *N. Engl. J. Med.*, **269**, 1060
61. Rosenblum, R., Tai, A. R. and Lawson, D. (1972). Dopamine in man. Cardiorenal hemodynamics in normotensive patients with heart disease. *J. Pharmacol. Exp. Ther.*, **183**, 256
62. Stoner, J. D., Bolen, J. L. and Harrison, D. C. (1977). Comparison of dobutamine and dopamine in treatment of severe heart failure. *Br. Heart J.*, **39**, 536
63. White, D. H., Crawford, M. H. and O'Rourke, R. A. (1979). Beneficial effects of prolonged low dose dopamine in hospitalized patients with severe refractory heart failure. *Clin. Cardiol.* **2**, 135
64. Maccannell, K. L., McNay, J. L., Meyer, M. B. and Goldberg, L. I. (1966). Dopamine

in the treatment of hypotension and shock. *N. Engl. J. Med.*, **275**, 1389
65. Talley, R. C., Goldberg, L. I., Johnson, C. E. and McNay, J. L. (1969). A hemodynamic comparison of dopamine and isoproterenol in patients in shock. *Circulation*, **39**, 361
66. Loeb, H. S., Winslow, E. B. J., Rahimtoola, S. H., Rosen, K. M. and Gunnar, R. M. (1971). Acute haemodynamic effects of dopamine in patients with shock. *Circulation*, **44**, 163
67. Holzer, J., Karliner, J. S., O'Rourke, R. A., Pitt, W. and Ross, J. (1973). Effectiveness of dopamine in patients with cardiogenic shock. *Am. J. Cardiol.*, **32**, 79
68. Brooks, H. L., Stein, P. D., Matson, J. L. and Hyland, J. W. (1969). Dopamine-induced alterations in coronary hemodynamics in dogs. *Circ. Res.* **24**, 699
69. Cobb, F. R., McHale, P. A., Bache, R. J. and Greenfield, J. C. (1972). Coronary and systemic hemodynamic effects of dopamine in the awake dog. *Am. J. Physiol.*, **222**, 1355
70. Lekven, J. and Semb, G. (1974). Effect of dopamine and calcium on lipolysis and myocardial ischemic injury following acute coronary occlusion in the dog. *Circ. Res.*, **34**, 349
71. Crexells, C., Bourassa, M. G. and Biron, P. (1973). Effects of dopamine on myocardial metabolism in patients with ischaemic heart disease. *Cardiovasc. Res.*, **7**, 438
72. Mueller, H. S., Evans, R. and Ayres, S. M. (1978). Effect of dopamine on hemodynamics and myocardial metabolism in shock following acute myocardial infarction in man. *Circulation*, **57**, 361
73. Warrell, D. A., Robertson, D. G., Newton Howes, J., Connolly, M. E., Paterson, J. W., Beilin, L. J. and Dollery, C. T. (1970). Comparison of cardiorespiratory effects of isoprenaline and salbutamol in patients with bronchial asthma. *Br. Med. J.*, **1**, 65
74. Poole-Wilson, P. A., Lewis, G., Angerpointer, T., Malcolm, A. D. and Williams, B. T. (1977). Haemodynamic effects of salbutamol and nitroprusside after cardiac surgery. *Br. Heart. J.*, **39**, 721
75. Sharma. B. and Goodwin, J. F. (1977). Beneficial effect of salbutamol on cardiac function in severe congestive cardiomyopathy: effect on systolic and diastolic function of the left ventricle.
76. Bourdillon, P. D. V., Dawson, J. R., Foale, R. A., Timmis, A. D., Poole-Wilson, P. A. and Sutton, G. C. (1980). Salbutamol in the treatment of heart failure. *Br. Heart J.*, **43**, 206
77. Stephens, J. D., Banim, S. O. and Spurrell, R. A. J. (1980). Haemodynamic effects of salbutamol alone and in combination with sublingual isosorbide dinitrate in patients with severe congestive cardiac failure. *Br. Heart J.*, **43**, 220
78. Fowler, M. B., Timmis, A. D. and Chamberlain, D. A. (1980). Synergistic effects of a combined salbutamol-nitroprusside regression in acute myocardial infarction and severe left ventricular failure. *Br. Med. J.*, **2**, 435
79. Timmis, A. D., Strak, S. K. and Chamberlain, D. A. (1979). Haemodynamic effects of salbutamol in patients with acute myocardial infarction and severe left ventricular dysfunction. *Br. Med. J.*, **2**, 1101
80. Dawson, J. R., Poole-Wilson, P. A. and Sutton, G. C. (1980). Salbutamol in cardiogenic shock complicating acute myocardial infarction. *Br. Heart J.*, (In press)
81. Yacoub, M. H. and Boyland, E. (1973). Cardiovascular effects of intravenous salbutamol after open heart operations. *Lancet*, **1**, 1260
82. Wyse, S. D., Gibson, D. G. and Branthwaite, M. A. (1974). Haemodynamic effects of salbutamol in patients needing circulatory support after open-heart surgery. *Br. Med. J.*, **3**, 502
83. Kho, T. L. (1979). The comparative cardiovascular effect of dopamine and

dobutamine in patients with myocardial infarction and with no cardiac output. *J. Drug Res.*, **4,** (Special Issue June 1979) p. 45

84. Stephenson, L. W., Edmunds, L. H., Raphaely, R., Morrison, D. F., Hoffman, W. S. and Rubis, L. J. (1979). Effects of nitroprusside and dopamine on pulmonary arterial vasculature in children after cardiac surgery. *Circulation*, **60,** I104–I110
85. Miller, R. R., Awan, N. A., Joye, J. A., Maxwell, K. S., DeMaria, A. N., Amsterdam, E. A. and Mason, D. T. (1977). Combined dopamine and nitroprusside therapy in congestive heart failure. *Circulation*, **55,** 881
86. Stemple, D. R., Kleiman, J. H. and Harrison, D. C. (1978). Combined nitroprusside dopamine therapy in severe chronic congestive heart failure. *Am. J. Cardiol.*, **42,** 267
87. Hess, W. Klein, W., Mueller-Busch, C. and Tarnow, J. (1979). Haemodynamic effects of dopamine and dopamine combined with nitroglycerin in patients subjected to coronary bypass surgery. *Br. J. Anaesth.*, **51,** (11) 1063
88. Stephens, J., Dymond, D. and Spurrell, R. (1978). Enhancement by isosorbide dinitrate of haemodynamic effects of dopamine in chronic congestive cardiac failure. *Br. Heart J.*, **40,** 838
89. Powles, A. C. P. (1978). Chlorpromazine and dopamine in shock. *Chest*, **74,** 319
90. Stephenson, L. W., Blackstone, E. H. and Kouchoukos, N. T. Dopamine vs epinephrine in patients following cardiac surgery: randomized study. *Surg. Forum*, **27,** 272
91. Rosenblum, R. and Frieden, J. (1972). Intravenous dopamine in the treatment of myocardial dysfunction after open-heart surgery. *Am. Heart J.*, **83,** 743
92. Holloway, E. L., Stinson, E. B., Derby, G. C. and Harrison, D. C. (1975). Action of drugs in patients early after cardiac surgery. I. Comparison of isoproterenol and dopamine. *Am. J. Cardiol.*, **35,** 656

33
Which electrolytes matter?

EUNICE LOCKEY

No-one would debate the need to correct a very low or a very high plasma potassium or a profound metabolic acidosis. Many problems in heart surgery are iatrogenic, however, and many can be prevented. The aim of this talk is to show how laboratory tests can be used to foresee and forestall problems and thus make cardiac surgery safer.

Nothing can replace being with the patient and using the human powers of critical observation, reasoning and common sense. The increasing use of computers and self-calibrating instruments has caused some workers to ascribe a degree of infallibility to these machines that is not justified. Any instrument can go wrong and the more sophisticated the instrument the less obvious this may be. Equally, the sample presented to the instrument may be faulty. Potassium measurement done by ion-selective electrode instruments measures the potassium in whole blood. This is very convenient and easy, but as there is no stage where the plasma is separated and looked at, haemolysis of the blood occurring after it has been drawn from the patient will not be noted, and a 'normal' answer may in fact mask a dangerously low one.

When grotesque plasma values are reported, we immediately repeat the test on a fresh sample. If the reported value is pleasing to us because it fits our preconceptions or is within the normal range, we accept it. Equally then, we must accept the slightly unusual answer and seek to explain it. It is such 'funny' values that may give us the first indication that some problem is present and enable us to short circuit it or prevent it from becoming serious. Equally, if we note patients at particular risk and monitor them carefully, we may prevent a problem arising.

Taking plasma potassium as an example, patients at particular risk of low levels are those who have had prolonged diuretic therapy; whose circulation has been much improved by surgery so that cells are repleting themselves with potassium; when an acidotic state is corrected, since alkalosis or even a relative alkalosis will put potassium into the cells; and when a lot of glucose is being given, since this similarly will move potassium into the cells. A profound diuresis after surgery may deplete the patient of potassium and is best avoided, but one must never make the assumption that a large urine volume contains a lot of potassium. This may not be so. Even if a lot of potassium is present in the urine remember that some of this comes from the dead and dying cells of the wounds to which it can never be returned. If perfusion is inadequate even grossly depleted cells will not accept potassium. If perfusion becomes a little less good, potassium will leak into the plasma and an iatrogenic cardiac arrest may result. High plasma potassium levels must be watched for, particularly in low cardiac output states therefore, and also in patients with renal insufficiency.

If we get an unexpectedly raised, but valid, level what should we consider? First, has the potassium supplement really been stopped, or are we giving 'hidden' supplements by transfusing old blood, injecting potassium penicillin etc. Second, is there a hidden extravasation of blood under the sternum or in the gut, or is the patient in non-oliguric renal failure. The latter patients are at particular risk after leaving the intensive care unit because the presence of a reasonable volume of urine may cause us, quite wrongly, to assume that the quality is also good.

Unexpectedly raised blood ureas are also good indicators of potential problems. Again, hidden extravasations of blood and non-oliguric failure must be considered. If both of these are excluded then the finding of a raised blood urea in the presence of urine containing a high concentration of urea, should suggest dehydration. Clinical dehydration can be very difficult to detect in heart surgery patients and many of the other standard biochemical parameters are unusable. The plasma proteins are diluted by the aqueous prime now commonly used; the red cells damaged by the pump disappear; and a hypokalaemic alkalosis may be present. Plasma sodium and chloride may not be particularly raised, especially if the patient was in severe heart failure before surgery. Thus the concerted rise in sodium, potassium, chloride, urea, proteins and haematocrit, seen in classical dehydration may be seen only as a plasma urea which is rather greater than expected in view of good urine urea concentration.

In oliguric states it is important to decide as soon as possible whether it is renal or pre-renal in origin. Examination of the urine before diuretics are given may bias one in a particular direction. In general, pre-renal causes produce urine of normal urea and potassium concentration, but low sodium content. Renal lesions, however, produce urines with low urea and potassium levels but raised sodium concentration. There is infinite gradation between the two of course, but measuring the sodium, potassium and urea in the urine may be of great diagnostic help and most certainly gives much more information than just measuring osmolality, since in urine, sodium and urea are major components (Table 1).

Plasma osmolality on the other hand is mainly due to sodium and chloride. Abnormally high urea and glucose levels will make a significant contribution, but normally these account for only about 10 mmol/kg out of a total of about 290. Unnatural compounds such as mannitol may make a significant contribution if they cannot be excreted by the kidney and in very small children too much contrast media may cause such profound hyperosmolar states that death ensues (Table 2).

Small children are also at particular risk from hypoglycaemia. They have

Table 1 Urine (illustrative values)

	Health	*Heart failure*	*Renal failure*
Na^+ mmol/l	80–160	0–10	30–100
Urea mmol/l	150–400	150–400	50–200

Table 2

Osmolalities	*(approximate)*
$NaHCO_3$ 8.4%	1800 mmol/kg
Dextrose 10%	650 mmol/kg
Dextrose 50%	3300 mmol/kg
Mannitol 25%	1500 mmol/kg
Conray 420	2100 mmol/kg

very small glycogen stores and if post-operatively they are in need of massive catechol-amine support these stores will quickly be exhausted. A constant check on the blood sugar levels in such situations will prevent fatal hypoglycaemia.

Finally, how one states a problem can have a profound effect on one's reaction to it. Jaundice appearing very soon after open heart surgery is almost always of the intrahepatic cholestatic type. The patient may have a very high bilirubin and be very yellow, but it is not a dangerous condition and he is not in liver failure. The defect is only in excreting bile and will resolve. If a term such as liver failure is used, however, steroids and neomycin are also likely to be used and apart from being unnecessary they may cause problems.

In conclusion, one must always remember that however abnormal the plasma chemistry may be, the patient is alive, if not well, and that these values may reflect the compensating mechanisms that are ensuring his survival. Conversely, normal plasma chemistry may be seen in patients whose whole body values are grossly abnormal.

What is certain is that a dead patient in electrolyte balance is infinitely worse off than a living patient in a biochemical mess. The art is in deciding which biochemical abnormalities need treatment and which are best ignored and in always trying to identify the patients at risk and wherever possible preventing a problem from arising.

34
Some applications of computers in postoperative care

S. RAO AND D. B. LONGMORE

INTRODUCTION

In the last two decades some advances have been made in the application of computers in medicine, although, overall, the application of computers has been disappointingly slow because of the problems of programming. The first mass-produced systems tended to be data-base systems which were expensive in terms of both money and man-power. These cumbersome systems were in the main confined to large hospitals for the storage and retrieval of patient data, storage and distribution of pathology data and for hospital administration needs. The subsequent availability of miniature electronic solid state components, particularly memories, meant that mini-computers could perform dedicated tasks at an economic cost and were ideally suited to the tasks of monitoring in intensive care. More recently, the sudden boom in microprocessor technology has meant that many of the computing tasks can now be performed at the bedside and hence the computer need no longer remain remote from the users, i.e. the clinicians and the staff. Although a wide variety of mini and micro-computer systems are available, their use in the post-operative care of cardiac patients in intensive care units is still not accepted as routine. There are several reasons for this. It is proposed in this paper to outline some of the problems involved in the use of computers for this purpose and to discuss a system which has been set up at the National Heart Hospital to aid patient management.

THE PRESENT STATUS OF PATIENT MONITORING AND ITS LIMITATIONS

The main objective in patient monitoring is to aid the clinician's assessment of the patient's condition so that he can make the appropriate therapeutic decisions based on the best possible information. In the case of patients who have undergone open-heart surgery, the 8 hour period immediately following surgery is very important and one during which all the vital systems try to attain stable conditions. An ideal patient monitoring system should not only give information about these essential physiological sub-systems but should also indicate the future trend of these systems. This is the philosophy behind the design of the system at the National Heart Hospital. The monitoring system should also be sufficiently sensitive to rfspond rapidly to any changes in the patient's condition and to give timely warning of any impending catastrophe.

In most intensive care units, the physiological variables monitored as trends are: systolic and diastolic values of arterial blood pressure, central venous pressure, left atrial pressure, central and peripheral temperatures. These are plotted at 15 minute intervals with other parameters, such as urine output, blood loss, the amount of blood given to the patient, recorded hourly. Respiratory function, such as ventilator settings and blood gases, concentrations of potassium etc. may also be measured usually when indicated by the clinical situation. Apart from these trends which are plotted on a chart, there are dynamic displays on the oscilloscopes of the blood pressure waveform and electrocardiogram.

As far as trend prediction is concerned, this is made visually from stored information. This procedure is satisfactory once a particular trend has been established, but when the patient has just been admitted to the Intensive Care Unit, there is very little information on which to draw. Apart from the drawback of relying on trends of indirect variables, such as using arterial systolic pressure as an index of cardiac output or the more general performance of the heart, important changes in cardiac rhythm can often be missed. At this stage the nurse is busy attending to the patient and connecting the pressure lines and drains etc. A computer system, because of its capability of processing information virtually instantaneously is ideally suited to carry out the monitoring functions automatically so that trends can be established quickly and constantly updated. Computer systems which accurately perform the function of automatic data acquisition can now be bought 'off the shelf' but at considerable cost. Such a system has been in routine use at the Medical Centre of the University of Alabama, Birmingham, USA[1] for more than 10 years.

AN INTEGRATED APPROACH INVOLVING NEW CONCEPTS IN DIAGNOSTIC TECHNIQUES

The previous section dealt with how computers are performing tasks and automatically producing trend records. However, one of the attractive features of a computer system is that because of its spread of processing data, it is capable of carrying out several tasks simultaneously. The first and the most obvious extension to the existing system is to use the computer to analyse physiological signals and to derive or extract from them more significant information. That is, firstly, to use techniques which involve mathematical methods on the dynamic information contained in the original signal and to obtain from the signal processing quantitative information about the patient's condition. Secondly, to use non-invasive methods to obtain information about the mechanical performance of the heart itself. A computer system has been set up at the National Heart Hospital which performs these functions as well as providing the traditional trend records.

SYSTEM DESIGN AND IMPLEMENTATION

Figure 1 is a diagram of the computer system and its peripheral devices. The computer itself consists of a 16-bit word Central Processing Unit with 24K electronic memory. This communicates with a double-disk drive with ample storage capacity of several mega bytes. Long-term storage of data can be accomplished, using the 7-track magnetic tape unit. The analogue-to-digital converter is fully programmable and software-controlled. The electrocardiogram goes through a specially built preprocessing unit which provides a timing pulse for each R-wave and all analyses use this timing pulse. The line printer (STATOS 31 series) operates electrostatically and in addition to the normal functions of a line printer, can be used to generate graphs. The operating system allows for two visual display units which can be used simultaneously. The main terminal is kept in the computer room while the second unit is stationed at the bedside. A special feature of this system is that drug dose rates also are automatically monitored. A special unit which interfaces directly with MVO Tekmar drip pumps has been designed and built. The operating system by which the user can communicate with the computer is called the Beta system. It is in effect a supervisory program, also referred to as an executive or real time executive program specifically designed for small systems. Beta contains routines which simplify the programming and use of peripheral devices such as the STATOS printer and colour television units. All the application programs for patient monitoring have been specially written in Fortran and assembler languages.

Starting the on-line suite of monitoring programs necessitates the opening of an index called POSTOP TREND. Two further indices are required for the creation of a unique file for each patient. Firstly, all information in the form of text, such as the name, age, sex and operation details, are contained in a file referenced by POSTOP TREND/TEXT, and all data resulting from the analysis of physiological signals are entered in a data file referenced by POSTOP TREND/DATA.

Finally, a response to the input 'Hospital number of the patient?' creates unique data and text files for a particular patient. The creation of such a file reserves enough space on disk corresponding to twelve hours of continuous trend recording, where the data is contained in a 19 × 96 data matrix. After the first 4 hours, the set of data relevant to this period is transferred to the permanent file and thereafter data transfer takes place automatically every 2 hours. Very few of the centres with an on-line monitoring facility store their data permanently and do not produce trends graphically on plotters. This is a reflection of the limited space available on disk and for a financial need to

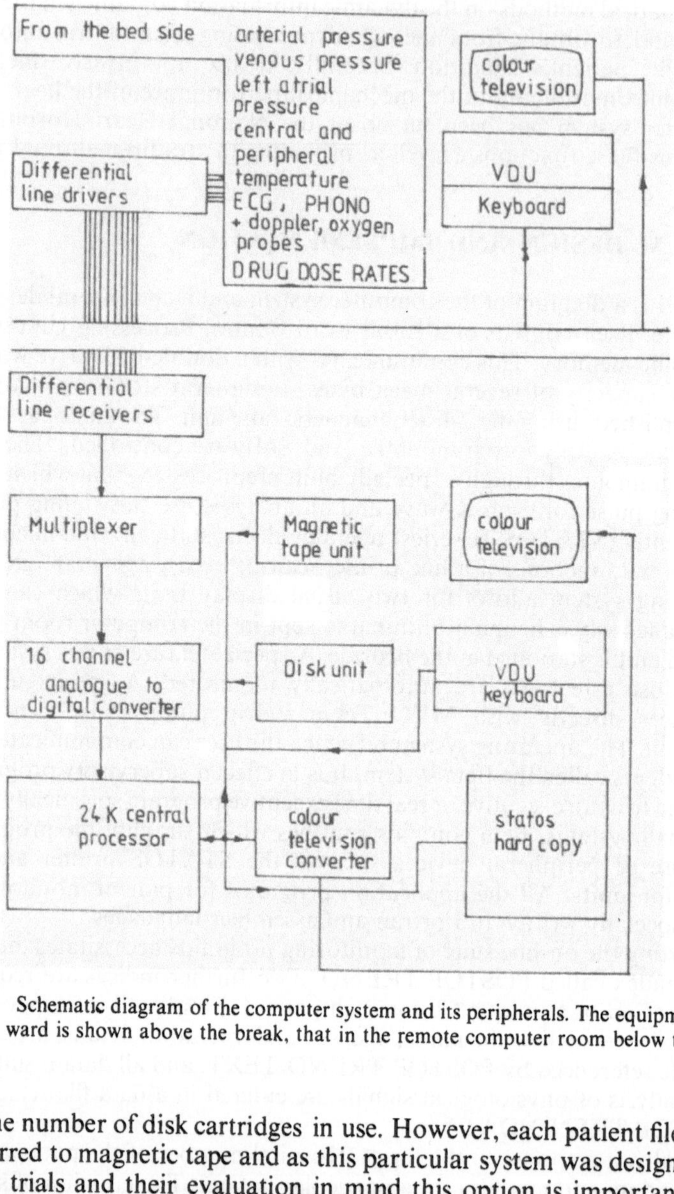

Figure 1 Schematic diagram of the computer system and its peripherals. The equipment in the recovery ward is shown above the break, that in the remote computer room below the break

limit the number of disk cartridges in use. However, each patient file can be transferred to magnetic tape and as this particular system was designed with clinical trials and their evaluation in mind this option is important in the retrospective statistical analysis of patient data.

Once the monitoring software has been set in motion, the whole process of signal analysis, data acquisition, storage and retrieval for display as trends on the colour television monitors is completely automatic. The use of the visual display unit by the bedside allows off-line entry of biochemical results from blood gas measurements, sodium and potassium levels, blood loss through the drainage tubes, the amount of urine produced and the amount of fluid given to the patient. These results are tabulated on the bedside display monitors and are readily available for examination. One further use for the bedside visual display unit is as a teaching device. As mentioned previously, this system is designed basically for the evaluation of diagnostic techniques and the derivation of new diagnostic indices. Therefore all such analyses are explained on the visual display unit so that the clinicians and nurses are aware of the nature of data being displayed on the television monitor screen. In fact, the television monitor itself is used as a teaching device by demonstrating exactly how the physiological signals are being analysed by showing intermediate steps in the analysis. Only 12 hour trends are stored in a permanent form as the most crucial period of recovery occurs during this period. However, the on-line monitoring proceeds indefinitely, giving reliable and accurate results over a long period, subject only to the freedom of the signals from random noise. The colour trends on the television screen are of 4 hours duration with the trends being updated every 2 hours. The most recent 2 hours of trend recordings are therefore always on display. Finally, all the information stored in a particular patient file can be printed on to paper. Although 12 hour trends are shown, any interval of time can be chosen for the examination of particular events. For example, a 1 hour period of instability can be plotted separately for special examination if the clinician requires it. Figure 2 shows some of the special software features which control the various peripheral devices in an integrated manner.

SYSTEM PERFORMANCE

Figure 3 shows typical 12 hour trends of haemodynamic variables obtained by computer analysis. Table 1 shows a computer printout of data that are entered manually from the laboratory. An example of a derived parameter from the blood pressure signal is the endomyocardial viability ratio[2]. A common occurrence in patients who have undergone coronary bypass graft surgery is sub-endocardial ischaemia. One cannot rely on systemic arterial and central venous pressure monitoring as sufficient evidence to indicate decreased sub-endocardial blood volume, which in turn could lead to a state of low cardiac output state. It has been shown that the myocardial oxygen requirements in the resting state relate to the area under the systolic part of the pressure curve and this area can be denoted as the time tension index (TTI). The amount of coronary flow available is directly related to the area below the diastolic part of the pressure curve, taking into account the left atrial pressure component (diastolic pressure time index) (DPTI). Figures 4 and 5 show beat-by-beat analysis of the ratio of DPTI and TTI. The general tendency is for an increase in this value as the patient recovers but little importance can be attached to the actual values.

Probably the most important measurements which are needed are those relating to cardiac output and general performance. These can be obtained in theory by several techniques[3]. Transcutaneous aortovelography is a very simple non-invasive method which can provide important information

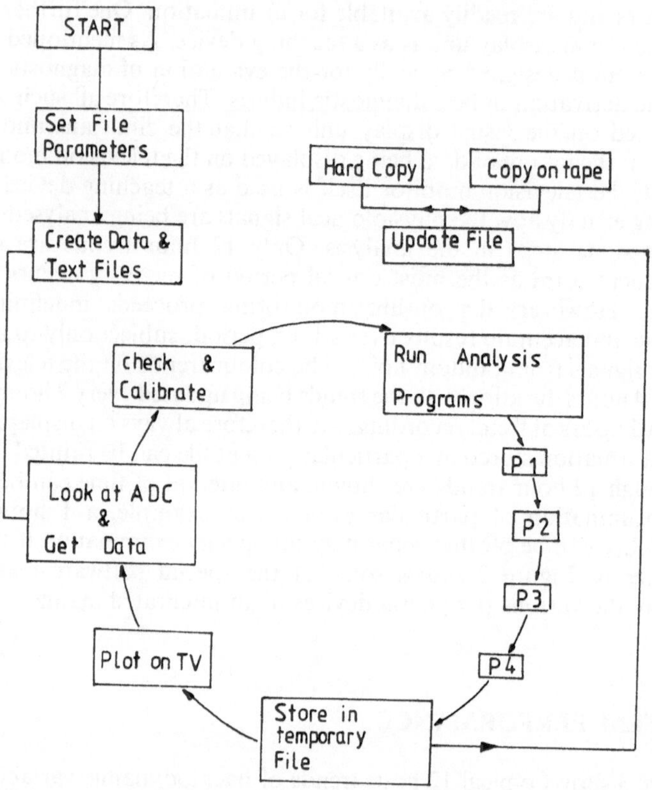

Figure 2 Block diagram showing how the software is organised so that data is collected, analysed and plotted continuously on the TV monitor

regarding blood flow from the heart, and the technique is currently undergoing evaluation using the computer system. Another possible application of the computer in intensive care is in the use of non-invasive diagnostic methods and signal analysis techniques. It has been postulated Longmore and Bass (unpublished results) that when the left ventricle is undergoing isometric contraction the resulting frequencies generated, i.e. in the first heart sound, are related to the tension in the left ventricle. They measured these by a manual technique and were able to confirm that there was a correlation. Hughes (unpublished results), using the same model applied a hopping fast Fourier transformation technique to derive estimates of the component frequencies and found good correlation with the rate of rise of left ventricular pressure recorded simultaneously as the first heart sound. The possible clinical applications of this method of characterising left ventricular function is currently being evaluated. Figure 6 shows the frequency/time plot below the left ventricular pressure which was obtained by analysis of the first heart sound shown on the top.

Table 1 An example of the computer system's off-line facility is shown. Blood gas results and fluid balance data are entered into the patient's file by using the second terminal in intensive care. As the level of potassium is a very important parameter to measure on patients in recovery, its value is also entered into the file.

BLOOD BALANCE/URINE OUTPUT

DATE:23.08.79
PATIENT'S NAME:WEST

TIME	HOURLY BLOOD DRAINAGE (TOTAL)	BLOOD IN	BALANCE	URINE OUTPUT (HOURLY)
4.00	430.0	2650.0	2220.0	20.0
5.00	460.0	2650.0	2190.0	60.0
6.00	470.0	2650.0	2180.0	450.0
6.00	470.0	2650.0	2180.0	500.0
8.00	480.0	2650.0	2170.0	140.0
9.00	500.0	2650.0	2150.0	200.0
10.00	510.0	2650.0	2140.0	140.0
11.00	520.0	2650.0	2130.0	50.0
12.00	520.0	2650.0	2130.0	50.0

...ALL BLOOD VOLUMES AND URINE OUTPUT ARE MEASURED IN MILLILITRES...

BLOOD GAS ANALYSIS RESULTS

DATE:23.08.79
PATIENT'S NAME:WEST

TIME	PO2	PCO2	PH	BE	SB	K+
17.30	111.0	32.0	7.4	-5.0	21.0	2.8
18.30	126.0	31.0	7.4	-6.0	20.5	3.4
21.00	119.0	30.0	7.5	-1.0	24.0	4.0
23.00	77.0	28.0	7.5	0.0	25.0	3.9

CONCLUSION

A mini-computer system has been set up in the intensive care unit at the National Heart Hospital. It has three main functions, the first of which is the automatic acquisition of traditional physiological variables in trend form. Secondly, it provides parameters which are derived from the dynamic sequel on-line as well as monitoring drug dose rates automatically. Thirdly, it is used to evaluate the information provided by non-invasive diagnostic techniques and to present all the results as trends on a colour television unit. The clinician thus has a wide variety of information about the patient's condition. Recently microcomputer-based information systems have become cheaper and easy to use since post-operative care does not end in intensive care, the long-term follow-up of patients is very important. The computer can play an important role in the statistical analysis of this follow-up data. In addition, it provides the opportunity to analyse data not only from the individual patient aspect but for research purposes in relation to the study of disease and assessment of the efficacy of therapeutic measures.

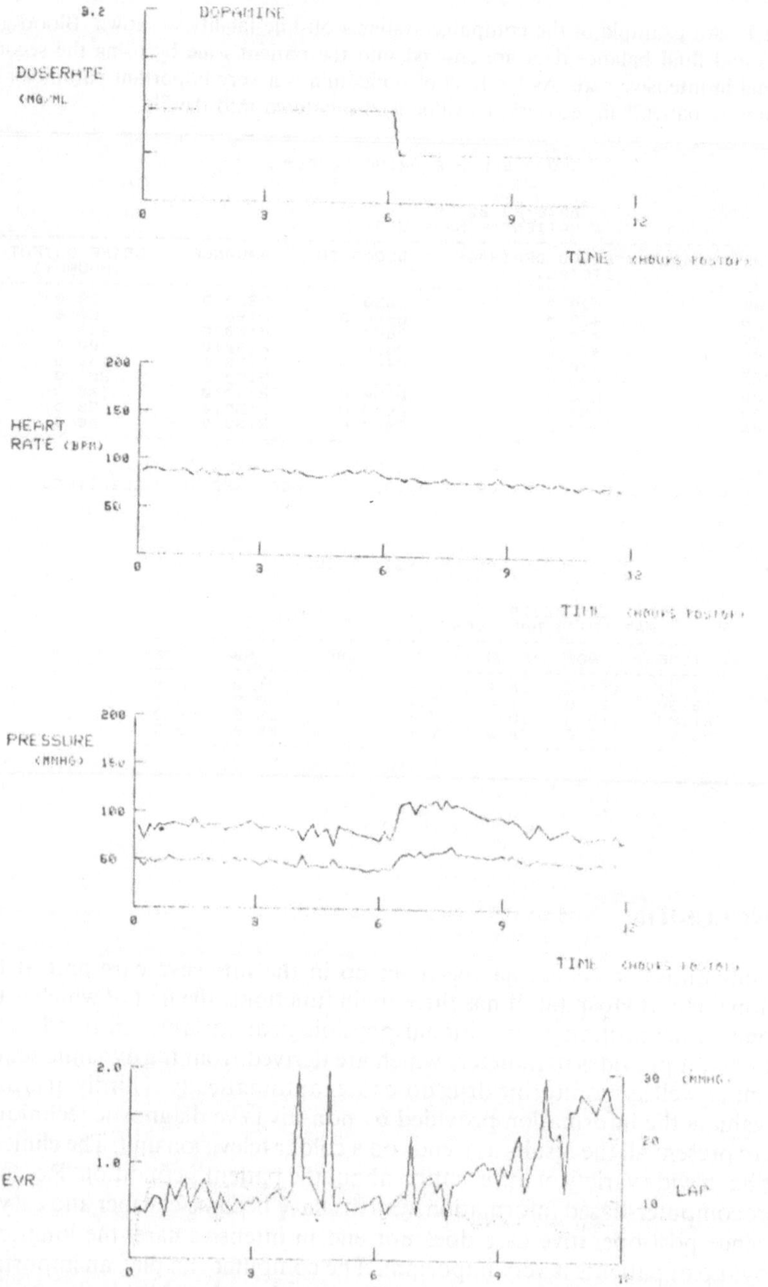

Figure 3 Consists of twelve hour trend plots of the heart rate, systolic and diastolic blood pressures and the endomyocardial viability ratio. The system also monitors drug dose rates so that the response can be seen at once in the patient when the dopamine doserate was halved. The blood pressure rose immediately and the EVR 'shows a steady increase from that time

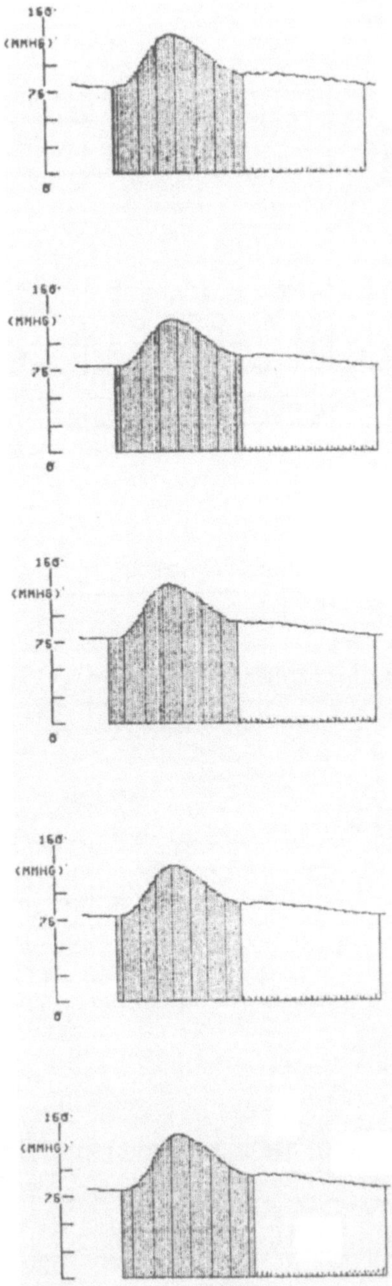

HEART	RATE	92
PRESSURE	SYSTOLIC	127
	DIASTOLIC	80
	TTI	29
	DPTI	22
	EVR	75

HEART	RATE	92
PRESSURE	SYSTOLIC	120
	DIASTOLIC	78
	TTI	27
	DPTI	23
	EVR	86

HEART	RATE	98
PRESSURE	SYSTOLIC	128
	DIASTOLIC	80
	TTI	29
	DPTI	25
	EVR	88

HEART	RATE	94
PRESSURE	SYSTOLIC	124
	DIASTOLIC	79
	TTI	28
	DPTI	25
	EVR	88

HEART	RATE	92
PRESSURE	SYSTOLIC	131
	DIASTOLIC	82
	TTI	30
	DPTI	24
	EVR	78

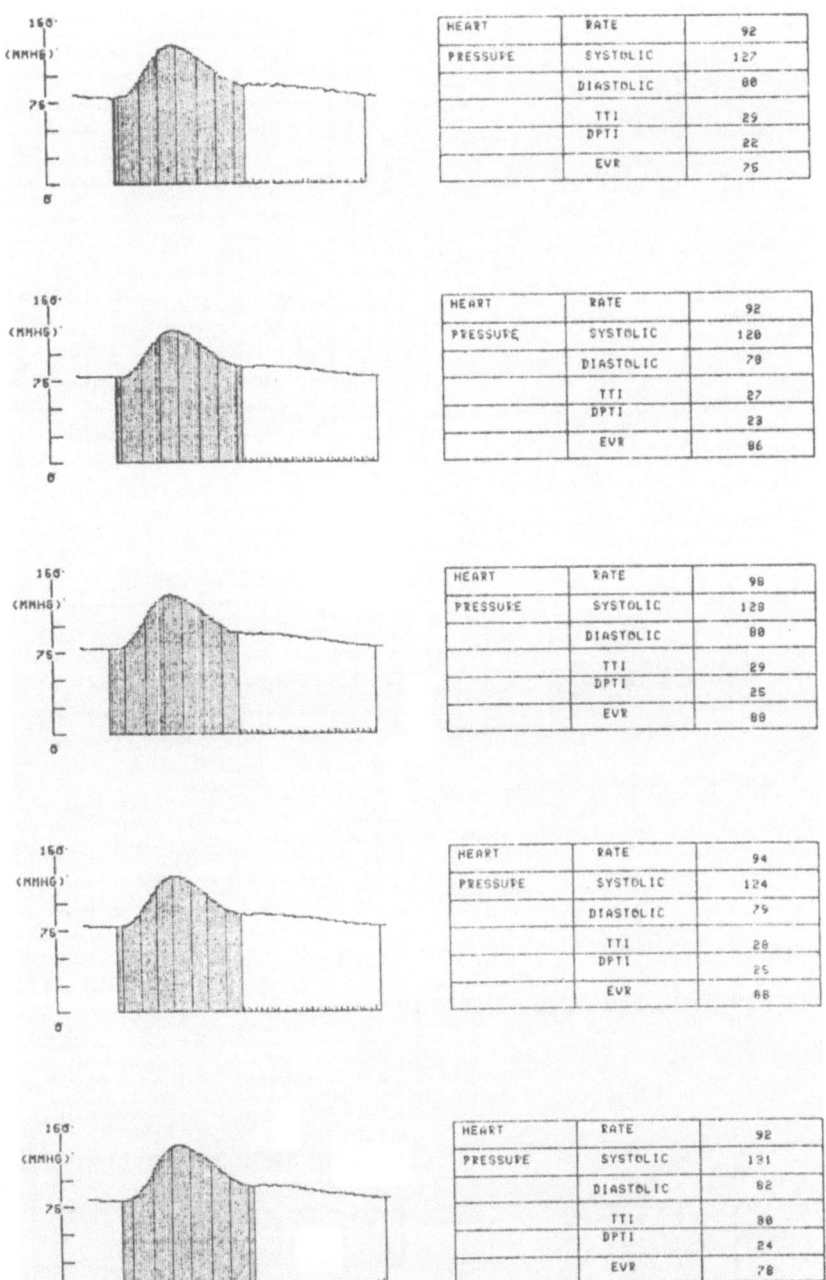

Figure 4 Plots of five consecutive pressure pulses analysed on-line, showing how the time tension index (TTI), diastolic pressure time index (DPTI) and the ratio (DPTI/TTI). The latter is called the endomyocardial viability ratio (EVR).

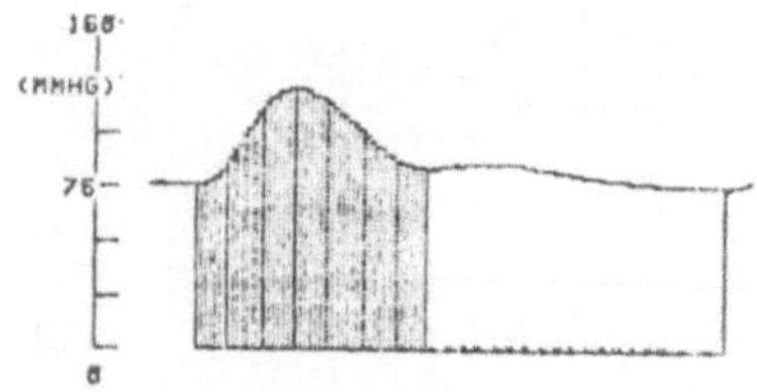

HEART	RATE	92
PRESSURE	SYSTOLIC	120
	DIASTOLIC	76
	TTI	25
	DPTI	26
	EVR	101

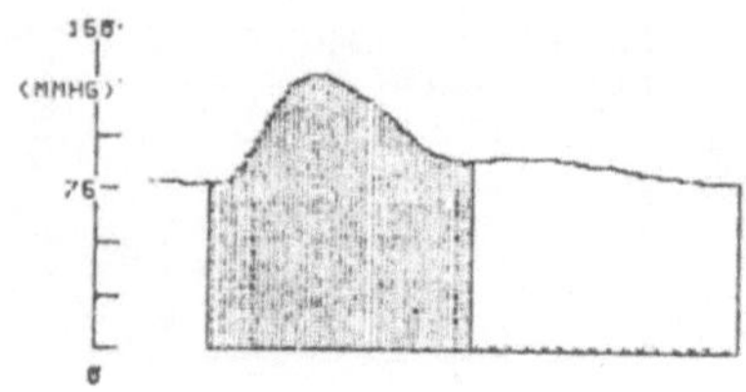

HEART	RATE	92
PRESSURE	SYSTOLIC	128
	DIASTOLIC	80
	TTI	28
	DPTI	23
	EVR	79

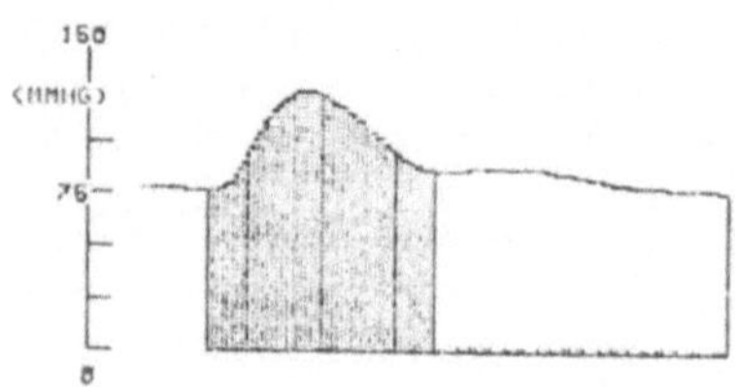

HEART	RATE	92
PRESSURE	SYSTOLIC	123
	DIASTOLIC	76
	TTI	25
	DPTI	25
	EVR	100

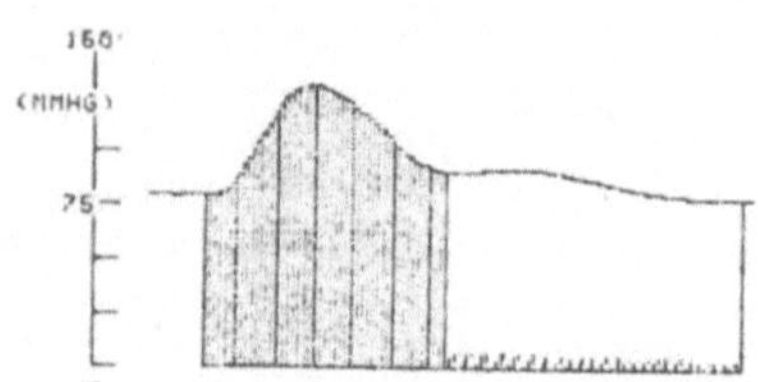

HEART	RATE	94
PRESSURE	SYSTOLIC	129
	DIASTOLIC	79
	TTI	28
	DPTI	25
	EVR	91

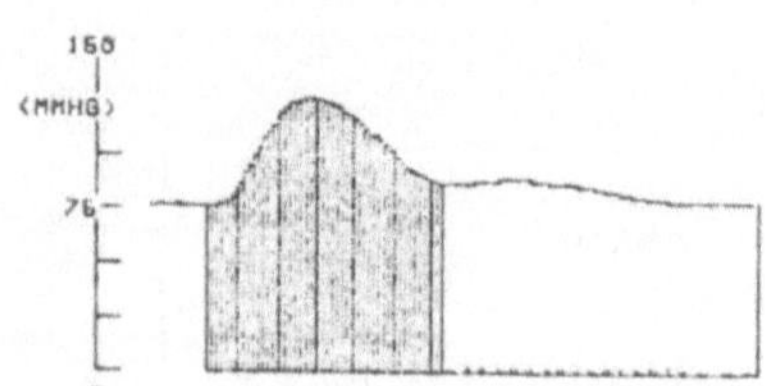

HEART	RATE	92
PRESSURE	SYSTOLIC	126
	DIASTOLIC	78
	TTI	26
	DPTI	28
	EVR	106

Figure 5 Five consecutive beat by beat analysis repeated two hours later on the same patient

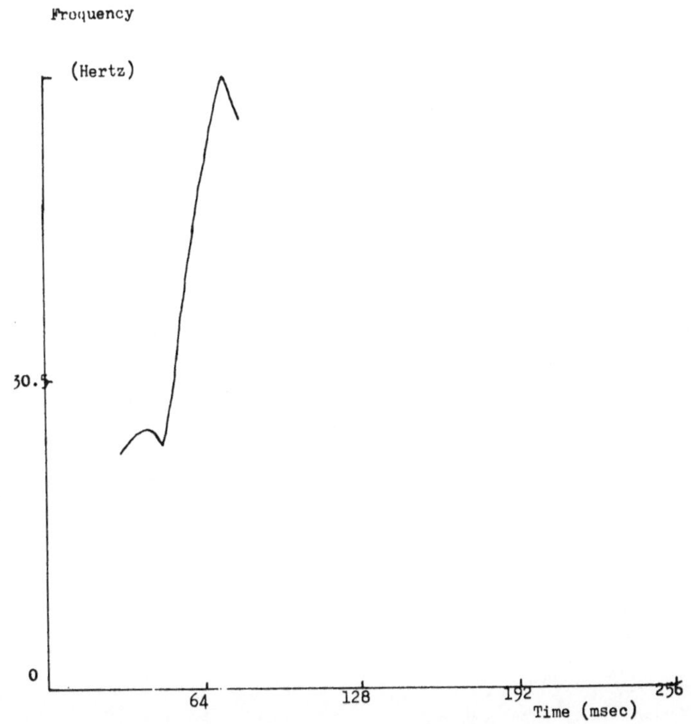

Figure 6 Plot of frequency-time curve derived by computer analysis, using the method described in text. Note the similarity of this curve with the rise in ventricular pressure during isovolumetric contraction

References

Hughes, T. (1979). Unpublished results

Light, L. H., Hanson, G. C., Sequeira, R. F. and Gross, G. (1980). Flow circulated information on the central circulation by transcutaneous aortovelography

Longmore, D. (1979). An introduction to non-invasive cardiodisgnostic techniques. In 'Non-invasive physiological measurements', Vol. I, (ed. P. Rolfe) pp. 1–19, Academic Press, London

Longmore, D. B. and Bass, R. W. (1973). Unpublished results

Philips, P. A. and Bergman, D. (1977). Intra-operative application of intra-aortic balloon counter pulsation determined by clinical pulsation determined by clinical monitoring of the endocardial viability ratio. *Ann Thorac Surg*. **23**, 45–51

Shepherd, L. C. and Kirklin, J. N. (1974). Cardiac surgical intensive care computer system. *Fed Proc*., **33**, 2326–8

35
Is red-cell potassium a prognostic indicator?

R. WYATT

Progress in cardiac surgery presents the anaesthetist with an increasing degree of sickness in patients, and with increasingly complex surgical procedures. One is perforce obliged to consider the patient's metabolic well-being in more detail; in particular a closer reflection of Na^+/K^+ pump activity (which accounts for 20% of total tissue energy consumption) would be desirable to monitor progress. Physiological 'protective' responses appropriate to a wounded animal in the wild are not necessarily beneficial to cardiac surgery patients, and having accepted the benefits of the abolition of 'fear' and 'flight' one should look again at more recondite responses such as carbohydrate intolerance, kalliuresis and hyponatraemia, whose ultimate manifestation is a 'sick cell' syndrome. Erythrocytes are readily biopsied and handled, are now recognized to have a not inconsiderable metabolic activity, and in slow-moving situations such as chronic diuretic therapy and geriatric inanition, red-cell potassium ($RBCK^+$) has been shown to be an accurate reflection of changes in total body potassium[1].

The author has measured total blood potassium (TBK^+) in totally haemolysed blood samples and calculated erythrocyte potassium from the formula

$$RBCK^+ = \frac{TBK^+ - (1 - PCV) \times \text{serum } K^+}{PCV}$$

Despite the use of bank blood and the introduction of other variables probably inevitable in the clinical situation, certain preliminary conclusions may be made:

(1) During bypass, and prior to bank blood administration, $RBCK^+$ falls.
(2) Large-dose narcotic anaesthesia, continuous potassium administration, and the use of a glucose/insulin infusion reduce, but do not abolish, this fall.
(3) In patients on large doses of propranolol, $RBCK^+$ leakage still occurs; it is the renal excretion of K^+ which is blocked.

(4) In cases with a satisfactory outcome $RBCK^+$ returns virtually to pre-bypass values within 12–18 h. In cases which do not prosper, it does not, and may be a better prognostic indicator of cell well-being than carbohydrate tolerance, as the latter is greatly affected by exogenous dextrose administration.

Reference

1. Bahemuka, M. and Hodkinson, H. M. (1976). Red blood-cell potassium as a practical index of potassium status in elderly patients. *Age and Ageing*, **5**, 24

36
Nursing management

JOAN E. BLUNDELL

The postoperative management of patients following cardiac surgery is unsatisfactory without a first-class recovery team. The skills of the nursing staff looking after the patients should include knowledge of the technical aspects of the equipment in use in addition to nursing care. Nurses working in such a unit should be highly trained in this speciality, in order to portray and uphold a cool, calm and effective outlook in all situations – come what may!!!

Before surgery, parents of children who are undergoing surgery are given an opportunity to visit the child. An explanation of the postoperative recovery is given to the adult patient at ward level, and this is reinforced if the patient visits the unit. The physiotherapist visits and explains what her role is in the recovery period. Bed is prepared in the recovery unit and taken to the theatre ready for the patient's return.

When the patient is ready for collection other patients are screened off, and the area is cleared for the returning unconscious patient. The patient is transferred on to his bed in theatre, attached to a portable ECG machine, a Tycos pressure gauge is attached to measure the arterial pressure. Drains are attached to drain-carriers and left on free drainage, any inotrophic support required is regulated by gate clamps on the drips. Providing the patient remains stable he sets off on his return journey escorted by the anaesthetist, who will hand-ventilate the patient; the nurse who will look after the patient in recovery, and a technician. On the return journey, the nurse is given a brief report of the operation, drains and lines *in situ*, support therapy, and any problems that may have occurred in theatre.

On admission to the unit a sister is at the bedside waiting to receive the patient. The anaesthetist attaches the patient to the ventilator, simultaneously the technician attaches the arterial trace and the left atrial line to the transducer, and the ECG to the monitoring system. Sister attaches and regulates the support lines to Tekmer infusion pumps, used in conjunction with a 100 ml buretrol infusion set with a safety valve. Meanwhile the nurse will start routine observations. Chest drains are transferred to floor stands re-zeroed and attached to suction. A rectal probe and a toe probe are attached for measuring the body temperature. A urinary catheter is attached to a urimeter, a nasogastric tube is left on free drainage. A space blanket is placed over the patient and the patient made as comfortable as possible. Routine blood tests are taken for gases and electrolytes, and the doctor's orders are written up. A continuous report is maintained of all treatment, nursing procedures, physiotherapy, doctors' visitations and relatives visitation. This is done in a special book, termed the 'Patient's Notebook'. This book holds together the minute-by-minute progress, care, and action whilst the patient remains in the intensive care unit. This record is kept primarily by the nurse looking after the patient, the doctors, and the physiotherapist, and remains their responsiblity. However, any person attending the patient can make notes in this book providing a narrative account of the patient's progress.

This book is invaluable in assessment of every patient. When the patient awakens he is reassured, told the day, date, time, what has happened, where he is, that he will be unable to speak because of the tube in his throat, and also that a nurse will be with him continually and if haemodynamically stable, sedated, according to doctor's instructions. Relatives are encouraged to telephone and, if they so desire, may visit.

We feel it is essential that relatives are kept well informed of the patient's condition. Quarter-hourly observations should be maintained until the patient is totally warm and well perfused, and only then are the observations reduced in number to allow the patient to rest maximally.

The physiotherapist treats the patient according to the stability of the patient's condition. Basic nursing care is a continuous process, to ensure the patient's comfort at all times. It involves endotracheal and oral suction, eye and mouth care, and pressure-area care particularly in the patient with a parlous circulation. All patients return from theatre on a ripple mattress and a sheepskin. Sedation is withheld on the morning following surgery, as it is planned to wean the patient off the ventilator and extubate, as soon as possible. Reassurance is given at all times. The anaesthetist assesses the patient, weans from the ventilator and extubates if possible. The patient is assessed regularly by the surgical team, who will give the day's instructions with regard to removal of lines, drains, and transfer out of the main unit. The patient is now given his first liquid refreshment. We feel it is psychologically important to transfer the patient from the main unit as soon as his condition permits. The patient remains in the progressive care area, which is still attached to the recovery ward, for a further 24 hours or longer if necessary. He should remain monitored, on ECG, one pressure line, and the urinary catheter should remain *in situ*. Continuous basic nursing care should be given, and adequate analgesia, at least 4-hourly. The patient is encouraged to eat and drink, and intense physiotherapy is continued. Chest wounds are inspected and left exposed to dry. Following further assessment by the surgical team, agreement is reached to transfer the patient to the ward, and all remaining lines and urinary catheter are removed.

PRIORITIES OF POST-OP MANAGEMENT

(1) Patient must never be left alone at any time.
(2) Standard of nursing care given should be as we would ask for any member of our family. A poor standard of nursing care is unacceptable.

(3) Good supervision, with an efficient and effective team and an approachable leader, who not only administrates but is very much involved at clinical level.
(4) Adequate analgesia!!
(5) Communication with patient: comfort; contact. Talking to patient, whether conscious or not.
(6) Relatives: making time to explain the clinical situation, honestly
(7) 'Nurses': consider stress; teaching to maintain standards; unit atmosphere; good communication with all departments; theatre, pathology, social worker, doctors and nurses.
(8) Tender loving care to patient and family is vital.

37
Nutritional care in cardiac surgery

R. K. WALESBY

INTRODUCTION

Chronic congestive cardiac failure in valvular heart disease is recognized[1] as a prelude to cardiac malnutrition (cardiac cachexia), the pathogenesis of which results from low cardiac output producing poor tissue perfusion and a-cellular hypoxia[2]. This, coupled with the induced hypermetabolic state required to maintain survival, produces the cardiac cachexic state, with general body-wasting especially of muscle protein and adipose tissue. The anorexia associated with the chronically sick induces additional weakness, dyspnoea, and gastric hypomotility, which is further insulted by therapeutic agents, digoxin, diuretics, and ionic supplements producing nausea and intensifying the anorexia. It is well recognized that nutritional depletion results in an increased morbidity and mortality from cardiac surgery irrespective of its technical excellence, and Moore *et al.*[3] have proposed that patients with a chronic loss of 30% or more of their health weight are unlikely to survive major surgery. However, in severely catabolic patients an acute loss of more than 15% of body weight is associated with a loss of immunological competence, poor wound-healing and increased morbidity and mortality[4]. The preoperative nutritional status is therefore of paramount importance and is likely to be better in ischaemic heart disease than in the more protracted illness of chronic valvular heart disease of multiple aetiology.

It is the aim of this chapter to discuss the identification and importance of patients in need of calorie/nitrogen nutritional support, to refer to the metabolic cost of cardiac surgery, and to propose a few regimes that can be clinically applied during the postoperative period.

ASSESSMENT OF THE NUTRITIONAL STATUS

The body comprises two main metabolic components, namely the fat mass and the lean body mass. The latter is made up of the muscle protein, liver glycogen, and bone. In the context of surgery, it is the extent of the lean body mass that determines metabolic survival, not the New York Heart Association classification grading of the patient. This functional assessment is based on history and examination only. There are naturally fewer survivors in operated grade IV than in grade II heart disease, but one cannot imply that all grade IV patients are nutritionally depleted or that those of grade II are nutritionally normal. Clinical impressions of the nutritional status are frequently unreliable. It is not uncommon for a thin patient to be nutritionally normal and have a normal lean body mass, while an obese patient may be nutritionally grossly depleted in muscle protein.

The nutritional assessment of patient's status may be documented along lines tabulated in Table 1.

Table 1 Criteria of nutritional depletion

Weight loss	greater than 10%
Triceps skinfold thickness	less than 10 cm (males) less than 13 cm (females)
Arm-muscle circumference	less than 23 cm (males less than 22 cm (females)
Serum albumin	less than 35 g/l
Serum transferrin	less than 1.5 g/l
Lymphocyte count	less than 1500/μl
Cell-mediated immunity	Candida, tuberculin or mumps skin tests negative

(1) Absolute weight loss of 10% on a previous health weight.
(2) Measurement of the fat mass from skinfold calipers using the method of Durnin and Wommersley[5]. Body weight is made up of a combination of the lean body mass plus the fat mass, so if the fat mass is derived from caliper studies, the lean body mass may be obtained by subtraction from the total body weight. Triceps skinfold thickness and arm-muscle circumference are used as gross indices of nutritional depletion of fat and muscle protein.
(3) Decrease in the protein binding as measured by transferrin and serum albumin. Low levels of these proteins indicate poor protein synthesis.
(4) Haematological assessment by a low lymphocyte count.
(5) Cell-mediated immunity as exemplified by a negative antigen test to Candida, tuberculin or mumps antigens.

More recently Walesby *et al.*[6] have measured the lean body mass of cardiac surgical patients using total body potassium (TBK) measured non-invasively with an accuracy of ±4% using a whole-body monitor. This measures the natural gamma emission of potassium 40 (K^{40}). This isotope of potassium 39 (K^{39}) occurs as a constant proportion of 0.012% of all potassium. In the non-acidotic patient, 98% of potassium is intracellular and only in the cells of the body cell mass. This measurement therefore indexes the nutritional status of the patient when compared with predicted total body potassium which is calculated from the regression formulae of Boddy *et al.*[7], and Goode and Hawkins,[8] based on height, weight, age, and sex. The results are shown in Figure 1 for valvular heart disease and Figure 2 for coronary artery disease. A patient with a measured total body potassium precisely the same as that predicted would lie along the vertical dotted line. If the total body potassium is in excess of that predicted the patient lies to the right of the line by up to 5, 10, 15, 20 %, etc. Similarly if he were depleted by 5, 10, . . . 25 % he would lie to the left of the line. Comparisons are given for each patient in relation to predicted total body potassium derived from the various aforementioned parameters. Depletion of total body potassium, and hence loss of lean body mass, is associated with an increase in mortality from cardiac surgery. The mortality appears proportional to the degree of depletion and is not specific to any particular type of valve disease (Figure 3).

Morbidity and mortality of nutritionally depleted patients has been assessed by comparing them with the nutritionally normal, where the nutritionally normal is defined as those with the total body potassium in excess

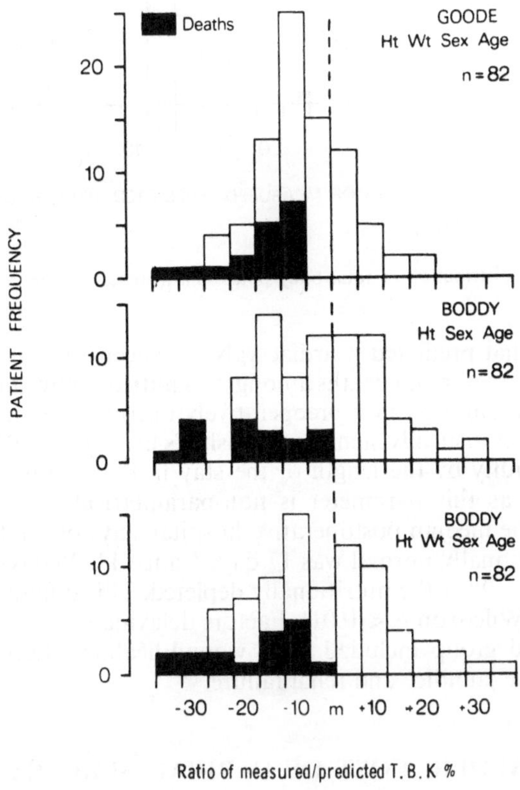

Figure 1 The distribution of total body potassium in patients undergoing cardiac valve replacement (n = 82)

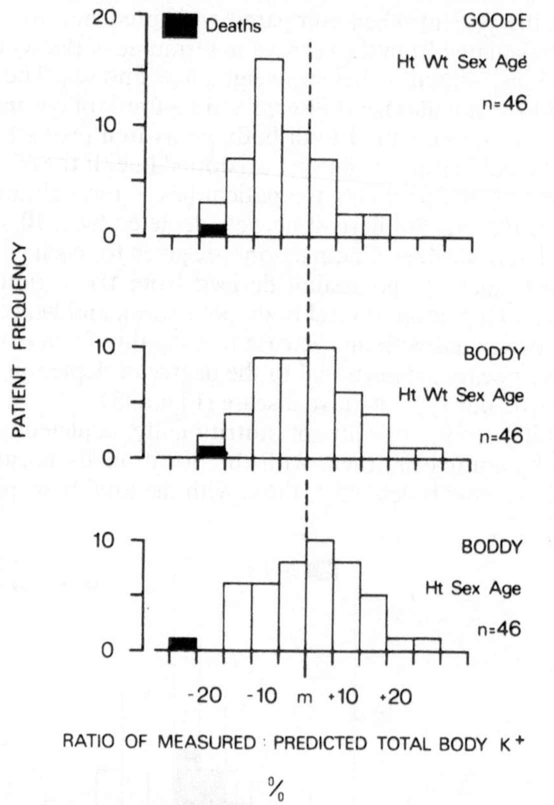

Figure 2 The distribution of total body potassium in patients with coronary artery disease ($n = 46$)

of 95 % of that predicted. Cardiac valve replacement was performed on 82 patients. There were no deaths amongst 28 nutritionally normal patients and 13 deaths amongst 54 in a preoperatively nutritionally depleted state. This difference is statistically significant (Fisher's exact $p < 0.01$). We have measured morbidity by the length of the stay in hospital in the postoperative period, but as this parameter is non-parametrically distributed we have compared the median postoperative hospital stays of the two groups. That of the nutritionally normal was 17 days (range 11–25 days) compared with 27 days (12–60) for the nutritionally depleted. This difference is statistically significant (Wilcoxon $p < 0.01$). Factors delaying recovery of the nutritionally depleted group included poor wound-healing, sternal disintegration, postoperative jaundice and renal failure.

THE METABOLIC COST OF CARDIAC SURGERY

All major surgical procedures incur a compulsory loss of nitrogen derived from breakdown of muscle protein in the postoperative period. There is not

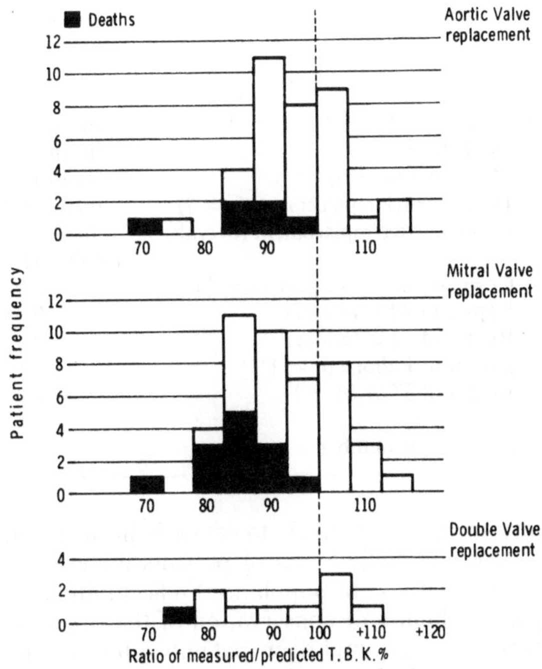

Figure 3 Total body potassium in valve surgery distributed according to individual valve (n = 92)

only an increase in breakdown of protein, but a failure to resynthesize proteins from amino acids. The metabolic loss incurred by an operation is expressed as negative nitrogen balance a day, and is the loss of nitrogen by the body less the nitrogen intake. Nitrogen losses can be measured precisely by a Kjeldahl technique on all body excreta, i.e. urine, faeces, perspiration, nasogastric aspirate and chest drainage. These analyses are technically very tedious and for ward purposes can be approximately measured from 24 h collections of urine to measure urinary urea. This accounts for approximately 80% of the total nitrogen excretion and can be converted into grammes of nitrogen lost a day (1 mmol of urea contains 28 mg of nitrogen). These measurements directly relate to changes in the lean body mass occurring with surgery. However, the assessment can be made indirectly from changes of total body potassium occurring with surgery, providing the acid–base status is normal at the time of each measurement. Manners[9] estimated the net metabolic cost of cardiac valve replacement as a negative nitrogen balance of 6.7 g of nitrogen a day over 7 postoperative days calculated from urinary nitrogen losses. Our sample of patients produced an almost identical result of 6.8 g of nitrogen a day over the same period, but when calculated from changes in total body potassium the losses rose to a mean of 9.7 and a median of 11.1 g of nitrogen a day negative nitrogen loss. The results are further divided in Table 2. They show that coronary artery surgery is far less of a metabolic demand on the body than single or double valve replacement and

Table 2 Metabolic cost of cardiac surgery
(From changes in total body potassium expressed as *negative* nitrogen balance/day over 7 postoperative days)

AVR ($n = 12$)	mean 7.7
MVR ($n = 13$)	mean 7.8
MV repair ($n = 5$)	mean 10.1
Double valve replacement ($n = 7$)	mean 14.4
Cardiac valve replacement (overall)	mean 9.7
	median 11.1
Coronary artery surgery ($n = 11$)	5.9
Repair of ASD ($n = 7$)	9.33
Repair of VSD ($n = 1$)	8.4
Repair of Fallot's ($n = 1$)	7.15
Repair of TGA ($n = 1$)	8.45

n = sample number

these patients are also more likely to eat early in the postoperative recovery phase. The high metabolic losses of patients undergoing closure of atrial septal defects (a relatively fit population) reflect a high lean body mass preoperatively and a failure of conservation of the tissues incurred by such a surgical procedure. In comparison patients who are already nutritionally depleted metabolize during surgical insult with more nitrogen and protein-sparing metabolic cycles, showing relative adaptation to their cachectic states.

The nitrogen and calorie intakes of a sample of patients following valve replacements has been made from weighed diets supplied to the patients in the postoperative period, and subtracting all returned foods. Allowance was made for the intravenous calorie intake in the immediate postoperative period. The mean daily calorie intake over 7 days was 662 ± 297 kcal a day (range 226–1178). Similarly nitrogen intake was 3.97 ± 1.79 g of nitrogen a day (range 1.2–6.7 g of nitrogen a day over 7 postoperative days), showing effective starvation of the patients in the first postoperative week. With fit patients this is probably effectively inconsequential, but, in already nutritionally depleted cardiac cachexia, it is more likely that a critical limit of 30% depletion, beyond which recovery is extremely unlikely, will be reached.

AIMS OF POST-OPERATIVE NUTRITIONAL CARE

Postoperative nutritional care should thus aim to:

(1) Identify the nutritionally malnourished. Once the nutritionally poor-risk patient has been identified in the preoperative period, if practical, operation should be withheld until the nutritional state is improved by diet supplements. These supplements can be administered at home under the guidance of the dietitian. The process necessarily takes 3–6 months and is applicable only to the chronically sick. Our preliminary

studies show this to be a promising policy and that it is possible to increase the lean body mass in chronic valvular disease without merely increasing weight by producing overhydration. To date we have too few patients to know if mortality and morbidity would be affected by such a policy.

(2) Minimise post-operative losses. We believe that a cardiac surgical patient who at any time during his surgery reaches a state of 30% depletion of his health weight will metabolically not withstand the surgery. Standard nutritional support consisting of unlimited dextrose or dextrose–saline is neither metabolically nor nutritionally beneficial. It counteracts the adaptive ketone response to starvation, thereby actually increasing metabolic demands and promoting protein catabolism. However, all too frequently a patient will remain ventilated and moribund in an intensive care unit for 5 days or more in the post-operative period on inotropic support before any suggestion of feeding is entertained. During this time not only are fluids restricted, but the associated hypermetabolic state may have produced net losses of up to 100 g of nitrogen (equivalent to 625 g of protein or 3 kg of muscle tissue loss). These are the patients least able to withstand losses, despite preoperatively having adapted to more protein-sparing metabolic pathways than the fit. Protein breakdown accelerates from the time of the initial incision reaching a maximum between 3 and 5 days post-operatively, but if the patient remains moribund or becomes septic, protein losses may continue at the maximal level of up to 20 g of nitrogen a day until resolution or death. It is probably impossible to make a sick cardiac surgical patient achieve a zero nitrogen balance in the postoperative period within the strict limits imposed by management of their attendant cardiac failure. However, any attempt at reducing the overall losses lengthens the time available in which cardiac recovery is still possible before a state of total body rot becomes established.

METHODS

Enteral feeding (oral or tube) is chosen if the bowel is functional. Parenteral feeding only if there is a good reason not to use enteral feeding. The two methods are complementary, not competitive. Many cardiac patients are unnecessarily managed by parenteral feeding, which is expensive and carries a significant mortality and morbidity. Figure 4 shows a suggested scheme for a patient's nutritional demands which should be worked through daily from the time of operation. If the patient can eat, make him eat; if he cannot, feed him!

Gut motility usually returns within 24–48 h after surgery and enteral feeding is the preferred route with minor attendant complications. Standardized hospital food or blended foods are best, but the large volumes required to blend such foods makes the diet unpalatable to patients and the fluid load unacceptable to cardiac surgeons. Standard enteric feeds are available in most hospitals; these comprise whole protein and a calorie source. They are supplied by the dietetics department to high standards, with added vitamins and minerals. Their main energy supply is caloreen, a polymer of glucose, but their main problem is that of maintaining sterility of the compound and a predisposition to reduce diarrhoea in patients once feeding is given in adequate quantities. However, by slowly introducing the feed, or by dilution of the feed, the chances of this are reduced.

Alternatively there are many excellent proprietary enteric feeds which infrequently give diarrhoea and in addition are guaranteed as sterile. Their introduction is aided by building up to an ideal quantity over a few days and can be given orally or by nasogastric tube. Enteric feeds can be administered by gravity infusion via fine-bore (1 mm) nasogastric feeding tubes inserted with a wire introducer into the stomach. The fine-bore tubes are more comfortable than the wide-bore tubes, and their use has not so far been associated with oesophageal erosions, ulcers, or strictures. Continuous gravity infusion saves a significant amount of nursing time and is associated with a much lower incidence of diarrhoea and vomiting than the bolus method. The preparation I have found most beneficial in cardiac surgery patients is Isocal (Mead Johnson Ltd) which is isosmotic and provides calories and nitrogen in an appropriate ratio to the postoperative period. It is also conveniently packaged in tins, requires no dilution and rarely gives diarrhoea. Clinifeed 400 (Roussel) is an excellent alternative but requires dilution before use and is more likely to produce diarrhoea unless introduced slowly. The relative efficiencies are shown below.

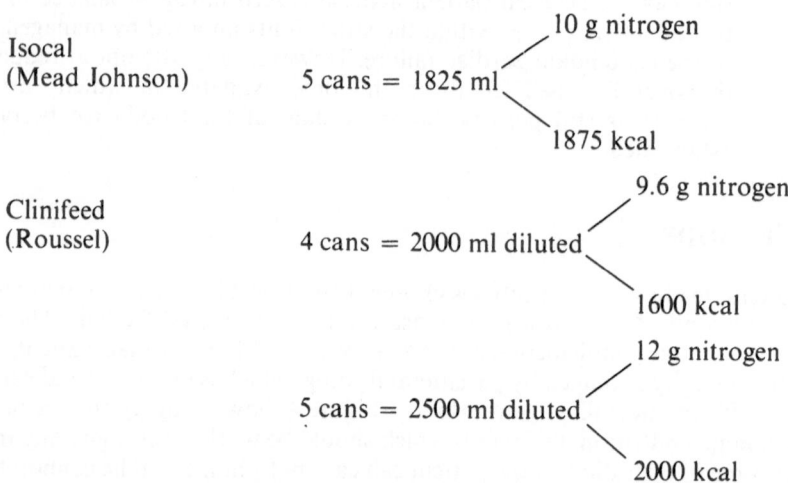

Isocal (Mead Johnson)	5 cans = 1825 ml	10 g nitrogen 1875 kcal
Clinifeed (Roussel)	4 cans = 2000 ml diluted	9.6 g nitrogen 1600 kcal
	5 cans = 2500 ml diluted	12 g nitrogen 2000 kcal

Both of these enteric feeds are complete in themselves, containing protein, fat, and carbohydrate. In addition there are mineral salts, trace elements with water and fat-soluble vitamins. Nutritional requirements are only sufficient if positive nitrogen balance is achieved. For this nitrogen input should daily exceed output by at least several grams, and if necessary the calorie to nitrogen

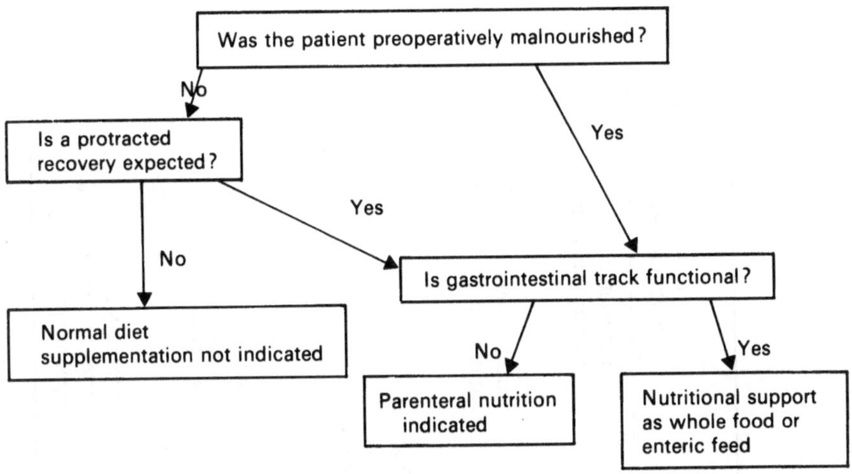

Figure 4 Daily flow chart for nutritional care

ratio may be increased with the addition of an energy source such as caloreen. A more comprehensive list is given in Table 3.

Flexical and Vivonex are low-residue (elemental) diets more applicable to bowel fistulae than cardiac surgery, but should not be overlooked when, occasionally, embolic diseases produce mesenteric occlusions requiring bowel resection and the production of the short-bowel syndrome. They can also be used in the prolonged abdominal ileus that may occasionally follow resections for coarctation of the aorta.

PARENTERAL FEEDING

This is instituted early if a long recovery is expected, or after 24–48 h in the absence of gastric motility.

General guidelines

(a) Use a central venous catheter aseptically introduced, used exclusively for feeding. No inotropes should be put through this line!

(b) Use dextrose as the principal calorie source. This directly enters the citric acid cycle for ready metabolism. Fats which are cleared rapidly from the blood require degradation to free fatty acids before becoming metabolically useful and rely on hepatic metabolism which is chronically impaired in longstanding valve disease. Tricuspid disease and valve disease producing pulmonary hypertension with chronic hepatic venous congestion are most frequently associated with hepatic malfunction. 500 cc of 10 % intralipid given twice weekly, or alternatively 1 unit of human plasma protein fraction given twice weekly are recommended, but continuous lipids tend to induce jaundice in cardiac patients.

Table 3 Palatable enteric feeds

Product	*Nitrogen source*	*Calorie/Nitrogen ratio*	*Advantages*	*Disadvantages*	*Approximate cost/10 g of nitrogen*
Complan	whole protein	100 : 1	—	inappropriately low calorie/nitrogen ratio	85p
Clinifeed 400 (Roussel)	whole protein	142 : 1	osmolarity 330; good general use	starter regime usually required to avoid diarrhoea	£3
Isocal (Mead Johnson)	whole protein	170 : 1	isosmolar; lactose-free; ready to use container; no starter regime required	—	£4
Flexical (Mead Johnson)	oligopeptides + free amino acids	256 : 1	lactose free; oligopeptides well absorbed	osmolarity 550; requires dilution and starter regime	£10
Vivonex (standard) (Eaton Labs)	free amino acids	286 : 1	lactose and fat-free	osmolarity 500; starter regime required: unpalatable	£11

Table 4

	g Nitrogen/l	kcal/l Na^+	Na^+	K^+	Mg^{2+}	PO_4^-	Cl^-	Zn^{2+}
Amino acid sources								
Synthamin 14	14	0	73	60	5	45	70	—
Synthamin 17	17	0	73	60	5	45	70	—
Aminoplex 12	12.4	0	35	30	2.5	—	67.2	—
Aminoplex 14	13.4	0	30	35	—	—	79	—
Vamin N	9.4	250	50	20	1.5	—	55	—
Amino acids with sugar								
Vamin – glucose	9.4	650	50	20	1.5	—	55	—
Sugar solutions with electrolytes								
Glucoplex 1000	0	1000	50	30	2.5	18	67	45.6
Glucoplex 1600	0	1600	50	30	2.5	18	67	45.6
Plain sugar solutions								
40 % dextrose	0	1500	0	0	0	0	0	0
50 % dextrose	0	1875	0	0	0	0	0	0

(c) In practice there are a number of commercially available amino acids, some with added dextrose, fructose, ethanol, or sorbitol as calorie sources. This allows the calorie/nitrogen ratio to be varied appropriate to the individual situation.

Table 4 contains a list of some of the more commonly used amino acid sources, together with their electrolyte concentrations. The more recently introduced sugar solutions with electrolytes may be particularly advantageous when combined with amino acid sources in cardiac surgery on account of the high potassium concentrations achieved. Nitrogen-sparing effects are best obtained by running amino acids and calorie sources synchronously by means of a '*Y*' connection drip-set, rather than administering the solutions alternately.

Table 5 contains tentative instructions for the introduction of parenteral nutrition in the postoperative cardiac surgery situation within strict fluid allowances. They are currently used by our staff and contain adequate electrolytes to make additional fluids unnecessary. The high sodium loads have infrequently proved a problem as the excess is usually excreted. Should one wish to reduce the daily sodium intake it is possible to replace the Glucoplex solution by 50 % dextrose throughout. It may then become necessary to give insulin by a slow infusion pump to maintain normal blood glucose levels. The high potassium content of Synthamin 14 (60 mmol/l) makes it most appropriate for postoperative use in cardiac surgery. A regime producing 200 kcal of energy for every gram of nitrogen supplied (6.25 g of protein) is appropriate to normal postoperative requirements, but in hypermetabolic states, or in sepsis, this ratio of calories to nitrogen should be increased to approximately 300 : 1. It is probably more important to keep the ratio correct

Table 6 What to monitor

Test	*Enteral feeding*	*Parenteral feeding*
Nitrogen excretion	daily	daily
Urinary glucose	twice daily	4–6-hourly
Blood glucose (dextrostix)	daily	4–6-hourly
Sodium Potassium Urea Creatinine Phosphate	twice weekly	daily
Liver function tests Clotting studies Haemoglobin White blood count	twice weekly	daily
Immune response	weekly	weekly

Daily urine nitrogen loss (g) = (urine output (L) × urea concentration mmol/l × 0.028 + 2 for non-urea nitrogen losses)

Table 5 Tentative parenteral nutritional introduction after cardiac surgery

	Fluid allowance ($ml\ m^{-2}\ h^{-1}$)		*Average daily volume for* $1{\cdot}5\ m^2$ *patient* (*cc/day*)		*Total daily intake*							
					Calories (*kcal*)	*Nitrogen* (*g*)	(mmol) Na^+	K^+	Mg^{2+}	Zn^{2+}	PO_4^-	Cl^-
Day 0 (operation)	30	=	1100	5 % dextrose or	206	0	—	—	—	—	—	—
				dextrose saline	165	0	33	33	—	—	—	—
Day 1	40	=	1400	1000 cc Glucoplex 1600 500 cc Synthamin 14	1600	7	86	60	5	45.6	33	102
Day 2	50	=	1800	1200 cc Glucoplex 1600 600 cc Synthamin 14	1920	8.4	104	72	6	55	40	122
Day 3	60	=	2200	1500 cc Glucoplex 1600 700 cc Synthamin 14	2400	10	126	87	7.3	68	48	150
Day 4	70	=	2500	500 cc Dextrose 50 % 1000 cc Synthamin 14 1000 cc Glucoplex 1600	2540	14	123	90	7.5	45.6	48	137
or Day 4	70	=	2500	1000 cc Synthamin 14 1500 cc dextrose 50 %	2800	14	73	60	5	0	30	70

Notes

1. Every third day replace 500 cc of the 50 % dextrose by 500 cc plasma (plasma protein fraction PPF) or by 500 cc 10 % intralipid with lipid-soluble vitamins, e.g. Vitlipid adult (Kabi Vitrium)
2. Daily add to formal regimes:
   (1) water-soluble vitamins one vial 'Solivito' (Kabi Vitrium)
   (2) trace elements, e.g. 'Addamel' (Kabi Vitrium)
3. Occasionally soluble insulin is required by infusion pump, or added to sugar solutions, to maintain normal blood glucose levels and avoid glycosuria

than to oversupply nitrogen with inadequate calories. This just produces degradation of the excess amino acids by deamination and entry of the products into the citric acid cycle.

Patients after cardiac surgery requiring enteral or parenteral feeding are necessarily acutely sick and intensively monitored. However, it is particularly important to know that not only is one doing the patient good by treating his nutritional state, but to know that one is doing no harm to his biochemistry. Table 6 provides a guideline of easily monitored parameters with suggestions on their frequency of monitoring. Remember that high urea concentrations in the blood generally represent hypermetabolism, whilst renal function is more closely monitored by creatinine clearance. Using Table 5 one can vary the regimes according both to fluid requirements and nitrogen excretion, in order to obtain the maximum benefit for an individual patient daily from his nitrogen losses over the preceding 24 h.

The preceding discussions are more tedius to describe than they are to implement, and it is the aim of this chapter to attempt to suggest basic regimes that can be administered with the minimum of effort and monitoring without endangering the patient.

References

1. Pittman, J. A. and Cohen, P. (1964). The pathogenesis of cardiac cachexia. *N. Engl. J. Med.*, **288,** 695
2. Abel, R. M., Fischer, J. E., Buckley, M. J., Barnett, G. O. and Austen, W. G. (1976). Malnutrition in cardiac surgical patients. *Arch. Surg.*, **111,** 45
3. Moore, F. D., Olsen, K. O., McMurray, J. D., Parker, H. V., Ball, M. R. and Boyden, L. M. (1963). *The Body Cell Mass and its Supporting Environments.* (Philadelphia: W. B. Saunders Co.)
4. Abel, R. M., Fischer, J. E., Buckley, M. J. and Austen, W. G. (1974). Hyperalimentation in cardiac surgery. *J. Thorac. Cardiovasc. Surg.*, **67,** 294
5. Durnin, J. V. G. A. and Womersley, J. (1974). Body fat assessed from total body density and its estimation from skinfold thickness: measurements on 481 men and women aged 16 to 72 years. *Br. J. Nutr.*, **32,** 77
6. Walesby, R. K., Goode, A. W., Spinks, T. J., Herring, A., Ranicar, A. S. O. and Bentall, H. H. (1979). The nutritional status of patients requiring cardiac surgery. *J. Thorac. Cardiovasc. Surg.*, **77,** 570
7. Boddy, K., King, P. C., Hume, R. and Wyers, E. (1972). The relation of total body potassium to height, weight and age in normal adults. *J. Clin. Pathol.*, **25,** 512
8. Goode, A. W. and Hawkins, T. (1978). Use of ^{40}K Counting and its relationship to other estimates of lean body mass. In Johnston, I. D. A. (ed.). *Advances in Parenteral Nutrition: an International Symposium.* (Lancaster: MTP Press)
9. Manners, J. M. (1974). Nutrition after cardiac surgery. *Anaesthesia*, **29,** 675

SECTION IV

Aspects of Postoperative Care (II)

38
Control of blood loss

H. H. BENTALL

In Section III a great deal of attention was given to electrolytes both scientifically and practically, but relatively little has been said on the control of haemorrhage. There are a few points, with respect to this important topic, which I hope may prove helpful. As has been emphasized elsewhere, what happens in the operating room has a profound bearing on the behaviour of the patient in the postoperative period. So let us first look at factors in the operating room which have a bearing on postoperative haemorrhage. As long ago as 1964 Blanca-Smith, Omeri, Melrose, Allwork and I drew attention to the relation of the size of the patient to perioperative haemorrhage, and suggested that it was useful to relate it to the surface area of the patient. It is useful to consider haemorrhage in three distinct periods: during the opening of the chest, during the bypass and in the postoperative period until the drains are removed. Only in this way can we compare patient to patient and usefully quantitate our results. The second most important factor that we learnt at that time was that the longer the bypass the greater the operative and postoperative haemorrhage. It is interesting to look back on the figures that were produced at that time, for all operations were done on the Mellrose Disc oxygenator using a whole-blood prime. The blood loss then was almost invariably more than we see at the present time in the uncomplicated coronary artery bypass operation, even when the perfusion period lasts more than an hour. I also draw attention to the discovery that the protamine which was used to neutralize the heparin, if given in excess, may itself become an anticoagulant. This hazard still holds good today, and we saw some figures to prove it. At that time using great care with haemostasis there was need to reopen around 10 % of the patients, a figure perhaps double that we find today using a more traumatic oxygenator and a clear fluid electrolyte prime. Bleeding from the edges of the sternum, especially in sick and elderly individuals, can still be a problem. The use of bone wax for its control is by no means satisfactory. A satisfactory commercial substitute for bone wax is not yet available. Reoperations still constitute something of a problem, and I wish wholeheartedly to concur with Professor Wheatley, and to agree that mobilization of the heart in reoperations should be confined to the minimum necessary to accomplish the technical procedures. The left ventricle should not be mobilized, especially posteriorly unless absolutely necessary. The operative blood loss is reduced by at least 500–1000 cc if this is done, and the danger of rupture of the posterial wall of the heart during mitral valve replacement in the elderly is largely avoided. One has to trade this of course with the inability to vent the left ventricle and therefore to devise more efficient ways of removing air from the left ventricle in the absence of a left ventricular vent. Our practice at Hammersmith is to pass a catheter through the replacement mitral valve. Gentle suction on this catheter after the heart is refilled but before beating is permitted removes most of the air. We use a stab wound in the aortic root controlled by a·purse-string suture to release air from the aortic root. We squeeze the heart and percuss the chest wall to dislodge entrapped air and we ask the anaesthetist to squeeze the lungs. In this way macroscopic air can be avoided. In practice the patients have been very much better off than after the ventricle has been mobilized in these reoperations. During the closure period, careful haemostasis is carried out without continually wiping away newly formed clot, and where possible the pericardium is closed, leaving only space for drainage in order to avoid inadvertent opening into the right ventricle during subsequent operations. Drainage of mediastinum, and where open, the pleura, is always carried out in the intensive care unit and we must not forget that there should be a small but steady blood loss for the first 6 h. Complete cessation of bleeding is not necessarily a good sign. If the patient starts to deteriorate, first manifested by an otherwise unexplained rise in pulse rate, cardiac tamponade should be suspected. Pulsus paradoxus is rarely seen, as in the kind of patient prone to this, cardiac output is insufficient to produce a truly paradoxical pulse. There may be a brief period when it can be appreciated in the femoral artery of the groin. Stuart Hunter can demonstrate a pericardial effusion of blood using his mobile ultrasound apparatus but I have no personal experience of this method. I am against empirical polypharmacy, an endeavour to control postoperative blood loss by means of drugs, platelet infusion, fresh frozen plasma and so on. I prefer wherever possible to try to identify the reason for bleeding. In an adult an early blood loss of a litre in an hour usually indicates the need for reopening the patient and securing the bleeding point surgically, rather than looking for some haematological cause. There are exceptions to this rule, especially in patients who have had division of multiple adhesions or who have had very long bypasses. In patients who are bleeding a great deal it should not be forgotten that the sick patient may be unable to metabolize the anticoagulant used in the bank blood, and the judicious use of regular small doses of calcium chloride may be necessary. Additional protamine is very rarely if ever required.

39
The horizontal dimension

A PATIENT FROM THE INTENSIVE THERAPY UNIT

I do not recommend you to seek three days as a patient in an ITU. But I strongly urge you to advance without fear to meet them if they come your way. They will constitute an experience which is unforgettable, at times deeply moving and difficult to describe adequately. I have forgotten nothing of my own encounter with the ITU which it was possible to remember and I still recollect some aspects of it with emotion. I will now tell you as best I can what seemed to me important about it.

In the first place, no forewarning of one's situation on recovering consciousness can adequately convey the sense of total dependence which the first moments of consciousness bring. One glimpses the dependence which the tetraplegic must feel. Ordinary bodily intakes and outputs are either in suspense or taken care of by tubes. Warm, naked and defenceless you realise fully for the first time the extent of your dependence for survival on the devotion and care of other human beings. I suppose there are those for whom this must be humiliating and harrowing. For my own part, after a short period of reflection, I felt a surge of warmth, affection and humility such as I had never known before. After the long years of struggle to make one's way, to support a wife and family and to be independent, the final surrender to the care of others seemed suddenly an act of faith in the essential goodness of the human race and I abandoned myself to it joyously.

But this emotion was followed swiftly, and I think naturally, by one which I think it may be important for you to note. I felt an intense desire to communicate. For this purpose one has effectively just the one free hand. Hands are quite effective means of communication, whereas feet are not. I waved my free hand from time to time in the hope that someone would grasp it: but no one ever did. Of course they could not have known how much I wanted that contact which in the conventional hand-clasp we daily take for granted. I wanted to use it to express my gratitude for a renewal of life and for the care I was receiving. I might have been able to write a note of thanks had I been given a pencil and paper, although that is doubtful. But it was contact that I was really after and the need seemed pressing.

I now remark on a few things which I thought were disagreeable during the long twilight hours between sleep and waking. First of all, as everyone knows, the sense of hearing seems to survive the lapse or suppression of all others. No doubt in primeval times it was necessary even in sleep to hear the approach of the dreaded dinosaur. I was surprised to hear someone say: 'Look at me', (calling me by my first name). 'Don't you recognise me?' My eyes must have been open for the surgical registrar (for he it was) to have addressed me so. But I could not see anything. I could hear him perfectly and recognise his voice but the brain was evidently unable to interpret the images which my eyes were forming. This was not particularly distressful but quite slight noises penetrated the light unconsciousness and seemed an exaggerated annoyance, especially at night. I recall resenting even the subdued conversation of the staff in the dimmed light at night and wishing they would stop. But by day I enjoyed the few words which were spoken to me

And now the ventilator. Conscious and in daylight, I had no trouble with this at all. But in the long hours of night, when semi-conscious, silent and terrible struggles took place. I leave it to you to discern the causes of this. I can only tell you the effects.

What happened was that I woke, as it seemed, in the process of suffocation. I could not breathe and the machine did not seem to be doing it for me. I became alert enough to think: 'I am trying to breathe spontaneously and am out of step with the ventilator.' So I tried to exhale more air in the hope of getting back into step. But no air came; perhaps the tube was blocked with secretions. Soon the sensation was that of the moments when an intravenous injection of thiopentone begins to take effect and I went gladly to meet the unconsciousness which I knew was coming. I had several of these episodes in the course of one night. Each occasion was unpleasant and frightening because I thought that I was going to die of it and wanted quickly to be released from the struggle. Whether in all this I made any sound or movement, I do not know but think rather not. I recall that it was daylight when I heard the anaesthetist say: 'I think you can manage better without this now.' The tube was removed and the relief was very great.

Sucking-out is not the ordeal that one account of it has claimed. I suppose a lot depends on the skill and delicacy of touch of the operator. I reckon that I was very fortunate in all things in the hospital where I was. And although there was some pain associated with the two or three suckings-out which I can recall, I would not describe it as significant.

The great thirst which succeeded the removal of the IT tube was a much more serious matter in my estimation. It began while I was breathing spontaneously but wearing an oxygen mask. It soon increased to the point where it became an overmastering obsession, making rest impossible. I know that at this stage I must have been a great trouble to the staff with my constant clamour for water. They told me that they had been instructed not to give me any fluids in order to reduce the load on the heart. I took this in, but my body plainly did not believe it and I reached the point where I felt that I would die of thirst anyway and would sooner die of heart-failure. An occasional tiny drink in a plastic measure was given, but this seemed rather to increase the desire for water than to relieve it. At last I heard someone say: 'The body knows best when it really needs water. Give him a glassful.' After these words of incredible wisdom came the most delicious relief. But the ordeal lasted over some considerable period of hours, some passed in evil dreams and imaginings and some in full awareness and I wonder if it was really necessary.

The removal of the major drains gave me no trouble, as I believe they have done to some others. There was, of course, some associated pain but it was greatly diminished by pethidine and of no consequence. Even so, at the end of the three-day sojourn, one feels considerably battered and scarred by the encounter. And as one's grip of life strengthens and the mind grows clearer, one looks around with a renewed interest in life and the people round about. Just as one gets close to making the most satisfying contact with the staff, one is returned to the ward and, in my case, to twelve hours of unpleasant nausea. But that is a small price to pay for survival.

I come now to the last and most difficult aspect of the experience about which I feel a strong urge to tell you. As the ensuing weeks and months went by, an increasingly strong sense of attachment to and dependence upon the hospital in general and the unit in particular gradually laid hold of me. I began to pause outside the ITU and to hope to be invited in or to talk to some doctor or nurse coming out. This was obviously not a desire which I could reasonably expect to be met and it was not. But reason had little to do with it, and the sense of attachment grew no less with the passage of time. Turning into the hospital now, after the lapse of almost exactly four years, I note a sudden rise in my heart-rate and I know that this sympathetic stimulation is one of pleasure and not of fear at returning to the place where life seemed to have begun again. I know from discrete enquiries of one or two other patients that I am not alone. I have often asked myself why I should have these abnormal feelings of dependence and attachment and whether I could or should try to get rid of them. Many of the good people who took such care of me have left but my attachment to the place itself grows no less. One day I asked myself on what other occasion I had lived through a period of oblivion, during which I was devoid of respiration and supplied with oxygenated blood from an external source, to emerge naked into a warm world, eyes open but unseeing, hearing and responding to sounds but unable to speak, yearning for contact, longing for a drink and totally dependent. Putting these circumstances together, it was no surprise to note from the newspapers how many people who have had open heart surgery followed by a spell in an ITU instinctively speak about being born again.

Thus I conclude what I have to tell you from the patient's viewpoint. Some will say that my latter remarks are fanciful and that the whole experience in the ITU is rather unpleasant and best forgotten. I do not agree and am sorry for those who think so. For them life must be just a meaningless burden and the experience in the ITU just another travail. Whereas for me the extraordinary gift of a further span of life coincided with a remarkable spiritual experience through which I am glad to have passed.

I am very glad to have had this chance to speak to you and through you to your colleagues to whom I owe so much. I am truly grateful for the wonderful care I was given in the hospital where I was and I know very well that I owe to them the fact that I am here today.

Footnote:
In the operation I was given a human aortic valve replacement and two coronary artery by-pass grafts. It took a long time. I was then 56 and am now 60. I am perfectly well and working very hard full-time. I do not normally think about myself as much as I had to do in order to write this paper. I am a lawyer by training. I am not religious.

40
Pulmonary problems after cardiopulmonary bypass

J. W. W. GOTHARD

INTRODUCTION

Lung biopsies taken in the period immediately after cardiopulmonary bypass show characteristic changes of interstitial oedema, swollen endothelial and alveolar cells (types I and II), and aggregation of abnormal leukocytes in relation to the endothelium of the pulmonary capillaries, arterioles and venules[1-3]. Intracellular damage also occurs with swelling and destruction of mitochondria and endoplasmic reticulum in the alveolar cells and a marked depletion of lysosomal bodies in the abnormal leukocytes.

These changes are particularly marked in patients with abnormal pre-bypass lung biopsies[3], Ratliff *et al.* being able to demonstrate only minimal histological changes in patients with normal pre-bypass biopsies. The degree of lung damage seen at an ultrastructural level is more marked after long bypass procedures and more evident in patients with pre-existing pulmonary hypertension[2,3].

Patients after cardiopulmonary bypass exhibit some degree of pulmonary dysfunction. Hypoxaemia breathing air is common and various studies[4-8] have demonstrated an increase in the alveolar–arterial oxygen gradient (A–a gradient), venous admixture (shunt) and dead space–tidal volume ratios (V_D/V_t), although the time course of these changes is variable. Functional residual capacity is decreased, as is compliance, so that the work of spontaneous respiration is increased. Diffusing capacity for carbon monoxide (Dco) is decreased after cardiopulmonary bypass (c.p.b.) and this probably represents a real change even allowing for a decrease in lung volume. Values obtained for extravascular lung water after c.p.b.[9-11] are conflicting in that some workers have demonstrated a rise whereas others have not. This may represent the limitations of available measurement techniques although a recent study[11], measuring extravascular thermal volume of the lung, demonstrated a rise in lung water after bubble-oxygenator bypass but not after membrane-oxygenator bypass.

Recent evidence[8] suggests that the majority of changes in pulmonary function after c.p.b. are little different from those observed after major non-bypass surgical procedures in patients with normal preoperative lung function. In this group lung damage due to c.p.b. is minimal unless bypass time is prolonged. The development of bypass techniques using improved oxygenators, blood filters, a non-haem prime and cardioplegic myocardial preservation has helped minimize pulmonary damage so that the condition known as 'the pump lung syndrome' is no longer seen. The majority of patients after c.p.b. therefore will require little respiratory support and many units advocate early weaning from mechanical ventilation in this group. However, certain categories of patient are still likely to have severe pulmonary problems after c.p.b. which require careful ventilatory management. To identify these groups in our present practice a simple retrospective study has been carried out.

REVIEW OF PATIENTS REQUIRING PROLONGED RESPIRATORY SUPPORT

A retrospective study has been carried out for the years 1974 and 1979 to establish the type of patient requiring prolonged respiratory support after cardiopulmonary bypass (3 days or more). Respiratory support consisted of mechanical ventilation via an endotracheal or tracheostomy tube in adults, and either mechanical ventilation or continuous positive airway pressure via an endotracheal tube in children. The duration of respiratory support in each group was recorded to the nearest day and was considered to have ended when adults were completely weaned from the ventilator or when children were successfully extubated.

RESULTS

The duration of respiratory support, in those initially ventilated for 3 days or more, is shown for adult cases in Tables 1 and 2, and for paediatric cases in Table 3.

The percentage of adult cases requiring prolonged ventilation decreased from 7.9% to 4.5% over the period reviewed ($p = 0.05$), and the mean duration of mechanical ventilation also decreased (8.6–7.8 days). The total number of coronary artery vein graft (CAVG) patients requiring prolonged respiratory support increased from 1974 to 1979 (see Table 2) but, because of an increase in workload, the percentage figures of 4.5% in 1974 and 2.5% in 1979 were not significantly different.

Patients undergoing valve surgery represented the major group requiring prolonged respiratory support in both years (27 cases in 1974 and 16 in 1979). However, the percentage of valve-surgery patients requiring prolonged mechanical ventilation decreased from 9.9% in 1974 to 5.1% in 1979 ($p = 0.05$), and this accounts for the overall drop in the number of patients requiring respiratory support.

Table 1 Adult bypass cases 1974 and 1979

	Total	*No. of cases on respiratory support 3 days or more*	*Mean duration of respiratory support (days) if > 3 days*
1974	393	31 (7.9 %)*	8.6
1979	551	25 (4.5 %)*	7.8

* $p = <0.05$

Table 2 Duration of respiratory support after coronary artery and valve surgery

	No. of cases	*No. on respiratory support 3 days*	*Mean duration of respiratory support (days) if ⩾3 days*
1974			
CAVG	66	3 (4.5 %)*	10.3
Valves	272	27 (9.9 %)†	8.1
1979			
CAVG	192	5 (2.6 %)*	8.8
Valves	312	16 (5.1 %)†	9.5

* $p = 0.05$
† Not significant

Table 3 Details of paediatric bypass cases requiring prolonged respiratory support

	No. of cases on respiratory support ⩾3 days	*Percentage of total*	*Mean duration on respiratory support (days) (if ⩾ 3 days)*	*Mean age (months)*	*No. of patients 1 year or less*
1974	62	24*	6.9	53.2	18
1979	60	28.5*	8.0	31.8	27

* No significant difference

The percentage of paediatric cases requiring prolonged respiratory support increased (24 % to 28.5 %) over the period reviewed, although this was not statistically significant. The mean duration of respiratory support was longer in this group of patients in 1979 (8.0 days) than in 1974 (6.9 days). However, the mean age of the patients was lower in 1979 (31.8 months) than in 1974 (53.2 months) and the 1979 figures include a greater number of infants (1 year or less).

DISCUSSION

This study confirms that there are three groups more likely to need prolonged ventilatory support after cardiopulmonary bypass, i.e. patients after valve surgery who have pre-existing pulmonary dysfunction, those with a low cardiac output, and infants after corrective surgery for congenital heart disease.

In the first category it is well known[4,5], that the degree of pulmonary dysfunction secondary to heart disease correlates well with functional classification. Mitral stenosis, in particular, raises pulmonary venous pressure causing an increase in extravascular lung water and a redistribution of pulmonary blood flow so that total lung capacity and vital capacity are decreased and the work of breathing increased. The degree of extravascular lung water present also correlates to some extent with functional classification[4]. It is not surprising, therefore, that patients in functional classes III and IV, and particularly those with pulmonary hypertension, are more likely to need prolonged ventilation after c.p.b.[12]. Many of these patients will have myocardial failure requiring inotropic support, and therefore can also be considered as part of the group requiring respiratory support because of a low cardiac output.

The improvement in figures in the valve surgery patients for duration of mechanical ventilation from 1974 to 1979 could solely be due to differences in case selection. However, it is interesting to note that the majority of cases in 1979 were carried out using a membrane oxygenator and cold cardioplegia, whereas the 1974 cases were carried out using a disc oxygenator and other methods of myocardial preservation.

Hypoxaemia after c.p.b. may not be due to primary pulmonary dysfunction. A low cardiac output resulting in a decreased mixed venous oxygen content can cause, and will certainly exacerbate, pre-existing hypoxaemia, as in the case of valve-surgery patients.

A low cardiac output accounts for the majority of patients requiring prolonged ventilation after CAVG surgery, many of these patients also requiring inotropic support, vasodilator therapy or intra-aortic balloon pumping in addition to intermittent positive pressure ventilation.

The final category of patients likely to need prolonged respiratory support after c.p.b. is of infants with congenital heart disease. Infants have a relatively large closing volume and airways closure can occur during normal tidal breathing. Postoperatively a decrease in functional residual capacity will exacerbate any hypoxaemia as a result of c.p.b.

Children with congenital heart disease also suffer from abnormalities within the pulmonary circulation. Pulmonary plethora, as occurs in a left to right shunt, decreases the compliance of the lungs and so increases the work of breathing. Some children develop pulmonary oedema as a result of the high flow so that defective gas exchange occurs too. Finally, functional and anatomical changes develop in the pulmonary circulation which result in pulmonary hypertension. Attempts at spontaneous ventilation can result in an increase in pulmonary artery pressure and, as shunt reversal cannot occur postoperatively when the defect has been closed, serious right ventricular failure results.

Those patients with oligaemic lung fields are cyanosed from birth and develop polycythaemia which predisposes to thrombosis within the pulmonary circulation as well as in other vascular beds. The pulmonary circulation remains underdeveloped in some of these children, and pulmonary hypertension is likely when the defect is closed. Damage to the pulmonary vessels can occur as a result of the high pressure which develops and defective matching of ventilation and perfusion is inevitable. Flow through bronchopulmonary anastomoses, which develop as a result of pulmonary oligaemia, also contributes to pulmonary congestion after repair of the cardiac defects.

Children in the categories described above, and other groups with abnormalities of pulmonary blood flow or ventricular failure, are likely to need considerable inotropic support, and possibly pulmonary vasodilator therapy. To ensure optimal arterial oxygenation they also require respiratory support either in the form of mechanical ventilation or CPAP.

As corrective surgery for congenital heart disease is now being carried out at a relatively early age respiratory care is likely to remain one of the major problems of postoperative management in children. Recent evidence[13,14], however, suggests that the use of profound hypothermia in cardiac surgery, particularly when induced by surface cooling, may decrease the incidence of respiratory problems in children.

FUTURE DEVELOPMENTS IN MANAGEMENT

The management of patients with respiratory failure after c.p.b. is well established and is reviewed elsewhere[15,16]. The majority of patients can be assessed on clinical criteria[17] and arterial blood–gas analysis. Some groups, however, have measured indices of lung function such as vital capacity, VD/Vt ratios, and peak inspiratory force in an attempt to assess the optimal time for weaning from respiratory support.

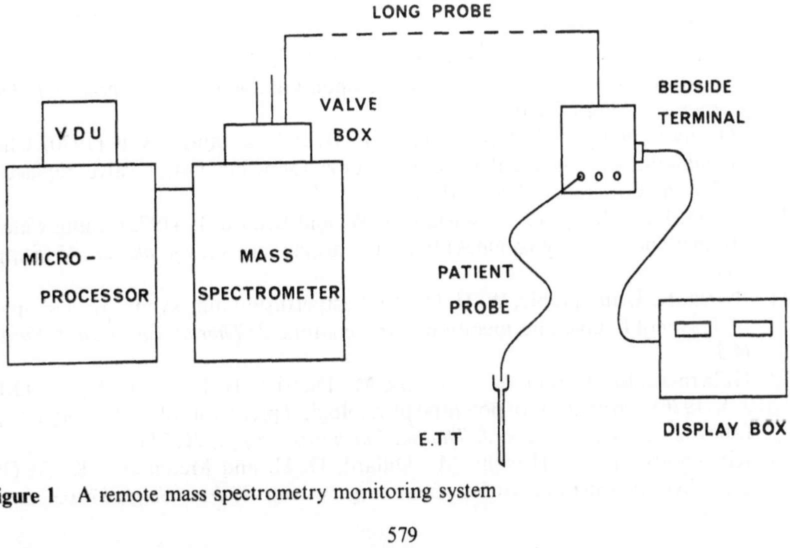

Figure 1 A remote mass spectrometry monitoring system

Respiratory mass spectrometers can now be used remotely to monitor several beds in an intensive care unit[18]. A system designed for this purpose, and shown in diagrammatic form in Figure 1, can be used to measure respired gas tensions, metabolic gas exchange, lung volume, pulmonary blood flow, and pulmonary tissue volume. The clinical role of such a system has yet to be defined but some workers[19-21] have found similar measurements useful in assessing the cardiopulmonary function of critically ill patients. If meaningful measurements can be made non-invasively and automatically in this way, respiratory mass spectrometry may well be useful in the management of the small proportion of cases that develop respiratory failure after cardiopulmonary bypass.

References

1. Wilson, J. W. (1972). Pulmonary morphologic changes due to extracorporeal circulation; a model for 'the shock lung' at cellular level in humans. In Forscher, B. K., Lillehei, R. C. and Stub, S. S. (eds.). *Shock in High- and Low-flow States*, pp. 160–71. (Amsterdam: Excerpta Medica)
2. Asada, S. and Yamaguchi, M. (1971). Fine structural changes in the lung following cardiopulmonary bypass. *Chest*, **59**, 478
3. Ratliff, N. B., Young, W. G., Hackel, D. B., Mikat, E. and Wilson, J. W. (1973). Pulmonary injury secondary to extracorporeal circulation. *J. Thorac. Cardiovasc. Surg.*, **65**, 425
4. Laver, M. B., Hallowell, P. and Goldblatt, A. (1970). Pulmonary dysfunction secondary to heart disease. *Anaesthesiology*, **33**, 161
5. Anderson, N. B. and Ghia, J. (1970). Pulmonary function, cardiac status, and post-operative course in relation to cardiopulmonary bypass. *J. Thorac. Cardiovasc. Surg.*, **59**, 174
6. Llamas, R. and Forthman, H. J. (1973). Respiratory distress syndrome in the adult after cardiopulmonary bypass. *J. Am. Med. Assoc.*, **225**, 1183
7. Turnbull, K. W., Miyagishima, R. T. and Gareim, A. N. (1974). Pulmonary complications and cardiopulmonary bypass: a clinical study in adults. *Can. Anaesth. Soc. J.*, **21**, 181
8. Rea, H. H., Harris, E. A., Seelye, E. R., Whitlock, R. M. L. and Withy, S. J. (1978). The effects of cardiopulmonary bypass upon pulmonary gas exchange. *J. Thorac. Cardiovasc. Surg.*, **75**, 104
9. O'Connor, N. E., Sheh, J. M., Bartlett, R. H. and Gazzaniga, A. B. (1970). Changes in pulmonary extravascular water volume following mitral valve replacement. *J. Thorac. Cardiovasc. Surg.*, **61**, 342
10. Parker, D. J., Karp, R. B., Kirklin, J. W. and Bedard, P. (1972). Lung water and alveolar and capillary volumes after intracardiac surgery. *Circulation*, **45** (Suppl. 1), 139
11. Byrick, R. J. and Noble, W. H. (1978). Postperfusion lung syndrome. Comparison of Travenol bubble and membrane oxygenators. *J. Thorac. Cardiovasc. Surg.*, **76**, 685
12. Hilberman, M., Kamm, M. S., Lamy, M., Dietrich, H. P., Martz, K. and Osborn, J. J. (1976). An analysis of potential physiological predictors of respiratory adequacy following cardiac surgery. *J. Thorac. Cardiovasc. Surg.*, **71**, 711
13. Rittenhouse, E. A., Hitoshi, M., Dillard, D. H. and Merendino, K. A. (1974). Deep hypothermia in cardiovascular surgery. *Ann. Thorac. Surg.*, **17**, 63

14. Barash, P. G., Berman, M. A., Stansel, H. C., Talner, N. S. and Gonau, L. H. (1976). Markedly improved pulmonary function after open heart surgery in infancy utilizing surface cooling, profound hypothermia and circulatory arrest. *Am. J. Surg.*, **131**, 499
15. Kouchoukas, N. T. and Karp, R. B. (1976). Functional disturbances following extracorporeal circulatory support in cardiac surgery. Pulmonary system. In Ionesau, M. I. and Woder, G. H. (eds.). *Current Techniques in Extracorporeal Circulation*, pp. 268–86 (London/Boston: Butterworth)
16. Gilston, A. (1979). Techniques and complications in cardiac surgery. In Langton Hewer, C. and Atkinson, R. S. (eds.). *Recent Advances in Anaesthesia and Analgesia*, pp. 72–8. (Edinburgh/London/New York: Churchill Livingstone)
17. Gilston, A. (1976). A clinical scoring system for adult respiratory distress syndrome. *Anaesthesia*, **31**, 448
18. Gothard, J. W. W., Busst, C. M., Branthwaite, M. A., Davies, N. J. H. and Denison, D. M. (1980). Applications of respiratory mass spectrometry to intensive care. *Anaesthesia*, (In press)
19. McAslam, T. C. (1976). Automated respiratory gas monitoring of critically injured patients. *Crit. Care Med.*, **4**, 255
20. Prakash, O. and Meij, S. (1979). Use of mass spectrometry and infrared CO_2 analyzer for bedside measurement of cardiopulmonary function during anaesthesia and intensive care. *Crit. Care Med.*, **5**, 180
21. Geisler, F. H., Farrell, E. J. and Siegel, J. H. (1978). A new noninvasive method for the simultaneous determination of cardiac output, VA/Qc disparity, and the magnitude of peripheral perfusion, suitable for use in the critically ill patient. *J. Trauma*, **18**, 751

41
The aetiology, pathogenesis, and prevention of prosthetic valve endocarditis

R. FREEMAN

Although patients recovering from open heart surgery are subject to all the usual postoperative infections, such as wound infection, pneumonia, urinary tract infection, and so on, one infection dominates all others in this field of surgery – prosthetic valve endocarditis (PVE). PVE is perhaps, a misnomer, since in the ensuing discussion it will embrace infection on prosthetic materials other than valves, but the term is one which will be understood in this context. This chapter aims to consider certain aspects of PVE with the hope of pointing out possible routes of investigation and management.

INCIDENCE

PVE and similar infections are known to be commoner, following implantation of an intracardiac prosthesis, than endocarditis complicating other intracardiac surgery. Endocarditis occurred in 1.3 % of patients undergoing repairs of congenital defects without prosthetic inserts but in 9.5 % of patients undergoing valve replacement with Starr–Edwards prostheses in one reported series[1]. Although the actual incidences will vary from series to series, the relative excess of endocarditis in patients receiving prosthetic material remains. Most series also demonstrate a predilection for PVE on aortic prostheses compared to mitral; the reverse is true of native valve endocarditis (NVE). Over the last several years better operative and perfusion techniques, combined with better postoperative management, have reduced the overall incidence of PVE to 2 %[2] or less in most modern centres, but the condition remains the most serious complication of cardiac surgery since it results at best in re-operation and at worst it kills the patient. The latter result after an elective operation is a tragedy.

PATHOGENESIS

Figure 1 illustrates the distribution of PVE relative to time after operation. It is, of course, diagrammatic but shows the most important point which is that PVE occurs in two distinct groups: early and late. The two groups differ in other fundamental ways. Thus early PVE is associated with organisms rarely found in classical endocarditis on natural valves, whereas late PVE

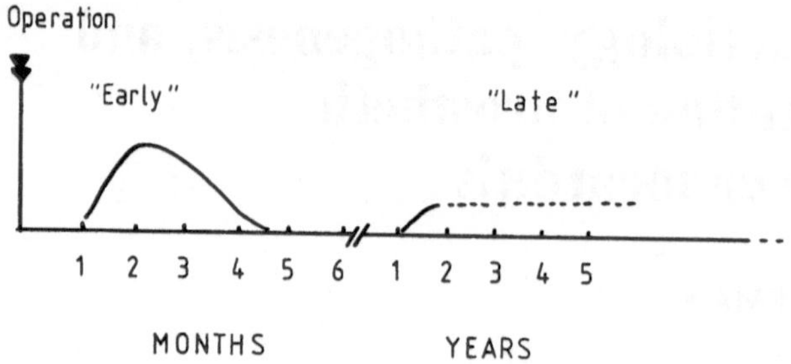

Figure 1 Occurrence of PVE

accords much more closely with the classical pictures of subacute bacterial endocarditis, both in causative organisms and clinical presentation.

Early PVE almost always presents within a few (usually 3) months of operation and has a high incidence of valve-related complications. The mortality rate is high, even with re-operation, and abscesses related to the annulus of the valve spreading to adjacent tissues are common. Late PVE presents with a more insidious picture, classical stigmata of SBE are common and although re-operation is often necessary it is usually for haemodynamic reasons. Abscess formation can and does occur, but not to the same extent or in such a fulminant manner as in early PVE. It is thought that late PVE represents a return to the risk of the haemodynamic lesion possessed by the patient with no additional risk due to the nature of the implant, and that the organisms (usually streptococci) reach the valve by the classical routes of NVE. Thus, dental prophylaxis and adequate management of genitourinary and gastrointestinal conditions are mandatory.

Early PVE, however, occurring as it does within 2–3 months of operation and being associated with organisms characteristic of the operative and postoperative periods (see below), is thought to represent a complication of the operation itself. It is therefore early PVE, with its high mortality and devastating results, which this account will concentrate upon.

Before leaving this discussion of the distinction between early and late PVE it must be said that overlap of the two conditions will occasionally occur. In particular, typical PVE may present much later than indicated above. This is often due to a delay in the expression of the disease occasioned by inadvertent partial treatment of the infection by short courses of antibiotics given for incidental infections, such as chest infections. In one of our cases of early PVE the organism was a penicillin-sensitive staphylococcus and the patient received several courses of penicillin-type drugs for minor infections in convalescence, resulting in a presentation with typical 'early' PVE at 8 months after operation. The final point related to pathogenesis is one which is fundamental to our understanding of the disease and therefore its prevention. In NVE it is known that although streptococci do not account for the majority of bacteraemias and septicaemias in susceptible patients, they nonetheless account for the vast majority of cases of endocarditis. It has been suggested that streptococci have a facility for adhering to cardiac endothelium not possessed by other organisms – at least not to the same extent[3]. Even among streptococci it is clear that some species adhere more easily than others, and it has been suggested that the mechanism may be associated with production of dextrans or 'bacterial gum'[4]. It is interesting to note that the re-emergence of the streptococci as the dominant organisms in late PVE coincides with the time interval during which the prosthesis becomes endothelialized, thus presenting a surface akin to that of a natural valve. If this is so, the obvious question becomes 'Does the newly implanted valve, in its un-endothelialized state, present a surface to which the organisms associated with early PVE have a facility to adhere?' To consider this question it is first necessary to look at the organisms so associated.

ORGANISMS ASSOCIATED WITH EARLY PVE

From Table 1 it is seen that early PVE is commonly caused by staphylococci – particularly the coagulase-negative variety, diphtheroids, and fungi, especially yeasts. Gram-negative bacilli such as *Escherichia coli*, *Proteus* and so on, also occur, but when their incidence is related to their preponderance in hospital-related sepsis and septicaemia, it is unlikely that they represent a group showing a facility to cause early PVE. Yeasts are of great interest, since it appears that they are the one group of organisms related to early PVE

Table 1 Aetiology of PVE, and interval between surgical procedure and diagnosis

Causative agent	*Early**	*Late*
Streptococcus species	5	27
Staphylococcus epidermidis	14	15
Staphylococcus aureus	9	8
Diphtheroids	7	2
Micrococcus	2	3
Gram-negative bacteria	9	5
Candida species	9	2
Aspergillus species	1	1
TOTAL	56	63

* Endocarditis occurring within 2 months of valve replacement.
Taken from Kaye, D. (ed.). (1976) *Infective Endocarditis*. (Baltimore: University Park Press)

for which a definite mechanism has been elucidated and for which specific successful measures have resulted. Thus, to digress for a short while, Evans has shown that patients receiving antibiotics will develop a build-up of yeasts within the gut and on mucosal surfaces[5]. This process is further aggravated in heart surgery patients by the stagnation of the gut which usually follows the operation. Evans invoked the concept of 'persorption'[6] in which it is shown that if a sufficient concentration of yeasts develops within the gut the organism will appear in the circulation. At lesser concentrations soluble antigen may circulate without intact organisms being released. It was further shown that this process probably explained the development of antibodies to yeasts in convalescence from heart surgery, the incidence of which had been up to 30%. Evans then attacked the problem by giving antifungal agents immediately preoperatively and peroperatively (using topical and non-absorbable agents) to reduce this reservoir. This technique was rewarded by a considerable reduction in both yeast counts in the gut and, more importantly, in the incidence of postoperative antibody levels (this latter both in incidence and titre[7]). Another important change in the same patients was the reduction in the amount of antibiotic given to the patients. Since the advent of this scheme *Candida* endocarditis has been virtually eliminated in the centres using it, occasional patients developing severe postoperative problems needing parenteral nutrition or peritoneal dialysis being the only ones still at risk. It is arguable that these latter patients would be at risk from *Candida* infection due to these techniques regardless of the heart surgery in any case.

Thus the evidence on yeast infection as a part of early PVE can act as a pointer to further studies on the other organisms. However, some of the arguments are not directly translatable; for instance fungal prophylaxis is organism-specific in a way not possible for bacteria. This apart, the yeast story reveals one important truth, which is that the first line of attack is to identify the organism, its reservoir, and its route of access to the valve.

Returning now to the original list of organisms it is seen that in those centres using fungal prophylaxis, narrow-spectrum antibiotic prophylaxis, and practising aggressive control of coliform infections in the postoperative phase, the two organisms remaining at the heart of the problem of early PVE are coagulase-negative staphylococci and diphtheroids. Since in most series, even those containing Gram-negative bacilli and fungi, these two organism groups are statistically the majority it is pertinent to concentrate on them.

Coagulase-negative staphylococci

One of the problems with these organisms in the past has been that one coagulase-negative staphylococcus has looked much like another. Although schemes for their subdivision have been devised, no scheme has been simple. A rapid technique (API-staph; API Laboratories) has become commercially available and we have been using this method in some of our studies. Table 2 shows the species into which it is possible to subdivide coagulase-negative staphylococci. It is important for further discussion to accept two premises

Table 2 The subdivision of coagulase-negative staphylococci using API-staph technique

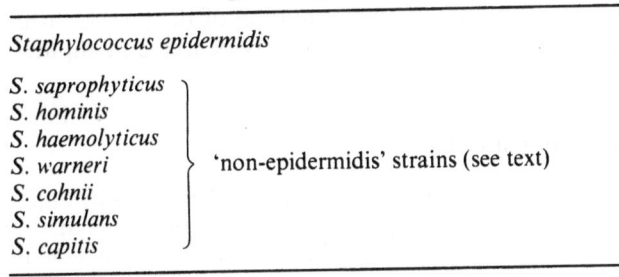

Staphylococcus epidermidis	
S. saprophyticus	'non-epidermidis' strains (see text)
S. hominis	
S. haemolyticus	
S. warneri	
S. cohnii	
S. simulans	
S. capitis	

The scheme is based on that devised by Kloos, W. E. and Schleifer, K. H. (1975). *J. Clin. Microbiol.*, **1**, 82–88.

about this technique. First, there is currently some debate among microbiologists about the validity of the species names and distinction. For the present purpose this does not matter since our use of API-staph depends on its ability to confirm or deny the identity of two or more isolates; the actual name allotted to the isolate is inconsequential. Secondly, whilst some of the names might be revised, the fundamental distinction within the scheme – the distinction between *Staphylococcus epidermidis* and the rest – is likely to remain. In order not to offend the purists the terms 'epidermidis' and 'non-epidermidis' will suffice for the present purpose. It will be seen that in the studies to be discussed these terms will be adequate. It is important to note at this stage that *Staphylococcus epidermidis* is used here as a specific epithet and not as a synonym for coagulase-negative staphylococcus. Thus, it is now possible to compare different isolates of coagulase-negative staphylococci in a useful, albeit limited, way.

Diphtheroids

Diphtheroids are members of the genus *Corynebacterium*, and their detailed identity is at the moment a task beyond the capabilities of most routine laboratories. Such schemes as there are for subdividing these organisms are cumbersome and not adaptable for rapid use. It is impossible so far even to accurately relate one isolate to another. Part of the problem is the slow-growing nature of the genus. Recently a technique has been devised whereby the chemical structures of different isolates can be compared for evidence of identity and this approach may be promising for our purpose (Noble, W. C., personal communication), but as yet the advent of a useful, rapid, and reliable method for dealing with these organisms is awaited.

If we therefore concentrate on these two groups of organisms the next question is to determine the reservoirs of them and, if possible, their route(s) of access to the prosthesis.

RESERVOIRS AND ROUTES OF ACCESS

Figure 2 is a diagrammatic representation of the possible routes and reservoirs relating coagulase-negative staphylococci and diphtheroids to the prosthesis.

Direct implantation with prosthesis

This has undoubtedly happened in the past. More recently improved methods of sterilization of prosthetic valves has largely eliminated the problem. Non-biological prostheses (e.g. Starr–Edwards type) can be adequately sterilized by physical means and, unless contaminated immediately prior to

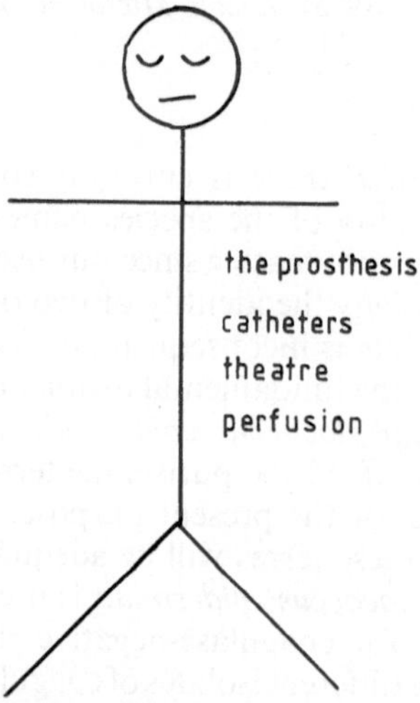

Figure 2 Some sources of PVE

insertion, present little problem. Biological prostheses present a different problem. They cannot be sterilised by standard physical means (e.g. heat) and reliance is usually placed on chemical methods. Unfortunately some chemical disinfectants are incapable of completely sterilizing the tissue and some others, capable of sterilization, will damage the tissue. One approach tried in the past was to use antibiotics[8] instead of disinfectants, but the results merely demonstrated that even mixtures of antibiotics will not approach the spectrum of a good chemical agent. Another approach was evident when it was found that glutaraldehyde has beneficial effects on the structure of biological material, improving its characteristics for use in prosthetic valves. It must be stressed that glutaraldehyde at the pH and concentration used for fixation is not reliably bactericidal, and that a further agent (usually formalin) will be needed to sterilize the fashioned valve. Formalin appears to be particularly suitable, having the ability to kill even spores and acid-fast bacilli such as *Mycobacterium fortuitum*[9] which has caused trouble in the past.

All in all, the implanted valve appears to be rarely the source of PVE and in the recent era, certainly not PVE due to staphylococci and diphtheroids.

Airborne contamination of the operative field

This possibility is one which has received curiously little attention. Both the common organisms with which we are concerned are found on human skin and it is vital that this possibility be investigated. Since we are now able to subdivide coagulase-negative staphylococci easily it should be possible to attempt correlation between theatre air samples and subsequent isolates from cases of PVE. This we intend to do, if for no other reason than the fact that reducing this route is a relatively easy task compared with some of the others. The recent innovation of cardioplegic solutions may be relevant, since these solutions contain no antibiotics and thus the arrested heart is partly bathed in a non-protective medium, even if the blood is full of antibiotic.

Perfusion apparatus

Perfusion blood cultures are routinely obtained at all operations in Freeman Hospital. Earlier reports indicated that coagulase-negative staphylococci and diphtheroids could be found in 7.5% and 9.8%[10] of such samples respectively. Initially we found that an organism could be obtained in 10.6%: coagulase-negative staphylococci in 6%, and diphtheroids in 3.4%. However, following the introduction of a broad-spectrum β-lactamase addition to the culture, whereby the prophylactic antibiotic being given was specifically neutralized, the overall isolation rate went up to 17.7%, that of coagulase-negative staphylococci to 10.8%, and of diphtheroids, 5.4%. Table 3 demonstrates this.

Thus perfusion blood is one reservoir from which both the putative causes of PVE can be isolated with ease. Table 4 shows the result of applying the API-staph method to the coagulase-negative staphylococci isolated and similar organisms found in the catheter tip cultures of the same patients, in an attempt to prove or disprove identity. The numbers are extremely small, but what evidence there is would suggest that the two reservoirs are not linked. It is tempting to accept perfusion blood as one source of PVE. However, of the two cases of PVE which have occurred in Freeman Hospital over the period in which perfusion blood cultures have been obtained, in neither case was the causative organism eventually isolated from the clinical disease found in the perfusion blood culture.

In one of these two cases no organism was isolated and in the second the disease was due to a coagulase-negative staphylococcus (*Staphylococcus epidermidis*), whereas perfusion blood taken at the time of operation yielded a diphtheroid.

Intravenous and intra-arterial catheters

Of all the possible sources of organisms likely to be associated with early PVE this reservoir has been under the greatest suspicion. One of the main

Table 3 The effect of routine addition of a broad-spectrum β-lactamase preparation to cultures of perfusion blood

β-Lactamase	No. of cultures	No. positive	Coagulase-negative staphylococci	Diphtheroids	Streptococci	Coliforms	Others
Not added	448	37 (8.3%)	20 (4.5%)	12 (2.7%)	5 (1.1%)	2 (0.4%)	0
Added	147	26 (17.7%)	16 (10.8%)	8 (5.4%)	2 (1.4%)	1 (0.7%)	2 (1.4%)

Effect of adding β-lactamase to perfusion blood cultures – overall isolation rate, and organism-specific isolation rates.

	Preliminary	Late
Lactamase not added (448 cultures)		
Coagulase-negative staphylococci	7	13
Diphtheroids	0	12
Streptococci	2	3
Coliforms	2	0
Others	0	0
	11 (2.45%)	28 (6.25%)
Lactamase added (147 cultures)		
Coagulase-negative staphylococci	5	11
Diphtheroids	1	7
Streptococci	2	0
Coliforms	1	0
Others	0	2
	9 (6.1%)	20 (13.6%)

Effect of β-lactamase addition on distribution of the isolates relative to time of laboratory incubation.

Table 4 **Analysis of the species of coagulase-negative staphylococcus isolated from cultures of perfusion blood, and their correlation with catheter tip cultures from the same patients**

Patient	*Antibiotic*	*Incubation*	*Result*	*Patient*	*Antibiotic*	*Incubation*	*Result*
1	Fluclox	late	*epiderm.*	13	Fluclox	late	*epiderm.*
2	Fluclox	preliminary	*epiderm.*	14	Fluclox	late	*epiderm.*
3	Fluclox	late	*epiderm.*	15	Fluclox	preliminary	*epiderm.*
4	Cephradine	late	*epiderm.*	16	Fluclox	late	*epiderm.*
5	Cephradine	late	*epiderm.*	17	Fluclox	late	*epiderm.*
6	Fluclox	late	*saproph.*	18	Fluclox	late	*epiderm.*
7	Fluclox	late	*epiderm.*	19	Fluclox	preliminary	*epiderm.*
8	Cephradine	late	*epiderm.*	20	Fluclox	preliminary	*epiderm.*
9	Lincomycin	late	*saproph.*	21	Fluclox	late	*epiderm.*
10	Fluclox	preliminary	*epiderm.*	22	Fluclox	late	*capitis.*
11	Fluclox	late	*epiderm.*	23	Fluclox	preliminary	*epiderm.*
12	Fluclox	late	*epiderm.*				

Results of speciation of 23 consecutive coagulase-negative staphylococci from perfusion blood cultures. (*epiderm* = *S. epidermidis*; *saproph* = *S. saprophyticus*; *capitis* = *S. capitis*).

			Positive cultures	
No. of patients	*No. of catheters*	*No. positive*	*Patient*	*Result*
23	35	4	No. 4	*S. saprophyticus*
			No. 6	*S. episermidis*
			No. 11	*S. epidermidis*
			No. 22	*S. epidermidis*

Correlation of perfusion blood cultures and positive catheter tip cultures on 23 consecutive occasions.

reasons is that some of the catheters concerned may directly overlie the newly implanted valve. Therefore, the left atrial line is particularly deserving of study.

We have embarked upon a detailed study of the organisms isolated from these catheters in open heart surgery patients, in an attempt to define the problem more precisely and possibly plan a rational strategy. From earlier work it is clear that organisms, particularly staphylococci, can be isolated from these catheters with ease, that the incidence of positive cultures is highest in catheters which have been in place some time (more than 2 days) and that the type of organism recovered changes with the time *in situ*. Thus, in an earlier series in which catheters were left in place for a mean time of 3.9 days organisms were found in 35%, whereas when strenuous efforts were made to remove central lines as soon as possible leading to a mean time *in situ* of 1.75 days, the isolation rate was only 8%[11]. Resistant organisms, and especially yeasts, are only found in catheters which have been in place for more than 5 days. These findings, taken together with improved postoperative care in recent years which will reduce the necessary time for catheter use, go some way towards explaining the fall in the incidence of early PVE.

Taking the catheter population as a whole (i.e. adding all results together, regardless of the type of catheter and its place of insertion), we have established several other parameters. In Table 5 the relationship of catheter isolations to age is seen. Not surprisingly, isolation rates are highest at the extremes of age. This table also shows that coliform organisms and streptococci figure in those two age groups but are rare in the intervening years. This latter finding would suggest that coliform septicaemias would occur more commonly in the postoperative stages in very young patients and in the elderly; a

Table 5 The relationship of the number and types of organisms isolated from catheter tips (all sites) and the patient's age

No.	*Age group (years)*	*Cns*	*Streps.*	*Diph.*	*Colifs.*	*Yeasts*	*Total organisms*
48	0–1	9 (18)	7 (14)	1 (2)	9 (18)	—	26 (54)
27	1–5	5 (18)	4 (15)	—	—	—	9 (19)
37	5–10	4 (11)	—	—	—	—	4 (11)
36	10–20	3 (8)	—	1 (3)	—	—	4 (11)
22	20–30	2 (9)	—	1 (4.5)	—	—	3 (13.5)
51	30–40	7 (14)	1 (2)	2 (4)	—	—	10 (20)
148	40–50	17 (11)	3 (2)	—	2 (1.3)	—	22 (15)
232	50–60	32 (14)	2 (1)	1 (0.5)	8 (3.5)	—	43 (18.5)
104	>60	22 (21)	4 (4)	—	7 (7)	1 (1)	34 (33)

KEY: Cns = coagulase-negative staphylococci
Streps. = Streptococci (all types)
Diph. = diphtheroids
Colifs. = Coliform bacilli
Figures in parentheses are percentages.

suggestion correlating with clinical experience. Detailed analysis of these results, relating the organism type to age and site of the catheter (a burdensome analysis which will not be reproduced here) reveals that coliform organisms and streptococci are found in the over-50 years groups in all line sites, but in the babies are predominantly in the arterial lines and venous lines. In particular, left atrial lines are not a source of these organisms in babies, whereas in older patients they may be CVP; and subclavian lines which are used in older patients are rarely used in babies. Having defined some simple general facts about catheters in open heart patients, the discussion will now centre on the two principal organisms of early PVE and their relation to individual catheter sites.

Table 6 shows the incidence of coagulase-negative staphylococci and diphtheroids in various specified catheter sitings. Two obvious facts emerge. First, diphtheroids are conspicuous by their absence. We suspect that this may be a technical factor, since most catheter studies (including our own)

Table 6 The isolation rate of coagulase-negative staphylococci and diphtheroids in various catheter sites

Catheter site	*No. of catheters*	*Cns*	*Diph.*	*Total*
Left atrium	154	12 (8)	1 (0.6)	13 (8.5)
Right atrium	21	—	—	—
Arterial lines	270	41 (15)	1 (0.4)	42 (15.5)
Venous lines	137	20 (14.6)	3 (2)	23 (16.7)
CVP lines (including subclavian and long-lines)	46	20 (43)	1 (2)	21 (45)
Peripheral lines	40	5 (12.5)	—	5 (12.5)

KEY: Cns = coagulase-negative staphylococci;
Diph. = diphtheroids
Figures in parentheses are percentages

have only incubated the material for 24–48 h, and diphtheroids are notoriously slow growers. We have now begun incubating the cultures for much longer periods and hope to thereby obtain a truer picture. If, however, no increase is found this would leave the perfusion bloods as the only known common source of these organisms and would, therefore, lead our attention back to the operating theatre. The second point is that the right atrial lines virtually never grow any organism whatsoever. Since this line is frequently handled and has drugs (for instance, isoprenaline) given through it, it is of interest that it is so uniformly free of organisms. In comparison the left atrial line yields staphylococci or diphtheroids in 8% of cases although this line is handled much less. The venous lines yield staphylococci or diphtheroids in 16% of cases and the arterial lines, very frequently handled and in an obvious site to suffer from skin and even faecal contamination, yield 15.5%. It may be that the effects of frequent handling are, to some extent, offset by the effect of a high flow rate, but even so the findings in the right atrial catheters remain a paradox. The findings in tips from CVP, subclavian and long-line catheters are no surprise since they are catheters used in patients in worse health, and in whom complications have occurred; such patients (and their lines) receive intensive handling. Table 7, in relating the percentage of the various catheters which yield coagulase-negative staphylococci and diphtheroids to age, reveals that, apart from arterial catheters, catheter-associated organisms are a feature of the older age groups. This might partly explain the observation that PVE more rarely complicates repair of congenital defects than valve insertions.

Table 7 The relationship between catheter site, age group, and the isolation rate of coagulase-negative staphylococci and diphtheroids combined (percentages)

Age group (years)	*LA*	*RA*	*AL*	*VL*	*CVP, etc.*	*Per*
0–1	0	0	33	27	no caths	0
1–5	0	0	23	33	no caths	0
5–10	0	0	10	9	no caths	0
10–20	0	0	7	20	33	0
20–30	0	no caths	17	12	no caths	no caths
30–40	9	0	12	20	60	20
40–50	10	0	13	11	9	16
50–60	8	0	15	21	31	0
>60	10	0	10	10	83	40

Note: In some of the categories only small numbers of catheters were used, so the results should be interpreted with caution.
KEY: LA = left atrium; RA = right atrium; AL = arterial line; VL = venous line; CVP, etc. = CVP lines, long-lines and subclavian lines; Per = peripheral lines

Another avenue of investigation which we have explored is that of examining the distribution of the various API-staph types in the different situations. Briefly, it was found that *Staphylococcus epidermidis* (the commonest variety on the skin) was the universal finding in contaminants obtained from blood cultures but that 44% of isolates from catheter tips were non-epidermidis (17% were the variety known as *S. saprophyticus*). Further investigation revealed that the non-epidermidis types were heavily associated with catheters which had been in place some time, whereas *S. epidermidis* strains were only found in catheters removed within the first few days (mean time *in situ* for those yielding *S. epidermidis*, 2.08 days; for those yielding *S. saprophyticus*, 5.88 days)[12]. We thus consider that the non-epidermidis strains have a possible facility for establishing themselves and adhering on to catheter material ('Teflon'). It is a logical step to postulate that if such strains can stick on to catheter prosthetic material, they may stick on to the un-endothelialized valve also.

We have recently taken the investigation a little further. Table 8 shows the results of applying API-staph typing to the coagulase-negative staphylococci found in the different catheter sites (for this purpose CVP lines, long-lines

Table 8 The relation of API-staph type to the site of the catheter

Catheter site	*No. of isolates tested*	*Epidermidis*	*Non-epidermidis*
Left atrium	10	6	4
Right atrium	—	—	—
Arterial lines	41	25	16
Venous lines	19	10	9
CVP, etc.	12	12	0
Peripheral	5	5	0

and subclavian catheters were grouped under one heading). A very clear distinction emerges. All the catheters which are specific to open heart surgery (left atrium, right atrium, arterial and venous lines) have a mixed population of *S. epidermidis* and non-epidermidis. In contrast all the lines which, although used here on heart surgery patients, are used throughout all forms of medicine (CVP, long-line, subclavian and peripheral lines) have a population which is exclusively *S. epidermidis*. An obvious argument is that the former group were in longer, bearing in mind our earlier findings, but in fact the CVP lines had a mean time *in situ* of 5.2 days. The explanation of this difference is not easy. Two possibilities have occurred to us: first, the LA, RA, arterial and venous lines are inserted in the theatre, whereas the others are inserted postoperatively. It may be that this possibility will again lead us to the theatre as the prime source of these organisms, although the increase in the incidence of non-epidermis types with time would be against this theory, or secondly it could be that *S. epidermidis* represents exogenous contamination of the catheters, whereas the non-epidermidis types represent endogenous seeding. Subclinical bacteraemias are well recognized, and their seeding of catheter tips has been described before. This would mean that, although the catheters acted as an intermediate reservoir, the primary source must be elsewhere in the patient's body. The gut is one possibility, other possibilities are the mucosal surfaces. The gut stasis which follows heart surgery might well increase the concentration of non-epidermidis staphylococci, just as was earlier demonstrated for yeasts. The event leading to dissemination is not difficult to pin-point: perfusion. This might explain some of the perfusion blood culture results, although as already mentioned, no identity was found in the few patients in which it was attempted.

These data lead us to five important conclusions:

(1) Both the principal organisms associated with early PVE can be isolated with ease from cultures of perfusion blood.
(2) Coagulase-negative staphylococci (and possibly diphtheroids when a better technique is employed) can be isolated from intravenous and intra-arterial catheters.
(3) There appears to be a subpopulation of coagulase-negative staphylococci (the non-epidermidis types) which may be particularly fitted to adhere to prosthetic material.

(4) Urgent work is needed to try and analyse diphtheroid isolations in a similar way.
(5) Urgent work is needed to define precisely the origins and routes of spread of non-epidermidis types of coagulase-negative staphylococci.

If some of these projects bear fruit, it should be possible to attack the reservoirs or design prophylaxis specific to the problem organisms, or both.

The mention of prophylaxis leads on to the final piece of work which it is relevant to consider. Whilst it will be better and more satisfactory to identify the reservoirs and routes of access of the causative organisms of PVE the present lack of knowledge forces us to rely on chemoprophylaxis as the practicable measure presently available.

CHEMOPROPHYLAXIS

The value of prophylaxis has never been established beyond question, although it is commonly accepted that it is valuable[13]. Since the problem organisms are Gram-positive the drugs used have tended to be iso-oxazolyl penicillins (such as cloxacillin) or cephalosporins. Recently a scheme involving the addition of gentamicin has been claimed to produce excellent results, in that no PVE followed 800 perfusions[14]. Our experience has been limited to the first two regimes, in that our routine prophylaxis is with flucloxacillin, but for a short while one group of patients received cephradine on a studied basis. Whilst studying this group we observed certain parameters which we think are worthy of further consideration.

Table 9 is a comparison of the flora found in the tracheal secretions of patients receiving antibiotic prophylaxis for heart surgery. The minor groups of patient on drugs other than cephradine or flucloxacillin can be ignored for the present purpose, although it is clear that in heart surgery patients receiving antibiotics additional to their routine prophylaxis (often for excellent reasons) the tracheal flora becomes more resistant. However, it is seen that flora changes on flucloxacillin are minimal, whereas on cephradine it is much more common to see the emergence of resistant Gram-negative bacilli such as *Proteus*, *E. coli* and so on. Although we have not studied the gut flora specifically, it is extremely likely that these changes are reflected in the gut. Thus, a broader-spectrum prophylaxis seems to change the bacterial flora of the patient towards a more antibiotic-resistant population, and specifically to encourage the emergence of Gram-negative bacilli ('coliforms'). Although this is not shown here, we were able to detect a similar change in the organism types isolated from the catheter tips of the same patients. Thus, we consider that widening the spectrum of prophylaxis exacts a price in the short term. The question posed by this is whether this price is translated into clinical problems. The final table (Table 10) reveals that a study of all patients perfused between April 1978 and December 1979 shows that of 814 cases (353 of which involved valve insertion) four cases of 'PVE' resulted. Of these four cases two were infections of prosthetic valves (both aortic; one due to *S. epidermidis*, one due to a diphtheroid) and two were infections of prosthetic material other than valves. Thus, the incidence of PVE is low,

Table 9 Incidence of isolation of various organisms from cultures of tracheal secretion in patients undergoing open heart surgery, related to the antibiotic being administered. (Apparent discrepancies in total are due to more than one organism being isolated from one specimen)

Antibiotic	*No. of patients*	*No. of specimens*	*No growth*	Haemophilus *species**	*Coliforms†*	*Yeasts*
Fluclox	90	91	57 (63)	30 (33)	5 (5.5)	—
Cephradine	46	49	26 (53)	13 (27)	11 (22)	—
Fluclox + Neomycin	3	15	4 (27)	1 (7)	11 (73)	—
Fluclox + Ampicillin	3	8	1 (12.5)	—	7 (87.5)	—
Ampicillin	2	16	4 (25)	—	11 (69)	1 (6)
Fluclox + Gentamicin	1	2	1	—	1	—
Ampicillin + Gentamicin	1	2	2	—	—	—
Ampicillin + Gentamicin + Fluclox	4	7	4	2	2	2
TOTAL	150	190	99 (52)	46 (24)	48 (25)	3 (1.6)

* Of the 46 *Haemophilus* species isolated 36 (78 %) were *Haemophilus parainfluenzae*, the remainder being *H. influenzae*.
† The term 'coliform' is used as a collective name for facultatively anaerobic Gram-negative bacilli, e.g. *E. coli*, *Proteus*, *Klebsiella*, *Pseudomonas*, and so on.

Table 10 Relating the operative throughput to prosthetic infection and postoperative septicaemias (April 1978–December 1979)

		Prosthetic infections	
Total perfusions	*Valves inserted*	*Of valves*	*Others*
814	353	2 (= 0.24 % perf. = 0.56 % valve)	2 (= 0.24 % perf.)
		Combined 4 (0.49 % of perfusions)	

Flucloxacillin prophylaxis 762	no. septicaemias during hospitalization 7 (3 children)	incidence 0.9 %
Cephradine prophylaxis 52	no. septicaemias during hospitalization 4	incidence 7.7 %

u

being either 4 per 800 perfusions (0.5 %), or 2 per 353 valves (0.6 %). None of these cases received cephradine.

During the same period our laboratory proved by blood culture isolation 12 cases of postoperative septicaemia. Of these 7 occurred in 762 patients given flucloxacillin (or lincomycin when penicillin-allergic) and 4 in 52 patients given cephradine.

We conclude that narrow-spectrum prophylaxis with flucloxacillin will result in an extremely low incidence of PVE. Use of a cephlosporin *might* reduce this further (52 patients is too small a number to decide this) but that this will result in an unacceptably high incidence of Gram-negative infections in the immediate postoperative period. This distinction relating to Gram-negative septicaemia becomes even more striking when it is realized that the flucloxacillin group contains all the babies and children, since they are a group particularly liable to develop such septicaemias. These statements, of course, take no account of other factors, but we consider it likely that most other variables were randomized.

All practitioners of medicine are painfully aware that there are no blacks and whites, only shades of grey. We suggest that narrow-spectrum prophylaxis produces an acceptable balance between long-term and short-term risks and should remain our policy whilst we continue to unravel the basic mechanisms of PVE. Hopefully, we will eventually prevent the disease by alternative methods.

References

1. Yeh, T. J., Anabtawi, I. N. and Cornett, V. E. (1967). Bacterial endocarditis following open heart surgery. *Ann. Thorac. Surg.*, **3,** 29
2. Weinstein, L. and Rubin, R. H. (1973). Infective endocarditis. *Prog. Cardiovasc. Dis.*, **16,** 239
3. Parker, M. T. and Ball, L. C. (1975). Streptococci associated with systemic disease in man. Pathological Society of Great Britain and Ireland. 113th meeting. (Preprinted abstracts)
4. Hehre, E. J. and Neill, J. M. (1946). Formation of serologically reactive dextrans by streptococci from subacute bacterial endocarditis. *J. Exp. Med.*, **83,** 147
5. Evans, E. G. V. (1976). Mycological aspects of open-heart surgery. In Ionescu, M. I. and Wooler, G. H. (eds.). *Current Techniques in Extracorporeal Circulation*, pp. 397–406. (London and Boston: Butterworth)
6. Krause, W., Matheis, H. and Wulf, K. (1969). Fungaemia and funguria after oral administration of Candida albicans. *Lancet*, **1,** 598
7. Evans, E. G. V. and Forster, R. A. (1976). Antibodies to Candida after operations on the heart. *J. Med. Microbiol.*, **9,** 303
8. Waterworth, P. M., Lockey, E., Berry, E. M. and Pearce, H. M. (1974). A critical investigation into the antibiotic sterilization of heart valve. *Thorax*, **29,** 432
9. FDA (1977). Morbidity and Mortality Report, Feb. 1977: *Isolation of Mycobacteria species from porcine heart valve prostheses*, pp. 42–3. (Centre for Disease Control, United States Department of Health, Education and Welfare)
10. Ankeney, J. L. and Parkney, R. F. (1969). Staphylococcal endocarditis following open-heart surgery related to positive ultra-operative blood cultures. In Brewer, L. A. (ed.). *Prosthetic Heart Valves*, (Springfield, Illinois: Charles C. Thomas)

11. Freeman, R. (1976). Microbiological aspects of open heart surgery. In Ionescu, M. I. and Wooler, G. H. (eds.). *Current Techniques in Extracorporeal Circulation*, (London and Boston: Butterworth)
12. Freeman, R. and Hjersing, N. (1980). Studies on the species of coagulase-negative staphylococci isolated from catheter tips from open-heart surgery patients. *Thorax*. (In press)
13. Jacoby, I., Mandell, L. A. and Weinstein, N. (1978). The chemoprophylaxis of infection. *Med. Clin. N. Amer.*, **62,** 1083
14. Newsom, S. W. B. (1978). Antibiotic prophylaxis for open-heart surgery. *J. Antimicrob. Chemother.*, **4,** 389

42
Prevention and treatment of renal failure

F. D. THOMPSON

INTRODUCTION

Any major surgical intervention, or indeed trauma of any kind, may result in a temporary, recoverable severe renal damage. This is particularly so with major cardiovascular surgery. The renal lesion first generally recognized as complicating wartime bombing casualties in Britain was referred to as the crush syndrome. Subsequently this has been given many names but that most widely used is acute tubular necrosis, although possibly better named acute tubular dysfunction, as histologically necrosis is most striking by its absence. It is primarily this renal lesion which is considered in this article. The occurrence of severe renal failure following trauma is assumed to have arisen in previously normal kidneys. In the presence of severe cardiovascular disease renal functional impairment or pathological lesions of the kidney are not a rarity. There is a strong argument in favour of a careful factual assessment of the renal status *before* any patient undergoes such major surgery.

PREOPERATIVE ASSESSMENT

There are many reasons why the patient with cardiac disease may have an associated impairment of renal function. Patients with congestive cardiac failure may well have a reduction in the glomerular filtration rate (GFR)[1], sodium and water retention[2] and a significant degree of proteinuria. Patients with subacute bacterial endocarditis may have the associated glomerulonephritic lesion[3] and those with long-standing cyanotic problems may also exhibit renal functional impairment. This last group exhibit histological changes in the glomeruli which consist of pronounced dilatation of the capillary tuft, mesangial cell proliferation and thickening of the basement membrane. In those reaching adult life, nitrogen retention, haematuria and heavy proteinuria have been described[4]. It is no surprise that patients with atheromatous involvement of the coronary vessels may have other vessels involved with a similar process, and the renal vasculature is no exception. This renal atherosclerosis often produces small, shrunken kidneys with an associated reduction in function. Patients with abdominal aortic aneurysms may have ureteric involvement, especially if leakage has occurred. The ureters may become encased in fibrous tissue causing obstruction, and this form of retroperitoneal fibrosis may require combined urological and vascular surgery. A sound case can be made therefore for an accurate preoperative assessment of renal function. In this respect the random blood urea is inadequate as nitrogen retention will not occur until almost two-thirds of overall function is lost. A more accurate measure of GFR is required and a creatinine clearance will suffice, but the isotopic techniques involving the clearance of ^{51}Cr-labelled EDTA eliminate the need for timed, accurate urine collections which may be a source of error[5]. The simultaneous estimation of the clearance of [^{131}I]-hippuran will measure the effective renal plasma flow. Now that the gamma camera is being used to assess cardiac function[6], it may well be possible to assess renal function at the same time. In addition to obtaining information relating to the anatomy of the renal tract it is also possible to measure renal blood flow and GFR and to assess individual kidney function[7].

During the preoperative assessment certain problems may arise. The use of contrast media during angiography presents the nephron with a high osmotic load and subsequent obligatory diuresis. In patients with polycythaemia secondary to cyanotic heart disease this may be harmful unless urinary losses of water and electrolytes are carefully measured and replaced. If this practice is not observed then further haemoconcentration occurs, which may lead to thrombotic complications and renal failure. Dietary sodium restriction and the long-term use of diuretics have often been used in the management of congestive cardiac failure. This may lead to abnormalities of renal function as hypovolaemia and a subsequent reduction in GFR can occur. The hypovolaemia triggers antidiuretic hormone release and hence water retention. The potent loop diuretics block the normal reabsorption of sodium in the ascending diluting segment of the distal nephron, and the ability to excrete free water is lost. At this stage hyponatraemia[8] and peripheral oedema develop and a case can be made for stopping the diuretics, measuring the plasma volume, and possibly considering haemodialysis and ultrafiltration. This will allow the patient to proceed to surgery in a more favourable state of sodium and water balance. Hopefully the accurate assessment of patients may reduce the incidence of acute renal failure across surgery.

PREOPERATIVE MANAGEMENT

Urine flow rates are carefully monitored across surgery, and if oliguria develops repeated injections of diuretics such as mannitol and frusemide are often given. No firm evidence exists as to the benefit of this technique and it may well be that to leave the diuretic challenge until the normal circulation has been established will prove to be equally beneficial. The composition of priming fluids is being discussed elsewhere and it is interesting to note that the composition of such fluids may affect overall function. Joekes *et al.* in the 1950s showed that the use of rheomacrodex across cardiac surgery exhibited an antidiuretic effect (personal communication).

POSTOPERATIVE MANAGEMENT

Recognition of renal failure

The management of oliguria (urine volume 0.5 ml/min or less) in the immediate postoperative period involves the distinction being made between prerenal failure due to hypovolaemia and acute tubular dysfunction due to ischaemia, antibiotics, septicaemia, etc. When a reduced urine flow is a response to hypovolaemia, this is a normal physiological response and the urine characteristics will reflect this. The osmolarity will be above 750 mOsm/l, the concentration of urea is greater than 320 mmol/l and, when compared to that of plasma, will give a U/P ratio of above 20:1. When renal tubular dysfunction is the cause of oliguria then the ability to pass a concentrated urine is lost. The osmolarity is below 600 mOsmol/l and approximates to that of plasma. The urinary urea concentration will be below 190 mmol/l and the U/R ratio in this instance is often well below 10:1. The osmolarity of urine should be interpreted with caution because if contrast has been injected for an intravenous urogram (IVU), mannitol given, or glucose and insulin used to lower the plasma potassium, then a falsely high reading may be obtained.

Some patients develop acute renal failure whilst maintaining a normal urine flow. Non-oliguric renal failure[9] may be missed as fluid overload and hyperkalaemia are not immediate problems. Their management involves careful fluid and electrolyte control and haemodialysis may be required.

Correction of prerenal factors and diuretic challenge

When tubular function is normal and oliguria is a physiological response to hypovolaemia then the obvious management is the prompt correction of the underlying condition. When tubular damage has occurred the use of a diuretic challenge may in one or two instances reverse the renal failure. The only reversals that we have seen in our unit have been with the use of mannitol 25 g given by rapid intravenous infusion. A positive response will soon be apparent as the urine flow will increase within 10–20 min of administration. Bolus injections of frusemide in doses ranging from 40 to 250 mg have been used and in some instances the urine flow rate has increased, which may be beneficial in the presence of severe fluid overload and hyperkalaemia. There is no evidence, however, that the course of renal failure is actually reversed.

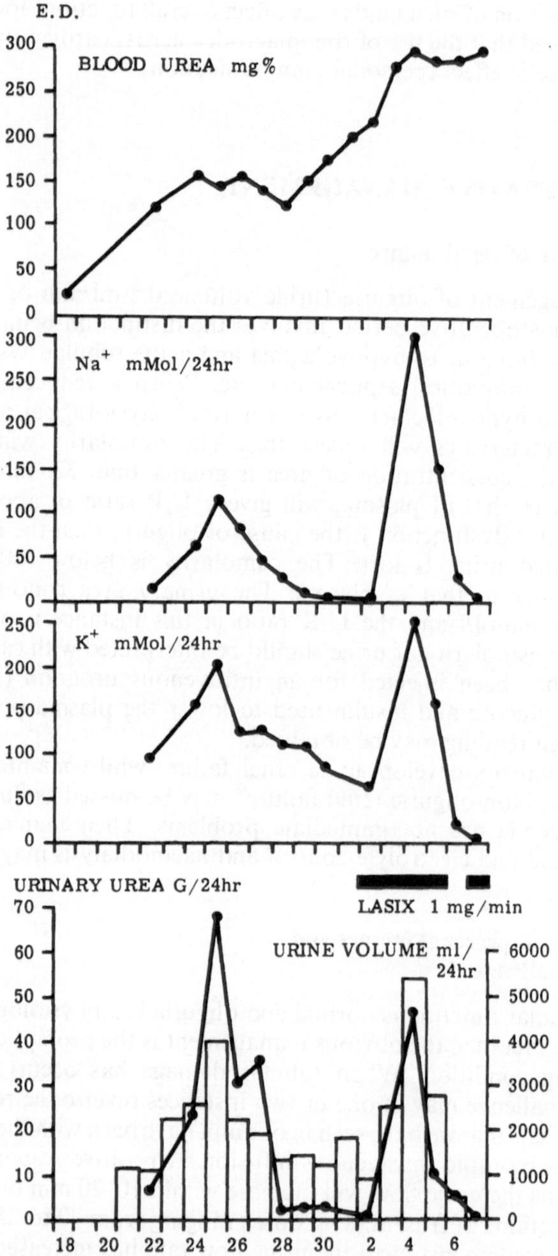

Figure 1 The urinary losses of sodium and potassium during an intravenous infusion of Lasix given at the rate of 1 mg/min

Infusions of frusemide in a dose of 1–2 mg/min have been used, but again no long-term benefit has accrued. Urinary losses of sodium and potassium are considerable (Figure 1) and may produce dangerous arrhythmias. The only benefit from frusemide infusion is the possible prevention of dangerous hyperkalaemia and fluid overload when intravenous inotropic support is needed.

Haemodialysis

There is no doubt that early, frequent haemodialysis is the treatment of choice, should this diuretic challenge fail. For this the patients may need to be transferred to a specialist unit capable of managing postoperative cardiac problems in addition to their routine management of acute renal failure. Haemodialysis machines are becoming more compact and therefore more readily portable, and on occasions dialysis can be carried out within the cardiac unit. The use of haemodialysis early in the course of renal failure may well prevent complications and certainly gives the patient the best chance of survival.

The indication for starting haemodialysis is simply the presence of renal failure. Nothing can be gained by waiting until the patient is unwell with a raised blood urea, severe hyperkalaemia and fluid overload. It is obviously desirable to keep the patient as fit as possible by starting dialysis early. The ideal is to dialyse for short periods on a daily basis if required as the problems of arrhythmias and hypertension tend to develop after 3 or 4 h of dialysis. This approach allows adequate calories to be given in the form of carbohydrate or lipids and gradually amino acid solutions and finally gastrointestinal feeding with protein can be introduced. During the catabolic phase it is expected that the patient should lose weight, and account has to be taken of the water produced by metabolism. Once the anabolic phase is entered the protein intake can be increased and from this point a slight, steady weight-gain can be expected.

The period of oliguria or anuria may last for up to 40 days and, generally speaking, acute tubular dysfunction is potentially reversible. Once the urine volumes increase they may do so in a dramatic fashion with the patient entering a diuretic phase where the urinary losses of sodium and potassium have to be carefully monitored and replaced if necessary. Some of these points are illustrated in Figure 2. This patient with Marfan's syndrome required emergency surgery for aortic dissection. This involved coronary vein grafts and replacement of his aortic valve and ascending aorta. The management of his postoperative renal failure included haemodialysis which was started on the third postoperative day. Dialysis was required for a further 13 days. The urine output returned on the eleventh postoperative day and reached 3.5–4.0 l by Day 14. Five years later the patient is fully active and has a creatinine clearance of 82 ml/min.

It is well known that major changes in the cardiovascular system occur during haemodialysis[10–12]. In a recent study conducted in our unit on 52 chronic haemodialysis patients, 42% had an increase in cardiac output (in some the output doubled) and in 58% there was a fall in cardiac output, the

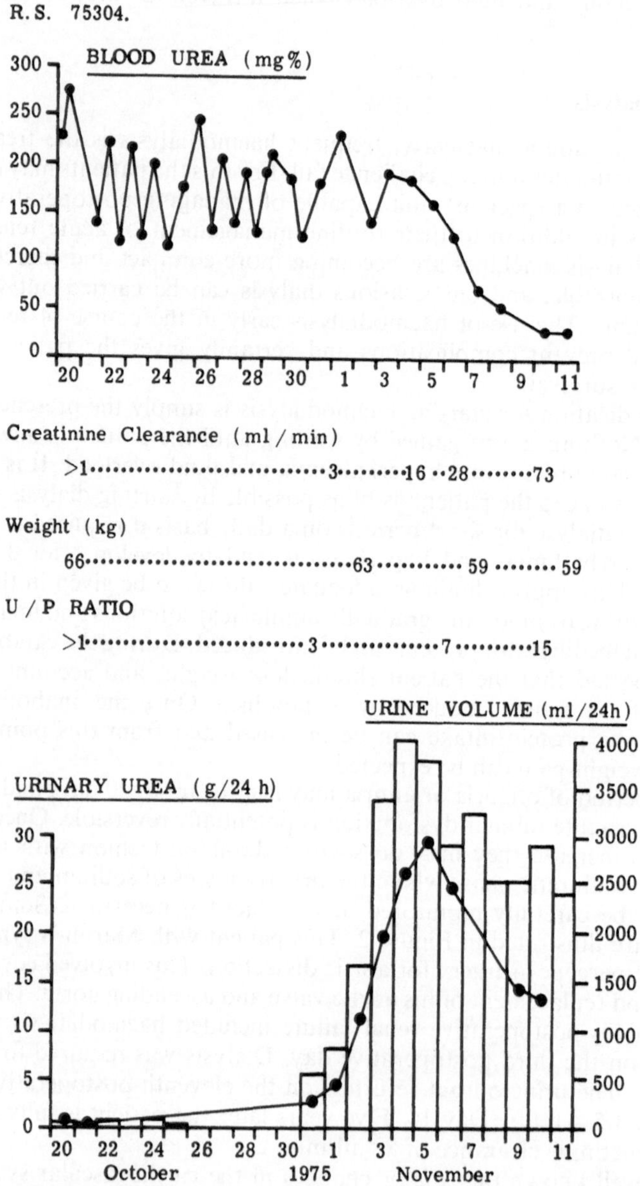

Figure 2 The postoperative course of a patient who developed acute renal failure after emergency surgery. The sharp drops in blood urea concentration represent periods of haemodialysis. The operative date was 18 October

greatest change being a drop of 70 %. Similar changes in pulse rate are seen and the major change in blood pressure is a tendency to fall. With more ambitious surgery being undertaken for congenital heart disease, these changes may be harmful in the early postoperative period, and in this situation peritoneal dialysis may be indicated in this early critical period when haemodynamic stability is of prime importance.

Peritoneal dialysis

In young children when haemodialysis can present technical problems, peritoneal dialysis may be adequate if catabolism is not severe. Figure 3 illustrates such a case of a young child who underwent surgery for Fallot's tetralogy and who was supported for over a week by peritoneal dialysis. This example is the exception as all too commonly peritoneal dialysis is not adequate to prevent the urea rising. The problems of 'splinting' the diaphragm when the abdomen is full[13], and the need to dialyse continuously for 24 h, obviously limit mobility. Therefore it cannot be too clearly stated that early, frequent, short periods of haemodialysis remain the treatment of choice and peritoneal dialysis should only be used if this support cannot be given.

Associated problems

Occasionally the state of the renal vessels is in doubt. In the case of aortic dissection the question of renal artery involvement often arises and in embolic disease renal arterial occlusion is a possibility. In such cases, when the overall renal perfusion is suspect, further investigations have to be considered. The presence of a nephrogram during an IVU confirms the presence of adequate blood supply. Gamma camera studies using [^{99}Tc]-DMSA may provide valuable information[7], but if doubt still exists then invasive angiography may be needed.

The anaemia of renal failure develops rapidly and excessive blood transfusion may lead to a rise in bilirubin. Blood may have to be given in the postoperative period for many reasons but the routine transfusion to maintain the haemoglobin at the preoperative level is to be avoided. Occasional profound jaundice is seen without hepatocellular damage and is thought to be a result of bile inspissated in the small canaliculi. No specific treatment is of value. However, when cellular damage results in liver failure, the prognosis is grave and if indicated special supportive measures will be needed.

Drug administration during the period of renal failure has to be carefully controlled[14]. Those agents such as digoxin and the aminoglycosides whose excretion is solely dependent upon glomerular filtration need to have their dosage drastically modified and the measurement of plasma concentrations will provide a guide to overall dosage.

The commonly used inotropic agents, adrenaline, noradrenaline, isoprenaline and dopamine, may well have adverse effects on renal blood flow. Renal blood flow and its distribution between cortex and medulla is affected by these agents[15–17]. Low dosage of dopamine 3 μg min^{-1} kg^{-1} may well

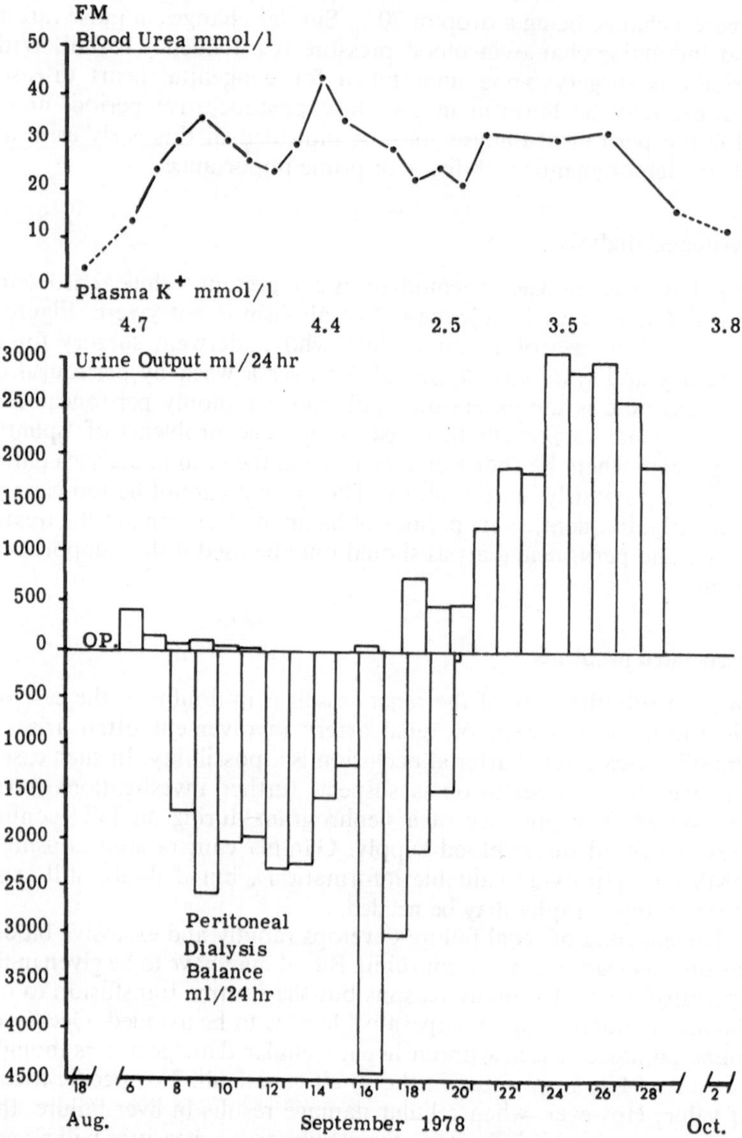

Figure 3 The use of peritoneal dialysis in a child who developed acute renal failure following surgery for Fallot's tetralogy

improve renal blood flow[18], but at high dosage this renal blood flow is curtailed and the price of cardiac support may be at the cost of reduced glomerular filtration. The presence of an aortic balloon for counterpulsation may alter renal blood flow. Some clinicians have suggested that it augments blood flow and improves renal perfusion and function, while others feel its presence impedes renal blood flow. The price for left ventricular support may be reduced renal function.

What developments can be envisaged in the immediate future? The incorporation of ultrafiltration units and dialysis modules within the bypass circuit are certainly possibilities, and with the addition of membrane oxygenators may provide short-term support for the critically ill patient. At present careful preoperative assessment and the early treatment of acute renal failure provides the best chance of salvaging some of these extremely ill patients.

References

1. Barger, A. C., Muldowney, F. P. and Liebowitz, M. R. (1959). Role of the kidney in the pathogenesis of congestive heart failure. *Circulation*, **20,** 273
2. Peters, J. P. (1952). The problem of cardiac edema. *Am. J. Med.*, **12,** 66
3. Boulton-Jones, J. M., Sissons, J. G. P., Evans, D. J. and Peters, D. K. (1974). Renal lesions of subacute infective endocarditis. *Br. Med. J.*, **2,** 11
4. Heptinstall, R. H. (1974). *Pathology of the Kidney*, 2nd Edn., Vol. II, pp. 1162–4. (Boston: Little Brown & Co.)
5. Constable, A. R., Hussein, M. M., Albrecht, M. P., Thompson, F. D., Philalithis, P. E. and Joekes, A. M. (1979). Single sample estimates of renal clearances. *Br. J. Urol.*, **51,** 84
6. Pachinger, O., Ogris, E., Probst, P., Joskowics, G., Sochor, H. and Kaindl, F. (1979). Assessment of left ventricular performance and myocardial viability using quantitative radioisotope techniques. *Br. Heart J.*, **42,** 205
7. O'Reilly, P. H., Shields, R. A. and Testa, H. J. (1979). *Nuclear Medicine in Urology and Nephrology*. (London: Butterworths)
8. Fichman, M. P., Vorherr, H., Kleeman, C. R. and Telfer, N. (1971). Diuretic-induced hyponatraemia. *Ann. Intern. Med.*, **75,** 853
9. Anderson, R. J., Linas, S. L., Berns, A. S., Henrich, W. L., Miller, T. R., Gabow, P. A. and Schrier, R. W. (1977). Non-oliguric acute renal failure. *N. Engl. J. Med.*, **296,** 1134
10. Cohen, M. V., Diaze, P. and Scheuer, J. (1979). Echocardiographic assessment of left ventricular function in patients with chronic uraemia. *Clin. Nephrol.*, **12,** 156
11. Bernstein, A., Zambrano, S. S., Morrison, R. S. and Spodick, D. H. (1975). Cardiac effects of haemodialysis: non-invasive monitoring by systolic time intervals. *Am. J. Sci.*, **269,** 189
12. Goss, T. E., Alfrey, A. C., Vogel, J. H. K. and Holmes, J. H. (1967). Hemodynamic changes during dialysis. *Trans. Am. Soc. Artif. Internal Organs*, **13,** 68
13. Goggin, M. J. and Joekes, A. M. (1971). Gas exchange in renal failure. *Br. Med. J.*, **2,** 244
14. Bennett, W. M., Singer, I. and Coggins, C. J. (1974). A guide to drug therapy in renal failure. *J. Am. Med. Assoc.*, **230,** 1544
15. Aviado, A. D. Jr., Wnuck, A. L. and de Beer, E. J. (1958). The effects of sympathomimetic drugs on renal vessels. *J. Pharm. Exp. Ther.*, **124,** 238
16. Spencer, M. P., Denison, A. B. Jr. and Green, H. D. (1954). The direct renal vascular effects of epinephrine and norepinephrine before and after adrenergic blockade. *Circ. Res.*, **11,** 537
17. Carriere, S. (1969). Effect of norepinephrine, isoproterenol, and adrenergic blockers upon the intrarenal distribution of blood flow. *Can. J. Physiol.*, **47,** 199
18. Hollenberg, N. K., Adams, D. F., Mendell, P., Abrams, H. L. and Merrill, J. P. (1973). Renal vascular responses to dopamine: haemodynamic and angiographic observations in normal man. *Clin. Sci. Mol. Med.*, **45,** 733

SECTION V
The Brain

43
Psychometric testing in the evaluation of the postoperative cardiac patient

D. W. BETHUNE

The first and obvious questions to be asked with regard to psychometric testing in the perioperative period is why does it need to be done? The situation can be considered to be analogous to many others that arise in clinical medicine. For example, if a patient presents with respiratory failure, a competent clinician can diagnose the fact that the patient has respiratory failure and can detail the underlying pathology and, almost certainly, give a diagnosis. Tests of lung function, on the other hand, can document the degree of failure of ventilation but will not decide the aetiology or the prognosis of the condition. I feel that the use of psychometric testing in the perioperative period is in a very similar position, and however sophisticated and precise the tests become they will never be as accurate or valuable as pre- and post-operative clinical assessment by interested psychologists and psychiatrists. The approach whereby trained psychiatric workers perform a pre- and post-operative evaluation has been used in the Hamburg study[1]. While the results of this study are uniquely valuable, the degree of commitment of trained personnel both in expertise and time makes such a study design impracticable for general use.

With their admitted failings psychometric tests still appear to have a useful role to play. They allow documentation and numerical scoring to plot a patient's recovery from anaesthetic and surgical procedures, they will give a numerical score for those patients identified as having some form of neuropsychiatric disturbance in the postoperative period, and analysis of the results allows a degree of differentiation between functional and organic based psychoses. A variety of different techniques and types of equipment, have been used to quantify the effects of changes occurring during the perioperative period[2]. The most impressive studies in this field are those by Aberg who used a modified (Swedish) intelligence test[3]. By careful analysis of the results of his initial studies he was able to identify and correct details in the surgical and perfusion procedures which had a deleterious effect and his later studies[2–4] demonstrate that this had resulted in measurable benefit. Aberg's series of studies demonstrate the beneficial effect of careful psychometric testing in improving the standard of patient care in one particular unit.

Tests used to evaluate the patient's neuropsychiatric function following anaesthesia and surgery have varied from the simple remembering of a short phrase through various standardized test procedures up to complicated test rigs such as the car simulator used by Green *et al.*[5]. The complexity of the test used by no means makes the results obtained more significant or valuable. It is interesting that in the experiments performed with a car simulator, looking at the recovery from anaesthesia, the experimenters noted that the subjects performance on the simulator had returned to normal when clinically they were still obviously under the influence of the anaesthetic agents. In looking for a suitable test to evaluate patients following open-heart surgery and to a lesser extent following general anaesthesia and surgery, it is important to determine which function should be examined. The clinical observation that, following open-heart surgery, patients who have obvious disturbance of conscious level without any localising signs, inevitably have a considerable degree of memory dysfunction suggested that memory function could well prove to be a valuable index of organic brain damage. The additional observation that occasional patients complain of varying degrees of memory loss after discharge and full physical recovery following an apparently uneventful surgical procedure with an unremarkable immediate postoperative course, further reinforced the idea that postoperative memory function should be examined and documented. The full recovery of memory function is also delayed in patients following general anaesthesia and surgery. Patients who have woken up shortly after the anaesthetic and have rationally answered questions either in the theatre corridor or on arrival in the recovery room will, on questioning some days later, say that they woke up in their beds many hours after the operation. This slow return of memory function in patients who are otherwise completely normal is frequently a source of some difficulty in the nursing care of the patient, as many of these patients will deny having received messages which were given to them shortly after surgery. This delay in full return of memory function after anaesthesia has obvious medico-legal implications and has been documented by Ogg *et al.*[6].

DESIRABLE FEATURES OF PSYCHOMETRIC TESTS FOR USE IN THE PERIOPERATIVE PERIOD

There are obviously desirable features that must be possessed by any test protocols that are adopted. One is that it should be comparatively uninfluenced by the patients age or by their general intelligence, otherwise the interpretation of results becomes more difficult. If it is to be used in the ward environment it should not involve the use of complicated equipment and it must be suitable for use with a patient in the condition to be expected at the time of the test. It is no use designing a test in which the patient has to stand when one is intending to evaluate patients who will probably still be confined to bed. An important point is that the test methods should not distress the patient. This is an interesting facet but with certain test regimes, particularly those which involve repetition and learning, the patient is prone to notice postoperatively that their performance is depressed beyond what they personally expect following the preoperative test. This knowledge will undoubtedly upset the patient and on occasion even cause an acute anxiety reaction. Ideally a test protocol should be short enough not to fatigue the patient and should be designed so that the tester can give the subject a sense of achievement and a sense of having satisfactorily completed the task at the end of the test.

TESTS OF MEMORY FUNCTION

Many tests of memory function have been described. These vary from simple tests such as the digit span where a series of unconnected numbers are read out in increasing sequences until the patient fails to repeat the sequence correctly. The test is given with the patient repeating numbers in the order given by the tester and then with the subject giving the numbers in reverse order. The sum of the forward and reverse scores gives a total digit span. This type of memory test appears to test an immediate memory recall and is very much akin to the memory level used when one looks at a telephone number in a directory and then immediately dials the number. Most people would have extreme difficulty in recalling that number a few minutes later. This type of test with immediate recall has proved very insensitive and scores have been unaffected even when clinically apparent organic brain dysfunction has occurred. It appears that other tests of short term memory such as the picture memory test as used by Aberg[3] has a similar inability to pick up significant degrees of organic brain dysfunction.

An assessment of personal memory and orientation in time and space can be obtained by using a standardized questionnaire and this can include simple memory tests relating to recent preoperative events.

Psychometric testing must be used in conjunction with a neurological history and our experience suggests that standard questions appear to be valuable and accurate in identifying acute changes in body image. Minor degrees of neurological dysfunction which can easily be missed on physical examination will be noted and reported by the patient in response to direct questioning.

A more formal memory test was developed by Dr Moyra Williams[7] initially in conjunction with an investigation into the effects of ageing on memory[8]. We have found this delayed visual memory test useful to quantify the degree of disturbance in patients who had some degree of organic dysfunction following open heart surgery[9] and also in assessing recovery following minor outpatient anaesthesia and surgery[6]. The original test has been modified to include two cards on each test occasion[10]. One of the cards is repeated on each occasion the test is given. The other card being a new card on each occasion. A card is shown to the patient and the objects on the card are identified with the patient and the patient is then given up to 1 minute to memorise the pictures. The second card, the one which is repeated on each test occasion, is then shown to the patient, the objects identified in the same way as with the first card. Other tasks are then performed for a period of approximately 8–10 minutes and the patient is then asked which objects they can recall spontaneously from the cards. For any objects not recalled spontaneously a verbal prompt is given and finally if there are still objects not recalled a visual prompt card is shown and the patient asked to identify the pictures on the visual prompt card which they recall seeing on the original card. From the results of the spontaneous recall, verbal prompting and visual prompting, a penalty test score is derived which gives an assessment of overall delayed memory recall. As there are four cards, the test can be repeated on three occasions using a fresh card as the initial card on each occasion. This visual delayed memory recall test apparently gives a reasonable assessment of the patients memory function. It is not particularly affected by the patient's intelligence. It satisfies the major criteria in that because of the progressive prompting the patient will always have a sense of achievement by the time the test is completed. It requires minimal equipment and can be performed with the patient in bed or sitting on a chair by the side of the bed. The results that we have obtained suggest that it can be used to quantify minor degrees of cerebral dysfunction in the postoperative period after open heart surgery and also to identify and quantify the transient memory loss which occurs after uncomplicated general anaesthesia and minor surgery.

CONCLUSIONS

The use of psychometric testing is valuable in quantifying the degree of dysfunction that the patient may have. It is not, however, a diagnostic tool and it appears at the present time that it is unlikely to be useful in distinguishing between groups of patients who have been managed in different ways during the perioperative period if their postoperative course on careful clinical assessment is identical. I would suggest that tests of psychometric function, and particularly memory testing, should be used when clinical evaluation of new equipment, methods or devices is being attempted. By using these tests it will be possible to pick up minor degrees of dysfunction and quantify them.

ADDENDA:

Following a meeting of an International Research Group in March, 1980, an attempt is to be made to design an internationally acceptable standard test instrument. Initially, the tests to be evaluated include the Figure Rotation and Figure Identification tests used by Aberg[2] in his extensive Swedish studies. The conceptual level analogy testing as used by Rabiner and Willner[12] in New York and the delayed visual recall test briefly described above. Initial studies are in progress to determine which parts of this formidable battery of tests should be incorporated in a final test protocol.

ACKNOWLEDGEMENTS

I would like to acknowledge assistance from East Anglian Regional Health Authority in funding a part-time Research Worker, Mrs. M. Sayers who carried out the psychometric testing and Astra Pharmaceuticals for assistance with data processing.

References

1. Dahme, B. and Gotze, P. (1980). Objective classification of psychopathological symptoms after open heart surgery. In Speidel, H. and Rodewald, G. (eds.) *Psychic and Neurological Dysfunctions after Open Heart Surgery*, p. 41. (Stuttgart: George Thieme Verlag)
2. Aberg, T. and Kihlgren, M. (1980). The use of psychometric testing as a quality criterion in open heart surgery. In Speidel, H. and Rodewald, G. (eds.) Psychic and Neurological Dysfunctions after Open Heart Surgery, p. 107. (Stuttgart: George Rhieme Verlag)
3. Aberg, T. (1974). Effect of open heart surgery on intellectual function. *Scand. J. Thorac. Cardiovasc. Surg*., Suppl. 15
4. Aberg, T., Kihlgren, M., Jonsson, L., Stjernlof, K. and Tyden, H. Improved cerebral protection during open heart surgery. To be published in Proceedings of the Second International Symposium on psychopathological and neurological dysfunction following Open Heart Surgery. Milwaukee 1980.
5. Green, R., Long, H. A., Elliott, C. J. R. and Howells, T. H. (1963). A method of studying recovery after anaesthesia. *Anaesthesia*, **18,** 189
6. Ogg, T. W., Fischer, H. B. J., Bethune, D. W. and Collis, J. M. Day Case Anaesthesia and Surgery. *Anaesthesia*, **34,** 784
7. Williams, M. (1953). Investigation of amnesic defects by progressive prompting. *J. Neurol. Neurosurg. Psychiatry*, **16,** 14
8. Simpson, B. R., Williams, M., Scott, J. F. and Crampton Smith, A. (1961). Effects of anaesthesia and elective surgery on old people. *Lancet*, 1961, **11,** 887
9. Bethune, D. W. (1980). The assessment of organic brain damage following open heart surgery. In Speidel, H. and Rodewald, G. (eds.) *Psychic and Neurological Dysfunctions following Open Heart Surgery*, p. 100. (Stuttgart: George Thieme Verlag)
10. Bethune, D. W. (1980). Test of delayed memory recall suitable for assessing post-operative amnesia. *Anaesthesia* (In press)
11. Second International Symposium on psychopathological and neurological dysfunctions following open heart surgery. Milwaukee, March 1980
12. Rabiner, C. J. and Willner, A. E. (1980). Differential psychopathological and organic mental disorder at follow up five years after coronary bypass and cardiac valvular surgery. In Speidel, H. and Rodewald, G. (eds.) *Psychic and Neurological Dysfunctions following Open Heart Surgery*, p. 237. (Stuttgart: George Thieme Verlag)

44
Brain damage following open heart surgery

G. RODEWALD, P. GÖTZE, J. GUNTAU, R. JANZEN,
H.-J. KREBBER AND H. POKAR

INTRODUCTION

Our group at Hamburg University has been working in the field of neurological and psychopathological disorders following open heart surgery since 1964[1,2]. Since 1974 there has been a permanent interdisciplinary group supported by the German Research Society.

The study presented here was designed to evaluate the incidence and causes of brain damage following open heart operations with extracorporeal circulation in order to find measures to prevent severe functional and structural changes.

METHODS OF EXTRACORPOREAL CIRCULATION

These investigations refer to adult patients with predominantly acquired-heart disease who were operated upon using extracorporeal circulation. Our perfusion unit consisted of roller pumps, a Rygg–Kyusgaard bubble oxygenator which had been modified to allow us to use gas-to-blood-flow ratios as low as 0.7/0.8 : 1.0. This reduces the number of microbubbles considerably. Bentley microporous filters were placed between the cardiotomy reservoir and the venous return line. The unit was primed with Ringer's lactate and whole blood when necessary diluting the patients hematocrit to 26–30 %.

Canulation was performed with separate canulae in i.v.c. and s.v.c. and the arterial return placed in the femoral artery in most cases.

Flow rates were about 2.4 l/min per m^2 B.S., mean arterial pressure was kept at 70–80 mmHg and venous pressure at 6–8 mmHg. Body temperature was lowered to 28–30 °C. Cardiac arrest was induced by cold cardioplegic infusion, a method described in detail elsewhere[3]. With this arrangement we were able to maintain extracorporeal circulation safely for 4–5 hours. Within this time limit we have been so far unable to detect a statistically significant relationship between duration of ECC and central nervous disturbances or damage to other organs.

PREOPERATIVE STUDY

Before discussing postoperative brain damage it is necessary to evaluate to what extent heart patients suffer from *neurological deficiency*. Nowadays, preoperative neurological examinations should be performed generally. For example, on patients with acquired valcular disease who may have encountered cerebral emboli or on older patients, especially those with CHD who may suffer from cerebral vascular disease[4 6].

In order to establish how often and how reliably neurological disturbances can be detected in our clientel we compared the results of a retrospective study of 230 surgical hospital charts from 1978 to 1979 with the results from a prospective study of 100 patients treated between 1975 and 1977.

The patients from the retrospective study were examined in the neurological clinic on a routine base. The patients from the prospective study[4] were investigated preoperatively by a neurologist of our group with the main purpose of finding postoperative disturbances.

It became evident that in the retrospective study in 13.5% out of 230 patients neurological findings were preoperatively present while in the prospective study in 27 out of 100 patients positive findings were present (Table 1).

A comparison of patients with coronary artery disease and with valvular disease in both groups is depicted in Table 2. Including central nervous dys-

Table 1 Preoperative central nervous dysfunction

	Retrospective study $n = 230 = 100\%$	*Prospective study* $n = 100$	
No findings	199 = 86.5%	48	
Positive findings	3 = 13.5%	52	25 in history
			8 physical examination
			19 hist. *and* phys. exam.

Table 2 Preoperative central nervous dysfunction

	Retrospective study			*Prospective study*		
Patients with	*n*	*Positive findings*	%	*n*	*Positive findings*	%
Valvular lesions	136	18	13.2	57	37	64.9
CHD	94	13	13.8	26	11	42.3

functions in history 65.9% of 57 valcular patients had positive findings in the prospective study while only 13.2% of 136 similar patients were positive in the retrospective study. A similar proportion was found in patients with coronary artery disease. One interesting point that emerged from the retrospective study was the fact that some patients forget their history of embolic events and only remember, when specifically asked about such an episode. Concerning the preoperative findings, we conclude that neurological routine examination is much less effective than a specifically aimed study. This is important from a legal point of view as well as from a therapeutical one and certainly also for the analysis of causes of postoperative disturbances.

POSTOPERATIVE EXAMINATIONS

We compared the results of a retrospective study with those of the aforementioned prospective study. Table 3 depicts on the left that out of all 583 adult patients with predominantly acquired-heart disease who were operated upon in 1978 and 1979 with extracorporeal circulation 21, that is 3.6% had postoperatively severe central nervous disturbances. These diagnoses were reached in consultation with the neurologists.

The analysis of the prospective study is some what more complicated. From the results presented on the righthand side of the table it can be seen

Table 3 Postoperative central nervous dysfunction

Retrospective study		*Prospective study*	
Total	$n = 583 = 100\%$	Total	$n = 99$
No findings	$562 = 96.4\%$	Preop vs. postop unchanged	60
Severe disturbances	$21 = 3.6\%$	Changed	39
		30 Mild	9 Moderate

that 60 out of 99 patients were unchanged postoperatively *vs.* preoperatively with regard to their neurological status, while in 39 *a change was present*, 30 mild and 9 moderate, that is epileptic seizures and cerebral nerve dysfunction respectively. Severe disturbances such as new hemiparesis or intracranial hemorrhage were not seen in this group. Out of the 39 patients 16 had a normal neurological status preoperatively. The patients included in the prospective study were not known to the surgeons. Neurologists were asked for an opinion when ever clinical signs were noted. This was true in three out of the nine moderate cases but in none of the remaining 30 mild cases. We refer to this last group later.

Changes to neurological status in the patients from the prospective study generally occurred at the first day postop., but sometimes not until the 3rd postop. day and persisted in 15 out of 39 patients for more than 4 days. In five patients the postoperative disturbances were still noted in the 3rd and 4th week postop. The relationship between time-since-operation and neurological disturbances implies that there must be some aetio-pathological influence from surgery. The fact that with the exception of a few cases the changes had disappeared after 3 or 4 weeks, demonstrates that we are dealing mainly with reversible functional cerebral defects rather than organic loss of cerebral substance.

The comparison of both studies reveals that to us, as heart surgeons, only moderate or severe cerebral dysfunction comes to our attention while a special investigation detects a considerably higher number of disturbances, most of them however not especially aggrevating.

HOSPITAL MORTALITY AND CENTRAL NERVOUS DISTURBANCES

Mortality following open heart surgery has decreased considerably in recent years.

The review of the hospital mortality is depicted in Table 4. After 583 consecutive open heart procedures in 1978 and 1979 in adults with predominantly acquired-heart disease, a total of 20 that is 3.4% of all operated patients died. The leading causes of death, that is the initial causes, are a result of cardiac surgery. Half of all death is caused for cardiac reasons. It is remarkable that the emergency patients all died of preoperatively existing reasons and displayed through surgery and the postoperative period continuing low

Table 4 Operative mortality (within 30 d postop) and leading cause of death following 583 open heart procedures (18–73 yrs. old, mainly acquired heart diseases)

Causes of death	*n*	*Scheduled procedure*	*Emergencies*
Exitus in tabula:	3		
Haemorrhage		1	–
Myocard. inf.(?)		1	–
Preop. L.C.O.		–	1
Cardiac:	9		
Arrhythmias		1 (c.d.)	–
Sudden death		2	–
Pre- and postop L.C.O.		–	5 (2× c.d.)
Pericard. tamponade		1	–
Intra/postop. AO-diss:	3	3	–
Katabolie, kachexie:	2	2 (1× c.d.)	–
Inoperable lesion:	1	1 (1× c.d.)	–
Duodenal ulcer:	1	1	–
Infection:	1	1	–
TOTAL	20	14	6

c.d. = cerebral damage

cardiac output. It is of interest that five of the 20 dead had central nervous dysfunctions during their course but in none was brain damage the leading cause of death.

INCIDENCE AND CAUSES OF CENTRAL NERVOUS DISTURBANCES

Table 5 lists the original causes that produced the postoperatively noted central nervous disturbances. In 20 out of 22 cases the disturbances were a sequela of reduced perfusion of the brain. This hypoperfusion was either *localized* in the brain or was found associated with *general* hypoperfusion, i.e. low cardiac output. According to the charts and the measured parameter

Table 5 Central nervous disturbances following open heart surgery (n = 22)

Sequelae	← *Initial cause*	*n*	*Died*	*Leading cause of death*
Localized disturbances of brain perfusion	Air embolism	6	1	Kachexia
	Embolism	1	–	
n = 9	Recurrence of symptoms of previous embolism	1	–	
	Cerebral vascular lesion *and* L.C.O.	1	–	
Disturbances of brain perfusion due to L.C.O.	Myocardial failure	3	2	Myocard. failure
	Arrhythmias	3	1	Arrhythria
L.C.O. caused by	Intraop. AO-dissection	1	–	
	Intraop. Haemorrhage	1	–	
n = 11	Pericard. Tamponade	2	–	
	Inoperable lesion	1	1	Inoperable
Postperfusion syndrome	ECC?	1	–	
Psychoorganic syndrome		1	–	
	TOTAL	22	5	

we tried to evaluate the underlying causes for the diminished perfusion. This was relatively easy in cases with localized hypoperfusion of the brain but much more difficult in those patients with generalized hypoperfusion.
Here are two examples:

(1) The three cases with severe arrhythmia lead to resuscitation with subsequent low cardiac output. The cause for the low cardiac output was not the resuscitation but the arrhythmia.

(2) A patient with acquired aortic and mitral valve lesion and idiopathic hypertrophic left ventricular outflow tract obstruction died despite valve replacement from low cardiac output, but the cause of this lethal development was the technical inoperability, or perhaps even a faulty diagnosis.

It should be noted that in nine cases a localized, and in 11 cases a generalized hypoperfusion resulted in central nervous complications.

The avoidance of some of the causes that result in localized disturbances of brain perfusion such as air embolism, which probably has a higher incidence than the 1% that was observed is still to be discussed. Causes for generalized hypoperfusion are always possible following open heart surgery but not always predictable and therefore not completely avoidable.

One out of 22 patients developed signs of the so called postperfusion syndrome with damage of almost all organs, and one a psycho-organic syndrome. These two patients had no intra- or postoperatively noted disturbances of body perfusion. Here still remains the question of the influence of extracorporeal circulation, which will be discussed later.

NEUROLOGICAL FINDINGS, CLINICAL DIAGNOSIS AND OUTCOME OF THE PATIENTS

Table 6 depicts neurological findings and diagnosis which are also supported by EEG and CT findings, where it was indicated. Groups 1 and 2 include the nine patients with localized hypoperfusion of the brain caused either by air embolism (which incidently were on the right side of the brain) or particulate emboli, which involved a region of arterial supply. The third group contains 13 patients, 11 of whom suffered from low cardiac output and 2 developed postperfusion syndrome or a severe psychoorganic syndrome.

As already mentioned, five of 22 patients died, but not primarily of brain damage. Out of eight survivors in the group with localized hypoperfusion of the brain five had no more symptoms 2–3 weeks following the event and three only had minor residuals. According to general neurological experience the long term prognosis is quite favourable in these cases. Out of nine survivors

Table 6 Central nervous disturbances following open heart surgery (n = 22)

Neurological findings	*Clinical diagnosis*		*n*
Transient hemiplegia, dysphasia, hemianopsia transient Jacksonian seizures	Syndrome of air embolism		*n*
Hemiparesis etc. Visual dysfunction etc. Dysarthria etc.	Syndrome of MCA* Syndrome of PCA* Syndrome of BA*	Distal ischemia of local perfusion	3
Psycho-organic syndrome, disturbances of consciousness (EEG: theta–delta-activity) Comatose state (EEG: delta–subdelta–activity)	Syndrome of global brain dysfunction		13

* MCA: medial cerebral artery
PCA: posterior cerebral artery
BA: basilar cerebral artery

with general non-localized brain damage seven were almost free of symptoms 2–3 weeks later, two had persisting symptoms even weeks later. This relatively benign outcome in this group should not mask the fact that the prognosis of general non-localized brain damage is completely uncertain, in contrast to the relatively good prognosis of the more localized disturbances.

PROBLEMS STILL TO BE SOLVED

When comparing our own earlier experience and the more recent communications of others with our data presented here, it becomes quite obvious that some progress has already been achieved. Out of 583 patients undergoing open heart surgery – including emergencies – 20 died within 30 days postop., that is 3.4%. None of them died primarily of brain damage. Out of these 583 patients 22 (3.6%) suffered from localized or general brain damage, and out of the 17 survivors only five, that is 85% of all patients operated upon presented themselves with persisting neurological symptoms. We as surgeons can find explanations for the central nervous disturbances, especially as neurological findings and diagnosis fit well together. Except for the annoying fact that all the disturbances occurred unexpectedly and it was therefore not possible to take measures against them and that the analysis had to be after the event we are satisfied with our longing for causality, but still there remains a problem unsolved.

That in the prospective study neurologists found among the 99 postoperative patients of nine cases with moderate brain damage, only three of them presented themselves to the surgeons with seizures, but there were 30 more patients who presented a change of their neurological status postoperatively *vs.* preoperatively. Although this group showed discrete signs of brain damage we could not find haemodynamic reasons retrospectively. Here other factors must have been active, which we do not know but are beyond doubt related to the surgical procedure. It is a disturbing conclusion that in the 22 patients with brain damage in the retrospective study *other* causes might have been present besides haemodynamic parameters.

Things become even more complicated when we realize that central nervous disturbances are often associated with psychopathological abnormalities. There were four patients in the prospective study who postoperatively became delirious and all of them developed central nervous symptoms as well. Out of four other patients with a severe postoperative psycho-organic syndrome three presented central nervous symptoms also.

On the other hand out of 49 patients with a psycho-pathological uneventful postoperative course only 13 presented central nervous symptoms.

According to our findings there is a connection between postoperative psychic disturbances and neurological disturbances or from the opposite point of view both disturbances may have the same cause.

Thiopental (Luminal) was given intraoperatively when periods of prolonged hypotension were present or whenever there was suspicion of cerebral damage, whatever the cause, and continued from 24 hours to several days postoperatively. This method has been described by Bleyaert *et al.*[7,8]

The importance of this last finding is that psychopathological disturbances have been found to affect the long-term result of otherwise successful heart operations.

CONCLUSIONS

(1) Meticulous preoperative neurological and psychiatric examinations of heart patients reveal far more neurological and psychiatric disturbances than a plain routine examination.
(2) Meticulous postoperative neurological and psychiatric examinations reveal far more disturbances as seen and diagnosed themselves by cardiovascular surgeons.
(3) Most of the postoperative neurological dysfunctions resolve, psychic disturbances however may affect the results for years.
(4) The low hospital mortality and the postoperative small incidence of severe neurological and psychopathological disturbances, which are also easily explained should not mask the fact that open heart surgery – despite the great successes – still has many problems.

References

1. Götze, P. (1980). *Psychopathologie der Herzoperierten.* (Stuttgart: Enke)
2. Speidel, H., Dahme, B., Flemming, B., Götze, P., Huse-Kleinstoll, G., Meffert, H. J. and Rodewald, G. (1979). Psychische Störungen nach offenen Herzoperationen. *Nervenarzt*, **50,** 85
3. Bleese, N., Döring, V., Pokar, H., Polonius, M.-J., Steiner, D. and Rodewald, G. (1978). Intraoperative myocardial protection by cardioplegia in hypothermia. *J. Thor. Cardiovasc. Surg.*, **75,** 405
4. Aquilar, M. J., Gerbode, F. and Hill, J. D. (1971). Neuropathologic complications of cardiac surgery. *J. Thor. Cardiovasc. Surg.*, **61,** 676
5. Branthwaite, M. A. (1972). Neurological damage related to open-heart surgery. *Thorax*, **27,** 748
6. Branthwaite, M. A. (1975). Prevention of neurological damage during open heart surgery. *Thorax*, **30,** 258
7. Bleyaert, A. L., Nemoto, E. M., Safar, P. *et al.* (1978). Thiopental amelioration of brain damage after global ischemia in monkeys. *Anesthesiology*, **49,** 390
8. Rockoff, M. A. (1978). Barbiturates following cardiac arrest. *Anesthesiology*, **49,** 385

THE SIR THOMAS HOLMES SELLORS LECTURE

45
Preservation of the myocardium: some biochemical considerations

WINIFRED G. NAYLER

Irrespective of our approach to the problem of preserving the myocardium – whether it be from the point of view of the physician treating patients with ischaemic heart disease or the cardiac surgeon introducing periods of ischaemic arrest to facilitate surgery – there are certain fundamental questions to be answered. For example, why do some hearts survive long episodes of ischaemia whilst others fail? Why does the reintroduction of coronary flow usually exacerbate the damage caused by the preceding episode of ischaemia? Why is the duration of the ischaemic episode so critical, and why can the administration of cardiac stimulants reduce the chances of salvaging ischaemic myocardium? Why is the presence of hyperthyroidism undesirable, and why should raised glucose levels confer protection? Before answering these and other questions relating to the preservation of the myocardium we need to review the factors which influence energy production and utilization in the myocardium.

ENERGY PRODUCTION AND UTILIZATION

Energy production

The heart is essentially an aerobic organ. It therefore requires a continuous and unfaltering supply of oxygen to generate the energy required for the maintenance of its cellular structure and function. This energy is made available as adenosine triphosphate (ATP) and its production is localized in the mitochondria. Normal, well-oxygenated heart muscle contains approximately 25 μmol ATP/g dry weight. In addition it may contain as much as 30 μmol creatinine phosphate (CP)/g dry weight. This CP serves as a reserve energy supply in the sense that should the rate of oxidative phosphorylation fall to such an extent that ADP is rephosphorylated slowly, and ADP therefore begins to accumulate in the cytosol, the phosphate moiety of CP can be transferred to ADP via creatine phosphokinase activity to generate ATP. It follows logically, therefore, that during conditions of reduced oxygen availability and ischaemia, CP depletion precedes ATP depletion (Figure 1). Nevertheless, when heart muscle becomes either hypoxic or ischaemic it is the depletion of the tissue stores of ATP that triggers the deterioration in structure and function which, if left unchecked, will result in tissue destruction (Figure 2) followed by cell death and necrosis.

Energy utilization

The overall effect of ATP depletion on the functioning of the myocardium can be most easily explained if it is considered in terms of the consequences of the failure of the various ATP-dependent systems.

The cell membrane

At the level of the plasmalemma ATP provides the substrate for two important enzymes – the Na^+K^+ ATPase[1], and a Ca^{2+}-sensitive ATPase[2].

The Na^+K^+ ATPase enzyme traverses the cell membrane (Figure 3), and its function is to transport Na^+ out of K^+ into the cell, against their relative concentration gradients. The activity of this enzyme is inhibited by toxic concentrations of the cardiac glycosides (Figure 3) and by substrate depletion – as occurs, for example (Figure 1) during an ischaemic episode. Failure of this Na^+K^+-activated ATPase enzyme results in a gain in intracellular Na^+

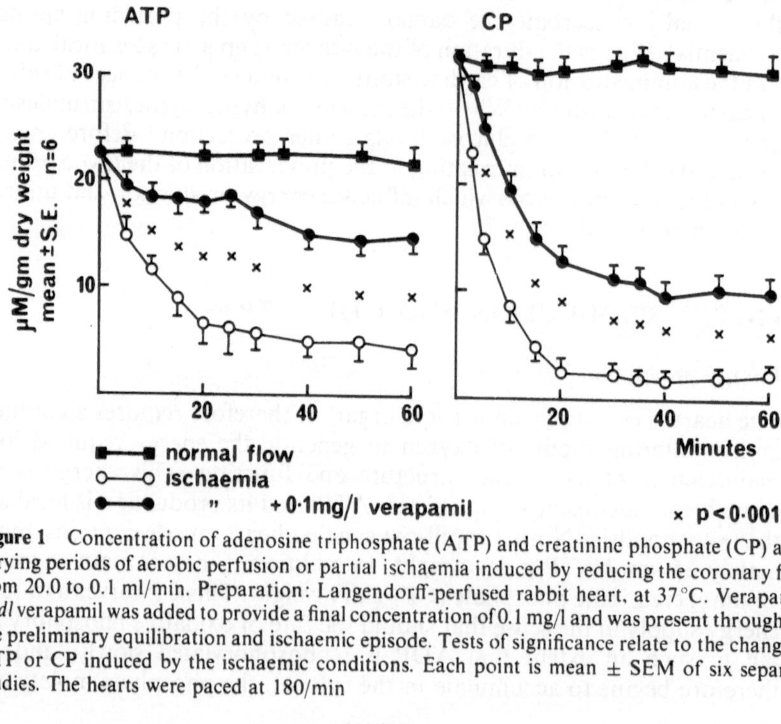

Figure 1 Concentration of adenosine triphosphate (ATP) and creatinine phosphate (CP) after varying periods of aerobic perfusion or partial ischaemia induced by reducing the coronary flow from 20.0 to 0.1 ml/min. Preparation: Langendorff-perfused rabbit heart, at 37 °C. Verapamil, as *dl* verapamil was added to provide a final concentration of 0.1 mg/l and was present throughout the preliminary equilibration and ischaemic episode. Tests of significance relate to the change in ATP or CP induced by the ischaemic conditions. Each point is mean ± SEM of six separate studies. The hearts were paced at 180/min

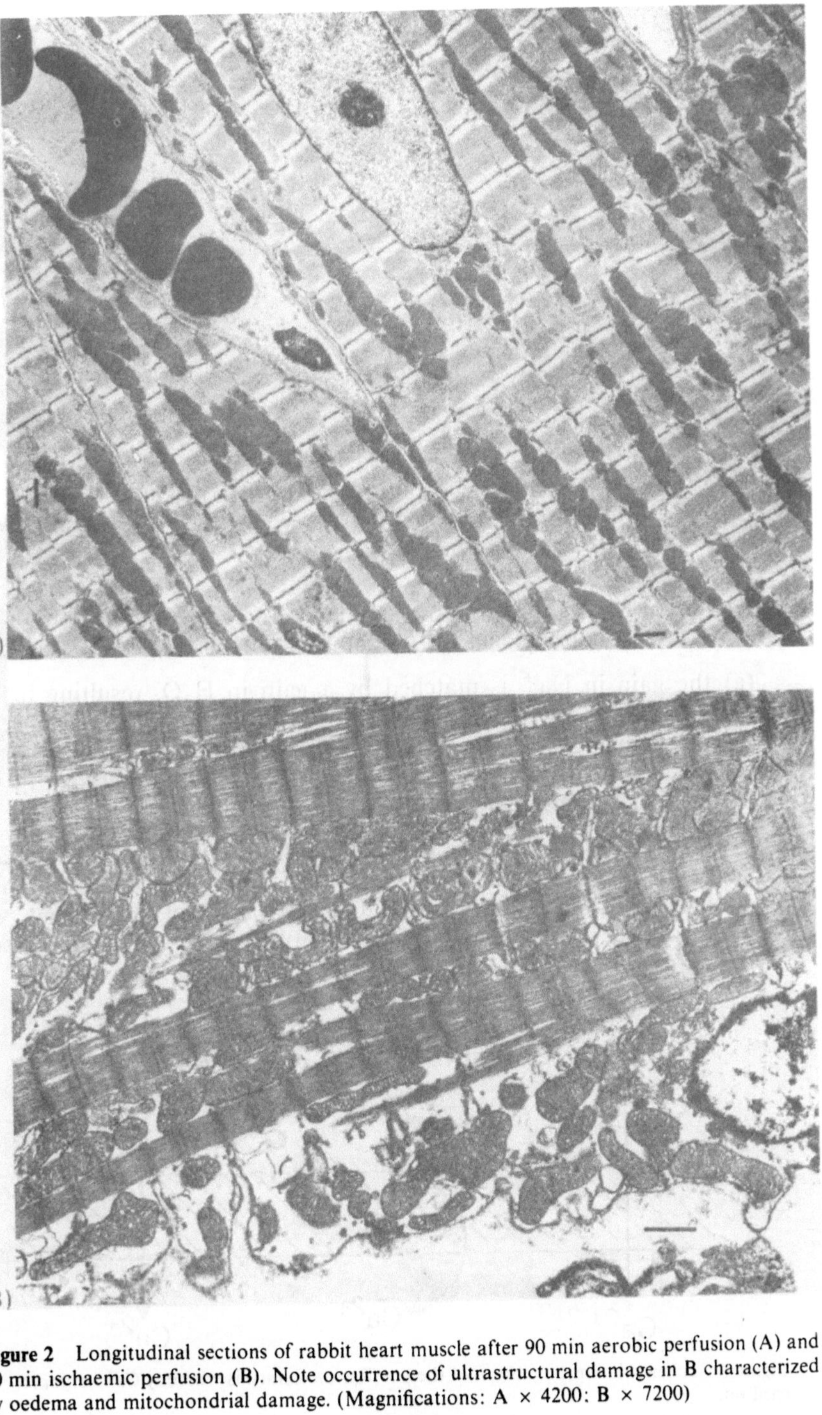

(A)

(B)

Figure 2 Longitudinal sections of rabbit heart muscle after 90 min aerobic perfusion (A) and 90 min ischaemic perfusion (B). Note occurrence of ultrastructural damage in B characterized by oedema and mitochondrial damage. (Magnifications: A × 4200: B × 7200)

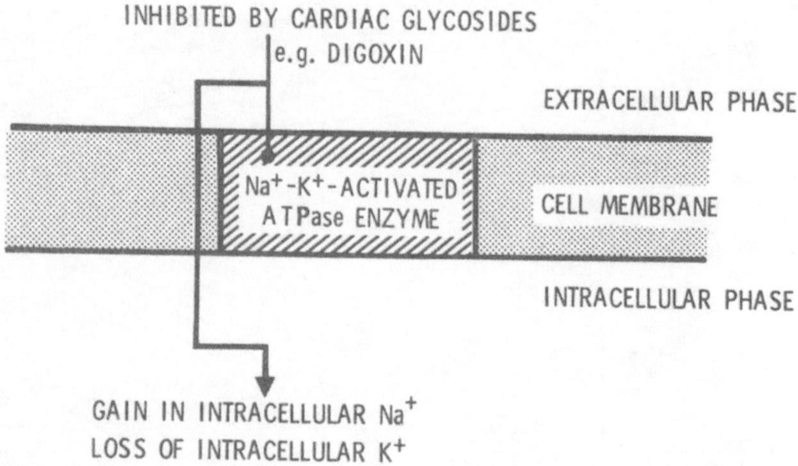

Figure 3 Schematic representation of the vectorial arrangement of the Na^+K^+ ATPase enzyme. Note that inhibition of this enzyme caused by substrate depletion causes a gain in intracellular Na^+ and a loss of K^+

and a loss of K^+, leading to ionic imbalance and electrical instability. There are two further consequences of the failure of the Na^+K^+ ATPase enzyme:

(a) the gain in Na^+ is matched by a gain in H_2O, resulting in tissue oedema;

(b) the gain in Na^+ triggers a $Ca^{2+}:Na^+$ exchange mechanism[3], the end-result of which is the transport of excessive amounts of Ca^{2+} into the cell in exchange for Na^+ (Figure 4).

The Ca^{2+} sensitive ATPase is located[4] on the inner surface of the plasmalemma and functions to transport Ca^{2+} out of the cell and hence against the concentration gradient for Ca^{2+} of 2000 : 1. Failure of this enzyme, which could result from an ischaemia-induced depletion of ATP, would result in the retention of Ca^{2+}.

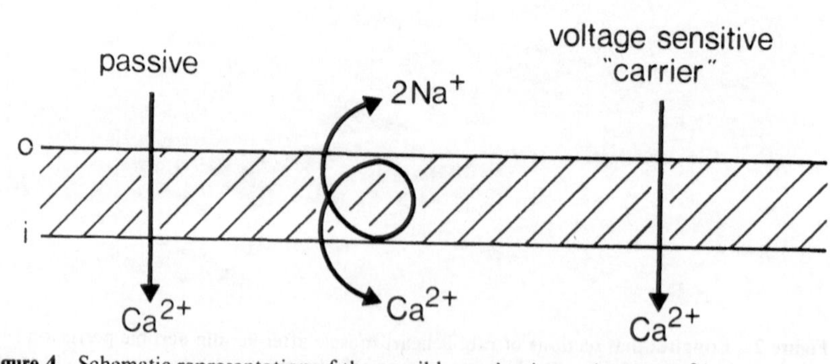

Figure 4 Schematic representation of the possible mechanisms whereby Ca^{2+} enters the myocardium

In summary, therefore, substrate-induced failure of the plasmalemmal Na^+K^+-activated and Ca^{2+}-activated ATPases will result in a net gain in tissue Ca^{2+}, Na^+ and H_2O, and loss of K^+.

The myofibrils and the supply of 'activator' Ca^{2+}

In cardiac, as in skeletal, muscle the activation of contraction depends upon the availability of energy for the formation and activation of the linkages between the actin and myosin components (Figure 5) of the myofibrils[5]. This energy is generated via the hydrolysis of ATP, the relevant ATPase enzyme being located in the terminal heads (Figure 6) of the myosin subunits. Accordingly, therefore, energy in the form of ATP is needed if the mechanical activity of the heart is to be maintained.

The activation of contraction in heart muscle is triggered by the delivery of a bolus of Ca^{2+} (Figure 5) to the myofilaments (Figure 6). Some of this Ca^{2+} enters from the extracellular phase, through voltage-activated, ion-selective channels (Figure 4) that require energy – presumably in the form of ATP – for the maintenance of their normal function[6]. Possibly energy (as

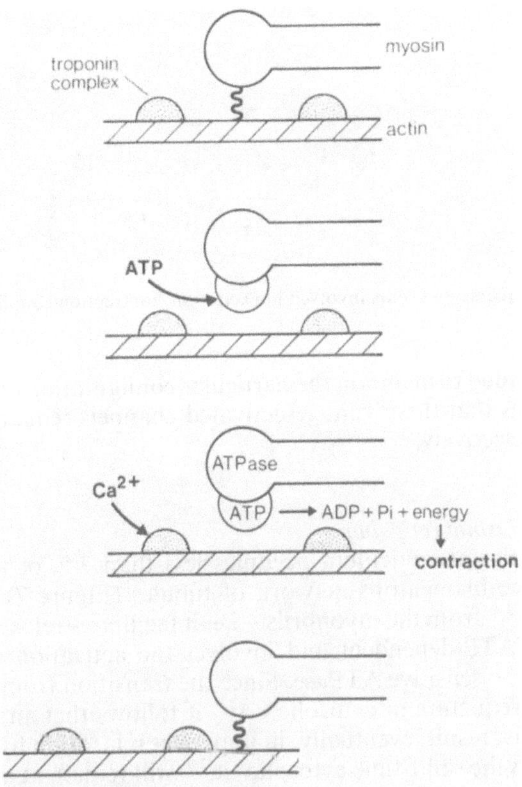

Figure 5 Sequence of events involved in the generation of energy to allow the displacement of actin filaments relative to the myosin filaments

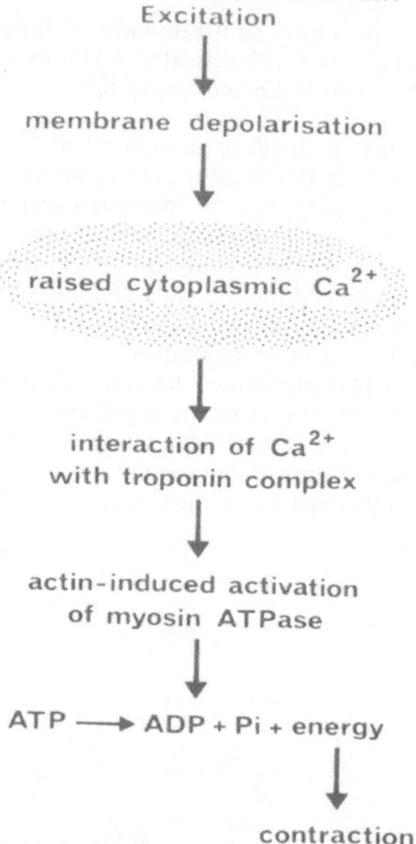

Figure 6 Sequence of events involved in excitation–contraction coupling in heart muscle

ATP) is needed to maintain the particular configuration of the cell membrane that ensures that these voltage-activated channels remain patent and retain their ion selectively.

The sarcoplasmic reticulum

The sarcoplasmic reticulum occupies less than 3% of the cell volume. It forms a fine filamentous network of tubules (Figure 7) and functions[7] to retrieve Ca^{2+} from the myofibrils – i.e. it facilitates relaxation. The retrieval process is ATP-dependent and involves the activation of a sarcolemmal-located Ca^{2+}-sensitive ATPase. Since the transition from systole to diastole requires a reduction in cytosolic Ca^{2+} it follows that an inadequate supply of ATP must result, eventually, in imperfect relaxation followed by arrest in systole[8]. At the same time cytosolic Ca^{2+} will remain at an abnormally high level.

If the inadequate supply of ATP is due to an impaired delivery of O_2 associated with a restricted coronary blood flow, then the failure of the myocardium to relax during diastole has important consequences: (a) because it will be accompanied by a reduction in the time available for flow through any collateral vessels that are still patent; and (b) because of imperfect relaxation, vessels which might otherwise have remained open may be 'squeezed' shut.

There are other consequences of the raised cytosolic Ca^{2+}, apart from imperfect relaxation. Thus: (a) latent Ca^{2+}-sensitive ATPases will be activated, resulting in 'wastage' of any remaining ATP; (b) latent Ca^{2+}-sensitive phospholipases and proteases will be activated, causing tissue damage, loss of selective membrane permeability and release of endogenous catecholamines; (c) since the mitochondria are avid accumulators[9] of Ca^{2+} they will begin to become overloaded with Ca^{2+}. Under these conditions, and as Figure 8 shows, the mitochondria are no longer capable of producing ATP even when they are placed in an ideal environment. Possibly it is at this stage (Figure 9) that the state of 'irreversible damage' is reached. In terms of ultrastructure this is characterized by the formation of contraction bands, disruption of the mitochondria and the presence of massive oedema (Figure 10).

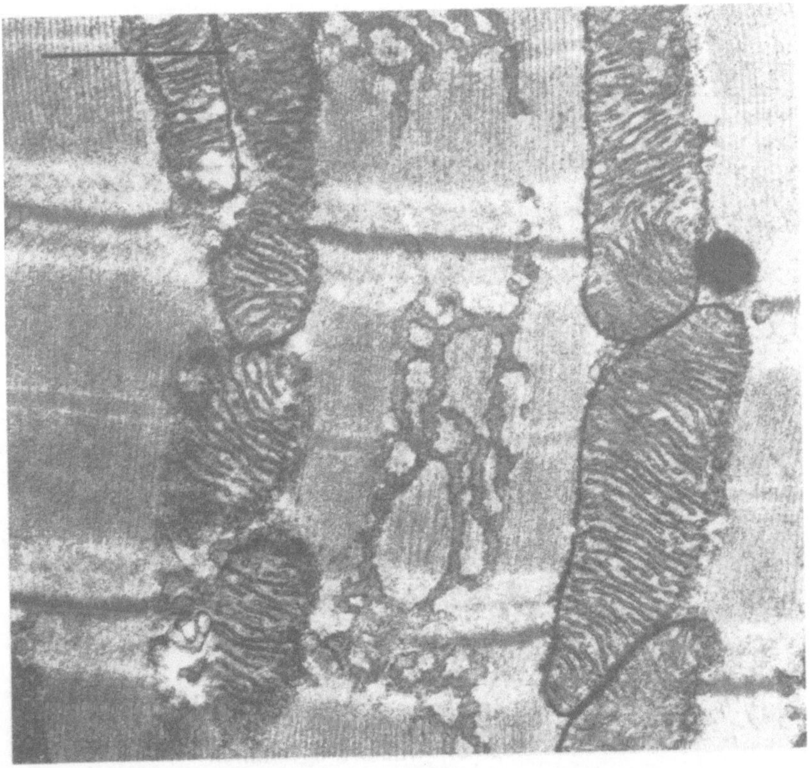

Figure 7 Longitudinal section of heart muscle showing myofibrils, mitochondria and the lace-like distribution of the sarcoplasmic reticulum. (Magnification: × 26 000)

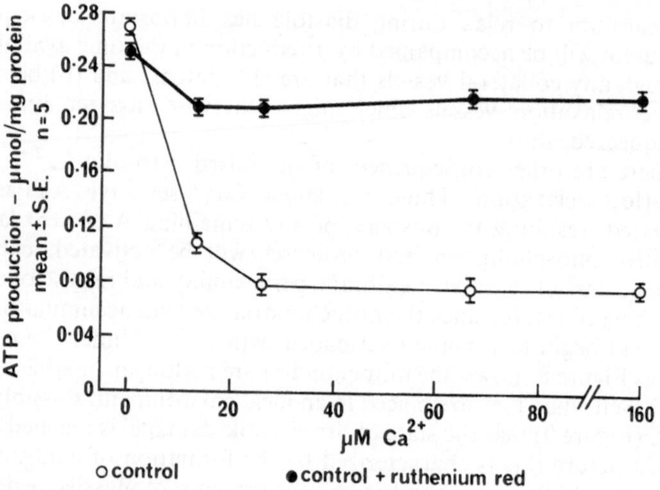

Figure 8 Effect of a raised Ca^{2+} concentration of the ATP-generating capacity of mitochondria. Note that ruthenium red, which prevents the mitochondria from accumulating Ca^{2+}, protected the mitochondria

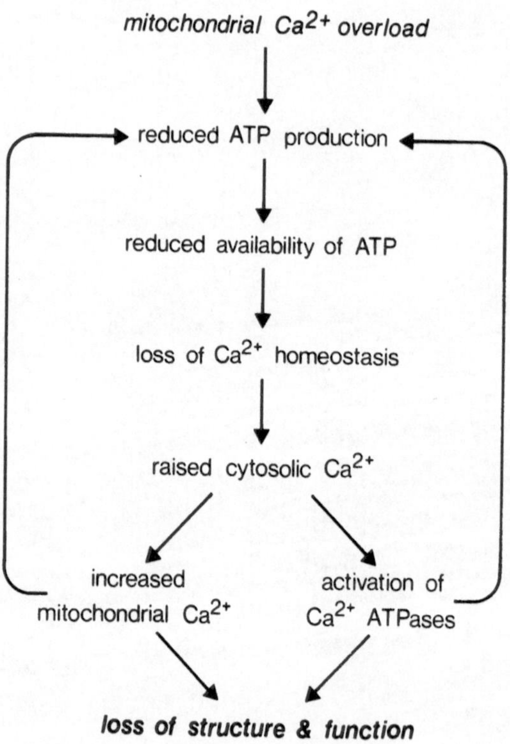

Figure 9 Schematic representation of the sequence of events involved in the onset of cell destruction following the occurrence of Ca^{2+} overloading

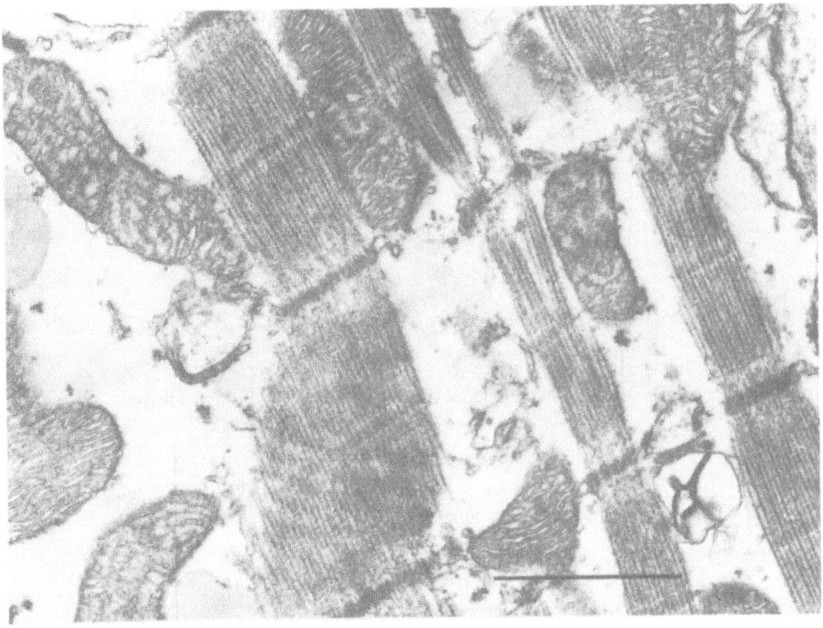

Figure 10 Longitudinal section of heart muscle showing the exacerbation of tissue damage during reperfusion after an ischaemic episode

THE EFFECTS OF ISCHAEMIA AND REPERFUSION

Figure 1 shows the effect of ischaemia, induced by total cessation of coronary flow, on the tissue level of ATP. In accordance with the foregoing discussion this reduction in the tissue stores of ATP (and CP) must result in a progressive loss of structure and function (Figure 11). The rate at which this progressive loss of structure and function develops will, according to our current hypothesis, depend upon the rate of depletion of the tissue stores of ATP, the availability of Ca^{2+}, and the avidity of the mitochondria for Ca^{2+}. The rate of depletion of the tissue stores of ATP, and the availability of Ca^{2+} in the cytosol will depend, in turn, upon many factors including age (the neonatal heart having higher reserves of ATP than the adult[10]), prior therapy – for example prolonged pretreatment with either reserpine or propranolol increases tissue reserves of glycogen and therefore will facilitate glycolysis, nitroprusside therapy promotes collateral flow and lowers peripheral vascular resistance[11], physical training enhances the Ca^{2+} accumulating activity of the sarcoplasmic reticulum[12]. Heart rate, contractility and peripheral vascular resistance are also of importance, since these are the main determinants of myocardial O_2 consumption and hence ATP utilization.

Having depleted the tissue stores of ATP (and CP) during the initial period of ischaemia (Figure 1) we are faced with the problem of explaining why reperfusion exacerbates the damage caused by the initial period of ischaemia[13–15]. There are two schools of thought: (a) it is the sudden readmission of O_2 that is deleterious, possibly because of the formation of free oxygen

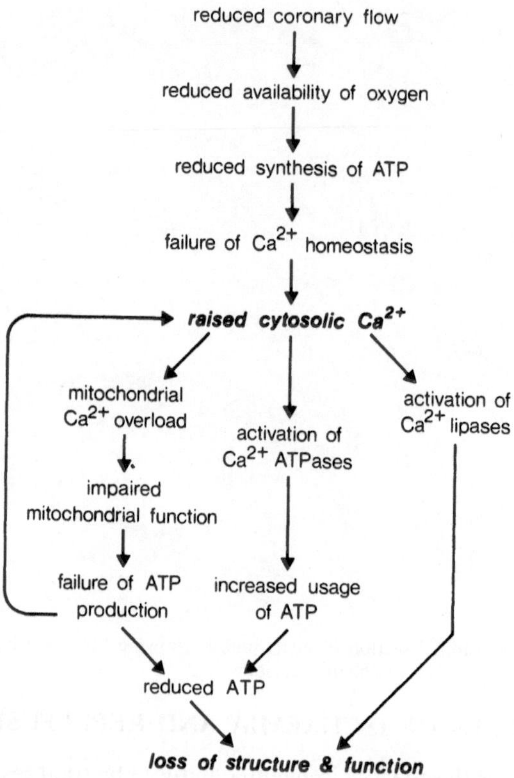

Figure 11 Sequence of events involved in ischaemic-induced damage to the myocardium

radicals and peroxides[16]; or (b) it is the sudden influx of an unlimited amount of Ca^{2+} through cell membranes made leaky during the preceding episode of ischaemic or hypoxia (Figure 2B). This massive entry of Ca^{2+} results in mitochondrial Ca^{2+} overloading, and this in turn leads to a reduced mitochondrial ATP-producing activity

Whatever its cause the sudden reperfusion of a previously ischaemic zone exacerbates the damage caused by the preceding ischaemic episode, the extent of the exacerbation being proportional to the duration and severity of the preceding period of ischaemia or hypoxia[14]. This exacerbation of damage can be quantitated in many ways, including enzyme leakage, increase in resting tension, gain in tissue Ca^{2+}, further deterioration in mitochondrial function and explosive destruction of the myocytes[15]

PROTECTION OF THE REPERFUSED ISCHAEMIC MYOCARDIUM

Although we are a long way from understanding all of the events that contribute to the destruction of mammalian heart muscle when it is made ischaemic and then reperfused, we can at least begin to establish a rationale for the development of protective procedures. Clearly these are aimed at preserving the tissue stores of ATP at a level which will ensure maintenance of homeostasis with respect to Ca^{2+}, thereby avoiding the phenomenon of 'Ca^{2+} overload' and the associated irreversible loss of mitochondrial ATP-producing activity (Figure 8). Various parameters can be used to quantitate the efficacy of a particular protective procedure, including the measurement of cardiac output, ST segment elevation, tissue and plasma CPK levels, rate of lactate formation, systolic time, intraventricular pressure, rate of relaxation, tissue electrolytes (Na^+, K^+, Ca^{2+} and Mg^{2+}), ultrastructure, tissue levels of ATP and CP, and mitochondrial function – quantitated in terms of their O_2 using and ATP-producing capacity.

During the past decade many therapeutic interventions have been introduced to slow or prevent the development of cell damage following periods of ischaemia and reperfusion. Potentially useful agents include β-adrenoceptor antagonists[16]; slow channel inhibitors; Ca^{2+} antagonists, e.g. verapamil[17]; vasodilators, including nitroprusside and nitroglycerine[11]; anti-oxidants, including α-tocopherol[6]; and metabolic substrates – e.g. glucose[18]. Obviously if drug therapy is to be used there are many factors which must be taken into consideration, including the time of drug administration, whether or not effective doses can be tolerated, and whether the drug has access to the affected cells. Even if drug therapy is effective it is often difficult to establish why. For example, in the case of slow channel inhibitors they could diminish the rate of ATP utilization because of their direct effect on slow channel Ca^{2+} entry into the myocardium[6], and the resultant negative inotropism. Alternatively they may be effective because they decrease peripheral vascular resistance, thereby reducing the energy requirements of the heart. Another possibility is that because they dilate the coronary vasculature they may, unless global ischaemia is present, improve oxygen availability in the affected area, at the same time as they increase substrate supply and facilitate the removal of metabolic waste. The same difficulty is encountered if we try to explain why β-adrenoceptor antagonists may be protective, provided that they are given early during the ischaemic episode[19] – they could reduce the rate of ATP depletion because of the decrease in heart rate. Alternatively it may be the establishment of β-adrenoceptor blockade that is of predominant importance. There is another possibility – that is, the β-antagonists may have a direct cellular effect. On the other hand pharmacological interventions may be unnecessary – for simple hypothermia may provide adequate protection.

HYPOTHERMIA

During open heart surgery requiring aortic cross-clamping, hypothermia, with or without chemically induced cardioplegia, is widely used to protect the heart against the deleterious effects of ischaemia and post-ischaemic reperfusion. If the arguments we have been considering above are valid, then we should be able to establish that hypothermia can be used to prevent Ca^{2+}

overloading and the accompanying loss of mitochondrial function. To test this hypothesis, isolated Langendorff-perfused rabbit hearts were made ischaemic for 90 min at either 37, 34, 28, 25 or 23 °C. At the end of the ischaemic episode the hearts were reperfused at 37 °C for another 30 min. At the end of the reperfusion process the mitochondria were harvested as previously described and assayed for Ca^{2+} content, ATP-producing activity, and respiratory function, assessed in terms of their capacity to utilize O_2, to convert ADP → ATP (QO_2), and the efficiency of that conversion, measured as the respiratory control index (RCI). Figure 12 shows that mitochondria which were obtained from hearts that had been made ischaemic at 28 °C or below and then reperfused at 37 °C maintained RCI, QO_2 and ATP-producing activity which was not markedly different from that obtained for hearts perfused at the same temperature (Figure 13) but under aerobic conditions. Figure 12 also shows that the mitochondria which were harvested from hearts that had been cooled to 28 °C or below during the 90 min of ischaemia retained an ATP-producing activity that was high relative to that obtained for mitochondria from hearts that had been maintained at 34 or 37 °C. Figure 14 shows that these same mitochondria that had a high ATP-producing activity and normal oxidative phosphorylation maintained relatively low

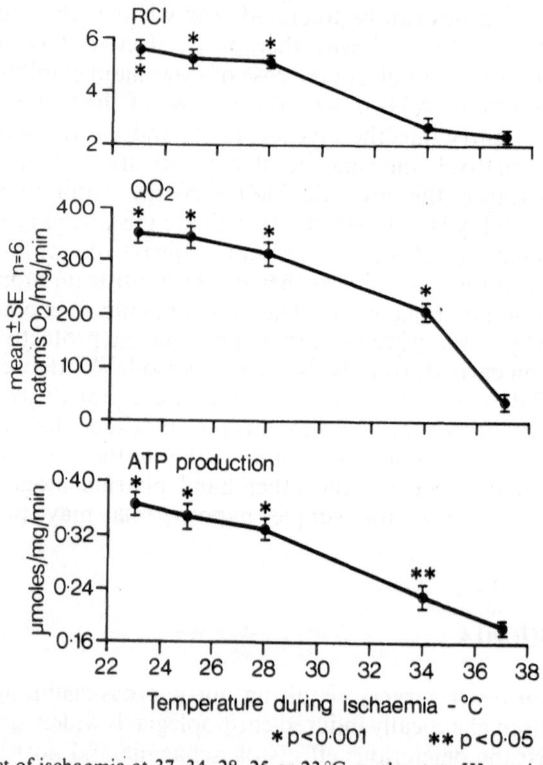

Figure 12 Effect of ischaemia at 37, 34, 28, 25 or 23 °C on the state III respiration, respiratory control index and ATP-producing activity of mitochondria incubated in the presence of glutamate substrate[15,19]. The mitochondria were isolated after 30 min reperfusion at 37 °C

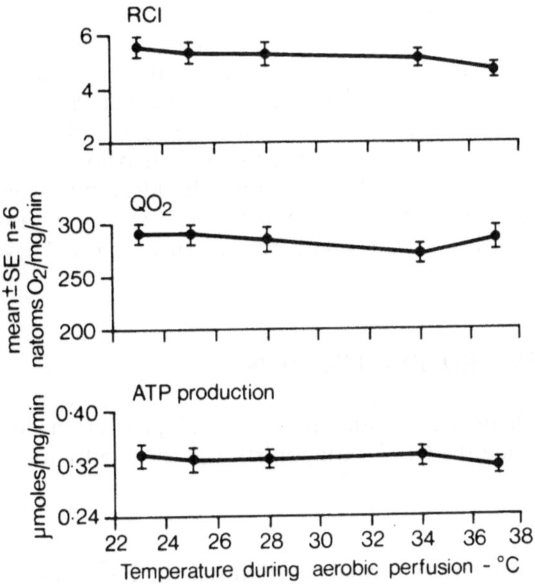

Figure 13 Effect of aerobic perfusion at 37, 35, 28, 25 and 22 °C on the oxygen-utilizing capacity, respiratory control index and ATP-producing activity of mitochondria isolated after 90 min perfusion

levels of mitochondrial Ca^{2+}. By contrast, mitochondria obtained from hearts that were reperfused after being maintained at 34 or 37 °C during the ischaemic episode were overloaded with Ca^{2+} (Figure 14). These data fit well with our hypothesis that overloading of the mitochondria with Ca^{2+} signals their failure to generate ATP. This failure to generate ATP parallels

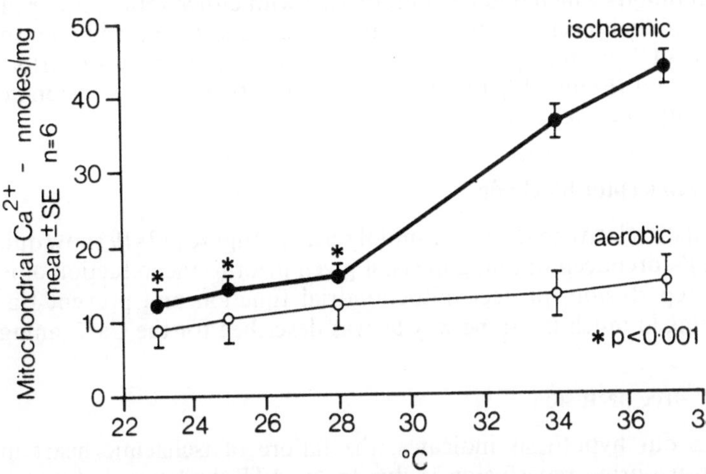

Figure 14 ATP-producing activity of mitochondria isolated after 90 min perfusion or total ischaemia at the indicated temperatures followed by 30 min reperfusion under aerobic conditions at 37 °C. For conditions of assay see reference 15

the inability of these hearts to exhibit active tension development during reperfusion. Thus, whereas hearts that were maintained at 37 °C during the 90 min of ischaemia failed to regain any active tension-generating capacity during reperfusion, hearts that were maintained at 28 °C regained about 70 % of their pre-ischaemic active tension generation. In conclusion, therefore, these data show that hypothermia to 28 °C or below can be used to protect the ATP-producing activity of the mitochondria in ischaemic heart muscle, and that this protection is accompanied by an improved recovery of active tension-generating capacity and the absence of Ca^{2+} overloading during reperfusion at 37 °C.

DRUG-INDUCED PROTECTION

Drugs which provide a similar pattern of protection described for hypothermia include the Ca^{2+}-antagonists and the β-adrenoceptor antagonists.

Ca^{2+}-antagonists

When administered to normal heart muscle the Ca^{2+} antagonists[20] including verapamil and nipedipine, restrict the entry of Ca^{2+} through the voltage-activated ion selective channels (Figure 15). Theoretically, therefore, these drugs should prevent ischaemic and reperfusion-induced damage because, by restricting the entry of Ca^{2+} they reduce the amount of Ca^{2+} available for interaction with the myofibrils, thereby reducing (Figure 16) the rate of ATP-utilization. In addition, in the intact circulation these drugs may have an ATP-sparing effect since they are all peripheral vasodilators. Figure 16 shows that one of these drugs – verapamil – does indeed have an ATP-sparing effect. The data shown in Figures 17–19 show that hearts excised from rabbits which had been pretreated with either verapamil or nipedipine prior to their excision and perfusion – these hearts retained their mitochondrial ATP-producing activity, the mitochondria were not overloaded with Ca^{2+} and (Figure 19) the hearts recovered their active tension-generating capacity upon reperfusion.

β-adrenoceptor blockade

The data relative to the propranolol series in Figures 17–19 show quite clearly that β-adrenoceptor antagonists, if given prior to the induction of ischaemia and reperfusion, protect mitochondrial function and prevent Ca^{2+} overloading in much the same way as was described for the Ca^{2+} antagonists.

Ca^{2+}-free perfusion

If, as our hypothesis indicates, the failure of ischaemic heart muscle to recover during reperfusion is due to an ATP-depletion induced failure to prevent the cells and particularly the mitochondria from becoming overloaded with Ca^{2+}, we are left with explaining why adequate protection cannot

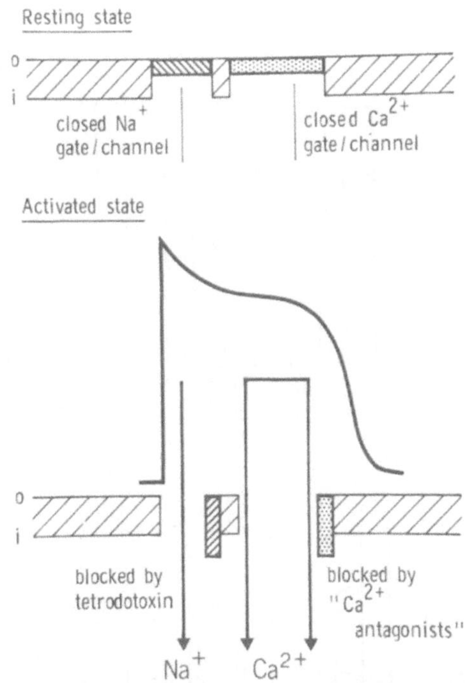

Figure 15 Schematic representation of the entry of Ca^{2+} through voltage-activated, Ca^{2+}-selective channels, and the inhibitory effect of verapamil. Note that during the rested state the 'channels' are closed

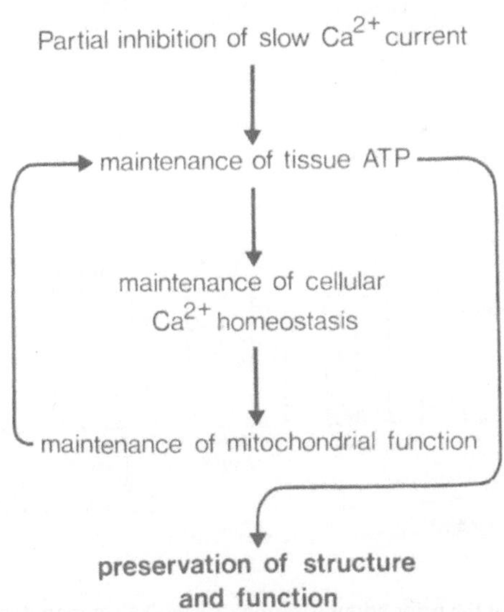

Figure 16 Schematic representation of the mechanism whereby Ca^{2+} antagonist drugs might protect the ischaemic heart, provided that they were administered prior to the onset of the ischaemic episode

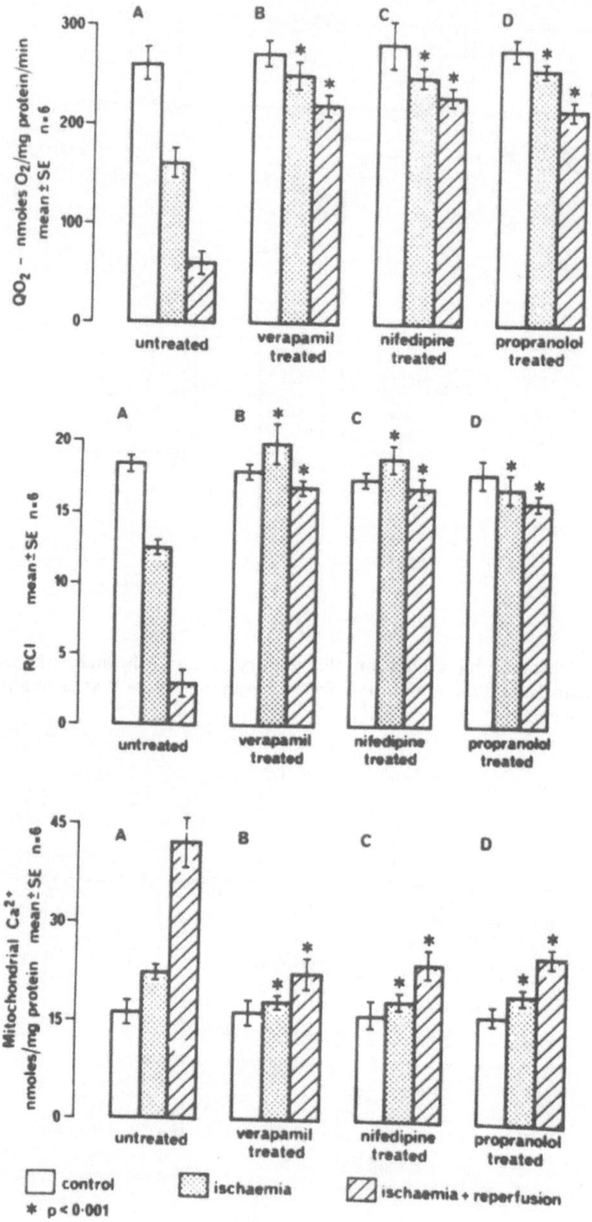

Figure 17 Effect of the prior administration of 1 mg/kg verapamil, nipedipine, or propranolol s.c. twice daily for 3–5 days on the respiratory activity and Ca^{2+} content of mitochondria isolated after 90 min ischaemia, with and without aerobic perfusion. Tests of significance relate to the protection afforded by the treatment

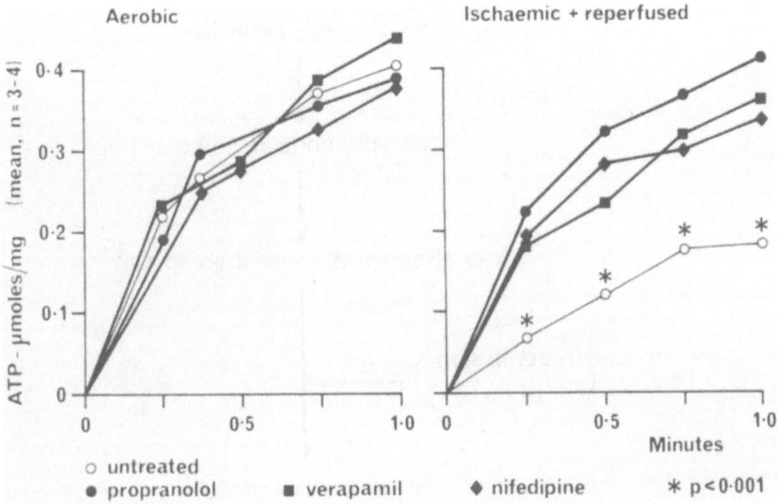

Figure 18 Effect of pretreatment for 3–5 days with verapamil, nipedipine, or propranolol on the ATP-producing activity of mitochondria isolated after 90 min ischaemia at 37 °C

be obtained simply by removing Ca^{2+} from the coronary perfusion circuit. Unfortunately, perfusion of mammalian heart muscle with Ca^{2+}-free solutions results in the destruction of the selective permeability properties of the cell surface, so that (Figure 20) when Ca^{2+} is readmitted these ions are free to

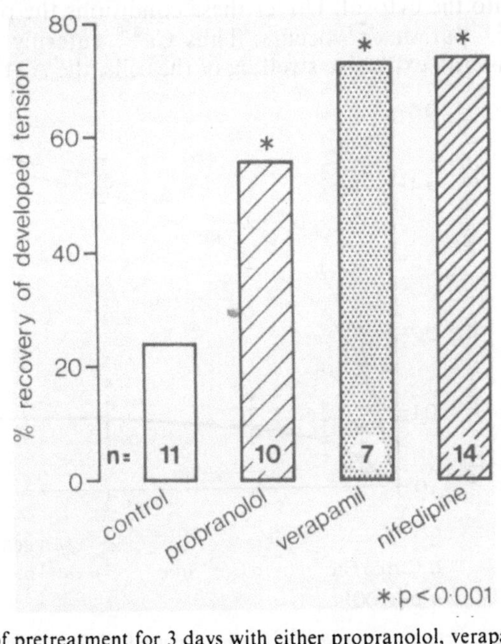

Figure 19 Effect of pretreatment for 3 days with either propranolol, verapamil, or nipedipine (1 mg/kg s.c. or i.p. twice daily) on the recovery of active tension generating capacity in heart muscle made ischaemic for 90 min at 37 °C and then reperfused

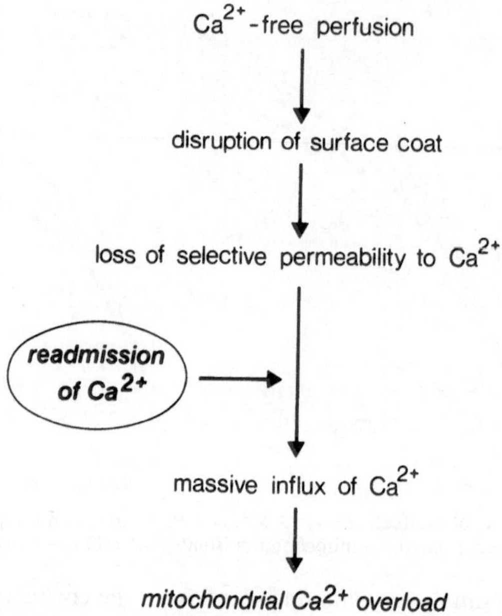

Figure 20 Schematic representation of the sequence of events induced by the readmission of Ca^{2+} after a period of Ca^{2+}-free perfusion

penetrate into the cytosol. Under these conditions the phenomenon known as the 'Ca^{2+} paradox'[21] occurs. Thus Ca^{2+} entering in an uncontrolled manner causes an explosive swelling of the cells, the ATP-producing activity

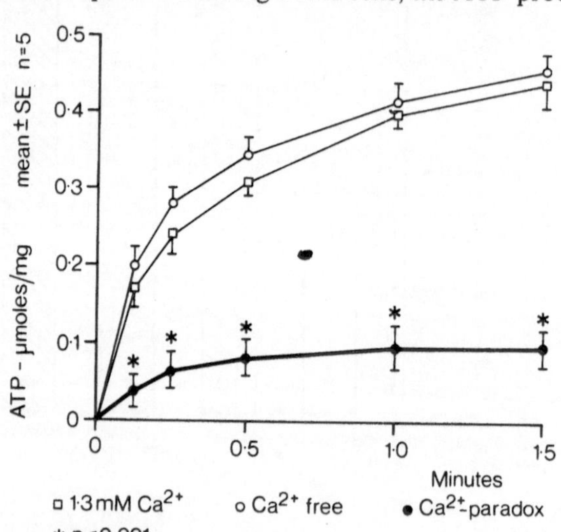

Figure 21 Effect of readmitting of Ca^{2+} after a period of Ca^{2+}-free perfusion on the ATP-producing activity of cardiac mitochondria. Ca^{2+} paradox refers to the readmission of Ca^{2+} after a period of Ca^{2+}-free perfusion

of the mitochondria declines (Figures 21 and 22) and the mitochondria become overloaded with Ca^{2+}. Under these conditions we can no longer expect a resumption of normal metabolic and mechanical activity.

CONCLUSION

Procedures which are known to protect heart muscle against the effect of ischaemic-induced damage and the exacerbation of that damage during reoxygenation and reperfusion include hypothermia and the administration of Ca^{2+} and β-adrenoceptor antagonists. These protective procedures have a common end-point: they all prevent the mitochondria from becoming overloaded with Ca^{2+}, so that the ATP-generating capacity of the mitochondria is maintained. These agents also have an ATP-sparing effect. The combination of an ATP-sparing effect and the preservation of the ATP-generating capacity of the mitochondria should ensure that sufficient ATP remains available, even after prolonged periods of ischaemia, to ensure the survival of the myocardium and the resumption of its normal mechanical, electrical, and metabolic activities upon reperfusion. To some extent the damage that occurs during reperfusion must be directly proportional to the degree of ATP depletion – thus the shorter the period of ischaemia the greater the chance of survival. Inotropic agents such as digitalis or isoproterenol may exacerbate ischaemic and reperfusion-induced damage because of their enhancement of ATP utilization and because they promote the entry of Ca^{2+} into the myocardium. Reperfusion with glucose-containing solutions should facilitate recovery, mainly because even if it is only metabolized anaerobically, it will ensure the production of some additional ATP to maintain intracellular homeostasis with respect to Ca^{2+}.

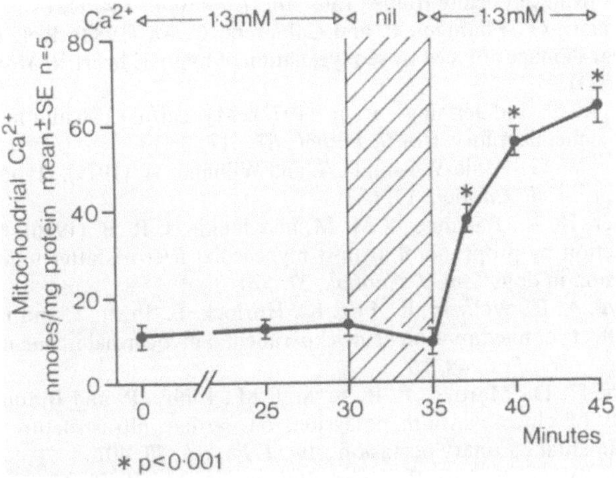

Figure 22 Effect of readmitting Ca^{2+} after a period of Ca^{2+}-free perfusion on the Ca^{2+} content of cardiac mitochondria

In general, therefore, protection of the ischaemic heart involves the introduction of regimes that will result in the maintenance of intracellular homeostasis with respect to Ca^{2+} so that the ATP-producing activity of the mitochondria will be preserved.

References

1. Matsui, H. and Schwartz, A. (1966). Purification and properties of a highly active, ouabain sensitive, Na^+K^+ dependent adenosine triphosphatase from cardiac muscle. *Biochem. Biophys. Acta*, **128,** 280
2. Mas-Oliva, J., Williams, A. J. and Nayler, W. G. (1980). Two orientations of isolated cardiac sarcolemmal vesicles separated by affinity chromatography. *Analytic Chem.* (In press)
3. Reuter, H. (1974). Exchange of calcium ions in the mammalian myocardium. *Circ. Res.*, **34,** 599
4. Nayler, W. G., Mas-Oliva, J. and Williams, A. J. (1980). Cardiovascular receptors and calcium. *Circ. Res.*, **46,** 161
5. Langer, G. A. (1973). Excitation contraction coupling. *Phys. Rev.*, **35,** 55
6. Sperelakes, N. and Schneider, J. A. (1976). A metabolic control mechanism for calcium ion influx that may protect the ventricular myocardial cell. *Am. J. Cardiol.*, **37,** 1079
7. Hasselbach, H. (1980). Quantitative aspects of the calcium concept of excitation – contraction coupling – a critical evaluation. *Basic Res. Cardiol.*, **75,** 2
8. Cooley, D. A., Reul, G. J. and Wakash, D. C. (1972). Ischemic contracture of the heart: stone heart. *Am. J. Cardiol.*, **29,** 595
9. Lehninger, A. L. (1974). Ca^{2+}-transport by mitochondria and its possible role in the cardiac contraction–relaxation cycle. *Circ. Res.*, **35,** Suppl. 111, 83
10. Jarmakani, J. M., Nakamishi, T. and Jarmakani, R. (1979). Effect of hypoxia or calcium exchange in neonatal mammalian myocardium. *Am. J. Physiol.*, **237,** H612
11. da Luz, P. C., Forrester, J. S., Wyatt, L., Tyberg, J. V., Chagrisulis, R., Parmley, W. B. and Swan, J. H. (1975). Effect of verapamil on regional coronary and myocardial perfusion during acute coronary occlusion. *Circulation*, **52,** 400
12. Bersohn, M. M. and Scheur, J. (1978). Effect of ischemia on the performance of hearts from physically trained rats. *Am. J. Physiol.*, **234,** H215
13. Guarnieri, G., Flamigni, P. and Caldarera, C. M. (1980). Role of oxygen in the cellular damage induced by reoxygenation of hypoxic heart. *J. Molec. Cell. Cardiol.* (In press)
14. Shen, A. G. and Jennings, R. B. (1972). Myocardial calcium and magnesium in acute ischemic injury. *Am. J. Pathol.*, **67,** 417
15. Nayler, W. G., Poole-Wilson, P. A. and Williams, A. (1979). Hypoxia and calcium. *J. Molec. Cell. Cardiol.*, **11,** 683
16. Reimer, K. A., Rasmussen, M. M. and Jennings, R. B. (1976). On the nature of protection by propranolol against myocardial necrosis after temporary coronary occlusion in dogs. *Am. J. Cardiol.*, **37,** 520
17. Selwyn, A. P., Welman, E., Fox, K., Horlock, P., Pratt, T. and Klein, M. (1979). The effects of nifedipine on acute experimental myocardial ischaemia and infarction in dogs. *Circ. Res.*, **44,** 16
18. Sybers, H. D., Maroko, P. R., Ashraf, M., Libby, P. and Braunwald, E. (1973). Effects of glucose–insulin–potassium on cardiac ultrastructure following acute experimental coronary occlusion. *Am. J. Pathol.*, **70,** 401
19. Nayler, W. G., Ferrari, R. J. and Williams, A. M. (1980). The protective effect of pretreatment with verapamil, nifedipine and propranolol on mitochondrial function in the ischaemic and reperfused myocardium. *Am. J. Cardiol.*, **46,** 242

20. Fleckenstein, A. (1970). Specific inhibitors and promoters of calcium action in excitation–contraction coupling of heart muscle and their role in the prevention and production of myocardial lesions. In Harris, P. and Opie, L. (eds.) *Calcium and the Heart*. p. 135 (New York: Academic Press)
21. Zimmerman, ANE, Daems, W., Hulsmann, W. G., Snijder, J., Wisse, E. and Durrer, D. (1967). Morphological changes in heart muscle caused by successive perfusion with calcium-free and calcium-containing solutions (calcium paradox). *Cardiovasc. Res.*, **1,** 201

Comment on Professor W. G. Nayler's lecture

H. J. BRETSCHNEIDER,
M. M. GEBHARD AND
C. J. PREUSSE

The attentive reader of this proceedings will not have failed to notice that between our arguments and the concepts of Professor Nayler, besides essential agreements, from the view of cardiac surgical practice there also are contradictions or, at least ambiguities. For safer cardiac surgery almost nothing is more hazardous than to repress uncertainties and contradictions. Since, following Professor Nayler's most impressive 'Sir Thomas Holmes Sellors Lecture', there remained no time for discussion, Doctor Holden has asked us to give a short letter of comment.

We would like to first point out the decisive, more or less explicitly formulated agreements between our two approaches:

1 Under completely ischaemic conditions the myocardium cannot indefinitely cover the energy demand of structure and function preservation.
2 In the anaerobic myocardium the decisive path of energy production is glycolysis.
3 Calcium ions are of central importance to the integrity of the outer cell membrane, to stimulation of metabolism, to activation of the contractile system as well as to ATP synthesis.
4 In connection with the central importance of the calcium ions, calcium-antagonistic as well as β-blocking agents can show a cardioprotective effect (presupposing a premedication well balanced in time and dosage).

Formulated and implied divergences follow from a differing quantitative analysis and another stressing of the factors decisive for the ischaemia tolerance of the heart. The proper emphasis on the various factors, however, is in any case the prerequisite for the adequate evaluation of the over-all effect of the protective measures.

On Point 1

The ratio 'energy production to energy demand' in the ischaemic anaerobiosis is not a natural constant, but can be shifted in a favourable or unfavourable direction by the ion composition of the cardioplegic solution. Moreover, even the absolute value of energy demand of the arrested heart – independent of temperature – can conveniently be decreased or inconveniently be increased. Reduction of the energy demand and amelioration of glycolytic energy production, at the same temperature and without a special premedication, can extend the reversible margin of an ischaemic anaerobiosis by a factor of 8; that is by up to 700 %.

On Point 2

The most effective way to ameliorate glycolytic energy production is by adequate extracellular buffering. In connection with an adjusted extracellular ion milieu, thereby the ratio 'glycolytic energy production to energy gain from the high-energy-phosphate reserves',

$$\frac{\Delta \text{ lactate} \times 1.5}{\Delta \sim P}$$

can be increased from about 2.2 to 4.5. This ratio too, therefore, can no longer be seen as a natural constant.

On Point 3

The calcium paradox is overrated by all investigators who experiment on small-animal hearts (guinea pigs, rats, rabbits), away from clinical conditions. Compared to dog hearts, which are much more similar to the human heart, small-animal hearts show considerable electrophysiological differences. Additionally, the ratio 'perfusion rate per weight unit' under usual experimental conditions is much higher; in the isolated guinea pig heart, for instance, it amounts to at least 2–3 times that of human or dog hearts. The initiation of calcium paradox is also decisively dependent on temperature, particularly ion composition, and pH of the calcium-free perfusate. The temperature coefficient of the calcium paradox is between 35 and 25°C very high: with our cardioprotective solution in the dog heart, even after a 60 min continuous perfusion at 25 °C we have not been able to evoke a calcium paradox. Under the prescribed application conditions of our almost calcium-free cardioplegic solution at 5–10 °C, in several thousand patients – even after repeated intraoperative application – a calcium paradox has never been described. Besides, it must be remembered that the critical calcium concentration in the perfusion system, beyond which a calcium paradox experimentally can be reproducibly evoked, i.e. below 20 μmol/l, is generally not reached in clinical practice. At the cell membranes of dog heart, during cold application of the calcium-free solution, the critical inferior calcium ion concentration is only attained after several hours of continuous perfusion.

On Point 4

The very impressive cardioprotective effects of calcium-antagonistic and β-blocking drugs in small-animal hearts are corroborated by the results from a group from our institute (V. A. Mezger and P. G. Spieckermann), but cannot be evaluated without consideration of the experimental conditions. The killing of the animals, the excision of the hearts, and the connection with the perfusion system all together bring about a massive adrenergic stress, which fortunately does not occur in such a degree for the human heart before artificial arrest, thanks to good anaesthesia. In experiments on large warm-blooded animals (dog, calf) the clinical conditions of a well-adjusted deep anaesthesia with controlled normoventilation can easily be simulated; under these conditions, according to our experiences, verapamil and propranolol, 'only' effect a prolongation of the tolerated ischaemia time of about 20%. The corresponding factor of 1.2, together with the factor resulting from an optimal cardioplegia, between 25° and 15°C results in a total factor of $8 \times 1.2 \rightarrow 10$, compared to a pure ischaemic heart arrest without special premedication but with a well-adjusted neurolept analgesia. A gain of 20% at a normothermic ischaemia tolerance of the human heart about 10 min is without practical relevance; at hypothermia of 15°C and myocardial protection with our new solution in the dog heart one can reach an ischaemia tolerance time of about 500 min without special premedication; under these conditions a premedication of calcium-antagonistic or β-blocking agents gives an impressive prolongation of the tolerated ischaemia time of about 20% that means of about 2 h.

Summarizing one can say:

(a) Calcium-antagonistic and β-blocking drugs act the more cardioprotectively, the stronger and more pathological a following pre-ischaemic adrenergic stress is.

(b) Under an optimal deep anaesthesia the cardioprotective action of β-blockers and calcium antagonists alone is not sufficient to insure a successful operation (even in a pre-damaged myocardium) within more than 15 min of aortic clamping at temperatures between 30° and 25°C without employment of a cardioplegic solution.

(c) Transfer of findings from small-animal hearts to clinical practice inevitably needs the intermediate stage of experiments on large warm-blooded animals under clinic-like conditions.

Reply to Professor Bretschneider

WINIFRED G. NAYLER

I feel I should thank Professor Bretschneider for his comments. In the main we agree. Certainly there are very many approaches that can be taken with respect to studies into the basic mechanisms that need to be delineated if we are to protect the heart against the effects of inadequate oxygenation, perfusion and subsequent reoxygenation and reperfusion. Professor Bretschneider and I both agree that control of the intracellular distribution of Ca^{2+} is of vital importance, and that a supply of energy is needed for this. We both agree that protection of the energy supply can be mediated in several different ways, including the use of cardioplegic solutions. Others favour the use of pharmacological agents. Whether or not Ca^{2+}-free perfusion is 'deleterious' or protective depends simply upon what is meant by Ca^{2+}-free. Most of the reagents used for preparing cardioplegic solutions contain enough contaminant Ca^{2+} to prevent the deleterious effect of Ca^{2+}-free perfusion (Ca^{2+} – paradox) from becoming manifest, unless very high flow rates are used.

Conclusions

M. P. HOLDEN

THE AIMS OF THE MEETING

(1) To emphasize to all the members of the clinical team that cardiac surgery is now very much a multi-disciplinary specialty, and that everyone working in such a department is a professional expert in his or her own right.
(2) To disseminate as much information as possible, precisely, concisely and without elaboration or pain, concerning current ideas and practices and aspirations for the future to all groups of personnel working in cardiac surgery.

STRUCTURE OF THE MEETING

In 1978, when it was suggested that I should organize an international symposium on cardiac surgery, I considered that it would be a welcome challenge, providing that the format was different from the multiplicity of meetings which currently exist around the world. There are now so many gatherings on the international circuits concerning the many aspects of the cardiac surgical discipline – for example, anaesthesia, pathological anatomy, intensive care, paediatric cardiology, myocardial metabolism, extracorporeal circulation, artificial organ engineering, to name but a few.

Consequently, for any member of the operating team, be they surgeon or monitoring technician, to attempt to keep up to date with current thought and developments would be a physical and intellectual impossibility, either to attend all these meetings or to read all the journals. In fact to attempt to do so, as many of us are discovering, leaves insufficient time to perform the clinical work for which we are employed. Some of the meetings are clinically orientated, and to use the current jargon, they are of the 'workshop' variety.

These are often excellent events, in that they offer current thoughts and expertise in a practical form. Many other meetings, be they local, national or international, frequently allow the presentation of incomplete data, often by junior members of the clinical research team who are there simply to practise the difficult art of public speaking, and often fail to keep within the prescribed time limits.

This system is quite laudable and is socially pleasing, but it is an inferior and expensive way of disseminating knowledge to busy clinicians and scientists. With the restrictions on travel allowances, precipitated by the present inflationary strictures, chronic 'conference-goers' will have to be far more selective in their choice of meetings.

How then can we justify yet another symposium? Simply on one premise, which is recognized by every successful manager. The premise is simply this: cardiac surgery is very much a team effort, and everyone must realize this fact, and accept it absolutely. Good team relationships are paramount in order to improve the efficiency and safety of teamwork.

It has become apparent during the last 5 years, although many surgeons have been reluctant to acknowledge this evolution, that all patients undergoing open heart surgery owe the safety of their lives, not just to the surgeon, but to a wide spectrum of individuals. For example, if the extracorporeal perfusionist allows the level in the oxygenator to fall below a critical point, or he sucks when he should pump, then the patient may die or almost certainly be crippled. If the nurse does not realize that the left atrial pressure line, whilst providing invaluable information, can severely disable the patient with air, thrombus or infection, then her immediate superiors and teachers are guilty of omission. If the anaesthetist does not collaborate totally with the surgeon regarding the perfusion pressure, then the subendocardial layer of the left ventricular wall can be irreversibly damaged. If the physiotherapist is not aware of the profoundly deleterious effects of prolonged anoxia during endotracheal suction, cardiac arrest can follow. If the resident is lulled into a false sense of security by the monitor pressure readings whilst the patient becomes vasoconstricted, cold, oliguric and increasingly acidotic an irreversible cycle may well ensue. These are some examples of the total dependence of the surgeon and his patient on the care and skill of other team members at all times.

We therefore considered that every person in the surgical team had to be made more aware of the multi-disciplinary approach and of their critical role. But this meeting was not simply a public relations exercise, although that aspect is very important in creating safer and more efficient units. Obviously with the present patient referral system the consultant cardiac surgeon has to acknowledge the full and overall responsibility for the patient's welfare, but the surgeon must also be aware, as a simple act of common sense relating to human nature, that far superior results will be achieved if all his or her colleagues are treated with genuine respect.

A critical analysis of our surgical results is always beneficial, and many of the better departments hold regular and frequent clinico-pathological meetings to assess where they are going wrong and how they may improve. At a national level in the United Kingdom we have all benefited from the advent of the Cardiac Surgical Register. Understandably, clinicians have felt it incumbent upon their professional virility to report only positive findings, even if these had no statistical or scientific merit. Much value to the specialty, and ultimately the patients, would be achieved if medical authors occasionally wrote about their mistakes and failures. Alas, we are all cognizant of the painful truths that it takes a great person to acknowledge their mistakes consciously and publicly, and the possibilities of American-style litigation are ever lurking. Nonetheless, this is an aspect of our publication life which we must reconsider with seriousness and diligence.

Another major consideration in the conception of this meeting, after the content, architecture and the audience had been decided, was the title which needed to demonstrate the overall aims and concept of the event. So many technical and scientific developments have been incorporated into the day-to-day practice of heart surgery, which have allowed its progress, in terms of complexity and success during the space of two decades, to explode. Yet patients still die unexpectedly, or receive crippling morbidity problems, often for no discernible reasons.

In an attempt to reassess the possible ways by which we could reduce the present mortality and morbidity figures still further, it was decided to examine all aspects of the operative procedure from the time the clinical diagnosis of cardiac pathology is suspected until the patient is completely rehabilitated in his or her former occupation after successful surgery. In essence, this exercise entailed scrutinization of all aspects of procedural safety. We were aware that open heart surgery can never be 100% safe, just as no aspect of human life can be 100% perfect in any sphere of activity. Therefore, it seemed logical that the title of the symposium should be 'Towards Safer Cardiac Surgery'.

There is an optimum time and duration of such meetings. The skill demonstrated, so often these days by the anaesthetists, nurses and intensivists in resuscitating patients, sometimes after suboptimal surgery, an exhaustive meeting. If a meeting is only of one day's duration, then the participants do not have the time to develop an empathy for the occasion, and if it is of greater length than three days they become saturated and exhausted, even if they managed to leave their seat of employment for this lengthy period. Consequently, we opted for one whole and two half days.

The format, or skeleton, was difficult to derive, because there is nothing more infurating than the current fashion of conferences where several series of lectures or seminars are progressing concurrently. Inevitably, one has to miss out on something, because often two important topics clash. To prevent this dilemma we decided to have only one lecture-room functioning. How then do we overcome the problem of congestion in the programme when there are so many 'burning issues' to discuss? Further, what is the optimum length of time for each presentation; should we have panel or individual discussion periods; and can we expect real and productive discussion from an audience of 350 people? I maintained that it was paramount that, primarily, we should hear what the clinical and scientific experts had to say, and then if there was available time, formal discussion could follow on a limited basis in the auditorium. Informal discussions could proceed afterwards, because almost everyone was living on the same campus of the delightful University of York. Just as there are 'chronic conference-goers', so there are 'chronic question-askers' who always seem 'just to have a few slides with them'. It was planned to prevent this phenomenon from occurring, and further, in order to give the presentations a fresh yet sound appeal, the speakers were carefully chosen, and the precise title of their paper was suggested to them, for example, 'Does the intra-aortic balloon pump augment safer cardiac surgery?' and 'Which electrolytes matter?' Without exception the speakers accepted this 'request' and challenge, and entered into the spirit of the opportunity with an enthusiasm and courtesy which I shall always appreciate. Surprisingly, most of them demonstrated their expertise by working within the deliberately short time available for their presentation. In order to maintain such an intensive programme 'on an even keel', we had to select chairmen who are recognized internationally for their clinical and scientific expertise and achievements, and also for their meticulous control and gentle authority of presence.

CONTENT OF THE MEETING

It will be appreciated that there was no logistic possibility of covering all aspects of the management of open heart surgery patients which might enable it to become a safer procedure. Therefore, many subjects which the participants and readers of this book will consider to be grievous omissions – for example, the value of pacing, or the management of bleeding – could not be included. Fortunately, we can rectify this problem when the second and subsequent Symposia are held, and their Proceedings are published.

The first section, which deals with technical matter of coronary artery, valvular and paediatric cardiac procedures, was kept deliberately short. This policy was adopted because the former two groups have been overexposed during the last decade, and on the whole they would benefit from less discussion and more prolonged clinical trials during the next decade. In view of the pleasing and increasing longevity of some homograft and xenograft valves which have the great advantages of near-normal haemodynamic characteristics, minimal noise levels and low thromboembolic rates without anticoagulants, it seemed appropriate to briefly comment on the present state of the art and the aspirations for the future. Whilst I am convinced that we will never have a perfect valve prosthesis of any kind, we can hope that some of the more promising bioprostheses, such as the pericardial type, may allow the patient 10–15 good years before further replacement is necessary.

There is now no question concerning the benefits of coronary artery bypass grafting. This operation relieves angina in the great majority of patients, when the surgery is performed meticulously and there is adequate revascularization within the limits of competence of the surgeon and the ability of the myocardium to withstand prolonged anoxia. Then the mortality is close to zero if the left ventricular function is reasonable, and there is no additional pathology. The haemodynamic superiority of the internal mammary artery over the saphenous vein will be pointlessly debated for some time to come. However, the greater versatility of the saphenous vein in the form of separate 'jump' graft makes this conduit the prime choice for most surgeons. It is now becoming apparent from the most recent trials (Professor D. G. Julian, personal communication, 1980) that the surgical treatment of all forms of coronary artery disease, except perhaps single-vessel problems, is superior to medical treatment in terms of symptomatic relief and increased life-expectancy at 5 years.

Congenital heart disease is a vast subject with a seemingly daily increase in the therapeutic repertoire as skilful surgical teams keep pace with the pathological anatomists. Therefore, it was considered appropriate that within the style of this meeting, an internationally respected speaker should present a review of the present state of the art with a philosophical and provocative look into the next 5 years.

Another major aspect of our daily operative routine, which has increased the safety by 'protecting' the myocardium to a greater extent against the surgeon's arrogance, has been the reincarnation of cardioplegic solutions. We are indebted to the West Germans, particularly, for their pioneering work involved in the successful reintroduction of these fluids which show a greater respect for the importance of pH and osmolality than did their forebears. Unfortunately, many opportunists, realizing that their fame and fortune was not to be found in the sphere of heart valve development, switched their oftimes unscientific attentions to the production of the ultimate elixir which would protect the myocardium indefinitely, and propel their reputations to even greater heights. It has been emphasized by a meeting recently held in North America, under the same sponsorship as this meeting, organised by Dr Robert Litwak, and reported with customary wisdom and perspicacity by Dr Dwight McGoon[2], that there probably are as many different solutions being used around the world as there are cardiac surgeons, and that the variety of the solutions greatly outnumbers the metabolic substrates and inorganic elements found within the myocardium! The analysis of their value is made virtually impossible, because each clinician has a different regime of application of a fluid containing a different cocktail from any other surgeon, and they are all using different parameters for this assessment.

Thus, it is only by the surgeons, the biochemists and other workers meeting together at such gatherings as this, that the problem will ever stand a chance of being unravelled. Suffice it to say that probably the two most important points that we must recognise until the ultimate solution arrives, which allows true suspended animation of the myocardium are:

(1) stop the heart beating as quickly as possible, so that its energy substrates are not wasted unnecessarily;
(2) the myocardial temperature should be reduced to 20–25 °C as soon and as safely as possible, and maintained there.

All other modifications to the procedural recipe must be made with the good sense of the clinician.

The greater part of the symposium was, therefore, given over to the two vast and extremely important areas of open heart surgery, namely,

(1) cardiopulmonary bypass;
(2) postoperative care.

By paying greater attention to these two aspects of management we may make advances during the next 5 years which will give us the opportunity of matching the incredible expertise of the scientific investigators who lectured during the first day. What an amazing thought that during the next 5 years nuclear magnetic resonance will, in all probability, have revolutionized the management and care of our patients as much as echocardiography has done during the preceding 5 years. This was a delightful glimpse into the future, and we are indebted to the speakers who ventured out of their own disciplines to explain, so explicitly, what they could offer our patients.

It would be unseemly, and unnecessary, to mention the subject material of every paper in detail, but let us briefly consider the problem of bleeding. It has been apparent to the surgeons for some time, particularly those who still close chests after the interesting part of the operation is completed, that, even though the anaesthetist emphasizes that 'the blood is clotting at his end', as assessed by the 'Haemochron' which has enabled much greater control of the heparin–protamine administration, and even though the surgeon may also 'see clots at his end', the patient continues to bleed. Further, the clots may then stop forming; we know not why. At the other end of the spectrum some patients mysteriously, but fortunately, cease haemorrhaging when the chest is closed. Is this due to slight, but adequate compression, or is it due to removal of the bleeding tissue–air interface? The clinical problem lies in the dilemma of 'knowing' which patients will stop bleeding when the chest has been closed, and those who will not. In Newcastle we have made a little progress in this area recently, although we have no idea of the mechanism of action. Those patients who continue to bleed three quarters of an hour after obtaining good 'Haemochron' control have their chests packed with swabs. This we have found extremely beneficial in a large department performing 800 open operations per year, in that it saves much time with no morbidity problems. It is difficult to prove the value of this working hypothesis scientifically. It is also apparent that children who have had an atrial or ventricular septal defect closed do not bleed, assuming surgical competence. The operative field is instantly dry, whereas a middle-aged double-valve replacement patient, and not necessarily a 're-do', may continue to ooze from every tissue in sight. This phenomenon occurs in patients with a 'so-called' normal full laboratory clotting profile. Thus, there is more to post-bypass bleeding than our present state of knowledge affords us. Fortunately the papers relating to prostacyclins, toxins, suction, gaseous emboli and other blood–gas interface situations with their important effects on thrombocytes and other haematological components offer us considerable hope. It is also becoming apparent that immunological phenomena may have a role in aspects of this surgery other than transplantation.

Less than a decade has elapsed since the intra-aortic balloon pump was being heralded in as the greatest advance in cardiac surgery after the discovery of oxygen, yet it is largely obsolete now, except in specific circumstances, such as unstable angina, left mainstem disease prior to operation, and as a last resort postoperatively. The reason for the sudden decline in usefulness of this expensive device is largely attributable to the use of cardioplegic solutions and the greater thoughtfulness for the well-being of the myocardium by surgeons, anaesthetists and perfusionists. There cannot be a better example of the rapidly changing nature of this surgery, and the need for us all to avoid being reactionary without falling into the hypnotic lure of new gimmicks. Relating specifically to the salutary paper presented by a patient, we learnt that physical contact and communication are essential, and that hearing is accentuated. This is obvious, when one ponders on the matter, but like all obvious and important considerations, we are always irritated that we had not thought of them ourselves. If only we stopped to reflect and occasionally put ourselves in the patient's situation! Naturally, no two patients are alike, and I recall one young man, following coronary artery surgery, who was driven to distraction by the rustle of the tinfoil which was supposed to be keeping him warm! Perhaps we should maintain a register of all major points raised by patients on the intensive care unit, and then modify our management accordingly. Following that, the use of sedatives may dramatically fall.

It becomes apparent that 'ICU' is a more suitable title than 'ITU', and that the emphasis should be on the central word 'care', which is an all-embracing word. I propose that we should 'care' primarily, and be 'intensive' constantly but cautiously. After all, what value are the recorded parameters, if the nurse is so preoccupied with her collection and documentation that she does not have the time to consider their significance or to look at the patient? The answer is simple: they are counterproductive and detrimental.

CONCLUSION

We have been aware for a quarter of a century that ours was an exciting specialty which offers us unrivalled opportunities of working on the edge of many new frontiers. Originally, it was a specialty for the surgical and rheological entrepreneurs. Without those apparently fearless, perceptive and of times ruthless clinical and intellectual pioneers, the first patients would never have been put on bypass. This meant a considerable increase in the mortality figures for atrial septal defect patients who had been very safely corrected with hypothermia and inflow occlusion.

To prevent the specialty going round in boring, fruitless orbit as gastric surgery has done for the last 200 years, only to have its monotonous and mutilating circuits broken by tablets of Cimetidine, we must realize that unless cardiac surgeons and all their clinical colleagues meet regularly with each other and the pure scientists, and listen to what the other has to say, then cardiac surgery will stagnate and ultimately fragment.

Our keywords towards safety should be:

Care, Common sense, Communication, Collaboration and Computers.

References

1. Editorial (1975). Organization of cardiac surgical services. *Br. Med. J.*, 609
2. Professor D. G. Julian, personal communication, 1980
3. McGoon, D. C. (1980). The quest for ideal myocardial protection. *J. Cardiovasc. Surg.*, **79**, 150

Index

accidents, perfusion-related 437–44
  causes 437
  human failure 437
  incidence 438
  and management 444, 445
acebutolol 269
acid citrate dextrose, blood pH 395
acidosis, glycolysis-induced intracellular 27
actin 386
adrenaline 519, 520
age
  and bypass surgery 82
  and risk in congenital heart disease 16, 17
air embolism 348, 368–71, 440, 441
  causes 372
allograft 57
American Institute of Ultrasound in Medicine (AUIM)
  clinicians guide 126
anaerobiasis
  and anaerobic perfusion 22
  energy supply 27
  factors affecting 31–3
  ischaemic of heart 22–6
anaesthesia 21, 94, 281
  and coronary artery surgery 267–77
  induction and maintenance 270, 271
  intravascular monitoring 270
  management 270
  pre-operative preparation 267–70
analgesia, neurolept 21
aneurysmectomy
  patient selection 237, 238
  and ventricular function 238–40
angina 84, 95, 193
  postoperative cardiac surgery 89, 92–4
  thallium scintigraphy 197
  unstable, nuclear imaging 185
angiocardiography 99–107
  aortic valve disease 100
  atrial septal defect 99, 100
  hazards 101–6
    and condition 101, 102
    and heart disease 102, 103
  importance 99–101
  multivalve surgery 100
  radionuclide *see* nuclear imaging technique
angiography
  percutaneous 103
angiograms, contrast and radionuclide 235
  sensitivity and echocardiography 74
angiotensin II 284
  and pulsation perfusion 489
antibiotics, prophylactic
  and prosthetic infections 596–8
  and tracheal infection 596, 597
aorta, coarctation
  transvenous aortography 105
aortic aneurysm 132
aortic incompetance 10
  and early death 11
aortic regurgitation
  echocardiography 147–9
  timing of surgery 148
aortic stenosis 132
  aetiology 147
  echocardiography 145–7
  subvalvar 146
  timing of surgery 96
aortic valve disease 100
  calcification, echocardiogram 131
arterial circulation, air bubble sources 328
arterial switching 15, 16
asymmetric septal hypertrophy 133
atenolol 269
ATP
  critical content of ischaemia 30, 40
  α, β and γ groups in muscle 161, 162
  heart, determinants 515
  in ischaemia 41, 43, 45
  ischaemic effects 635, 636
  ischaemic stress indicator 46, 48
  monocyte utilization 386, 387
  and NMR imaging 161
  and perfusion time 628
  pre-ischaemia, determination 28
ATPase
  calcium sensitivity 633, 634

$Na^+ K^+$ – arrangement 630
atrial myxoma
diagnosis 143
left, echocardiography 130
atrial septum
defect 99, 100
defect closure 96
atrial spasm 96
Australia antigen screening 401
autograft 57
autolysis 57

balloon atrial septostomy 15
balloon catheter aortogram 102
balloon inflation system 491
bioassay
fetal heart for toxin 450–71
biological materials
clinical problems 65–8
sources 65
Blalock shunt 102
blood
citrated, storage changes 402
embolization products 374
gases in postoperative hypothermia 285
loss, control 569, 570
osmometry 409–14
perfusion, disadvantages 402
rheology 403–9
shear stress 405
tonicity 409, 410
vessel distribution, Doppler echocardiography 123
brain damage 287
and open heart surgery 619–26
postoperative causes 376
preoperative causes 366
and pulsatile perfusion 486, 487
buffer
cardioplegia 40
histidine/histidine HCl 28
myocardial extracellular space 27, 29
bypass *see also* cardiopulmonary
veno-arterial 477, 478, 480
veno-venous 477, 478, 480

calcification 67
mitral valve 139–41
calcium
activator 631
antagonists 640
entry, myocardium 630
-free perfusion 640, 643, 644, 651
importance 648, 649
readmission, effects 644, 645
release, myocardial 31
withdrawal 35
Candida sp. endocarditis 585, 586
carbon-11 209
carbon dioxide
and hypothermia 284, 285
and protons 394
cardiac arrest
elective 263
ischaemic 34
methods of artificial 35
post-ischaemic heart rates and solutions 46
post-ischaemic oxygen uptake 47
cardiac surgery, metabolic cost 556–8
cardiogenic shock 106
cardiogram-dimension relations
normal, apex 76
cardioplegia 21, 249
methods, pros and cons 36
perfusion time and energy 36, 37
perfusion time and oxygen 37, 38
potassium 209
procaine and 35, 36
use in London Chest Hospital 84
in vein grafting 84, 94
cardioplegic solution 29
and ATP content 48
Bretschneider 40–5, 49
and emboli 369
Hamburg 40
Kirklin 40, 41, 48
Papworth 272
properties 36
St Thomas' 40, 41, 48
cardioprotective solution
cations and buffers 40
osmolality 32
reperfusion 44
cardiopulmonary bypass
accidents 437–44
air embolism 368–73
aortotomy size 299
biochemical disturbances 375
β-blocker comparison 275
blood damage 461, 462
blood loss, perfusion and transfusion 300
blood viscosity 406
cardiotomy suction 313–22
circuit, scheme 340, 341
complications, causes 293–9, 575–80
cooling, 272, 273 *see also* hypothermia
contraction coordination 75
critical time 271
developments 1951–3 260, 261
emergency drill 445
equipment 261, 361, 430–5
erythrocyte counts 294–9
filters, SEM of 362, 363

haematological values after 314
haemodynamic management 271
heat exchanger 337, 432
and heparin 359–63
high flow–low flow 262
hypotension 375–7
infections 310
maintenance haematocrit 420
and myocardial revascularization 272–5
organ damage 367, 368, 409
oxygenator comparison 297, 298, 301–7, 429–33
oxygen damage and perfusion flow 408
platelet counts 294–9, 301, 373
priming fluids 420
prostacyclin use 355–77
prostaglandin effects 307, 308
protein denaturation 462–8
and pulmonary function 575–80
pulsatile flow 483–96
pumps 434, 435
safety 427–45
safety organization 435–7
towards safer 293–310
cardiotomy reservoirs 338–48, 433, 434
and gaseous microemboli removal 341–3
low pressure vacuum 442
and microemboli size 344–6
suppliers 350, 351
types 341–3
cardiotomy suction
blood/air in suction line 320
extracorporeal circuits 314, 315
haematological changes, dogs 317
haematological effects 313–22
laminar shear stresses 319–21
and microemboli 339
plasma haemoglobin 316, 318
and pumps 316, 317
platelet counts and 316, 319
screen filtration and air 318
system 339
turbulent shear stresses 321
catecholamine synthesis 519
catheter
balloon 102
infected 589, 591–5
and thrombosis 104
tip deflector 104
cavitation 124, 125
central nervous system
causes 623, 624
disorders 290
postoperative 621, 622, 624, 625
preoperative 620, 621
hypotensive damage 290
and mortality in open heart surgery 622, 623
cerebral blood flow
disturbance and neurological disorders 290
in extracorporeal circulation 289
factors affecting 288
measurement 287, 288
publication review 288, 289
cerebral dysfunction 505 *see also* central nervous system
aetiology and open heart surgery 326, 428
cerebral perfusion, cardiac bypass 287–91
circulatory arrest
paediatric 281–6
procedure 281–3
and temperature 283
circulatory subsystem, control 19
circumflex artery 195
occlusion, arteriogram 106
clinical observation, reappraisal 95–7
closed heart procedures 7
collateral vessels 196
colloids 414–8
adverse reactions 417
dextran 416
gelatins 416–8
priming fluids 415
computers
design and peripherals 537–9
and diagnosis 536, 537
monitoring results 542–5
pressure pulses 543
twelve hour trend plots 542
in postoperative care 535–45
software organization 540
system performance 539–41
congenital heart disease 13–20
and age and size 16, 17
data analysis 20
disease assessment 15, 16
echocardiography 132, 133, 135
operative procedure 17, 18
paediatric diagnosis 135
postoperative care 18, 19
survival adaptation 19
congestive cardiomyopathy 145, 146
contrast media 211, 532, 533
and hazards 101, 102, 105, 106
hyperaemia 211
operator inexperience and 105
cornea 67
coronary artery
anomalous 245
bypass, potassium in urine 274
coronary artery disease 195
atresia, thallium scan 200
mortality 82
pressure–dimension loop 74
severity, assessment 244, 245

and stress radionuclide ventriculography 243, 244
coronary artery stenosis 210
coronary artery surgery
bypass graft
and age, sex 82, 83
arteriogram 199
associated operations 83
exercise test 96
graft number 84, 85
mortality 81
postoperative follow-up 89, 92–4
preoperative state 84
and diffuse disease 84
technique changes 81–93
coronary atherosclerosis 96
coronary perfusion 8
coronary vein grafting 2
Corynebacterium spp, endocarditis 585, 587
creative phosphate
and contractile inactivation 28
in ischaemia 41, 43, 45
CT *see* tomography, computed

Dacron tubes 65
data analysis 20
death *see also* mortality
causes 2
initiation 22
deBakey cannulae 8
deBakey pump 434
degeneration 57
dextrans 416
dextrose 5%, composition 412
diastole abnormalities 75
diatrizoate 106
diazepam 271
disease assessment and safety 13
diuretics 286
dobutamine 518–21
structure 520
dopamine 519, 520, 521
Doppler effect 118 *see also* echocardiography
cardiology applications 136, 137
doxorubicin 243
drugs
α-blocking 283, 284
β-blocking 31, 267–70, 275, 640–4
calcium antagonism 31
cardiotoxic 243
inotropic 513–24
operation pretreatment 31, 32
postoperative 509
and ventricular function 240–3
dura mater patch 56
dyskinesia 135
echocardiogram
cross-sectional 140, 142
echo and apex 72
ischaemic heart disease 70
M-mode 69, 71, 72, 78, 112, 113, 131
normal subject 71, 72
shortening fraction 70
echocardiography 109–38
A-scope 110, 111
access to heart 127
aortic regurgitation 147, 148
aortic stenosis 145–7
B-scope 112–8
cardiology role
Doppler techniques 135–7
invasive techniques 138
two dimensional scanning 134, 135
cavitation effects 124, 125
congenital heart disease 132, 133
digitized, computer output 146
Doppler diagnostic methods 118–23
blood flow 136, 137
continuous wave 119, 120, 123
directionally sensitive systems 121, 122
imaging 122, 123
pulsed system 120, 121
resolution 122
electronically scanned linear 115
fast mechanical scanner 115
frame freeze 117
hazards 124–6
heart valve studies 128–32
image display 116
invasive techniques 124
linear array, real time 116
M-mode recording 112, 113
microbubbles 124
mitral valve disease 139–45
oesophageal scanning 138
preoperative diagnosis 139–50
pulse-echo diagnostic methods 109–18
multiple reflections 112
resolution 110–2
pulse-echo: Doppler combined imaging 123
real-time scanning methods 114–6, 134, 135
safety contribution 126–38
swept gain 110
transducer array and electronic steering 115–7
two-dimensional B-scanner 113, 114
and ventricular function 69–78, 133
ECMO *see* oxygenation, long term membrane
ejection fraction
and akinesis 236
calculation 228, 229
and drugs 240, 241

postoperative 239
regional 231
electrocardiogram 97
calcified aortic valve 131
and saphenous vein graft surgery 188, 189
electrolytes, importance 531–3
endartectomy
patency rate 84
site of 84–7
success 87
endocarditis
infective, echocardiography 148–50
prosthetic valve 583–98
chemoprophylaxis 596–8
incidence 583, 584
organisms 585–7
pathogenesis 584, 585
sources 586–96
energy reserves and myocardial protection 28
energy turnover
ischaemic heart 23–6
and ischaemic tolerance 27, 30
myocardium 514–7, 627–35
enzymes and cardiac surgery 385
ergometrine 97
erythrocyte counts
damage and oxygenators 301, 302
and rotor pump 296
and venous perfusion 294, 295
erythrocyte potassium and prognosis 547, 548
Escherichia coli endocarditis 585
ethylene chlorohydrin 449
ethylene oxide sterilization 448–50
exercise scintigraphy
and disease detection 194
and obstructive coronary artery disease 193–201
protocol 194
exercise test 96
ventriculography 243
extracorporeal apparatus
hazard bioassay 450–71
extracorporeal circulation 21
methods 619

Fallot repair 9
fascia lata, frame mounted
complications 61, 66
fetal heart
drug effects 460
and operation plasma 463, 465
and oxygenation prime 464–8
and plasma from dead patients 463, 464
toxic gas detection 468–70
toxicity 367
and tubing types 468, 469
variation 470
fetal heart bioassay
baselines of performance 459, 460
beating rate and temperature 457, 459
circadian rhythm 460
cultural changes 453
culture time 459
fetus removal 452, 454–7
organ culture 450
sensitivity to toxin 451
survival time 454, 458, 459
variability of method 452
fibrinogen 377
fluorocarbon 419
freon 449
sniffing 450
toxicity 469–71

gamma camera 180, 181, 607
limitations 203
mobile 190
gamma irradiation 450
gas microemboli
in arterial line of oxygenator 333
cardiotomy reservours 338–48
carotid artery 328, 329
gas exchanger role 336, 337
heat exchanger 337
intraoperative recording 329
and micropore filters 347–9
in open heart surgery 325–50
from oxygenators 330–7
from priming blood recirculation 332
and roller pump 338
size profile 344–6
surgical sources 327, 328
ultrasonic detection 326, 327, 339
glomerular filtration rate 601, 602
glutaraldehyde 58, 59, 67
glycolysis
in anaerobic myocardium 648, 649
myocardial 27

haematocrit
optimal 405–8
and vascular resistance 404–6
haemodynamic effects, pulsation perfusion 487–90
haemoglobin, heterologous stroma, free 419
Haemophilus spp.
in trachea 597
halothane 271
HAM *see* microspheres, human albumin
heart block 8
early death 11
heart
aerobic and anaerobic energy demands 24–6

cannulation and microemboli 327, 328
energy demands 23
excitation–contraction coupling 632
inactivation and ATP, CP reserves 28
ischaemic tolerance, methods 35–8
lactate and ATP in ischaemia 25
-lung machine, first 261
rate, effects of 515
reanimation 22
section 633
heat exchanger 337, 432
calcium deposition 449
heparin 359
therapy monitoring 349, 439
hepatitis 401
heterograft 57
homograft
cadaver, problems 66
survival probability 60
homograft conduit 56, 57
hospital, patient attachment 573
Hounsfield numbers 168
hydrogen ions *see also* proton
origin and cycling in surgery 391–9
and pH 391
hydroxy ethyl starch 418, 419
5-hydroxytryptamine 308
hypertrophic cardiomyopathy (HCM) 129, 130
diagnosis and echocardiography 145, 146
hypotension
causes 375
during bypass 375–7, 409
effects 409
hypothermia 2, 8, 35, 261, 395, 396
bicarbonate disposal 397
circulatory arrest, paediatric 281–6
and carbon dioxide 284, 285
procedure 281–3
and renal function 396, 397
profound 242
protection 637–40
proton-potassium homeostasis 397
hypoxia
and myocyte in open heart surgery 382, 385
and myocyte structure 381

immunosuppression 68
indium-113 210
infarct avid agents 182
inotropic stimulation 513–24
and cardiac surgery 523, 524
drug effects 519–23
drug structures 520
and heart energetics 515–8
objectives 514
and renal blood flow 607, 608
intensive therapy unit (ITU), patients viewpoint 571–4
investigation techniques 95
iodine
^{123}I in nuclear imaging 202, 203
^{123}I 210
iopamidol 106
ischaemia 22–6
ATP phase 31
biochemical analysis 41, 43, 45
CP phase 31
and energy demand 30
non-ischaemic differences 30, 31
prolongation of tolerance 27
tolerance and energy 27, 30
ischaemic heart disease, ventricular function 76
isoprenaline 519, 520

jugular bulb thermovelocity probe 289
jump grafts 86, 87, 90, 91

kidney *see also* renal
preservation 34
krypton-81m 209
kinetics 212
scintigraphy 213
krypton-85 224

labetolol 269
β-lactamase, effect on perfusion blood 590
lactate
in ischaemia 41, 43, 45
myocardial concentration 25, 28
leaflets, deformed 140
leukocyte aggregates 294
leukocytopenia 308
line scan imaging 157
lipid metabolism and ischaemic tolerance 32
LVEDP *see* ventricular and diastolic pressure
lysolethicins 32

mannitol, 10% 413, 532, 533
composition 412
mass spectrometry monitoring 579, 580
memory function 615, 616
metoprolol 269
metrizamide 106
microaggregates 209–11
and dysrhythmias 210
microemboli in open heart surgery 35–50
micropore filters 347–9
precautions 348
microspheres 209–11
HAM scintigraphy 210–2
human albumin (HAM) 210
safety 212

mitral stenosis 10, 75
ausculatory features 96
echocardiogram 129, 130
mitral valve
abnormal, echocardiogram 129–33, 139–41
calcification 139
normal, echocardiogram 128
replacement, echocardiogram 144
mitral valve disease 75
disturbance, assessment 142
echocardiography diagnosis 143
regurgitation 129, 130
rheumatic, echocardiography 144, 145
preoperative echocardiography 139–44
surgery and angiocardiography 100
mitral valve prolapse 96
echocardiography 129, 130
morbidity
and cardiac output 17
causes 287
determinants 13
ECMO 480, 481
open heart surgery 428
pulsatile perfusion 492, 494
mortality rate 2, 11
and cardiac output 17
cardiovascular disease 355, 356
causes 287, 356
congenital ventricular septal defect 9, 10
coronary artery blockage 355–7
coronary artery bypass graft 81
coronary artery disease 82
coronary vein grafting 2
determinants 13
ECMO 478–80
ischaemic heart disease 358
nutrition depletion 555
open heart surgery 276, 427, 428, 503, 504, 622, 623
perfusion accidents 427, 439
pulsatile perfusion 492, 494, 495
murmur, Austin-Flint 131, 147
muscle, heart after perfusion 627, 628
Mustard venous inflow redirection 15
myocardial blood flow
xenon-133 scintigraphy 213, 214
myocardial cell
contraction and energy supply 387, 388
stressed, biochemistry 385, 386
myocardial cooling 273
myocardial equilibration
during perfusion, factors affecting 39
myocardial infarction
changes and NMR 155
nuclear imaging 181–7
perioperative 185, 186
radionuclide ventriculography 234–7
subendocardial 184, 185
transmural 183, 184
myocardial ischaemia, kinetics 515
myocardial perfusion
determinants 517, 518
invasive assessment 209
non-invasive scanning 187–93
nuclear imaging assessment 187
positron assessment 208, 209
myocardial preservation 8, 21–51, 277, 627–46
definition 21
drugs and 640–5
energy production 627–35
in ischaemia 648, 649
and hypothermia 637–40
phases 21, 22
and reperfusion 366, 367
myocardial protection 263, 272
advantages 50, 51
disadvantages 49, 50
drug-induced 640–5
methods and ischaemia tolerance 42
optimization 27, 28
pH effect 33
six method comparison 38–49
solution osmolality 32
temperature effects 33, 34
myocardium
calcium entry 630
energy turnover 514–7, 627–35
ischaemia effects 635–7
overdilatation 49
oxygen demand and temperature 24
reperfusion effects 635–7
stress–strain measurements 77
temperature reduction 657
myocytes, cardiac
biochemical relationship 397, 398
features in culture 379–89
and hypoxia 381–5
isolated 379, 380
protein balance 388, 389
stressed, events in 385–9
structure 380
myofibrils 631

neurological complications *see also* central nervous system, cerebral
in bypass hypotension 409
in open heart surgery 619–26
New York Heart Association clinical classes 238, 239
nifetipine 640, 642, 643
nitrogen-13 208, 209
kinetics 208

nitroglycerine and ventricular function 240, 241
NMR *see* nuclear magnetic resonance
noradrenaline 519, 520
nuclear cardiologist 179
nuclear imaging techniques 179–214
  coronary artery atresia 200, 201
  coronary artery disease 243–5
  coronary artery stenosis 210, 211
  coronary artery-vein graft assessment 197–9
  coronary collaterals 196
  dynamic imaging 223–49
    historical 223, 224
    principles 224, 225
  imaging equipment 180, 181
  infarcted myocardium 181–7
    cold spot scanning 181, 182
    infarct avid agents 182
    pyrophosphate scans 182–7
  microaggregates 210, 211
  multiple gated acquisition 225
    advantages 226, 227
    disadvantages 226, 227
    first pass studies 225, 226
    gated blood pool imaging 225, 226
  myocardial infarction 234–7
  myocardial perfusion
    non-invasive 187–93
    normal image 189, 190
    views used 191, 192
  obstructive coronary artery disease 193–202
  postoperative studies 211, 212
  pseudoaneurysm 240
  radiation dose 227
  regional wall motion 229–31
  shunt detection 246, 247
  thallium-201 scintigraphy 187–202
  three dimensional imaging 203–9
  and transplantation 249
  transit times 231–3
  triple vessell disease 196, 197
  valvular heart disease 196, 197
  vein grafts 245
  ventricular aneurysm 237
  ventricular function 248
  ventricular volumes 232
nuclear magnetic resonance
  body imaging 153
  echo planar imaging technique 159
  line scanning images 156–60
  nuclei and isotopic abundance
  perioperative value 160–3
  phosphorus imaging 161–3
  principles 154, 155
  and tissue water content 155, 156
  ultra-high speed cardiac imaging 160
  whole body electromagnet 158, 159
nursing
  postoperative management 549–51
  priorities 550, 551
nutrition
  amino acid sources 563, 564
  depletion criteria 554
  enteric feeds 560, 562, 563
    costs 562
  monitoring 564, 566
  parenteral feeding 561, 565
  postoperative 553–66
    aims 558, 559
    methods 559–61
    paediatric hypothermia 286
  status assessment 553

obstructive coronary heart disease 193–201
occlusive coronary vascular disease 2, 3
  symptomless 4
Omnopon 270, 271
open heart procedures 7, 262
  and brain damage 619–26
  gaseous microemboli 325–50
  and neurological disorders 325, 326
  toxins in 447–72
operation
  procedures 17
  risk factors 17
  safe, definition 13
osmotic pressure
  blood 409–14
  colloid 414–8
oxprenolol 269
oxygen, systemic transport and haematocrit 407
oxygenation, long term membrane extracorporeal (ECMO) 475–81
  acceptance 477
  circuitary 477
  particle generation 479
oxygenators 297–305, 330
  bubble 331, 336, 370, 429, 430, 443
  contamination 310
  disc 331
  failure 442–4
  membrane 331, 370, 429, 431
    advantages 304, 334
  type and microemboli 330–5
  type and platelet counts 297–303, 306, 307
  venous assistance 443
  venous obstruction 441

pain relief 509
parenteral feeding 561

particle embolization 371–3
  causes 373
perfusion *see also* pulsatile perfusion
  and endocarditis 589
  β-lactamase effects 590
  safety precautions 436, 437
  Staphylococcus spp. in 591
perfusion scintigraphy 191
pericardial baffle 56
pericardium
  effusion 133
  living in reparative surgery 65
phenergan 270
phenoxybenzamine 284
phonocardiogram 71
phosphocreatine in ischaemia and NMR 162
phosphorus, NMR image of tissue 161–3
pindolol 269
platelet activation
  ADP-induced and oxygenators 306, 307
  and damage 294
platelet counts
  and cardiotomy suction 316, 319
  and membrane types 298
  and oxygenators 297, 298, 301, 303
  and prostaglandin: heparin 363–5, 376
  and rotor pump 294, 297
  venous perfusion 296
platelet function
  in bypass grafting 301
  and oxygenators 303, 306, 307
platelet loss in surgery and open heart
    disorders 359
poloxalkol 419
positron *see also* tomography
  emission 206
  and myocardial perfusion assessment 208,
    209
  nature 206
postoperative assessment
  coronary bypass 89, 92–4
  echocardiography 127
  nuclear imaging 211–212
postoperative care 18, 19, 293, 503–609
  bleeding 503
  cardiac output 510
  cerebral complications 505, 511
  and clinical assessment 503–12
  complications, management 510–2
  computer use 535–45
  electrolyte/fluid problems 505
  and endocarditis 583–98
  and haemorrhage 569, 570
  hypothermia in infants 285
  infection 505, 506, 512
  inotropic stimulation 513–24
  invasive techniques 19
  nursing 549–51
  nutritional care 553–66
  and outline and monitoring 506–10
  patient monitoring 535, 536
  psychometric testing 613–7
pulmonary complications 504, 505, 511
  and renal failure 505, 511
  and return to activity 509, 510
potassium 531
  distribution and coronary artery disease 556
  red cell and prognosis 547, 548
  status and valve replacement 555, 557
  urinary and coronary artery bypass 274
potassium citrate arrest 7, 35
practolol 269
preoperative procedures
  β-blockade 31, 94, 267–70
  causes of brain damage 366
  echocardiography 127, 139–50
  exercise testing 269
priming fluids 401–20
  colloids 414–8
  composition 420
  crystalloids 411–4
  experimental 418–20
  tonicity 409, 410
  in UK use 420
procaine
  in cardiac arrest 35, 36
  toxicity 36
propranolol 269, 274
  and cardiac failure 276
  and myocardial protection 640, 642, 643
  and ventricular function 241, 242
prostacyclin (PGI_2) 304
  and air embolism 371
  and bleeding time 307
  in cardiopulmonary bypass 355–77
  discovery 357
  and fetal heart toxicity test 367
  filter SEM and 364
  -heparin combination 360
  and particle emboli 373
  platelet inhibition 307, 308, 359, 366, 376,
    377
  properties 358
prostaglandin E_1 (PGE_1)
  and bleeding time 307, 308
  bypass pretreatment 306
prosthetic materials 55–62
  autolysis 55
  calcification 61
  contamination 57–9
  degeneration 57, 59
  fixation 57, 58
  immunological rejection 59
  infected 596–8

echocardiography 151
rejection 57, 59
sterilizaiton 58
protamine chloride 299, 306, 365
protein denaturation 374, 375
and cardiopulmonary bypass 462–8
protein loss, postoperative 556, 557
proton regulation and pump primes 394, 395
proton release
and carbon dioxide 394
energy rich phosphates 393
glycolysis based 392
respiratory chain 393, 394
pseudoaneurysm 240
angiography 242
psychometric testing 613–7
and memory function 615, 616
perioperative 614, 615
pulmonary atresia 101
pulmonary dysfunction after cardiopulmonary bypass 575–80
pulmonary hypertension and early death 11
pulmonary oedema 103
pulmonary vascular disease in infancy 14
pulmonary venography 101
pulsatile assist devices (PAD) 491
pulsatile perfusion 18
arterial, concept 483
and baroceptor effects 484, 485
and brain function 486, 487
cardiac index 488, 491
in cardiopulmonary bypass 483–96
clinical safety 490–6
haemodynamic effects 487–90
hormonal effects 486, 487
and kidney function 485
metabolic effects 485
and microcirculation 484
and mortality 492, 494, 495
pulsatile system
Cobe–Stockert 492–4
haemolysis index 492
pump-lung syndrome 10, 401
pumps 434, 435, 476
pyrophosphate scan 182–7
role 187

radiocardiography, quantitative 231
radioisotopes
emission 180
half-life 180
number 179
radium C 223
rejection 57
renal failure 2, 505, 601–8
diuretic challenge 603, 604
frusemide and electrolyte loss 604, 605
haemodialysis 605, 607
peritoneal dialysis 607, 608
postoperative course 606
postoperative recognition 603
renal function
in hypothermia 396, 397
monitoring 601–8
preoperative assessment 601, 602
and pulsatile perfusion 485
renografin, iodine-131 label 224
reperfusion solution 44
respiratory support 576–8
revascularization surgery 245
and cardiopulmonary bypass 272–5

St Jude prosthesis 144
salbutamol 519, 520
in heart failure 522
salt solutions
balanced composition 412
Hartmans' 412
Plasmolyte-148 412
saphenous vein 56, 57
sarcoidosis 199
sarcoplasmic reticulum function 632, 633
Sci-Med lung 295
Senning technique of venous redirection 15
serum, osmotic constituents 410, 411
sex
and coronary bypass graft 82, 83
and organ survival 459–61
shunts detection and quantification 246, 247
silicone rubber membrane, clot on 360
Society of Computed Body Tomography 176
sotalol 269
Staphylococcus spp. endocarditis 584–6
from catheters 594, 595
in perfusion blood 590, 591
Starr–Edwards caged ball prosthesis 61
Swank's screen filtration, pressure technique 314
systemic vascular resistance and cardiopulmonary bypass 307, 308
systole, velocity of circumferential fibre shortening (VCF) 72
ultrasonic measurement 133
systolic pressure time interval (SPTI) 268

tachydysrhythmia 269
technetium-99m 180, 190, 205, 226
infarct avidity 182
in myocardial perfusion scanning 190
-stannous pyrophosphate 182, 183
temperature and myocardial preservation 33, 34
tetralogy of Fallot 100, 247, 608
clinical conditions 14

operative procedures 263
and predictability 14
transannular patch enlargement 15
thallium-201 206
and angina 197–200
body dose 208
distribution quantification 193
distribution and stress 194
non-coronary reliability 198
thallium perfusion
heart distribution 189
in myocardial perfusion scanning 187–201
imaging 202, 203
prospects 202, 203
scan projections 192
thallium scintigraphy
and disease extent 195, 196
indications 201
limitations 201
thiopentone 271, 281
thirst, postoperative 572
thrombocyte *see* platelet
thrombocytopenia 308, 309
thyrotoxicosis 460
timolol 269
tissue characteristics in NMR 155
tomography, computed (CT)
dynamic spatial reconstructor 173
gating methods 174–6
hazard 171, 172
heart 168–75
and motion 171
partial volume effect 169, 170
radiation dose 171, 172
ideal scanner 172, 173
method 167
pencil-beam scanner 168
resolution 171, 172
rotate only scanner 169
gating 174, 175
rotate-translate scanner 169, 175
gating 174, 175
and thoracic interfaces 170
tomography, emission (ECAT)
anterior infarction 205
single photon scanning 204, 205
tomography, positron 206, 207
toxins
bioassay 450–70
extracorporeal apparatus 374
in open heart surgery 447–72
tracheostomy 11
transcutaneous aortovenography 136
transit times 231–3
transplantation, assessment of cardiac 249
transposition of great arteries 15, 16
with large ventricular septal defect 16
tricuspid atresia 104
tricuspid valve, echocardiography 132
triple-vessel disease 196, 197
tropomyosin 386
troponin 386
tubing types 294–7
PVC, toxicity 447, 448
sterilization 448–50
toxicity 469, 470
d-tubocurarine chloride 281

ultrasound *see also* echocardiography
biological effects 125
echo contrast enhancement 124
frequency choice 119
gas microemboli detection 326, 327, 339
hazards 124–6
speed 109
urine
electrolyte loss and frusemide 604, 605
electrolytes 533
osmolality and solute excretion 411
osmotic constituents 410, 411

valve
aortic, cadaver 66
durability 61, 62
mechanical 67
mitral, complication probability 61
prosthetic, echocardiogram 131, 132, 148, 151
pulmonary, echocardiogram 132
replacements, tissue culture 58
survival probability 60, 61
xenograft 56, 57
valvular heart disease assessment 245, 246
vascular resistance
and pulsatile perfusion 489, 490
and viscosity 405
VCF *see* systole
vein grafts
artery bypass 65
dynamic imaging 245
particle injection 211
perfusion scan 198, 199
scintigraphy assessment 197, 198
ventilation, artificial, problems 10, 11
ventricle
left, hypertrophy 75
pseudoaneurysm 240
ventricular aneurysm, detection 237
ventricular clots 135
ventricular and diastolic pressure, left (LVEDP) 517, 518, 520
ventricular function
contractility index 232–4
dimension changes 74–7

drug effects 240–2
filling and diastole 75–7
following aneurysmectomy 238–40
left, echocardiography 69–78, 133
cavity size 69–71
contraction coordination 73–5
normal 71
wall movement 71, 72, 171
pressure-dimension loop 73
and heart disease 74
right, nuclear imaging 190, 191
right, radionuclide ventriculography 248, 249
ventricular septal defect 9
mortality and complications 9, 10
ventricular wall movement 71, 72, 171
and diastolic volume 516, 517
radionuclide measurement 229–31
ventriculography
ejection fraction measurement 228–30
exercise first pass 243
radionuclide and function 227–49
stress radionuclide and coronary artery disease 243, 244
volumes 232
verapamil, myocardial protection 640, 641
virus, rabies in corneal graft 59
viscosity function, blood 403
and bypass 406
and perfusion pressure 408, 409
and temperature 407

water, transcapillary movement 414

xenograft 57
antigenicity 59
xenon-133 196
and myocardial blood flow 213, 214
X-ray 100 *see also* angiocardiography, tomography
tomography 163

yield stress, blood 403, 404